Medical Center Occupational Health and Safety

Medical Center Occupational Health and Safety

Editor

Robert J. McCunney, M.D., M.P.H.
Director, Environmental Medicine
Massachusetts Institute of Technology
Cambridge, Massachusetts
Lecturer on Medicine
Harvard Medical School
Boston, Massachusetts
Staff Physician
Massachusetts General Hospital
Boston, Massachusetts

Associate Editor

Cheryl S. Barbanel, M.D., M.B.A., M.P.H., F.A.C.O.E.M.
Assistant Professor of Medicine
Boston University School of Medicine
Chief of Occupational and Environmental Medicine
Boston Medical Center
Director of Boston University Occupational Health Center
Boston University Medical Center
Boston, Massachusetts

LIPPINCOTT WILLIAMS & WILKINS
A **Wolters Kluwer** Company
Philadelphia • Baltimore • New York • London
Buenos Aires • Hong Kong • Sydney • Tokyo

Acquisitions Editor: Joyce-Rachel John
Developmental Editor: Sonya L. Seigafuse
Production Editor: Thomas Boyce
Manufacturing Manager: Kevin Watt
Cover Designer: Meryl Lavavi
Compositor: Lippincott Williams & Wilkins Desktop Division
Printer: Edwards Brothers

227 East Washington Square
Philadelphia, PA 19106-3780 USA
LWW.com

Printed in the USA

Library of Congress Cataloging-in-Publication Data

Medical center occupational health and safety / editor, Robert J. McCunney, associate editor, Cheryl S. Barbanel.
p. cm.
Includes bibliographical references and index.
ISBN 0-7817-2198-9
1. Medical personnel—Health and hygiene. 2. Medical centers—Health aspects. 3. Medical center—Safety measures. I. McCunney, Robert J. II. Barbanel, Cheryl S.
[DNLM: 1. Health Facility Environment—standards. 2. Occupational Diseases—prevention & control. 3. Occupational Health. 4. Safety Management—standards. WX 27.1 M489 1999]
RC965.M39M43 1999
363.11'93621—dc21
DNLM/DLC
For Library of Congress 99-14496
CIP

Care has been taken to confirm the accuracy of the information presented and to describe generally accepted practices. However, the authors, editors, and publisher are not responsible for errors or omissions or for any consequences from application of the information in this book and make no warranty, expressed or implied, with respect to the currency, completeness, or accuracy of the contents of the publication. Application of this information in a particular situation remains the professional responsibility of the practitioner.

The authors, editors, and publisher have exerted every effort to ensure that drug selection and dosage set forth in this text are in accordance with current recommendations and practice at the time of publication. However, in view of ongoing research, changes in government regulations, and the constant flow of information relating to drug therapy and drug reactions, the reader is urged to check the package insert for each drug for any change in indications and dosage and for added warnings and precautions. This is particularly important when the recommended agent is a new or infrequently employed drug.

Some drugs and medical devices presented in this publication have Food and Drug Administration (FDA) clearance for limited use in restricted research settings. It is the responsibility of the health care provider to ascertain the FDA status of each drug or device planned for use in their clinical practice.

10 9 8 7 6 5 4 3 2 1

To my family—
my wife Marilyn, son Robby, and daughter Kelsey.
To them, I am indebted for the pleasure and respite they provide me
from the rigors and demands of professional life.

Contents

Contributing Authors

Elisha H. Atkins, M.D.
Medical Director of Occupational Health Service
Massachusetts General Hospital
Chelsea
151 Everett Avenue
Chelsea, Massachusetts 02150

Daniel E. Banks, M.D.
Professor of Medicine
Section of Pulmonary and Critical Care Medicine
West Virginia University School of Medicine
Morgantown, West Virginia 26506

Cheryl S. Barbanel, M.D., M.B.A., M.P.H., F.A.C.O.E.M.
Assistant Professor of Medicine
Boston University School of Medicine
Chief of Occupational and Environmental Medicine
Boston Medical Center
Director of Boston University Occupational Health Center
Boston University Medical Center
D-203
88 East Newton Street
Boston, Massachusetts 02118

Edward Joseph Bernacki, M.D., M.P.H.
Associate Professor of Medicine
Director
Division of Occupational Medicine
Executive Director, Health, Safety and Environment
The Johns Hopkins University
Billings Administrative Room 129
600 North Wolfe Street
Baltimore, Maryland 21287

Perry D. Cooper, B.S.
The Johns Hopkins University
Homewood Safety Campus
103 Macauley Hall
3400 North Charles Street
Baltimore, Maryland 21218

Alain J. Couturier, M.D.
Medical Director
St. Joseph Mishawaka Health Services
Corporate Health Services
270 East Day Road, Suite 270
Mishawaka, Indiana 46545

Walter G. Diaz, R.N., C.S.P.
MIT Safety Office
Massachusetts Institute of Technology
77 Massachusetts Avenue, E19-207
Cambridge, Massachusetts 02139-4304

Louis Joseph DiBerardinis, M.S.
Associate Director
Environmental Medical Service
Massachusetts Institute of Technology
77 Massachusetts Avenue, 56-235
Cambridge, Massachusetts 02139-4307

Brian G. Forrester, M.D., M.P.H.
Medical Director, Occupational Health Services
Regional FirstCare
485 Highway 29N
Athens, Georgia 30601

Mitchell S. Galanek, C.H.P.
Radiation Protection Department
Massachusetts Institute of Technology
77 Massachusetts Avenue, 16-268
Cambridge, Massachusetts 02139-4307

Arun Garg, Ph.D., C.P.E.
Professor and Director
Ergonomics Laboratory
Industrial and Manufacturing Engineering
EMS E314
University of Wisconsin-Milwaukee
P.O. Box 784
Milwaukee, Wisconsin 53201

Richard W. Gilpin, Ph.D., R.B.P., C.B.S.P.
Biosafety Officer; Director, Biosafety Division
Department of Health, Safety and Environment
Assistant Professor of Occupational Medicine
Department of Medicine, School of Medicine
The Johns Hopkins Institutions
2024 East Monument Street
Suite 2-700
Baltimore, Maryland 21205-2223

Donald L. Haes, Jr., M.S., C.H.P.
Massachusetts Institute of Technology
Assistant Radiation Protection Officer
Environmental Medical Service
77 Massachusetts Avenue, 16-268
Cambridge, Massachusetts 02139-4304

Philip Harber, M.D., M.P.H.
Professor of Medicine
Director, Occupational and Environmental Medicine
University of California at Los Angeles
10911 Weyburn Avenue #344
Los Angeles, California 90024-7027

Kurt T. Hegmann, M.D., M.P.H.
Associate Professor
Department of Preventive Medicine
Medical College of Wisconsin
Milwaukee, Wisconsin 53226

Geoffrey A. Kelafant, M.D., M.S.P.H., F.A.C.O.E.M.
Medical Director
Sarah Bush Lincoln Occupational Health
P.O. Box 372
1000 Health Center Drive
Mattoon, Illinois 61938

Timothy J. Key, M.D., M.P.H.
University of Alabama
Division of Occupational and Environmental Medicine
930 20th Street South
Birmingham, Alabama 35294-2042

Ronald S. Leopold, M.D., M.B.A., M.P.H.
Medical Director
MetLife Disability
Building 2, 4th Floor
628 Hebron Avenue
Glastonbury, Connecticut 06033

Daniel F. Liberman, Ph.D.
Associate Director, Environmental Affairs and Safety
Boehringer Ingelheim Pharmaceuticals, Inc.
900 Ridgebury Road/ P.O. Box 368
Ridgefield, Connecticut 06877-0368

James A. MacLean, M.D.
Division of Allergy
Massachusetts General Hospital
Chelsea
151 Everett Avenue
Chelsea, Massachusetts 02150

Frank X. Massé, C.H.P., C.M.P.
Officer and Director of Radiation Protection Programs
Massachusetts Institute of Technology
77 Massachusetts Avenue, 16-268
Cambridge, Massachusetts 02139-4307

Robert K. McLellan, M.D., M.P.H.
Medical Director
Center for Occupational and Environmental Health at Exeter Hospital, Inc.
P.O. Box 1050
Exeter, New Hampshire 03833

Michael A. Mueller, M.D., M.P.H.
Assistant Professor
Division of Occupational and Environmental Medicine
University of Alabama at Birmingham School of Medicine
121 Community Health Services Building—20th
930 20th Street South
Birmingham, Alabama 35205

Karin D. Myerson, R.N., COHN-S
Myerson Occupational and Environmental Medicine, P.C.
10507 Greenacres Drive
Silver Spring, Maryland 20903

Ross S. Myerson, M.D., M.P.H.
Myerson Occupational and Environmental Medicine, P.C.
10507 Greenacres Drive
Silver Spring, Maryland 20903

Jon T. O'Neal, M.D., M.P.H.
Consultant in Occupational and Environmental Medicine
2305 Shoal Creek Boulevard
Austin, Texas 78705

Randy A. Roig, Ph.D.
STC Consulting
6016 Canning Street
Oakland, California 94609

Victor S. Roth, M.D., M.P.H.
Assistant Clinical Professor
M-Works
University of Michigan Occupational Health Services
2098 South Main Street
Ann Arbor, Michigan 48103-5827

Jonathan Silver Rutchik, M.D., M.P.H.
426 West Broadway, 6C
New York, New York 10012

John A. Schaefer, C.I.H., H.E.M.
Assistant Professor of Medicine
Division of Occupational Medicine
Environmental Health Officer
The Johns Hopkins University
2024 East Monument Street
Suite 2-700
Baltimore, Maryland 21205

Samuel Skarote, M.D.
Assistant Professor of Medicine
Section of Pulmonary and Critical Care Medicine
West Virginia University School of Medicine
Morgantown, West Virginia 26506

Lynn Stansbury, M.D., M.P.H.
Myerson Occupational and Environmental Medicine, P.C.
10507 Greenacres Drive
Silver Spring, Maryland 20903

Kevin C. Staudinger, M.D., M.P.H.
Medical Director, Occupational Medicine Clinics
Baptists Health Center, Inc.
3500 Blue Lake Drive
Birmingham, Alabama 35243

Carol A. Sulis, M.D.
Associate Professor of Medicine
Boston University School of Medicine
Director, Epidemiology Unit
Boston Medical Center
The Maxwell Finland Laboratory for Infectious Diseases
774 Albany Street
Boston, Massachusetts 02118-2393

Linda B. Wolfe, B.S., S.M. (N.R.M.), C.B.S.P.
Director of Environmental Health and Safety
Whitehead Institute for Biomedical Research
Nine Cambridge Center
Cambridge, Massachusetts 02142

Michael H. Ziskin, C.H.C.M., C.H.M.M.
Field Safety Corporation
Guilford, Connecticut 06437

Preface

Hospitals and other health care facilities can be just as hazardous as some industrial settings with both traditional and unique occupational health and safety risks. In fact, hospitals, medical centers, and various health care facilities have undergone increased scrutiny of their occupational health risks within the last ten years. In the late 1980s, the impact of HIV and Hepatitis-B in particular on health care workers prompted serious review of the potential hazards associated with the delivery of health care. Radiological, biological, and chemical materials became targets of prevention programs in response to both scientific and regulatory developments. Although, over the years, hospitals have appropriately focused on patient care, there has been scant recognition given to hospital hazards inherent in delivering care and the corresponding employee health issues.

This book is intended to provide a comprehensive perspective on occupational health and safety at the modern medical center with applications to numerous types of health care facilities. Although the term "medical center" may imply a high-powered academic institution, it was chosen for the book's title because of the wide-ranging nature of its mission: patient care, teaching, and research—all of which may have pertinence in preventing illness and injury among health care workers. The subjects covered in this text are likely to be valuable for physicians, nurses, and other professionals called upon to protect the health care worker. Topics range from specific hazards, such as latex, disinfectants, and chemotherapeutic agents, to plant operations and organization of an occupational health program. Research, laboratory, and autopsy operations are addressed, along with guidance on conducting indoor air quality evaluations and employing the Internet for specific medical center-related issues. Chapters are designed to be practical and address common challenges and responsibilities that face occupational health professionals at health care facilities. It is hoped that these goals have been met and the readers will find the book useful and of value well into the future.

RJM
Cambridge, MA

Acknowledgments

A book of this nature requires the help and guidance of many—staff, colleagues, and friends—without whom it would never have been completed. In particular, I have valued the guidance and "extra pair of eyes" of my associate editor and friend, Dr. Cheryl Barbanel. Reviewing more than 30 chapters requires diligence as well as skill in ensuring accuracy, appropriateness, and consistency in the material. She performed her tasks with thoroughness and insight. As a result of Cheryl's efforts, the final product is clearly better than it would have been otherwise.

My colleagues at Lippincott Williams & Wilkins have also played a major role in this book. With the guidance and support of publishing professionals such as Joyce-Rachel John, the publication reached the quality to which editors and authors usually strive. Credit is due the authors who suffered through critical reviews of their early manuscripts and responded professionally to the suggestions that Dr. Barbanel and I offered. Without their willingness to deliver quality work, this book clearly never would have been possible.

Most importantly, however, thanks are due to Bonnie Pires, my administrative assistant at MIT, who kept the book on track and the authors informed—no easy task, but one essential to the completion of this book. My thanks to all of the above.

Medical Center Occupational Health and Safety

Medical Center Occupational Health and Safety,
edited by Robert J. McCunney
Lippincott Williams & Wilkins, Philadelphia © 1999.

1

Medical Center Occupational Health and Safety

Cheryl S. Barbanel

Department of Medicine, Boston University School of Medicine, and Department of Occupational and Environmental Medicine, Boston Medical Center, Boston, Massachusetts 02118

The mission of medical centers has been to provide excellence in teaching, medical research, and clinical care. In today's rapidly changing health care environment, the balance among these three goals is being driven by financial restraints. This observation is underscored by the short-term basis on which medical establishments are currently valued and are summed-up by the marketplace claims of "high quality, low cost." Although medical centers have played a role in the delivery of occupational medical services in the United States, they have been rather slow to address the occupational health and safety risks to their own employees. A well-organized and comprehensive hospital-based occupational health and safety program, however, can reduce injuries and illnesses among employees, generate revenue by providing occupational safety and health services to external clients, and market its other health care services to employers (1).

This chapter reviews the history of occupational medicine, the role of the hospital in the provision of occupational medical services, the development of the early medical centers in the United States, and the current challenges of the medical center. The chapter also provides an overview of the risks to health care workers and the organization of health, safety, and environmental programs.

HISTORY OF OCCUPATIONAL MEDICINE AND THE ROLE OF THE MEDICAL CENTER

Observations related to increased rates of illness and mortality among miners date back to Roman times and are attributed to the more feeble conditions of workers who were slaves (2). It was not until the late seventeenth century when an Italian physician, Bernardio Ramazzini (1633–1714), known as the father of occupational medicine, published *De Morbis Artificum Diatriba* (Diseases and Occupations), that physicians were formally urged to pay attention to the role of work in the development of certain illnesses (3). In the seventeenth century, the economy in the American colonies was based on farming, fishing, maritime activities, and a few manufacturing industries. Little is known of diseases caused by work during this time (4). Throughout the next two centuries, periodic reports described illnesses associated with exposure to a variety of substances (5).

Occupational medicine was slow to develop in the United States because of the indifference of corporations to cheap immigrant labor and lack of unions to organize workers (6). In about 1814, Lowell Hospital in Massachusetts, sponsored predominantly by local industry, provided medical services for sick mill workers. Late in the nineteenth century, industrial interest in providing medical services surfaced. In 1882, the Northern Pacific Railway Beneficial Association, an employee-sponsored mutual benefit association, developed a program of complete medical care and other benefits financed by employer-employee payments. Medical care was provided through group practice in the Northern Pacific Hospital in St. Paul, Minnesota, and through arrangements with physicians in communities along the railroad (4).

Access to clinical teaching was the first goal for the establishment of university hospitals. The next goal was control over the quality of the instruction. By the 1880s and 1890s, a corresponding site for clinical research became important as well. At the end of the nineteenth century, Americans viewed the hospital as a philanthropic organization that existed to do good for the community. Funding was expected to come from philanthropy, the university, and the government, but not from patient care. The many advances that arose from university-based research convinced people who could afford to pay that hospital care had something to offer. Today income from patient care revenues is central to any medical center, including academic teaching facilities (7).

The University of Michigan organized its medical department in 1850 and was followed by the University of Pennsylvania and Johns Hopkins University. At this time, clinical instruction was not considered appropriate for an institution of higher learning. In 1868, after much debate, the University of Michigan opened the first university hospital in the United States, a 20-bed hospital intended as a teaching site for students. Johns Hopkins Hospital opened in 1867 and the Hospital of the University of Pennsylvania in 1874. To address the tensions that existed between medical schools and their affiliated hospitals, Johns Hopkins Hospital explicitly linked clinical care, postgraduate education, and medical research. Excellence in clinical care, teaching, and research has remained the model for the academic medical center for most of the twentieth century. Hospitals have been able to adapt to a changing environment by altering the importance of the three core values—excellent teaching, medical research, and clinical care (7).

Teaching of industrial health was initiated in 1905 at the Massachusetts Institute of Technology by Dr. Charles-Edward A. Winslow in the department of biology and public health. One year later, the medical department of the University of Pennsylvania, in conjunction with its doctoral program in public health, emphasized industrial hygiene with attention to plant inspections, in-plant emergency medical service, and the occupational disease clinic of the university hospital (4).

Physical examinations had begun to appear as an early component of occupational health efforts. In 1906, Massachusetts required by law the physical examination of all children applying for an employment certificate. Characterizing the early years of the twentieth century was the appearance of clinics designated specifically for the diagnosis of occupational diseases. The first of these clinics began as the outpatient department of the Cornell Medical School in New York City in 1910. It was followed by the Sprague Memorial Institute of the University of Chicago and by the Rush Medical College (4).

With the growth of industrialization in the early years of the twentieth century, the introduction of hazardous materials with potential for affecting the workforce increased (4). A rising number of employee-directed suits against employers for work-related injuries prompted the development of state workers' compensation statutes (1909–1911) (8). The workers' compensation system essentially established a no-fault insurance program such that any injured worker would be guaranteed compensation for medical bills, time lost from work, and permanent impairment or death. In return, employers were granted immunity from further legal action by the worker for work-related illnesses or injuries (2). In 1914, the United States Public Health Service established the Office of Industrial Hygiene and Sanitation, principally for worksite surveys and research in the field of occupational health, which is now the National Institute for Occupational Safety and Health (NIOSH) (6).

Alice Hamilton (1869–1970) was the first American physician to devote her life to the practice of industrial medicine. She was also the first woman to be appointed to the faculty of Harvard School of Medicine, where she taught from 1919 to 1935 (6). She wrote *Industrial Poisons* in the United States in 1925 and *Exploring the Dangerous Trades*, her autobiography, in 1943. Hamilton is considered the matriarch of American occupational medicine (9). In *Exploring the Dangerous Trades* Hamilton pointed out that American medical authorities had never taken industrial diseases seriously and that workers accepted the risks of working as part of the price for being poor. One of Hamilton's important lessons was that the most effective means of reducing excessive exposure is through control of the environmental sources (10).

In 1950, the University of Pittsburgh conferred the degree of doctor of industrial medicine on three graduates, and the American Medical Association (AMA) approved the establishment of residency in industrial medicine at Saginaw General Hospital in Michigan. In 1955, the Council on Medical Education and Hospitals of the AMA authorized the American Board of Preventive Medicine to create a subspecialty and examination and certification in occupational medicine. It was recognized that residencies in occupational medicine could be established in certain industrial or government facilities approved and that hospital training, characteristic of nearly every other medical specialty, was unattainable and inappropriate at the time (4).

The American Association of Industrial Physicians and Surgeons, founded in 1916, was later renamed the Industrial Medical Association, and finally the American Occupational Medicine Association (AOMA). In 1988, AOMA and the American Academy of Occupational Medicine, consisting primarily of board certified specialists in the field, merged into what is now the American College of Occupational and Environmental Medicine (ACOEM) (6).

Most important to the health of the worker was the passage of the Occupational Safety and Health Act of 1970, in which full cognizance was taken of the many needs for the workers' safety and health. The Occupational Safety and Health Act was passed to "assure safe and healthful working conditions for working men and women" and mandates that "each employer shall furnish to each of his employees employment and a place of employment which are free from recognized hazards that are likely to cause death or serious physical harm to his employee." The result has included increased legislation, education, research, training, and surveillance of workers at risk. Despite increased research in the areas of toxicology, epidemiology, and clinical occupational medicine, effects of harmful work exposure continue (4).

OPPORTUNITIES AND CHALLENGES

Medical centers face challenges of transforming medical education and medical care as profoundly as ever before in their history. Despite the emphasis now on ambulatory care services, strategic alliances, and group practices, the university hospital remains central to the academic medical center. The strength of the university hospital has been its ability to change and assume different functions throughout the century of its existence (7).

Funding and governance continue to be a subject of controversy. In the late nineteenth century, hospitals were seen as philanthropic institutions with funding expected to be provided by the university or the state. Since income from philanthropies and government grants has become uncertain, patient care revenue has become the primary source of income. In addition, public consensus on providing supplemental income for academic institutions for the social good of training physicians is eroding. The focus on generating income from patient care services has spurred the development of larger networks and increased attention on ambulatory care (7).

Medical centers are threatened by for-profit market forces, and systems for the delivery of health care are changing rapidly. These changes include large managed care organizations and large for-profit hospital chains, not-for-profit hospitals, and insurance companies that are converting to for-profit status. For-profit institutions accumulate profits, compete on price, and assume risk for defined populations. The number of physicians in solo practice has diminished, the physician's central role in making medical decisions has been taken over by mandated managed care practices. Marketplace demand for physicians continues to decrease, especially for specialists, whereas the demand for family physicians is rising (11).

Benefits of managed care include a stated focus on prevention and health promotion and control of health care costs, both of which are consistent with goals of occupational health and safety programs (12). Most managed care companies, however, have avoided financing education, research, and provision of large volumes of charity care, the traditional functions of urban academic medical centers. Many predict the pendulum will shift away from this stance with more legislation controlling health maintenance organizations (HMOs) and other for-profit ventures (13).

The increasing corporatization of medical centers has led to struggles for personal and institutional survival. Decreased governmental support in recent years has led to increased competition for federal funding and an emphasis on academic and industry joint ventures. Because of financial pressure, institutions that formerly collaborated are now competing to the detriment of scientific and clinical advancement. Scientists are considered business assets and training opportunities proprietary. Much medical and scientific capital is misdirected toward configuring competitive business strategies and hospital-to-hospital corporate warfare. Medicine, however, is not a commodity well suited for an uncontrolled marketplace, except in a quest of short-term gain rather than long-term societal advances. The substitution of business ethics for medical ones does not appear to be an appropriate way for medical centers to operate in the long-range view (14).

Medical centers have reconfigured their teaching programs and repriced clinical services to more effectively compete in the marketplace. Some of the strategies to compete include lowering costs to market levels, developing a primary care base beyond the traditional faculty practice, becoming leading players in managed care, and developing clinical centers of excellence. This is a radical change for traditionally conservative academic medical centers that never addressed competitive issues (15).

Medical schools have responded to the changing marketplace with an increasing focus on outpatient primary care. As hospital patient stays have decreased, patient care and training have shifted to outpatient treatment facilities. In addition to providing the most current diagnostic and treatments, teaching programs are incorporating concepts of quality assurance, evidence-based practice, management, business, and health organization.

The care paradigm of the medical center is another area that needs to be redesigned. The focus has to be shifted from diagnosis, therapy, and cure to prevention. Clinical care delivery has to be population-based and integrated; public health issues of the community have to be served. Patient encounters must be viewed not as visits but as part of a covered lives concept. Coordination of hospital care has to be considered beyond the hospital walls (16). Although this concept is new to the academic medical center, epidemiology, a public health orientation, population-based care, prevention, and health promotion are central tenets to the practice of occupational medicine.

Litigation involving academic medical centers increased in the last half of the twentieth century. The frequency and range of issues litigated since 1985 reflect the expanding complexity of administering policies over many departments and the growing responsibilities in education, clinical practice, and research. Litigation involving research has increased since the 1980s. The increase parallels federal policy initiatives designed to stimulate collaboration between industry and academia and the growth of regulations designed to monitor research policy. Litigation by community residents has involved environmental hazards generated from research facilities, such as the production of waste (17).

As legislation expands in environmental and occupational safety, conflicts may involve biomedical research projects that pose risk to study subjects, personnel, or the environment. Identifying, quantifying, and managing risk to research subjects, personnel, and the environment should be a continuous process not only to deter litigation but also to foster the advancement of biomedical science. Educating administrators and faculty on the need to formulate policies that can withstand judicial scrutiny will be key to reducing the risk for litigation related to environmental health and safety (17).

ORGANIZATION OF HEALTH, SAFETY, AND ENVIRONMENTAL PROGRAMS

Few workplaces are as complex as hospitals. Medical centers, in providing education, research, and medical services, also provide food services, waste disposal, maintenance, engineering, plumbing, carpentry, landscaping, and housekeeping, among other services, needed to operate the facility. Health care workers are at risk for many health and safety hazards. They are at more risk than other service workers and are at equal or greater risk than in some industrial jobs (18).

For many years, despite evidence of the hazards present in hospitals, hospital-based health and safety programs did not progress. One explanation was the traditional focus of hospitals on the management of disease rather than its prevention. It also was assumed that health care workers could take care of themselves and that staff medical problems could be handled in an informal manner, such as the proverbial corridor consult. Other factors included the high turnover rate among hospital staff, expense, and a tradition of health care workers' acceptance of certain risks as part of patient care (19).

The first industry-wide recognition of the importance of hospital employee health and safety programs came in 1957 when the AMA issued a report of the Joint Committee on Health Programs for Hospital Personnel that outlined elements of a comprehensive program (18). Fifteen years later NIOSH conducted the first comprehensive survey of health programs and services for hospital workers. In 1977, NIOSH published guidelines for evaluating occupational safety and health programs in hospitals. Only 8% of the hospitals reporting in the 1972 survey (NIOSH 1974–1976) met all nine criteria for a comprehensive hospital safety and health program (20).

In 1988, NIOSH published Guidelines for Protecting the Safety of Health Care Workers (19). Table 1-1 summarizes the steps for developing safety and health programs to identify and control occupational hazards in the hospital setting (21). As knowledge concerning these hazards has increased, a revised guideline is planned to include recent recommendations. The revised guidelines include, for example, Centers for Disease Control and Prevention (CDC) recommendations for protecting health care workers from tuberculosis and NIOSH recommendations for respiratory protection.

Medical center employees constitute more than 40% of more than 9 million health care workers in the United States and almost 4% of all workers (22). According to Bureau of Labor and Statistics data from 1995, hospital workers [Standard Industrial Classification (SIC) 806] averaged 10.1 nonfatal workplace injury and illness cases per every 100 full-time workers. This figure is compared with an average of 8.1 nonfatal injuries for all private industry and an average of 6.4 nonfatal injuries for all service workers. In 1995, hospitals had the second highest number of nonfatal injuries for industries with 100,000 or

TABLE 1-1. *Checklist for developing a hospital safety and health program*

Item	Component tasks
Administrative support	Form a safety and health committee. Appoint a safety officer, employee health director, and other responsible personnel. Allocate funds to evaluate and monitor hazards, implement controls, and conduct health examinations.
Hazard identification	Conduct periodic walk-through inspections. Obtain material safety data sheets (MSDSs) and other information on potential hazards. Maintain a log of hazardous chemicals and materials that are used or stored in each department.
Hazard evaluation	Conduct safety inspections and industrial hygiene monitoring of potential hazards and determine need for hazard controls. Conduct medical evaluations. Select appropriate medical surveillance programs.
Training	Develop and begin a training program for workers based on job responsibilities.
Controls	Select appropriate control measures and implement controls and medical surveillance programs as determined in the hazard evaluation.
Program review	Review results of periodic safety inspections, industrial hygiene monitoring, and medical surveillance programs to identify patterns of hazards, to measure the success of the safety and health program, and to determine the effectiveness of controls. As new hazards are identified or new procedures introduced, change the safety and health program.
Recordkeeping	Maintain records of results for all surveys, evaluations, monitoring corrective actions, and worker medical examinations. Records must be maintained in accordance with applicable regulations.

more employees (22). According to the Bureau of Labor Statistics 1995 incidence rate data on lost-time nonfatal work injuries in hospitals, overexertion (45%), especially involving lifting, was the leading event causing the greatest number of injuries. This was followed by injuries resulting from contact with an object or equipment, falls, and activities involving bending, climbing, reaching, and twisting, exposure to harmful substances, and assault. Strains and sprains accounted for about 58% of all injuries followed by bruises and contusions and pain. The back was most frequently affected. The leading source of injury involved a patient, contact with the floor, and worker motion or position (22).

The number and variety of hazards in hospitals include radiation, toxic chemicals, biologic agents, ergonomic stressors, violence, stress, and physical hazards, including heat and noise. Other risks are latex allergy, lacerations, electrical mishaps, slips, falls, back injury, shift work, and exposure to disinfectant, sterilants, hormones, antineoplastic agents, waste anesthetic gases, and infectious diseases. Table 1-2 is an overview of the complexity of occupational hazards according to hospital location (22) (see Chapter 2 for a more detailed description of medical center workers' compensation issues).

Biohazard and musculoskeletal risks are the most common potential hazards, although chemical exposures are increasingly reported, in part because of passage of right-to-know legislation. In research facilities of academic medical centers, large numbers of toxic chemicals can be found. In a study reviewing chemical exposures in an academic medical center, housekeepers were identified as the occupational group at highest risk followed by maintenance workers (23). Chemical exposure occurred most often by the dermal route, mainly to disinfects, cleaning compounds, and solvents (23). In a study of injuries and illness in an academic medical center, the five occupational groups with the greatest number of lost days per claim were animal caretakers, housekeepers, clinical aides, maintenance workers, and phlebotomists (24).

Every medical center should establish and maintain a comprehensive occupational safety and health program to monitor and protect the health of employees (25). The Occupational Safety and Health Act of 1970 is an attempt to assure safe and healthful working conditions free from recognized hazards that

TABLE 1-2. *Hospital occupational hazards by location*

Location	Hazard
Central supply	Infectious organisms
	Ethylene oxide
	Broken equipment (cuts)
	Soaps, detergents
	Steam
	Flammable gases
	Noise
	Asbestos
	Mercury
Dialysis units	Infectious organisms
	Formaldehyde
Dental service	Mercury
	Ethylene oxide
	Anesthetic gases
	Ionizing radiation
	Infectious organisms
Food service	Wet floors
	Sharp equipment
	Noise
	Soaps, detergents
	Disinfectants
	Ammonia
	Chlorine
	Solvents
	Drain cleaners
	Oven cleaners
	Caustic solutions
	Pesticides
	Microwave ovens
	Steam lines
	Ovens
	Heat
	Electrical hazards
	Lifting
Housekeeping	Soaps, detergents
	Cleaners
	Solvents
	Disinfectants
	Glutaraldehyde
	Infectious organisms
	Needle punctures
	Wastes (chemical radiation, and infectious)
	Electrical hazards
	Lifting
	Climbing
	Conditions conducive to slips and falls
Laboratory	Infectious organisms
	Toxic chemicals
	Benzene
	Ethylene oxide
	Formaldehyde
	Solvents
	Flammable and explosive agents
	Carcinogens
	Teratogens
	Mutagens
	Cryogenic hazards
	Wastes (chemical, radioactive, infectious)
	Radiation
Laundry	Wet floors
	Lifting
	Noise
	Heat
	Infectious organisms
	Needle punctures
	Detergents, soaps
	Bleaches
	Solvents
	Wastes (chemical and radioactive)
Maintenance and engineering	Electrical hazards
	Tools, machinery
	Noise
	Welding fumes
	Asbestos
	Flammable liquids, solvents
	Mercury
	Pesticides
	Cleaners
	Ammonia
	Carbon monoxide
	Ethylene oxide
	Freon
	Paints, adhesives
	Water treatment chemicals
	Sewage
	Heat stress
	Cold stress (refrigeration units)
	Falls
	Lifting
	Climbing
	Conditions conducive to strains and sprains
Nuclear medicine	Radionuclides
	Infectious organisms
	X irradiation
Office area and data processing	Video display terminals
	Air quality
	Ergonomic, body mechanics problems
	Chemicals
	Ozone
Operating rooms	Anesthetics, antiseptics
	Methyl methacrylate
	Compressed gases
	Sterilizing gases
	Infectious organisms
	Electrical devices
	Sharp instruments
	Lifting
Pathology	Infectious organisms
	Formaldehyde
	Glutaraldehyde
	Flammable substances
	Freon
	Solvents
	Phenols
Patient care	Lifting, pushing, pulling
	Conditions conducive to slips and falls
	Prolonged standing
	Infectious organisms

TABLE 1-2. *Continued.*

Location	Hazard	Location	Hazard
Patient care *(cont.)*	Needle punctures		Mercury
	Toxic substances		Conditions conducive to slips and falls
	Chemotherapeutic agents		
	Radiation	Print shop	Inks
	Radioactive patients		Solvents
	Electrical hazards		Noise
	Latex (allergy)		Fire
	Shift work	Radiology	Radiation
	Violence		Infectious organisms
Pharmacy	Pharmaceutical agents		Lifting
	Antineoplastic agents		Pushing, pulling

Adapted from ref. 21, with permission.

are capable of causing or are likely to cause death or serious physical harm to employees. This is accomplished by preventing, recognizing, and treating occupational illness and injury. An occupational safety and health program, in addition to ensuring a safe workplace for employees, can ensure regulatory compliance with requirements and guidelines of multiple national agencies as well as state and local regulations.

In addition to state and federal regulations of the Occupational Safety and Health Administration (OSHA), the Joint Commission on Accreditation of Health Care Organizations sets standards to protect employee health and safety. OSHA has promulgated a number of standards that directly affect hospital employees, including regulations related to formaldehyde, ethylene oxide, blood-borne pathogens, control of tuberculosis in health care facilities, and other regulatory requirements for research in biotechnology, certain laboratory areas, and cleanup of spills of hazardous materials. Standards in Title 29 of the Code of Federal Regulations (CFR) describe exposure limits and program requirements for general industry, which includes hospitals. The Food and Drug Administration, the Nuclear Regulatory Commission, the National Institute of Health, the CDC, and workers' compensation regulations also may affect medical center operations (26). The Americans with Disabilities Act assists occupational medical services and employers in determining disability, essential job functions, and identifying reasonable accommodations.

Program Elements

A comprehensive occupational health and safety program promotes the recognition, evaluation, and control of hazards to hospital employees. The goal of the occupational health program is to promote healthy workers and a healthy workplace through assessing potential hazards to workers, preventing occupational illness and injuries, and providing early treatment to facilitate recovery.

A hospital must have an occupational health program, and supervisors, employees, and management all need to be involved in safety and health issues. An effective occupational health and safety program requires the commitment and leadership of management. Management should communicate the goals of the program to the organization, assign responsibility, and provide the resources to achieve the program goals. Employee involvement is important to the success of the program. Involvement motivates employees to meet the goals of the program. Encouraging employees to report hazards, unsafe practices, and illness and to make safety suggestions, without fear of reprisal, is important. Follow-up on these reports and suggestions is necessary (27).

Another element of an occupational health and safety program is a document that describes the hospital's health and safety policies, objectives, actions, and personnel responsibilities. A multidisciplinary safety committee should be established to include the departments of industrial hygiene, occupational health nursing, occupational medicine, ergonomics, physical therapy, infectious control, and safety engineering. The committee should be led by an occupational health and safety professional. The committee reviews and analyzes reports related to health and safety program activities, makes recommendations to develop, implement, and revise the program, and reports to upper-level management on a regular basis (27).

Occupational Health Services

Occupational health services can prevent injury and illness by assessing the actual and potential hazards to workers and developing and managing programs that promote safety and health. An occupational medicine program should assist the medical center in complying with legal, ethical, and regulatory requirements for monitoring the health of employees involved in jobs with potential exposures. A comprehensive program addresses both risk management and regulatory issues. The occupational health services of a hospital should be managed preferably by an occupational health physician with experience in management. Guidelines for essential and elective components of an occupational medicine practice have been published by the ACOEM (28) (Tables 1-3, 1-4). The ACOEM section on medical center occupational health has posted on the Internet unofficial guidelines for employee health services in health care facilities (http://www.occenvmed.net/) with many links to useful additional resources.

Medical Surveillance Programs

Medical surveillance programs, including preplacement, baseline, periodic, postexposure, and exit examinations, should be organized on the basis of information from the worksite analysis and applicable OSHA and other standards. Examples of baseline examinations are audiometric examinations if noise exposure is a hazard (29 CFR 1910.95) and pulmonary function tests if a respirator is needed for one's work (29 CFR 1910.134). There must be established policy and procedures to provide postexposure evaluation and management of needle-stick injuries, and arrangements must be made for continued serologic testing if the employee leaves the in-

TABLE 1-3. *Essential components of occupational and environmental health programs*

Health evaluation of employees
Before assignment
Medical surveillance
After illness or injury
Diagnosis and management of occupational and environmental injuries or illnesses, including rehabilitation
Emergency management of nonoccupational injury or illness
Education of employees when potential occupational hazards exist
Implementation of programs for personal protective equipment
Evaluation, inspection, and abatement of workplace hazards
Toxicologic assessments, including advice on chemical substances that have not had adequate toxicologic testing
Biostatistical and epidemiologic assessments
Maintenance of occupational medical records
Immunization against possible occupational infections
Medical interpretation and participation in governmental health and safety regulations
Assistance in rehabilitation of employees with alcohol or drug dependency and those with emotional disorders

Adapted from ref. 28, with permission.

TABLE 1-4. *Elective components of occupational and environmental health programs*

1. Palliative treatment of nonoccupational disorders
2. Repetitive treatment of nonoccupational conditions prescribed and monitored by personal physicians
3. Assistance and control illness-related job absenteeism
4. Assistance and evaluation of personal health care
5. Immunizations against non-occupational infectious diseases
6. Health education and counseling
7. Termination and retirement administration
8. Participation in and planning an assessing of the quality of employee health benefits
9. Participation and systematic research

Adapted from ref. 28.

TABLE 1-5. *Safety and health program assessment worksheet*

Safety and Health Program Assessment Worksheet

Instructions: This form is for project use when assessing an employer's safety and health program. Maintain the completed form in the casefile. **Column 1:** Essential elements and sub-elements of effective safety and health programs. **Column 2:** Indicators that elements and sub-elements are present at the workplace (core requirements which must be present for an exemption to be granted are in **bold type**). **Column 3:** Consultant's judgment on whether the elements and sub-elements operate in ways which are adequate and appropriate for the workplace. **Column 4:** Use to record how the determination of effectiveness was made and what improvements are needed. Rectangular block may be used to record correction date.

Employer Name (State Option) | Visit Number | Consultant ID | Date

Elements	Indicators (Core Requirements **bold**)	In Place? Yes	No	How were you able to identify and verify their adequacy? What if any improvements are needed?
I. Management Commitment and Planning				
A. Policy and objectives for worker safety and health.	**1.) Established policy and objectives, communicated to employees.**	☐	☐	☐
B. Authority and accountability for safety and health protection.	**2.) Responsibilities defined and authority assigned.**	☐	☐	☐
	3.) Supervisor performance evaluated, and rewarded or corrected.	☐	☐	☐
C. Commitment of resources to workplace safety and health.	**4.) Adequate company resources allocated for safety and health (in staff, equipment, safety promotion, etc.)**	☐	☐	☐
D. Management involvement in employee safety and health concerns.	5.) Clear lines of communication for safety and health concerns.	☐	☐	☐
	6.) Management sets example on safe and healthful behavior.	☐	☐	☐
II. Hazard Assessment				
A. Hazard assessment.	**7.) Completion of comprehensive safety and health surveys.**	☐	☐	☐
	8.) Periodic self-inspections, conducted by qualified person.	☐	☐	☐
B. A reliable procedure for employees to report possibly hazardous conditions	**9.) Employees know how and whom to notify, fear no reprisal, and receive timely and appropriate responses.**	☐	☐	☐
C. Review of accidents or near-miss incidents and injury/illness experience.	**10.) Procedures to identify causes and needed corrective action.**	☐	☐	☐

III. Hazard Correction and Control				
A. Means of eliminating or controlling hazards.	**11.) Engineering and PPE controls in place, as appropriate.**	☐	☐	☐
	12.) Administrative controls, including safety and health rules and safe work procedures, established and implemented.	☐	☐	☐
	13.) Procedures for timely correction/control of newly-identified hazards.	☐	☐	☐
B. Disciplinary action or reorientation for supervisors or employees who break rules or disregard work or emergency procedures.	**14.) System for rule enforcement and discipline established and carried out.**	☐	☐	☐
C. Equipment maintenance program.	15.) Ongoing monitoring and maintenance of equipment.	☐	☐	☐
D. Emergency planning and procedures.	16.) Preparation, with training and drills as needed, for emergencies requiring PPE, medical care, emergency egress, etc.	☐	☐	☐
	17.) Emergency telephone numbers, exit routes, etc., visible to all.	☐	☐	☐
IV. Safety and Health Training				
A. Supervisors should understand the hazards associated with a job, their potential effects, and the supervisor's role in ensuring that employees follow the rules, procedures and work practices for controlling exposure to them	**18.) Supervisors can explain rules, procedures and work practices for hazard control, and how they teach and enforce them.**	☐	☐	☐
B. Employees are taught hazards and safe work procedures to protect themselves at the same time they are taught to do a job.	19.) Employees can explain how and why to do their jobs safely.	☐	☐	☐
	20.) Training is reinforced or repeated as necessary.	☐	☐	☐
C. Where personal protective equipment is required, employees know when, why and how to use it, its limitations and maintenance.	**21.) Employees use PPE when necessary.**	☐	☐	☐
	22.) Employees know why, how, limits and maintenance of PPE.	☐	☐	☐

PPE, personal protective equipment.

Source: Assistant Secretary for Occupational Safety and Health, U.S. Department of Labor. *The Integrated Management Information (IMIS) Consultation Forms Manual.* OSHA Instruction ADM 1-1.29. Washington, DC, Office of Management Data Systems, 1992.

stitution before completing the evaluation (29 CFR 1910.1030).

Rehabilitation

Rehabilitation involves facilitating an employee's recovery to the state before the injury or illness. Case management is a strategy of working with the employee to facilitate complete and timely recovery. Return-to-work assessment should be conducted for employees who have been absent from work because of injury or illness. The purpose of the assessment is to determine whether employees are well and able to perform all their job tasks, whether they need accommodations or restricted duties, or whether they pose a risk to coworkers or patients.

Informed Consent

Informed consent should be obtained from employees before they undergo health assessments or medical procedures. Employees have a right to refuse to participate in health services. Neither the employer nor OSHA can compel an employee to undergo any health assessment. If a hospital's employee policy states that the test results are a condition of employment, refusal may mean loss of the job (27).

Medical Records

Medical records must remain confidential. Employee personal health information is confidential and cannot be shared with management, supervisors, or coworkers without consent. The health care provider can share only information regarding work restrictions and information needed to ensure the health and safety of affected employees and their coworkers. The OSHA standard, Access to Employee Exposure and Medical Records (29 CFR 1910.1020), permits direct access to employer-maintained medical records only by the employee and his or her designated representative or by OSHA. Employees have the right to know the results of their health assessment and medical surveillance. Results should be provided directly and confidentially to individual workers (27).

Review

OSHA recommends review of occupational health and safety program operations at least annually to evaluate meeting the stated goals of the program. Trend analysis and program effectiveness also should be reviewed. Data should be compiled from activities related to the worksite analysis, hazard prevention and control, training and education, and record keeping. The results of the evaluation should be revealed to hospital management and all members of the hospital community through the safety and health committee. Table 1-5 is a safety and health program assessment worksheet (27).

WORKSITE ANALYSIS

The worksite analysis consists of a literature review, identification of hazard categories, worksite surveys, and analysis of trends. On the basis of a literature review, potential hazard categories can be identified in the hospital environment and control strategies can be developed. Worksite analysis should be conducted on an ongoing basis; frequency depends on the level of risk. Worksite analysis should take place when there are changes in procedures, equipment, or processes. Hazards can be categorized into biologic, ergonomic, chemical, psychologic, and physical (Table 1-6) (27).

After the potential health and safety hazards in the hospital are identified, a worksite survey should be performed. A worksite survey includes a walk-through, hazard analysis, and exposure monitoring. The purpose is to evaluate actual and potential hazards in a specific worksite. OSHA recommends worksite surveys to establish comprehensive health hazard inventories. The purpose of the walk-through is to observe work processes, methods, and practices, engineering and administrative controls in place, personal protective

TABLE 1-6. *Categories of potential hazards in hospitals*

Hazard category	Definition	Examples in the hospital setting
Biologic	Infectious or biologic agents, such as bacteria, viruses, fungi, or parasites that may be transmitted by contact with infected patients or contaminated body secretions or fluid	Human immunodeficiency virus infection, hepatitis B virus infection, tuberculosis
Ergonomic	An attempt to fit the job to the employee rather than the worker to the job; the study of human behavioral and biologic characteristics for the appropriate design of the living and working environment	Lifting, standing for long periods of time, poor lighting
Chemical	Various forms of chemicals that are potentially toxic or irritating to the body; including medications, solutions, and gases	Ethylene oxide, formaldehyde, glutaraldehyde, waste anesthetic gases, cytotoxic agents, pentamidine, ribavirin
Psychologic	Factors and situations encountered or associated with one's job or work environment that create or potentiate stress, emotional strain, or other interpersonal problems	Stress, shift work
Physical	Agents within the work environment that can cause tissue trauma	Radiation, lasers, noise, electricity, extreme temperatures

equipment used, and health problems among workers. A list such as that in Table 1-7 can be used as a guideline for conducting a facility walk-through (1).

Hazard analysis is conducted if further assessment of hazards of specific jobs or processes is needed. After all the steps in the work process are recorded and potential safety and health risks are identified, recommendations are made. Frequency and severity of accidents or illnesses, potential for injuries or illnesses, and any changes in equipment, processes, or operations are recorded. Recommendations may include substitution of a less hazardous chemical, facility alterations, equipment and material selections, or redesign of the job task.

When a comprehensive worksite analysis identifies existing and potential health hazards, exposure monitoring is used to evaluate the workers' level of exposure while performing the job. If the monitoring results exceed the exposure limit, some action or controls must be implemented. OSHA sets exposure limits for specific air contaminants and the duration of employee exposure.

Exposure monitoring includes environmental monitoring, a program of observation and measurement to determine levels of exposure to specific substances in the workplace; and biologic monitoring, the measurement of a chemical, its metabolite, and nonadverse biochemical effect in a person to assess exposure.

TABLE 1-7. *Guidelines for conducting a facility walk-through*

1. Are substances used in the workplace for which established Occupational Safety and Health Administration standards exist?
2. Are carcinogenic substances used?
3. Are policies in effect for certain issues such as alcohol or drug abuse?
4. Are accommodations or modified duty assignments available?
5. Are collective bargaining agreements in place that may affect delivery of medical care?
6. Are material safety data sheets available?
7. What is the level of existing first aid services?
8. Is a disaster plan in place?
9. What is the nature of control measures, such as engineering controls and personal protective equipment?
10. What staff members are responsible for health and safety measures?
11. Are current facilities adequate, especially storage of medical records?

Adapted from Weisberger BC, Gray DC. The establishment of an occupational heath program. In: McCunney RJ, ed. *Handbook of Occupational Medicine.* Boston: Little, Brown, 1988:47–60.

Specimens used are blood, urine, or exhaled air. Analysis of trends involves use of data to describe past trends or use of symptom surveys, questionnaires, or screening to identify current trends in problem areas.

Hazard prevention and control is accomplished with engineering controls, workplace practice controls, use of personal protective equipment, and emergency preparedness. Engineering controls are most effective and should be used whenever possible. An example of an engineering control is scavenging of waste anesthetic gases at their source. Emergency preparedness is an essential part of hazard control. It includes planning for emergency response operations to handle releases of hazardous substances (29 CFR 1910.120).

The purpose of training and education is to inform management, supervisors, and employees about their roles, responsibilities, and rights in establishing a safe work environment. Documentation of training is required by OSHA and the effectiveness of training should be evaluated. Accurate record keeping is essential to a comprehensive occupational health and safety program. Record keeping is important for providing continuity of care, for legal purposes, and for analysis of trends. An employer must complete OSHA Form 200 and OSHA Form 101 within 6 days of learning of a work-related injury (29).

REFERENCES

1. McCunney RJ. Providing high quality occupational medical services. *J Ambulatory Care Marketing* 1990;4:9–39.
2. McCunney RJ. Occupational medical services. In: McCunney RJ, ed. *A practical approach to occupational and environmental medicine*. Boston: Little, Brown, 1994.
3. Rammazzini B. Diseases of workers. In: *De morbis artificum diatriba*, 1713. New York: Hafner, 1964. Wright WC, translator.
4. Felton JS. Historical development of occupational medicine in the United States. In: Felton, ed. *Occupational medical management*. Boston: Little, Brown, 1990.
5. Raffle PAB, McCallum RI, Lee WR, Murray R. *Hunter's diseases of occupations*, 7th ed. Boston: Little, Brown, 1987.
6. Rom WN. The discipline of environmental and occupational medicine. In: Rom WN, ed. *Environmental and occupational disease*, 2nd ed. Boston: Little, Brown, 1992.
7. Martin SC, Howell JD. Creating university hospitals: rationales and realities. *Acad Med* 1995;70:1012–1016.
8. Felton JS. 200 years of occupational medicine in the U.S. *J Occup Med* 1976;18:809.
9. Hamilton A. *Exploring the dangerous trades*. Boston: Little, Brown, 1943.
10. Lippman M. 1989 Alice Hamilton Lecture: lead and human health: background and recent findings. *Environ Res* 1990;51:1–24.
11. Seifer SD, Troupin B, Gordon D, Rubenfeld GD. Changes in marketplace demand for physicians: a study of medical journal recruitment advertisements. *JAMA* 1996;276:695–699.
12. Kassirer JP. Is managed care here to stay? *N Engl J Med* 1997;336:1013–1014.
13. Ginzberg E, Ostrow M. Sounding board, managed care: a look back. *N Engl J Med* 1997;336:1018–1020.
14. Schnipper LE. As medical titans battle, what happens to the patients? *Boston Globe* April 3, 1997; Editorial section.
15. Vavala D. The new academic medical center hybrids: part business, part academic. *Physician Executive* 1996; 22:5–10.
16. Eliastrom M. The need for a new model of care: revisiting the archetype. *Physician Executive* 1996;22:11–13.
17. Helms LB, Helms CM. Litigation involving medical faculty and academic medical centers, 1950–1991. *Acad Med* 1993;68:7–19.
18. Lewey R. Organization and conduct of a hospital occupational health service. *Occup Med* 1987;2:618.
19. Guidelines for protecting the safety and health of health care workers; 1988; DHHS publication no (NIOSH)88-119.
20. Hospital occupational health and safety; 1977; DHEW publication no (NIOSH)77-141.
21. Hospital Occupational Service Study. Vols. I–VII; 1974–1976; DHEW publication nos (NIOSH)75-101, 75-154, 76-107, 76-115, 76-115A, and 76-116.
22. Department of Labor, Bureau of Labor Statistics. Survey of occupational injuries and illnesses, 1995. Summary 97-7. Washington, DC: US Government Printing Office, May 1997.
23. Weaver VM, McDiarmid MA, Humphrey FE, Schaefer JA. Occupational chemical exposures in an academic medical center. *J Occup Med* 1993;35:701–706.
24. McGrail MP, Tsai SP, Bernacki EJ. A comprehensive initiative to manage the incidence and cost of occupational injury and illness. *J Occup Med* 1995;37: 1263–1268.
25. Guidelines for employee health services in health care institutions. *J Occup Med* 1986;28:518.
26. Howard J. Medical center occupational health. In: McCunney RJ, ed. *A practical approach to occupational and environmental medicine*. Boston: Little, Brown, 1994.
27. US Department of Labor. Occupational Safety and Health Administration. Framework for a comprehensive health and safety program in the hospital environment. Washington, DC: US Government Printing Office, 1993.
28. Scope of occupational and environmental health programs and practices: report of the Occupational Medical Practice Committee of the American College of Occupational Medicine. J Occup Med 1992;34:436.
29. US Department of Labor. Bureau of Labor Statistics. Record keeping guidelines for occupational injuries and illnesses. Washington, DC: US Government Printing Office, September 1986.

Medical Center Occupational Health and Safety,
edited by Robert J. McCunney.
Lippincott Williams & Wilkins, Philadelphia © 1999.

2

Workers' Compensation Principles for Medical Centers

Ronald S. Leopold

MetLife Disability, Glastonbury, Connecticut 06033

Medical centers, including hospitals and nursing homes, account for a large sector of the workforce. These centers, like all places of employment, are required to maintain workers' compensation coverage for all employees. As the petroleum, construction, aerospace, and mining industries each have inherent and specific risks and hazards, so does health care. Characteristics concerns about workers' compensation in a medical center setting are (a) the relatively high incidence of occupational injuries; (b) the unique set of exposures in this setting, most notably to infectious agents; and (c) the numerous potential complicating factors that occur with work-related injuries and illnesses when coworkers and supervisors also are health care professionals.

PURPOSE OF WORKERS' COMPENSATION

Workers' compensation provides income benefits, medical payments, and rehabilitation payments to workers injured on the job and to survivors of workers who have been fatally injured (1). In 1911, the first workers' compensation laws passed in the United States. These laws and those that followed were enacted to spare the injured worker the burden of proof of employer negligence and to protect the employers from nuisance liability claims (2). Workers' compensation laws enacted a mandatory no-fault disability insurance system for injured workers. Employees, under workers' compensation law, are automatically compensated for injuries and illnesses sustained at work, regardless of fault (2).

Under workers' compensation laws, each stakeholder (employer and employee) essentially surrenders certain rights while being guaranteed certain benefits. Employers are required to pay all workers' compensation premium costs as a cost of doing business, and employees are obliged to participate and automatically surrender their right to take legal action against their employer for work-related injuries and illnesses (2). Most state workers' compensation laws share the following characteristics: (a) benefit formulas are prescribed in state legislation; (b) medical care and rehabilitation expenses are fully covered; (c) lost wages are partially reimbursed; (d) employers are legally responsible for maintaining workers' compensation insurance; and (e) it is a no-fault system (1).

STATE-BY-STATE VARIATION

Workers' compensation laws are state laws. There are therefore 50 state and three federal workers' compensation jurisdictions, each with its own statutes and regulations (1). Full- and part-time employees of hospitals and nursing homes are by and large fully covered and protected by individual state workers' compensation regulations. In all states, workers are entitled to full medical benefits for injuries and illnesses sustained on the job. Each state legislates the type and amount (often a formula) of lost wages that the employer (or insurance carrier) must pay a worker who misses work as a result of a work-related injury or illness. Specific benefits vary widely from state to state.

WORKERS' COMPENSATION INSURANCE RISK FOR THE HEALTH CARE SETTING

Underwriting of workers' compensation insurance requires a calculated analysis of the risks to a prospective customer. This includes a thorough understanding and recognition of the risks, hazards, and experiences of the individual industry. For example, an underwriter needs to consider the average threats of loss or claims in a nursing home and consider what special and individual hazards are likely or possible in the typical or not typical nursing home. One widely used source, *Best's Underwriting Guide* (3) offers a summary of average exposures to the principal hazards on an industry-wide basis and provides a consensus of seasoned underwriters regarding the inherent hazards of each industry.

HIGH COSTS OF WORKERS' COMPENSATION

The financial impact of workers' compensation claims are twofold—the costs of medical treatment and the costs of replacement wages (indemnity costs). The financial ramifications, therefore, of a work-related illness or injury leading to missed work are considerable, given that indemnity payments range anywhere from 50% to 150% of medical payments in a lost-time case. Some of the causes for high workers' compensation costs are (a) inapplicability of cost-control measures such as copayments and deductibles to curb medical expenditures; (b) difficulty in achieving medical fee discounts because of restricted ability to direct where injured workers can receive medical care; (c) rampant litigation in the workers' compensation system, which can complicate medical care and delay recovery; 4) perverse incentives for employees and their agents that might magnify injury severity (1).

WORKERS' COMPENSATION IN THE MEDICAL CENTER SETTING

Health care ironically has been slow to recognize the breadth and depth of work-related injuries and illnesses among its own. "The health care industry has a much longer history of treating, rehabilitating, and curing patients than it does in preventing injuries and illnesses, among its own workers" (4). Among the most common hazards are musculoskeletal and needle-stick injuries, followed by work-related illnesses such as infection with hepatitis B virus (HBV) or human immunodeficiency virus (HIV) and tuberculosis. Chemical hazards include asbestos and nitrous oxide, among others (4). Specific exposures for health care include lifting; exposure to waste anesthetic gases; laboratory chemical exposures; handling and disposal of radioactive materials; exposure to communicable diseases; assaults on employees; flammable gas use and storage; and arson (3). The medical center as employer functions in a dual capacity as employer and provider of medical treatment (3). The incidence of work-related injuries and illnesses places substantial burdens on health care organizations and medical centers, many of which are already contending with ongoing financial woes.

Incidence of Injury in the Health Care Setting

In 1990, according to the Bureau of Labor Statistics, 282,400 hospital workers suffered work-related injuries, and 168,200 nursing home and personal care workers were injured on the job (4). In 1994, the Bureau of Labor Statistics published data indicating 311,700 nonfatal occupational injuries among hospital workers and 217,200 nonfatal occupational injuries among workers in nursing and personal care facilities (5). Hospital safety and health administrators estimate that approximately 80% of workers at a health care facility are at high risk for one or more occupational injuries or illnesses. These people include health professionals, clinical support staff, technicians, housekeeping, food service, maintenance, and support staff (4).

The incidence of work-related injuries [(number of injuries ÷ total hours worked by all employees during the calendar year) × 200,000] was 10.3 for hospital workers and 16.6 for nursing and personal care facilities. This places health care workers at risk similar to that among workers in traditionally high-injury settings, such trucking and courier services (14.8), hotels and motels (10.0), and grocery stores (10.8) (Table 2-1) (5). The National Safety Council tracks similar data for members participating in its Occupational Safety/Health Award Program. Hospitals had 8.40 cases per 100 employees, and health services had 8.28 cases per 100 employees. In cases involving days away from work and deaths hospitals had 2.19 cases per 100 employees and health services had 2.16 compared with all industries, which had 1.64 (7).

In the 1995 National Safety Council study, both hospitals and health service companies averaged 25 days away from work for every 100 full-time employees (incidence per 100 full-time employees with 200,000 employee hours as the equivalent). This figure exceeded construction (23 days), mining (21 days), and petroleum and coal products (17 days) but was less than the number of days for all industries (36 days). Of note, for self-reported carpal tunnel syndrome, hospitals ranked ninth for all industries. Health assessment and treating occupations ranked second for all occupations (7).

Of particular concern is the high rate of low-back injuries among nurses aides and nurses. The National Council on Compensation Insurance examined back claims from its Detailed Claim Information database for 1981–1990 (8). The council reported that most back claims are caused by lifting. This is the likely reason that the three leading industry classifications are in health care. The highest category was for nursing homes.

Risk by Occupation

Approximately 80% of workers in a health care facility are at high risk for one or more occupational injuries or illnesses. These include clinical staff, technicians, housekeepers, food service workers, maintenance workers, and support staff. Any worker whose day-to-day duties focus on patients is at risk (4). In one study, workers' compensation records for back injury were reviewed for a large university hospital for a 2-year period. The 2.0% per year incidence of lost-work-time back injury among nurses was exceeded only by the 3.5% incidence among physical plant staff. In the same study, nurses' aides had an injury rate 3.3-fold higher than that among registered nurses and licensed practical nurses and higher than that among any other occupational group (Table 2-2) (9). The 1996–1997 *Bureau of Labor Statistics Occu-*

TABLE 2-1. *Incidence of nonfatal occupational injury per 100 full time workers classified by industry, 1994*

Industry	Total no. of cases	No. of lost day cases	No. of lost day cases
Services	6.1	2.7	3.5
Health services	**8.8**	**3.7**	**5.1**
Business services	4.6	2.2	2.4
Legal services	0.9	0.3	0.6
Auto repair, services, and parking	6.8	2.9	3.9
Hotel and other lodging	9.9	4.6	5.3
Retail trade	7.7	3.2	4.5
Finance, insurance, real estate	2.4	0.9	1.4

From ref. 6.

TABLE 2-2. *The ten occupations with the largest number of injuries and illnesses involving days away from work, shares of case and employment totals, 1994*

Occupation	No. of cases	Total no. of workers (,000)	Percentage of total cases	Percentage of workers
All occupations	2,236.6	92,973	100.0	100.0
Total for 10 occupations	728.7	14,636	32.6	15.7
Truck drivers	163.8	2,438	7.3	2.6
Laborers, nonconstruction	147.3	1,137	6.6	1.2
Nursing aides, orderlies	101.8	1,359	4.6	1.5
Janitors and cleaners	60.6	1,407	2.7	1.5
Laborers, construction	55.7	674	2.5	0.7
Assemblers	53.0	1,167	2.4	1.3
Carpenters	37.4	869	1.7	0.9
Stock handlers and baggers	37.2	1,121	1.7	1.2
Cooks	36.3	1,838	1.6	2.0
Cashiers	35.6	2,626	1.6	2.8

From ref. 10.

pational Outlook Handbook (11) includes a comprehensive listing of working conditions for individual job titles in all industries, including health care workers. These descriptions reveal many of the stresses and hazards associated with each of these professions. What follows are entries from that handbook.

Registered Nurses

Most nurses work in well-lighted, comfortable medical facilities. Home health and public health nurses travel to patients' homes and to schools, community centers, and other sites. Nurses may spend considerable time walking and standing. They need emotional stability to cope with human suffering, emergencies, and other stresses. Patients in hospitals and nursing homes need 24-hour care; nurses in these institutions may work nights, weekends, and holidays. They may also be on call. Office, occupational health, and public health nurses are more likely to work regular business hours.

Nursing has its hazards, especially in hospitals, nursing homes, and clinics, where nurses may care for persons with infectious diseases such as hepatitis and acquired immunodeficiency syndrome (AIDS). Nurses must observe rigid guidelines to guard against these and other dangers, such as radiation, chemicals used for sterilization of instruments, and anesthetics. In addition, they face back injury when moving patients, shocks from electrical equipment, and hazards posed by compressed gases (11).

Radiologic Technologists

Most full-time radiologic technologists work about 40 hours a week; they may have evening, weekend, or on-call hours. Technologists are on their feet for long periods and may lift or turn disabled patients. They work at radiologic machines but may also do procedures at patients' bedsides. Some radiologic technologists travel to patients in large vans equipped with sophisticated diagnostic equipment.

Radiation therapists who treat cancer patients are prone to emotional burnout because they treat extremely ill and dying patients on a daily basis. Although they exist in this occupation, potential radiation hazards have been minimized through the use of lead aprons, gloves, and other shielding devices and through use of instruments that monitor radiation exposure. Technologists wear badges that measure radiation levels in the radiation area, and detailed records are kept on their cumulative lifetime dose, according to Nuclear Regulatory Commission Standards (11).

Medical Records Technicians

Medical record technicians generally work a 40-hour week, although overtime may be required. In hospitals where medical record departments are open 18 to 24 hours a day, 7 days a week, technicians may work day, evening, and night shifts. They tend to work in pleasant and comfortable offices. Medical record technician is one of the few health occupations in which there is little or no contact with patients. Accuracy is essential, and this responsibility demands concentration and attention to detail. Medical record technicians who work at video display terminals for prolonged periods may experience eyestrain and muscle pain (11).

Nursing Aides and Psychiatric Aides

Most full-time aides work about 40 hours a week, but because patients need care 24 hours a day, some aides work evenings, nights, weekends, and holidays. Many work part time. Aides spend many hours standing and walking. Because they may have to move partially paralyzed patients in and out of bed or help them stand or walk, aides must guard against back injury. Nursing aides often have unpleasant duties; they empty bed pans and change soiled bed linens. They also care for disoriented and irritable patients. Psychiatric aides must be prepared to care for patients whose diseases may cause violent behavior. Although their work can be emotionally demanding, many aides gain satisfaction from assisting those in need (11).

Cardiovascular Technologists and Technicians

Technologists and technicians generally work a 5-day, 40-hour week, which may include Saturdays and Sundays. Those in catheterization laboratories tend to work longer hours and evenings. They may also be on call during the night and on weekends. Cardiovascular technologists and technicians spend a great deal of time walking and standing. Those who work in catheterization laboratories may face stressful working conditions, because they are in close contact with patients who have serious heart ailments. Some patients, for example, may have complications from time to time that have life-or-death implications (11).

Emergency Medical Technicians

Emergency medical technicians (EMTs) work both indoors and outdoors in all kinds of weather. Much of their time is spent standing, kneeling, bending, and lifting. They may risk noise-induced hearing loss from ambulance sirens and back injuries from lifting patients. EMTs may be exposed to diseases such as hepatitis B and AIDS and to violence from drug overdose victims. The work is physically strenuous and stressful—not surprising in a job that involves life-or-death situations. Nonetheless, many people find the work exciting and challenging. EMTs employed by fire departments often have about a 50-hour work week. Those employed by hospitals frequently work between 45 and 58 hours a week, and those in private ambulance services work between 48 and 51 hours. Some EMTs, especially those in police and fire departments, are on call for extended periods. Because most emergency services function 24 hours a day, EMTs have irregular working hours that add to job stress (11).

Clinical Laboratory Technologists and Technicians

For clinical laboratory workers hours and other working conditions vary according to the size and type of employment setting. In large hospitals or in independent laboratories that operate continuously, technologists and technicians usually work the day, evening, or night shift and may work weekends and holidays. Laboratory personnel in small facilities may work on rotating shifts rather than on a regular shift. In some facilities, laboratory personnel are on call, available in case of an emergency, several nights a week or on weekends. Clinical laboratory personnel are trained to work with infectious specimens. When proper methods of infection control and sterilization are followed, few hazards exist. Laboratories generally are well lighted and clean; however, specimens, solutions, and reagents used in the laboratory sometimes produce odors. Laboratory workers may spend a great deal of time on their feet (11).

Physicians

Many physicians work long, irregular hours. About one-half of all full-time physicians in 1994 worked 60 hours a week or more. In general, as they approach retirement age, physicians may accept fewer new patients and tend to work shorter hours. Physicians who are on call may make emergency visits to hospitals. A large percentage of physicians practice in groups or health care organizations that provide back-up coverage and allow time off. Many physicians must travel frequently between office and hospital to care for their patients (11).

Risk by Setting

Hospitals and nursing homes account for the largest work setting for health care workers. Nursing homes are one of America's fastest growing industries. Today, nursing homes and personal care facilities employ approximately 1.6 million workers at 21,000 worksites. By the year 2005, industry employment levels are expected to rise to an estimated 2.4 million workers (12).

Best's Underwriting Guide (3), described earlier in this chapter, offers a hazard index for each type of insurance on a per industry basis. This hazard index considers variables such as rate of filed workers' compensation claims per 1,000 employees, severity of claims (medical and lost wage expenditures), and industry-specific experience. Health care industries typically rank medium to high (Table 2-3). The rates listed are for 1989 and do not reflect recent increases in risk for exposure to infectious agents.

Free-standing Emergency Centers

In emergency departments and freestanding "urgi-centers" the main potential sources of workers' compensation claims are exposure to ionizing radiation and exposure to infectious disease. Those who operate radiographic equipment need training and monitoring for irradiation exposure. Viral hepatitis is the most serious and frequent disease hazard. Tuberculosis is a prominent concern. Eczema of the hands, forearms, and face is common. Slips and falls, sprains and strains, cuts and burns from autoclaves and sterilizers, and needle sticks also occur. Staff members may suffer fatigue and stress (3).

Home Health Services

Home health aides often find themselves in a variety of situations and settings that predispose them to workers' compensation claims. They work in uncontrolled surroundings, usually without backup from coworkers. Sprains

TABLE 2-3. *Hazard index for health care providers*

Industry	Best's Hazard Index[a]	Underwriting comments
Emergency centers (freestanding)	5	Varies with attitude of management
Health maintenance organizations	4	—
Home health services	7	Lifting injuries common
Hospice facilities	4	
Hospitals (General care)	8	Frequency of injury a problem
Medical laboratories	6	Severe exposure may be present
Nursing homes	8	Frequency of injury a problem
Surgical centers (outpatient)	5	—
X-ray laboratories (medical)	5	Personal monitoring and shielding are essential

[a]Low, 1–3; medium, 4–6; high, 7–9, very high, 10.

and strains from lifting or assisting patients in personal care or while lifting heavy medical equipment are extremely common. Disoriented or violent patients may injure home health aides, and slips and falls occur, particularly when the aide is not familiar with the home. Transmission of communicable disease from the patient to the health care worker is another major concern. Needle sticks are a notable risk and may occur more often in unfamiliar surroundings (3).

General Care Hospitals

Strains and sprains from lifting or handling patients and heavy objects, such as refuse, laundry sacks, oxygen cylinders, and medical equipment, account for most hospitals' overall workers' compensation claims. Falling and slips represent the second most common cause of hospital injuries. Needle sticks for nursing, housekeeping, laundry and laboratory personnel remain a serious problem. Shift-work fatigue is believed to contribute to accidents involving health care professionals. The potential for assault on hospital employees is an important concern. Injuries also may be caused by high-voltage medical equipment. Waste anesthetic gases in the operating room are a primary occupational exposure. These gases are flammable and have been associated with high rates of spontaneous abortions among female workers. Ethylene oxide, ionizing radiation, and antineoplastic agents are notable concerns (3).

Nursing Homes

According to 1994 Bureau of Labor Statistics data, nursing home workers face the third highest rate of occupational injuries and illnesses among all U.S. industries that have 100,000 or more nonfatal injury or illness cases a year; there were 221,000 cases in 1994 alone. Only meat products processing and motor vehicle and motor vehicle equipment manufacturing ranked higher. Nursing home workers suffered most injuries (51.2%) when handling residents. Fifty-eight percent of the injuries were strains and sprains. Although back injuries accounted for 27% of all injuries in the private sector, in nursing homes they accounted for 42% of all injuries. More than half of all nursing home injuries and illnesses were related to handling residents, and 42% were back injuries. Back injuries averaged more than $8,400 each in workers' compensation expenses alone (12). Other notable injuries include sprains and strains from lifting patients, injuries inflicted by disoriented patients, shocks and burns from use of high-voltage medical equipment, accidental puncture by syringes (with concomitant infectious disease transmission risk), and cuts from sharp medical instruments or broken glass (13).

INDUSTRY RISKS AND ISSUES FOR HEALTH CARE WORKERS

Every industry has its own portfolio of occupational hazards; many of these are often specific to a particular industry. Patient care and delivery of medical services is not without its own risks and hazards.

Infectious Disease

Health care workers are at risk for tuberculosis, hepatitis B and C viruses, and HIV infection. Occupational Safety and Health Administration (OSHA) guidelines on bloodborne pathogens require a comprehensive program for management of occupationally exposed workers at all health care institutions (14).

Medical centers have developed infection control programs to address the risk of work-related infectious exposure (that is, HIV infections and hepatitis B) and the consequent workers' compensation ramifications. Infectious illnesses contracted on the job are unquestionably compensible illnesses. That is, the medical center employer is required to pay for full medical benefits and to cover all lost wage costs, according to state regulations.

Medical centers have developed infection control programs to proactively address these issues (15). Since HIV was first identified in the early 1980s, at least 30, and perhaps as many as several hundred workers, have been infected with HIV, which causes AIDS (4). More recent data indicate that among the 4.4 million health care workers in the United States, 800,000 needle-stick or sharp-object injuries occur each year. Among these incidents, it is estimated that 16,000 persons are contaminated with HIV and even more with HBV and hepatitis C virus. The rate of HIV transmission is 0.3% per HIV-contaminated needle-stick injury (16).

In one study, 81 needle-stick injuries in a pediatric hospital over a 1-year period were evaluated. Disposable needles and intravenous devices accounted for 83.8% of the injuries. Thirty injuries occurred during procedures (withdrawal, insertion, taping, and other), and 51 occurred after procedures (disposal of loose sharp instruments, recapping, disassembly, and handling sharp instruments). Highest rates of injury were reported in the burn unit, infant-toddler unit, neonatal intensive care unit, and operating room. Staff nurses and nurse specialists sustained 59 of the injuries. Injuries also were reported by housekeeping staff, physicians, unit secretaries, and phlebotomists and laboratory technicians (17).

The Centers for Disease Control and Prevention recently estimated that in 13% of U.S. hospitals at least one worker contracts tuberculosis. Recent outbreaks of multidrug-resistant strains of *Mycobacterium tuberculosis* have prompted the National Institute for Occupational Safety and Health (NIOSH) to recommend that potentially exposed health care workers use powered air-purifying respirators with high-efficiency particulate filters (4). Other infectious agents can be transmitted from patient to health care worker, posing a direct threat to worker health and increasing workers' compensation costs. These include enteric pathogens that cause acute diarrhea, hepatitis A virus, herpes simplex virus, *Staphylococcus aureus,* group A and B streptococci, varicella-zoster virus, cytomegalovirus, *Neisseria meningitidis, Cryptosporidium, Bordetella pertussis,* the mites that cause scabies, and influenza virus (15).

Violence on the Job

Abuse-related injuries to health care workers, especially in an urban hospital, occur with remarkable prevalence, are serious, and can be costly in terms of time off work and compensation. Underreporting of these incidents, especially among physicians, has been described as likely (18). Service workers in general are at especially high risk for nonfatal assaults. They account for more than two fifths of lost workday cases resulting from assaults but for only one eighth of the workforce. Nursing aides and orderlies account for more than half of all assaulted service workers. They and other workers in health and residential care occupations (nurses and social workers, for example) are assaulted primarily by patients who resist help or residents who are prone to violence (10).

Of 242 reported abuse-related injuries in one study from Canada (18), 194 (80.2%) occurred among the nursing personnel. Nurses in medical units filed most (33.1%) of the reports. Although psychiatric nurses filed fewer reports (35; 14.5%), they had the highest rate of injuries per 100,000 paid hours among the nursing staff. Not surprisingly, security officers were at highest risk; 53.5% reported an abuse-related injury for a rate of 16.8 such injuries per 100,000 paid hours. Male staff members had a higher injury rate than their female counterparts in all occupational groups (18).

Bruising or crushing was the most frequent type of assault-related injury (126 cases); next most frequent were cuts and lacerations (47 cases) and human bites and exposures to blood or body fluids (23 cases). However, sprains and strains resulted in the largest amount of time lost (18). In all, more than 8,000 hours were lost because of abuse-related injuries, and more than $76,000 was paid in workers' compensation benefits (18). Concurrently, 646 incidents of verbal abuse and threatening behavior were reported. Only three abuse-related injuries and two incidents of verbal abuse were reported by physicians.

Substance Abuse

Chemical substance abuse is the third leading health problem in the United States. It is estimated that approximately 7 million workers are addicted to chemicals (19). There is a relation between chemical abuse and poor job performance (decreased productivity and efficiency, tardiness) and excessive use of sick time, disability, and workers' compensation (19). Chemical dependency among health care workers is higher than in the general population (15). Job stress and easy drug availability make chemical dependency one of the most frequent occupational illnesses to affect the medical center professional (15). The incidence of chemical dependency among hospital workers is high, possibly contributing to the number of on-the-job accidents (3). It may be difficult for health care workers to recognize the chemical dependency of a colleague because the affected worker usually protects his or her job performance over other life activities (15).

Exposure to Chemicals and Physical Agents

Although the risks of exposure to certain chemical agents in the hospital environment are well known, problems associated with the entire spectrum of chemicals used are not (20). Acute and chronic workplace exposures can represent costly problems for medical centers. In one study, the chemical groups to which workers were most likely to be exposed were disinfectants (25.9%), solvents (16.8%), and cleaning compounds (12.1%). Exposure by the dermal route was most common (37.9%). Thirteen percent of the exposures resulted in lost time and a similar percentage was reported on the OSHA log. Medical treatment was obtained by 53% of workers. Implications for hazard communication, record keeping, and prevention are discussed in the report (20). Other adverse health effects among health care workers include antineoplastic agents, anesthetic gases, sterilants such as ethylene oxide, and disinfectants (15).

In another study investigators analyzed incident reports related to chemical exposures, workers' compensation clinic logs, and the OSHA 200 log forms for an academic medical center to assess medical follow-up care and severity of the ailment. A total of 253 ex posures occurred from 1988 through 1990. The overall incidence rate was 8.0 per 1,000 person-years. Exposure rates by job title were highest for housekeepers (60.1 per 1,000 person-years) followed by maintenance workers (18.6) and laboratory technicians (13.1) (20).

WORKERS' COMPENSATION CHALLENGES IN MEDICAL CENTER OCCUPATIONAL HEALTH

Medical centers have unique resources to prevent illnesses and injuries that may arise in the delivery of health care.

Proper Lifting Techniques

The prevention of back injuries is worthy of serious attention and effort because of the high prevalence of these injuries and the corresponding disability. One difficulty is identification of equipment, job responsibilities, and work practices that put people at risk (4). Efforts have been tailored around modifying behavior and practices. One study showed that a 95% reduction in lost-time injuries could be obtained if a professional lifting team, rather than nurses, were to lift clients. The individual composition of the team would include persons already engaged in the movement and transport of patients. Secondary benefits to the lifting team approach are that morale improves among nursing staff, recruiting tasks become easier if nurses do not have to lift, and additional time is available for nursing care (21).

Needle-Disposal Programs

Several economic concepts related to the cost effectiveness of infection control may be applied for decision-making purposes. Determination of a base cost of a needle-stick injury was necessary for the analysis. Decision analysis of experience-based data aggregated from participating institutions showed the expected cost of needle-stick injury to be $363 (22). Continued efforts are needed to track needle-stick injury trends as new products are introduced in an attempt to minimize risk to health care workers (17).

To provide immediate assessment of injuries related to sharp objects, one medical center established a 24-hour hotline staffed by clinicians. These clinicians provided risk assessment at the time of the call. A 24-hour pharmacy service with an anonymous system to protect the confidentiality of the worker can provide prophylaxis within 5 minutes for workers potentially exposed to HIV. Hepatitis prophylaxis focused on hepatitis B immunization and administration of hepatitis B immune globulin to exposed workers. Medical management involved monitoring the adverse effects of postexposure prophylaxis, ensuring that workers received workers' compensation benefits, providing pretest and posttest counseling for exposed workers, and appropriate documentation. Confidentiality is essential for worker participation in the program. Institutional policies and procedures must address all the components of postexposure care and the issues related to HIV and HBV infection of health care workers. Sufficient staffing and funding, confidentiality, and prevention are the keys to a successful program (14).

Regulatory Initiatives

The U.S. Department of Labor launched its Worker Safety and Health, Employer Assistance Program for Nursing Homes in 1996. The secretary of labor unveiled a seven-state initiative to protect workers in more than 5,000 nursing homes and personal care facilities, one of the nation's fastest growing industries. According to the document (12), "Nationwide there are 1.6 million nursing home workers in more than 21,000 facilities. Our initiative emphasizes helping employers reduce injuries and illnesses through effective safety and health programs. The outreach effort will focus on common hazards found in nursing homes.".

In September 1996 in seven states OSHA began offering free, comprehensive safety and health seminars designed for nursing home employers. The OSHA seminars address nursing home risks, including back injuries from incorrect or strenuous lifting of residents, slips and falls, workplace violence, bloodborne pathogens, tuberculosis, and other infectious diseases (12).

Assistant secretary of labor for OSHA Joseph A. Dear described how nursing home employers implemented safety and health measures and achieved dramatic results. "In one case, an employer's workers' compensation costs dropped from $750,000 a year to $184,000, after he implemented a program to handle residents safely," said Dear (12). "The key to reducing injuries and illnesses is an effective safety and health program. Solutions to problems need not be expensive. Many hazards can be eliminated through simple, commonsense measures or low-cost equipment" (12).

CONCLUSION

Workers' compensation is a critical concern for medical centers. State regulations also challenge employers to minimize work-related injury and illness through prevention. The following checklist is drawn from *Best's Loss Control Engineering Manual* (13) and offers important steps in mitigating the personal, institutional, and financial consequences of occupational disorders:

- Management should buy into the importance of safety and health among workers and recognize the inherent risks of the industry.
- Training programs in safe work practices and observance of good occupational hygienic practices should be in place for all personnel.
- Employees at risk should be instructed in proper lifting techniques and given periodic

reviews on how to handle patients and operate equipment.

- Facilities and equipment should be inspected regularly.
- All new employees should undergo an orientation training program.
- Preplacement and annual medical examinations should be performed for all employees, especially those with patient contact. Employee medical records should be accurate and maintained appropriately.
- All employees should be appropriately immunized against infectious diseases.
- All medical personnel should be trained in the safe operation, storage, and use of medical equipment and supplies.
- All employees should be trained and retrained in universal precautions.
- Scheduling practices should be evaluated regularly.
- Employees should be instructed to report defective equipment and other conditions that are hazardous.
- Proper procedures for use of needles and sharp instruments should be in place.
- Appropriate employees should be trained in proper techniques for cleaning hazardous spills.
- Patient care employees should be taught the proper use of patient restraints to control potentially dangerous patients.
- The use of sophisticated electrical equipment should be limited to authorized personnel.
- Radioactive materials should be appropriately handled. Formalized training and retraining and monitoring programs should be in place.

REFERENCES

1. Boden L. Workers' compensation. In: *Occupational health: recognizing and preventing work-related disease*. Boston: Little, Brown, 1995.
2. Guidotti T, et al. The role of workers' compensation. In: *Occupational Health Services*. Chicago: American Medical Association, 1989.
3. Krolin G, et al. *Best's underwriting guide*. Oldwick, NJ: AM Best, 1993.
4. LaBar G. A healthy dose of worker protection. *Occup Hazards* 1992;54:21–26.
5. Nonfatal occupational injuries: number of cases and incidence rates, per 100 full-time workers, for industries with 100,000 or more injury cases, 1994. Workplace Injuries and Illnesses in 1994. USDL-95-508. Washington, DC: US Government Printing Office.
6. Nonfatal occupational injury incidence rates per 100 full time workers by industry, 1994. Workplace Injuries and Illnesses in 1994; USDL-95-508. Washington, DC: US Government Printing Office.
7. Accident facts. Itasca, IL: National Safety Council, 1996.
8. Workers' compensation back claim study. Boca Raton, FL: National Council on Compensation Insurance, 1993.
9. Fuortes L, et al. Epidemiology of back injury in university hospital nurses from review of workers' compensation records and a case-control survey. *J Occup Environ Med* 1994;36:1022–1026.
10. The 10 occupations with the largest number of injuries and illnesses involving days away from work: shares of case and employment totals, 1994. Characteristics of Injuries and Illnesses Resulting In Absences from Work; 1994;USDL-96-163. Washington, DC: US Government Printing Office.
11. Bureau of Labor Statistics. *1996–97 Occupational outlook handbook*, 22nd ed. Washington, DC: US Government Printing Office.
12. Labor Department Launches Worker Safety and Health, Employer Assistance Program for Nursing Homes. News Release USDL: 96-326, Washington, DC: US Government Printing Office, 1996.
13. Iannaccone M, et al. Best's loss control engineering manual. Oldwick, NJ: AM Best, 1995.
14. Fahrner R. Implementation of a hospital policy for health care workers exposed to hepatitis or the human immunodeficiency virus. *Am J Hosp Pharm* 1993;50: 269–275.
15. Howard J. Medical center occupational health. In: *Practical approaches to occupational and environmental medicine*. Boston: Little, Brown, 1994:428–444.
16. Tereskerz P, et al. Occupational exposure to blood among medical students. *N Engl J Med* 1997;335: 1150–1153.
17. Jackson MA, et al. Needlestick injuries in a pediatric hospital. *Pediatr Infect Dis J* 1994;13:318–320.
18. Yassi A. Assault and abuse of health care workers in a large teaching hospital. *Can Med Assoc J* 1994;151: 1273–1279.
19. Callery Y. Chemical abuse rehabilitation for hospital employees: examination of benefit usage when referred by an employee assistance professional. *AAOHN J* 1994;42:67–75.
20. Weaver V, et al. Occupational chemical exposures in an academic medical center. *J Occup Med* 1993;35: 701–706.
21. Charney W, et al. The lifting team: a design method to reduce lost time back injury in nursing. *AAOHN J* 1991; 39:231–234.
22. Laufer F, et al. Application of cost-effectiveness methodology to the consideration of needlestick-prevention technology. *Am J Infect Control* 1994;22:75–82.

Medical Center Occupational Health and Safety, edited by Robert J. McCunney. Published by Lippincott Williams & Wilkins, Philadelphia, 1999.

3

Bloodborne Pathogens

Jon T. O'Neal

Consultant in Occupational and Environmental Medicine, Austin, Texas 78705

PART 1. THE BLOODBORNE PATHOGENS STANDARD

On December 6, 1991, the Occupational Safety and Health Administration (OSHA) published its Occupational Exposure to Bloodborne Pathogens Standard, intended to prevent infections in workers who have contact with blood or blood products. With the exception of the Hazard Communication Standard (HAZCOM), which became effective a few years earlier and affected mainly hospital administrative and safety personnel, the requirements set forth in the Bloodborne Pathogens Standard (BBPS) were the first time most health-care workers (HCWs) were personally affected by an official OSHA regulation. The BBPS required workers to change their healthcare procedures and practices, a difficult undertaking, and compliance with the standard was estimated to cost the healthcare industry approximately $800 million a year.

OSHA spent over five years researching, gathering information, and formulating the Bloodborne Pathogens Standard. They received over 4,000 comments, exhibits, and testimonials from interested parties during the creation of the standard, at the time the largest input in the 20 year history of OSHA standard making. The final BBPS was based on consideration of information gathered from many different sources, and the resulting regulation is a mixture of preventive medicine, politics, and compromise.

The Bloodborne Pathogens Standard has two main goals: (1) to **prevent exposure** to bloodborne pathogens; and (2) to **prevent disease** if exposure occurs. OSHA seeks to achieve these goals by mandating two main requirements: (1) compliance with **universal precautions**; and (2) offering **hepatitis B vaccination** to employees. Universal precautions (Appendix B) is an approach to infection control that assumes all blood is infectious. Universal precautions had been merely recommendations from the Centers for Disease Control until the BBPS officially made the recommendations into enforceable requirements.

The hepatitis B vaccination series had also been only recommended for HCWs with occupational exposure to blood, and many at-risk employees did not have the vaccinations because of the cost involved (around $100 for the complete series). The BBPS officially required all employers to offer the hepatitis B vaccination series at no charge to employees with occupational exposure.

The BBPS is a precisely worded document, that requires specific actions of employers and employees. What follows in this chapter is an extremely simplified general overview of those requirements. The information presented here should not be regarded as a substitute for the actual requirements of the BBPS, the complete regulatory text of which is included as Appendix A. In all cases of practical interpretation, refer to the actual regulatory text.

HEPATITIS B VIRUS

HCWs have been known for many years to be at increased risk for acquiring hepatitis. But it was not until the development of hepatitis B antigen and antibody tests that the true risk was defined, and that HBV was identified as a relatively common infection. Hepatitis studies done in the 1970s showed that workers exposed to blood had a prevalence of HBV infection several times that of non-exposed workers in the general population, that the prevalence of HBV infection was related more to the degree of blood exposure than to patient contact, and that lab workers who had minimal patient contact had a high HBV infection rate. Studies have shown that HBV can survive for at least 1 week dried at room temperature on environmental surfaces, and that reported injuries do not account for the majority of HBV infections in HCWs. The majority of patients who are HBV-infectious are unrecognized as being infectious at the time of treatment, further emphasizing the need to follow universal precautions. These findings emphasize the importance of disinfection and sterilization as well as use of personal protective equipment (PPE) and HBV vaccination in case of PPE failure.

The CDC estimated in the late 1980s that approximately 8,700 HCWs were occupationally infected with hepatitis B virus (HBV) each year, with about 2,100 of those developing symptoms of acute infection, and 400 requiring hospitalization. OSHA estimated, before the implementation of the BBPS, that between 200 and 300 HCWs would die each year as a result of occupationally acquired hepatitis, and that compliance with the procedures set forth in the standard would prevent approximately 190 deaths from HBV infections.

Recent data show a dramatic decrease in the number of HBV infections in HCWs, with a decrease from an estimated 17,000 HBV infections in HCWs per year in 1983 to 400 infections in HCWs per year in 1995*. In 1983, the estimated incidence of HBV in HCWs was more than 3 times higher that the incidence of HBV in the general population (386 per 100,000 for HCWs vs. 122 per 100,000 for the general population). By 1995, the incidence of HBV infections in HCWs had dropped by 95% (9.1 per 100,000) and was over 5 times lower than the incidence of HBV infections in the general population (50 per 100,000). It is truly amazing that in just 12 years, with the institution of Universal Precautions and the Bloodborne Pathogens Standard, that the risk of HCWs contracting HBV has fallen so precipitously.

There has been considerable debate over the need for HBV vaccination booster doses. However, at this time, no studies have shown that booster doses are indicated after a successful initial HBV vaccination series and booster doses are not routinely recommended. If future studies show that HBV vaccination booster doses are indicated and are recommended by the Centers for Disease Control and Prevention, OSHA would require the employer to pay for the booster doses.

*Mahoney F, Stewart K, Hu H, Coleman P, Alter MJ. Progress toward the elimination of hepatitis B virus transmission among healthcare workers in the United States. *Arch Intern Med* 1997;157:2601–2605.

HEPATITIS C VIRUS AND HEALTH-CARE WORKERS

The BBPS barely mentions hepatitis C virus (HCV) and the risk to HCWs, mainly because HCV was not identified until 1989, after the vast majority of information had already been gathered for and the same year OSHA published the first draft of the standard (called the Notice of Proposed Rule Making). To fully address the HCV problem in HCWs, OSHA would have had to re-open the public comment period, delaying the implementation of the standard by probably years. However, since there is currently no protective HCV vaccination and no recommended post-exposure prophylaxis for HCV, the measures set forth in the BBPS that protect us from HIV and HBV infection, should also help decrease the risk of work-related HCV infections.

An estimated four million Americans are infected with HCV (through non-occupational routes) and about one million are infected with HBV. Though too early after the recent identification of HCV for comprehensive studies, and because HBV infections in HCWs have greatly decreased, HCV may now be regarded as the most important bloodborne exposure in HCWs.

HUMAN IMMUNODEFICIENCY VIRUS AND ACQUIRED IMMUNODEFICIENCY SYNDROME

During the first decade and a half of the AIDS epidemic (through June 1997), there were 52 confirmed cases, and 114 more reported cases of possible occupational HIV infection in HCWs. This contrasts sharply with an estimated tens of thousands of occupational HBV infections and thousands of occupationally related HBV deaths in HCWs during the same time. In absolute numbers, then, occupational HBV infection is more of a risk than occupational HIV infection. There has not been a single documented case of physician-to-patient HIV transmission in the United States. However, it was the fear of HIV and AIDS in workers and patients in the early 1990s that brought about the political climate necessary to allow OSHA to complete the necessary work and publish the Bloodborne Pathogens Standard.

OSHA ENFORCEMENT

During the first year of enforcement (March 1992 to February 1993), federal OSHA (not including states with their own OSHA plans) performed 984 inspections relating to its BBPS, including 371 hospitals, 103 dentists' offices, 87 doctors' offices, and 23 funeral homes. Political and congressional pressure has recently resulted in a more "user friendly" OSHA that focuses more on advising employers instead of aggressively inspecting for fines. From October 1997 through September 1998, federal OSHA performed only 564 inspections in all industry classifications, and only 213 inspections were in industries classified as health services (26 hospitals, 29 doctors' offices, 22 dentists' offices, 6 funeral homes, and 111 nursing homes were inspected during this period). Citations (653) were issued during these 213 inspections, resulting in an average 3.1 citations per inspection (average penalty was $719 per citation). The 26 hospitals inspected received 70 citations, resulting in an average 2.7 citations per inspection (but the average penalty for hospital citations was $2,589!). It appears that federal OSHA is now inspecting fewer hospitals than the first year of enforcement, though the average penalty for a hospital citation is still relatively expensive.

SCOPE AND APPLICATION

The BBPS applies to all occupational exposure to blood or other potentially infectious material.

DEFINITIONS

Bloodborne Pathogens: Disease-causing organisms carried in the blood, including HBV and HIV, HCV, malaria, syphilis, babesiosis, brucellosis, leptospirosis, arboviral infections, relapsing fever, Creutzfeld–Jakob disease, human T-lymphotropic virus type 1, and viral hemorrhagic fever.

Exposure Incident: Specific eye, mouth, mucous membrane (lip, nose, anus), nonintact skin, or parenteral (under-the-skin) contact with blood or potentially infectious materials. Nonintact skin includes skin with dermatitis, hangnails, cuts, abrasions, chafing, etc.

Occupational Exposure: Contact or reasonably anticipated contact between blood or other potentially infectious material and the eye, mouth, mucous membrane, nonintact skin, including parenteral contact occurring as a result of performance of work duties.

Other Potentially Infectious Materials (OPIM): Body fluids other than blood, and tissues, organs, or cells that may contain bloodborne pathogens, including semen; vaginal secretions; saliva in dental procedures; any body fluid visibly contaminated with blood; any unidentified body fluid; cerebrospinal, synovial, pleural, pericardial, peritoneal, and amniotic fluids; tissue or organs from living or dead persons; HIV- or HBV-containing cells, cultures, mediums, or solutions; and blood, organs, or tissues from experimental animals infected with HIV or HBV. Sweat, tears, and urine not visibly contaminated with blood are not OPIM.

Source Individual: A person (living or dead) whose blood/OPIM is the source of occupational exposure. An exposed employee is a person who has contact with a source individual's blood/OPIM.

EXPOSURE CONTROL

Employers who have employees with occupational exposure must establish a written **exposure control plan (ECP)** that, at least, contains the following:

- Exposure determination;
- Implementation plans;
- Procedures for evaluating exposure incidents.

The exposure control plan must also be accessible to employees, reviewed and updated at least annually or when new occupational exposures are possible, and available to OSHA personnel. The exposure determination identifies job classifications where workers may have occupational exposure. The exposure determination should contain a list of jobs in which all employees have occupational exposure and a list of jobs in which some employees have occupational exposure. OSHA does not require a list of jobs in which employees have no occupational exposure, and the worker exposure determination must be made without consideration of PPE usage. The purpose of the exposure determination is require the employer to identify and document those employees who must comply with and be educated about the Bloodborne Pathogens Standard.

METHODS OF COMPLIANCE

The first sentence in this paragraph is the most important sentence in the Standard, it states simply: "Universal precautions shall be observed to prevent contact with blood or other potentially infectious materials." The next sentence states that if one cannot tell what type of body fluid it is, consider it to be potentially infectious.

Engineering and Work Practice Controls

Engineering controls reduce exposure by either removing the hazard or isolating the employee from exposure. Needleless lines, self-sheathing needles, and sharps disposals are all considered engineering controls. Work practice controls reduce exposure by changing human behavior. Not recapping needles, handwashing, wearing gloves, actually using sharps disposals are all considered work practice controls.

Engineering controls must be reevaluated on a regular schedule, though the standard does not define a regular schedule. For example, some sharps boxes that are filled quickly should be changed daily, or twice a day, while some may need changing every other month. OSHA says reevaluate work practice controls as needed.

Employers must

- Provide readily accessible hand-washing facilities (if not feasible as in an ambulance, antiseptic hand cleanser and clean towels must be available);
- Ensure that employees wash their hands promptly after removing gloves or other PPE;
- Ensure that employees wash their hands/skin with soap and water, or flush mucous membranes with water promptly following contact with blood/OPIM;
- Provide appropriate containers (puncture resistant, labeled or color-coded, and leak-proof on sides and bottoms).

Employees must NOT

- Bend, recap, remove, or break contaminated needles or sharps;
- Eat, drink, smoke, apply cosmetics or lip balm, or handle contact lenses in areas with a reasonable likelihood of exposure;

- Keep food or drink in refrigerators, freezers, shelves, cabinets, or on countertops or benchtops where blood/OPIM is present;
- Perform mouth pipetting or suctioning of blood/OPIM.

Equipment that may be contaminated with blood/OPIM must be examined and decontaminated before servicing or shipping. Parts that remain contaminated must be labeled as such, and workers or servicing representative must be informed of the hazard.

Personal Protective Equipment

Even with engineering and work practice controls, risk may still exist, and in these cases personal protective equipment (PPE) should be used. PPE is special equipment or clothing worn to protect against a hazard, including gloves, gowns, face shields and masks, goggles and other eye protection, respirators, mouthpieces, resuscitation bags, and laboratory coats or other protective clothing. Work clothes, such as uniforms, pants, shirts, or blouses not intended to provide protection from bloodborne pathogens, are not considered PPE. Employers must

- Provide appropriate PPE, at no cost to the employee
- Ensure that employees use appropriate PPE
- Ensure that PPE is easily accessible and in appropriate sizes, and that hypoallergenic gloves, glove liners, or similar alternatives must be provided to employees who are allergic to normally used gloves
- Clean, launder, repair, replace, and dispose of PPE at no cost employees.

A worker whose PPE that is penetrated by blood or OPIM must be removed promptly prior to leaving the work area. An employee may, under rare and extraordinary circumstances, decline to use PPE when, in the employee's professional judgment, use of PPE would prevent the delivery of care or pose a hazard to the safety of the employee. When this occurs, the circumstances surrounding the incident must be investigated and documented to ensure similar incidents do not recur.

Gloves must be worn if hand contact with blood/OPIM is reasonably anticipated, when hands may contact mucous membranes or nonintact skin, and when handling or touching contaminated items or surfaces. Disposable gloves intended for single use may not be washed or decontaminated for reuse. Masks, eye protection, and face shields must be worn whenever splashes, spray, spatter, or droplets of blood/OPIM may be generated and eye, nose, or mouth contamination may be reasonably anticipated. Gowns, aprons, and other protective body clothing must be worn in occupational exposure situations. Surgical caps or hoods and/or shoe covers or boots must be worn when gross contamination can be reasonably anticipated (as in deliveries, or surgery).

Housekeeping

Employers are responsible for maintaining, cleaning, and sanitizing the workplace. They must prepare a written schedule for cleaning and decontamination that ensures routine and appropriate cleaning is performed. OSHA makes no reference to specific brands or types of cleaning/disinfecting agents, leaving that to the discretion of the employer. The standard simply states: "All equipment and environmental and working surfaces shall be cleaned and decontaminated after contact with blood or other potentially infectious materials." Environmental surfaces are areas such as floors, walls, and ceilings.

Contaminated work surfaces and protective coverings used to cover equipment must be decontaminated after the completion of procedures, promptly when there is a spill, at the end of the work shift if the surface or covering may have become contaminated since the last cleaning. Items that may become contaminated must be inspected and decontaminated on a regularly scheduled basis, and when visibly contaminated. Broken glassware that may be contaminated should be cleaned up using mechanical means, not picked up directly by hands.

Regulated waste and contaminated sharps must be promptly placed in a container that is closable, puncture-resistant, leakproof, labeled or color-coded, and closed before removal. Containers for contaminated sharps must be easily accessible and located as close as feasible to the area where the sharps are used; be kept upright, be replaced routinely, and not be allowed to overfill. Reusable containers should not be opened, emptied, or cleaned in a manner that would expose employees.

Contaminated laundry must be handled as little as possible. Workers who do handle contaminated laundry must wear appropriate PPE. Contaminated laundry should be placed in a bag or other container at the point of use but not sorted or rinsed there. Contaminated laundry should be transported in labeled or color-coded bags or containers and placed in leakproof bags or containers if wet.

HIV AND HBV RESEARCH LABORATORIES AND PRODUCTION FACILITIES

Two of the first 19 reported occupational HIV infections occurred in laboratory workers, and OSHA recognizes the increased hazard these employees face working with highly concentrated HIV/HBV by devoting a separate paragraph to these workplaces. The specific requirements of this section are presented in paragraph (e) of the regulatory text. A **research laboratory** is defined as a facility producing or using small quantities of highly concentrated HIV/HBV, and a **production facility** as a place that produces large quantities of highly concentrated HIV/HBV. Facilities that used unconcentrated blood as the only source of HIV/HBV, such as routine hospital laboratories, do not have to follow the added requirements of paragraph (e).

HEPATITIS B VACCINATION

The Occupational Safety and Health Act of 1970, which created OSHA, firmly established that employers were directly and financially responsible for the safety and health of their workers. This paragraph of the BBPS sets specific employer responsibilities, the most important probably being that: **The employer must make HBV vaccination available to all employees who have occupational exposure, at no cost to employees.** HBV vaccination must be made available to employees within 10 working days of initial assignment to jobs with occupational exposure. Before the vaccination series is started, however, employees must receive training, as outlined in paragraph (g). HBV vaccination does not need to be provided if the employees has previously received the complete HBV vaccination series, antibody testing shows that the employee is already HBV-immune, or vaccination is contraindicated for medical reasons.

There is considerable debate about the usefulness of HBV vaccination prescreening programs. Some employers feel prescreening identified employees who are already immune and do not need vaccination, while others feel the money spent on prescreening could be used to vaccinate more employees. The standard states that employees may not be required to participate in a prescreening program before receiving HBV vaccination. Employers may still offer a prescreening program, but employees have the right to decline prevaccination testing and yet still receive HBV vaccination.

All employees with occupational exposure must be offered HBV vaccination. Those that accept should have documentation of the completed series; those that decline must read and sign an HBV vaccination declination statement (see appendix to regulatory text). In essence, OSHA requires employers to provide documentation of either HBV vaccination, immunity, contraindication of HBV vaccination, or employee declination of vaccination. HBV vaccination documentation and exposure control plans are two of the most important pieces of documentation that will be asked for if your facility has an OSHA inspection.

POST-EXPOSURE EVALUATION AND FOLLOW-UP

The employer is responsible for providing and paying for all post-exposure evaluations and follow-up after exposure incidents. The Standard specifically states that the employers must

- Pay the bills
- Make vaccinations and evaluations convenient for employees (make available at a reasonable time and place)
- Ensure that evaluations and treatment are performed by licensed physicians or healthcare professionals
- Ensure that evaluations and treatment are provided according to current U.S. Public Health Service recommendations
- Ensure that laboratory test are performed by an accredited laboratory.

OSHA recognizes the dynamic nature of medical knowledge relating to bloodborne pathogens and wisely does not specify medical treatment in the Standard, but defers to other agencies, like the USPHS, the specific details of post-exposure evaluation and treatment. Though the BBPS only refers to HIV/HBV testing and evaluation (again, since the final draft was written before identification of HCV), HCV testing and evaluation should be included in post-exposure evaluation and follow-up. Once an exposure incident has been reported, an employer must immediately provide the exposed employee, at no cost to the employee, with a confidential medical evaluation and follow-up to include documentation of the route and circumstances of the exposure, identification of the source individual, testing of blood for HBV and HIV status, post-exposure prophylaxis, counseling, and evaluation of reported illnesses. Post-exposure prophylaxis guidelines from the CDC recommend starting HIV prophylaxis within a few hours of an exposure incident [*MMWR Morb Mortal Wkly Rep* 1998; 47(RR-7)].

Consent must be obtained from the exposed employee before testing of his/her blood for HIV/HBV status. Consent should also be obtained, if possible, from the source individual, before testing of blood. If consent is not obtained from the source individual, the employer should document this. Some states do not require consent from the source individual for post-exposure testing, and procedures for this practice should be referred to state medical and legal authorities.

Exposed employees have the right to decline post-exposure HBV/HIV testing, however, they would lose legal standing if they decline baseline testing and were later to claim they were infected by the exposure.

Results of a source individual's HBV/HIV testing results must be provided to the exposed employee, however, the exposed employee must be informed about confidentiality laws, in order to protect the source individual's privacy rights. Employers must pay for the source individual's testing, and provide the results to the exposed individual. However, even though it is not specifically stated in the Standard, the employer does not have the right to know the results of the source individual's or exposed employee's testing. A confidentiality conflict may occur when the employer is also the healthcare professional evaluating and treating the exposed employee. OSHA provides no specific guidance in this instance, but says only that matters of consent and confidentiality are extremely important in this setting.

Information Provided to the Health Care Professional

The employer must make sure the health care professional (HCP) responsible for the HBV vaccination program and post-exposure evaluations has a copy of the Standard, and must ensure the HCP performing post-exposure evaluations is provided with a description of the exposed employee's duties relating to the exposure, documentation of the circumstances of the exposure, the source individual's blood test results, and all relevant medical records. The employer is responsible for maintaining employee HBV vaccination and post-exposure records, however, the employer does not have a specific right to know the results of the source individual's blood testing or confidential medical information contained in the employee's medical records.

The Health Care Professional's Written Opinion

The employer must be provided with a "written opinion" from the healthcare professional treating or evaluating an employee. The employer has a right to know information contained in this written opinion, however, OSHA limits the HBV vaccination written opinion to stating whether HBV vaccination is indicated or has been received, and limits the post-exposure evaluation written opinion to stating that the employee has been informed of the evaluation results and has been told about any medical conditions that may result from the exposure. The HCP's written opinion should contain no other medical findings or diagnoses.

COMMUNICATION OF HAZARDS

Employers must tell employees about the hazards of bloodborne pathogens through the use of labels, signs, information, and training.

Warning labels must

- Be affixed to regulated waste containers, refrigerators, or freezers containing blood/OPIM
- Include the word "biohazard" and the biohazard symbol
- Be fluorescent orange or orange-red with lettering and symbol in contrasting colors
- Be affixed on or close to the container by a method that prevents loose or unintentional removal.
- Be affixed to contaminated equipment, and the parts that are contaminated must be identified on the label.

There are exceptions to biohazard labeling requirements. Red bags or containers may be substituted for labels if employees are trained about the meaning of red bags. Containers of blood or blood products that are labeled for release for transfusion or clinical use do not require biohazard labeling. Individual containers for blood/OPIM that are placed in a labeled container for storage or transport do not require individual labeling. Regulated waste that has been decontaminated does not require labeling or color-coding.

Signs are only required at the entrance to work areas in HIV/HBV research or production facilities, and must be fluorescent orange or orange-red with contrasting lettering and symbols and must bear the word *biohazard* and the biohazard symbol, the name of the infectious agent, special requirements for entering the area, and the name and telephone number of the laboratory director of other responsible person.

Information and Training

Employers must ensure that all employees with occupational exposure participate in a bloodborne pathogens training program. The training program must be provided at no cost to the employee, during working hours, at the time of initial assignment to tasks with occupational exposure, and at least annually thereafter. Training sessions should be presented in vocabulary and content appropriate to the employee's education level, literacy, and language. Annual training must be provided to employees within one year of their previous training. Additional training is required when new or modified tasks affect an employee's occupational exposure. A bloodborne pathogens training program must explain the following elements:

- The regulatory text, a copy of which must be accessible to the employees.
- The epidemiology, symptoms, and modes of transmission of bloodborne diseases
- The exposure control plan and how to obtain a copy
- Ways to recognize tasks or activities that may involved exposure to blood/OPIM
- The use and limitations of methods that prevent or reduce exposure, including engineering controls, work practices, and PPE.
- The types, proper use, and appropriate selection of PPE
- HBV vaccination, and that it will be provided at no cost to the employee

- The appropriate actions to take and person to contact in an emergency involving blood/OPIM
- The procedures to follow after an exposure incident
- The post-exposure evaluation and follow-up that an employer must provide after an exposure incident.
- The required labels, color-coding, or signs.

The training program must also offer an opportunity for **interactive questions** and answers with the **person conducting the training session.** The person conducting the training session must be knowledgeable in the preceding matters as they relate to the workplace, which means that employers cannot simply show a general videotape on bloodborne pathogens, without having someone trained and knowledgeable about the specific workplace present to answer questions.

RECORD KEEPING

Employee medical records must include the following:

- The employee's name and Social Security number
- Information on HBV vaccination status
- Dates of all HBV vaccinations
- Medical records relative to HBV vaccination
- All post-exposure evaluation results, testing, and procedures
- The healthcare professional's written opinions
- Information provided to the healthcare professional after an exposure incident.

The employer must maintain employee medical records for at least the duration of employment and 30 years. Employers also must maintain training records, which must include dates of training sessions, contents or summary of the training sessions, names and qualifications of trainers, and the names and job titles of persons attending the training sessions. Training records must be maintained for 3 years from the date of training.

If an employer ceases to do business and there is no new employer to keep the records for the required time, the employer must notify the National Institute of Occupational Safety and Health (NIOSH) at least 3 months prior to the disposal of the records, and then transfer the records to NIOSH, if they so request.

EFFECTIVE DATES

All the requirements of the Bloodborne Pathogens Standard have been in effect as of July 6, 1992, and OSHA has been inspecting workplaces and fining for non-compliance with the Standard since then.

PART 2. POST-EXPOSURE MANAGEMENT AND PROPHYLAXIS[1]

CDC defines an "exposure"[2] that may place a health-care worker (HCW) at risk for bloodborne viral infections as:

A percutaneous injury (e.g., a needlestick or cut with a sharp object)

Contact of mucous membrane or nonintact skin (e.g. chapped or abraded skin, or skin with dermatitis)

Contact with intact skin when the duration of contact is prolonged (i.e., several minutes or more) or involves an extensive area, with blood, tissue, or other body fluids.

Any direct contact (i.e., without barrier protection) to concentrated virus in a research laboratory or production facility.

---

[1]The information in this section is taken mainly from the following recent CDC reports and these reports, or the most current CDC reports on post-exposure management and prophylaxis, should be referred to for more specific or timely information:

Centers for Disease Control and Prevention. Public health service guidelines for the management of healthcare worker exposures to HIV and recommendations for post-exposure prophylaxis. *MMWR Morb Mortal Wkly Rep* 1998;47(RR-7).

Centers for Disease Control and Prevention. Immunization of health-care workers—recommendations of the Advisory Committee on Immunization Practices (ACIP) and the Hospital Infection Control Practices Advisory Committee (HICPAC). *MMWR Morb Mortal Wkly Rep* 1997;46(RR-18):1–42.

Centers for Disease Control and Prevention. Recommendations for follow-up of healthcare workers after occupational exposure to hepatitis C virus. *MMWR Morb Mortal Wkly Rep* 1997;46:603–606.

[2]OSHA calls these "exposure incidents."

Note: Exposure to *nonbloody* saliva, tears, sweat, urine or feces is not considered a risk and does not require post-exposure follow-up.

Medical Centers (and all healthcare organizations) should have in place written protocols for prompt reporting, evaluation, treatment, and follow-up of occupational exposures that may place HCWs at risk for bloodborne infection. OSHA requires employers to have exposure-control plans, including post-exposure follow-up and incident reporting.

Clinicians should be available *during all working hours*, including nights and weekends, to provide post-exposure care, and anti-retroviral agents for post-exposure prophylaxis (PEP) should be available for timely administration (ideally within a few hours of exposure.) HCWs should be educated to report exposures immediately after they occur, in order to implement PEP, if indicated, as soon as possible after the exposure. HCWs who are at risk for occupational exposure to bloodborne pathogens should be taught, as part of job orientation and ongoing job training, the principles of post-exposure management (PEM), including options for PEP.

EXPOSURE REPORT

If an exposure occurs, the circumstances and post-exposure management should be recorded in the HCW's confidential medical record. Relevant information includes the following:

Date and time of exposure;

Details of the procedure being performed, including where and how the exposure occurred, and if the exposure was related to a sharp device, the type of device and how and when in the course of handling the device the exposure occurred;

Details of the exposure, including the type and amount of fluid or material and the severity of the exposure;

Details about the exposure source, and if the source is infected with HIV or other bloodborne pathogens, and if the source is HIV-infected, the stage of disease, history of antiretroviral therapy, and viral load, if known;

Details about counseling, post-exposure management, and follow-up.

EXPOSURE SITE TREATMENT

Wounds and skin sites that have been in contact with blood or other potentially infectious material should be washed with soap and water; mucous membranes should be flushed with water. There is no evidence that the use of antiseptics for wound care or expressing fluid by squeezing the wound further reduces the risk for virus transmission. However, the use of antiseptics is not contraindicated. The application of caustic agents (e.g., bleach) or the injection of antiseptics or disinfectants into the wound is not recommended.

SOURCE INDIVIDUAL EVALUATION

The source individual, if identified, should be informed of the exposure incident. If indicated and consent is obtained, a blood sample should be drawn from the source individual and tested for hepatitis B surface antigen (HBsAg), antibody to human immunodeficiency virus (anti-HIV, or HIV antibody), and antibody to hepatitis C virus (anti-HCV). Samples need not be re-drawn if the source individual is already documented as having HIV-antibody or anti-HCV, or being currently infectious with HBV, HCV, or HIV.

Some states allow testing of previously obtained blood samples for post-exposure evaluation if consent is not obtained from a source individual. If a blood sample is not already available and the source individual does not give consent, drawing blood for post-exposure evaluation may be considered battery (unauthorized touching.) Therefore, local and state laws regarding consent for testing source individuals should be followed, and policies should be available for testing source individuals in situations where consent cannot be obtained (e.g., unconscious patients). Confidentiality of the source individual should be maintained at all times.

Many source individuals have medical records with information available at the time of exposure (e.g., laboratory test results, admitting diagnosis, or past medical history) that may suggest or rule out possible bloodborne pathogens infections. Information to be considered when evaluating a source individual for possible HIV infection include prior HIV testing or CD4+ count, clinical symptoms suggestive of primary HIV infection or undiagnosed immunodeficiency disease, and history of possible HIV exposures (such as IV-drug use, sexual contact with a known HIV-positive partner, unprotected sexual contact with multiple partners, or receipt of blood or blood products prior to 1985). If the source individual is known to have HIV infection, information about stage of infection (i.e., asymptomatic or AIDS), CD4+ T-cell count, viral load testing, and current and previous antiretroviral regimen, should be gathered for consideration in choosing appropriate PEP.

EXPOSED HEALTH-CARE WORKER EVALUATION

If indicated and if consent is obtained, baseline and follow-up testing of the exposed HCW for HBV, HCV, and HIV should be performed. Exposed HCWs have the right to decline baseline testing, however, they would lose legal standing if they declined baseline testing and were later to claim that they were infected by the exposure.

Post-exposure testing for exposed HCWs should include baseline and follow-up HBV testing, anti-HCV testing, and HIV-antibody testing. During all phases of post-exposure evaluation and follow-up, confidentially of the exposed HCW should be protected.

Post-exposure and follow-up HBV evaluation of the exposed HCW must be individualized because many HCWs are already immune to HBV, either as a result of successful vaccination or prior HBV infection. Though CDC has published guidelines for HBV PEP (see Table 3-1), they do not specifically address HBV follow-up testing.

- Baseline Anti-HBs testing may be done on exposed HCWs, unless they have recently been found to be known responders[3].
- If a previously vaccinated (or infected) HCW is a known responder, follow-up HBV testing is not indicated because the individual is considered to be immune.
- If a HCW is previously vaccinated and does not know his/her response; is a known non-responder; or is unvaccinated, follow-up HBV testing should include a baseline anti-HBs. If baseline anti-HBs shows the exposed HCW is a responder, no further HBV follow-up testing is indicated.
- If baseline anti-HBs shows the exposed HCW is a non-responder[4] or has no anti-HBs, follow-up HBV testing may be indicated (e.g., at 3 and 6 months). However, since HBV vaccination (or revaccination) is recommended as PEP for these individuals, they would be expected to test anti-HBs positive at follow-up testing because of vaccination. Therefore, other HBV testing (such as HBeAg, IgM anti-HBc, or HBsAg) may need to be considered to evaluate possible active HBV infection as a result of an exposure. Referral to an internist or infectious disease specialist may be indicated in these cases for individualized follow-up if the source of the exposure is high-risk for being HBV infectious.

Baseline and follow-up (e.g., at 6 weeks, 3 months, and 6 months) HIV-antibody testing of an exposed HCW is indicated if the source person is HIV-antibody positive, has AIDS, or is high-risk for HIV infection. It is unclear whether follow-up HIV-antibody testing is indicated at one year because only three in-

[3]Responder is defined as a person with adequate levels of serum antibody to hepatitis B surface antigen (i.e., anti-HBs >/= 10 mIU/mL).

[4]A non-responder has an inadequate response to vaccination, defined as serum anti-HBs <10 mIU/mL.

TABLE 3-1. *Recommended postexposure prophylaxis for percutaneous or permucosal exposure to hepatitis B virus, United States*

	Treatment when		
Vaccination and antibody response status of exposed person	Source HBsAg positive	Source HBsAg negative	Source not tested or status unknown
Unvaccinated	HBIG[a] × 1; initiate HB vaccine series	Initiate HB vaccine series	Initiate HB vaccine series
Previously vaccinated known responder[b]	No treatment	No treatment	No treatment
Known nonresponder	HBIG × 2 or HBIG × 1 and initiate revaccination	No treatment	If known high-risk source, treat as if source were HBsAg positive
Antibody response unknown	Test exposed person for anti-HBsAg If adequate,[b] no treatment If inadequate,[b] HBIG × 1 and vaccine booster	No treatment	Test exposed person for anti-HBsAg If adequate,[b] no treatment. If inadequate,[b] initiate revaccination

[a] HBIG dose 0.06 mL/kg intramuscularly.
[b] Responder is defined as a person with adequate levels of serum antibody to HBs (i.e., anti-HBs ≥10 mIU/mL); inadequate response to vaccination is defined as serum anti-HBs <10 mIU/mL.
HBsAg, hepatitis B surface antigen; anti-HBs, antibody to hepatitis B surface antigen; HBIG, hepatitis B immune globulin; HB, hepatitis. [Data from: Centers for Disease Control and Prevention. Immunization of health-care workers—recommendations of the Advisory Committee on Immunization Practices (ACIP) and the Hospital Infection Control Practices Advisory Committee (HICPAC). *MMWR Morb Mortal Wkly Rep* 1997;46(RR-18):1–42.]

stances of HIV seroconversion in HCWs delayed greater than six months have been reported[5–7]. Two of the delayed seroconversions were associated with simultaneous HCV exposure, however, it is not known whether HCV directly influences the risk for or course of HIV infection. CDC believes the infrequency of this occurrence does not warrant adding to the HCW's anxiety by routinely extending the duration of post-exposure follow-up to one year. Though not specifically recommended, it might be prudent to consider HIV-antibody follow-up testing at greater than 6 months (e.g., one year) for HCWs at risk for simultaneous HCV exposure. Also, CDC does not generally recommend routine use of direct HIV virus assays to detect infection in exposed HCWs.

If the source individual is seronegative for HIV, baseline testing or further follow-up of the exposed HCW normally is not necessary. However, if an HIV-seronegative source individual has recently engaged in behaviors that are associated with a risk for HIV transmission, baseline and follow-up HIV-antibody testing of the exposed individual should be considered.

For purposes of considering HIV PEP, the evaluation should also include information about medications the HCW may be taking and any current or underlying medical conditions or circumstances (i.e., pregnancy, breast feeding, or renal or hepatic disease) that may influence drug selection, and pregnancy testing should be offered to all women capable of becoming pregnant whose pregnancy status is unknown.

Baseline and follow-up (e.g., at 6 months) anti-HCV and alanine aminotransferase test-

[5] Ciesielski CA, Metler RP. Duration of time between exposure and seroconversion in healthcare workers with occupationally acquired infection with human immunodeficiency virus. *Am J Med* 1997;102(suppl 5b):115–116.

[6] Ridzon R, Gallagher K, Ciesielski C, et al. Simultaneous transmission of human immunodeficiency virus and hepatitis C virus from a needle-stick injury. *N Engl J Med* 1997;336:919–922.

[7] Gerberding JL. San Francisco General Hospital, unpublished data, May 1997.

ing of an exposed HCW is recommended if the source of the exposure is anti-HCV positive or high-risk for being HCV infectious. Alanine aminotransferase activity may be used as a surrogate marker for early hepatitis infection.

HEPATITIS C VIRUS POST-EXPOSURE PROPHYLAXIS

There is no vaccine currently available to prevent hepatitis C, and immune globulin is not recommended for post-exposure prophylaxis. However, in the absence of effective prophylaxis, persons who have been exposed to HCV may benefit from knowing their infection status so they can seek evaluation for chronic liver disease and treatment.

CDC and the Hospital Infection Control Practices Advisory Committee recommend considering implementing policies and procedures for follow-up for HCV infection after percutaneous or permucosal exposures to blood. At a minimum, such policies should include the following:

For the source, baseline testing for antibody to HCV (anti-HCV);

For the person exposed to an anti-HCV-positive source, baseline and follow-up (e.g., 6-month) testing for anti-HCV and alanine aminotransferase activity;

Confirmation by supplemental anti-HCV testing of all anti-HCV results reported as repeatedly reactive by enzyme immunoassay (EIA);

Recommending against post-exposure prophylaxis with immune globulin or antiviral agents (e.g., interferon)[8]; and

Education of HCWs about the risk for and prevention of bloodborne infections, including hepatitis C, in occupational settings, with the information routinely updated to ensure accuracy.

Counseling recommendations to prevent transmission of HCV to others are that persons who are anti-HCV-positive should refrain from donating blood, organs, tissues, or semen, and that household contacts should not share toothbrushes and razors. However, there are neither recommendations against pregnancy or breastfeeding nor recommendations for changes in sexual practices among HCV-infected persons with a steady partner. Although HCV sometimes can be transmitted from persons with chronic disease to their steady sex partners, the risk for transmission is low despite long-term, ongoing sexual activity. Infected persons should be informed of the potential risk for sexual transmission to assist in decision-making about precautions.

HEPATITIS B VIRUS POST-EXPOSURE PROPHYLAXIS

Post-exposure prophylaxis with hepatitis B immune globulin (HBIG—passive immunization) and/or vaccination (active immunization) should be used when indicated after an exposure incident (Table 3-1). HBV PEP should be considered for any percutaneous, ocular, or mucous membrane exposure to blood in the workplace and is determined by the HBsAg status of the source individual and the vaccine response or antibody status of the exposed HCW. Needlestick or other percutaneous exposures of unvaccinated persons should lead to initiation of the hepatitis B vaccine series (if not contra-indicated), regardless of the HBsAg status of the source individual, in order to protect the worker from future exposures.

If the source individual is HBsAg-positive and the exposed HCW is unvaccinated, HBIG should also be administered as soon as possible after exposure (preferably within 24 hours) and the vaccine series started. The effectiveness of HBIG when administered greater than 7 days after percutaneous or permucosal exposures is unknown.

[8]Several studies suggest that interferon treatment begun early in the course of HCV infection is associated with a higher rate of resolved infection. However, there are no data indicating that treatment begun early during the course of chronic HCV infection is less effective that treatment begun during the acute phase of infection (i.e., there is evidence that interferon may be effective during early infection, but no evidence that it works as prophylaxis against infection).

To simplify HBV PEP:

If the exposed HCW has adequate levels of anti-HBs, no PEP is indicated.
If the source individual is HBsAg negative, PEP is not indicated (unless the exposed HCW has not yet been vaccinated).
If the source individual has a positive or unknown HBsAg status, and the exposed HCW is unvaccinated or has inadequate levels of anti-HBs, PEP may be indicated.

POST-EXPOSURE COUNSELING

HIV-exposed HCWs should have access to persons who are knowledgeable about occupational HIV transmission and post-exposure counseling. In order to prevent secondary HIV transmission, especially during the first 6–12 weeks after an exposure, HIV-exposed HCWs should be advised to:

Use sexual abstinence or condoms to prevent sexual transmission and avoid pregnancy.
Refrain from donating blood, plasma, organs, tissue, or semen.
Consider discontinuation of breast feeding.

There is no need to modify a HCW's patient-care responsibilities to prevent HIV transmission based solely on an HIV exposure, however, if HIV seroconversion does occur, CDC's recommendations for HIV-infected HCW's should be followed.[9]

Exposed HCWs should be advised to seek medical evaluation for any acute illness that occurs during the follow-up period. Symptoms such as fever, rash, myalgia, fatigue, malaise, or lymphadenopathy, may indicate acute HIV infection but also may indicate a drug reaction or other medical conditions.

Exposed HCWs who chose to take HIV PEP should be advised of the importance of completing the prescribed regimen, and should be provided with information about potential drug interactions and the potential side effects of the prescribed drugs. Measures that maybe used to minimize side effects and monitoring for toxicity during follow-up should also be discussed. Evaluation of certain symptoms during a PEP regimen should not be delayed (i.e., back or abdominal pain, pain on urination or blood in urine, or symptoms of hyperglycemia such as increased thirst and/or frequent urination).

If the source individual's virus is known or suspected to be resistant to one or more of drugs in the HIV PEP regimen, other PEP drugs to which the source individual's virus is unlikely to be resistant are recommended. It is strongly recommended that PEP be started regardless of the resistance status in the source virus, and a third or fourth drug may be added to the regimen if resistance is known or suspected, until consultation with a clinical expert in the treatment of HIV infection can be obtained and the PEP regimen possibly modified. The National Clinicians' post-exposure Hotline (888-448-4911) may be contacted for information on HIV PEP.

HUMAN IMMUNODEFICIENCY VIRUS POST-EXPOSURE PROPHYLAXIS

There is no currently available and effective HIV vaccination; however, anti-viral medications that have been found effective in the treatment of HIV-infected individuals are now recommended as HIV PEP for high risk exposures. The decision to recommend HIV PEP depends upon a risk assessment of the nature of the exposure and the amount and type of blood or body fluid involved in the exposure. Since new anti-viral drugs and drug combinations are being introduced quite rapidly, the most recent CDC recommendations on HIV PEP should be referenced for the most timely information. The information presented here is based on the HIV PEP guidelines set forth by CDC in the MMWR, May 15, 1998/Vol. 47/No. RR-7.

CDC bases their PEP recommendations on a risk assessment determined by an **Exposure Code (EC)** and an **HIV Status Code**

[9]Centers for Disease Control and Prevention. Recommendations for preventing transmission of human immunodeficiency virus and hepatitis B virus to patients during exposure-prone invasive procedures. *MMWR Morb Mortal Wkly Rep* 1991;40(RR-8).

(HIV SC). The Exposure Code assesses the source material (i.e., blood, body fluid, OPIM) and the type of exposure (i.e., percutaneous, mucous membrane, skin). The HIV Status Code assesses the HIV status of the exposure source. HIV PEP recommendations are based on assessing both the EC and the HIV SC.

1. Determining the HIV Exposure Code (EC)

If the **source material** is **NOT** blood, bloody fluid, or other potentially infectious material (OPIM)[10], or an instrument contaminated with one of these substances, HIV **PEP** is **NOT indicated.** (EC is 0.)[11]

If the **source material IS** blood, bloody fluid, OPIM, or an instrument contaminated with one of these substances, HIV **PEP MAY BE indicated** based on the type of exposure.

Determining the Type of Exposure

If **intact skin** only was exposed, HIV **PEP** is **NOT indicated**[12]. (EC is 0.)

If **mucous membranes** or **skin with compromised integrity**[13] was exposed, the EC is based on the **volume** of exposure. If a **small volume** of source material was involved (e.g., a few drops for a short duration), the **EC** is **1.** If a **large volume** of source material was involved (e.g., several drops, major blood splash and/or longer duration—i.e., several minutes or more), the **EC** is **2.**

If the exposure was **percutaneous,** the EC is based on the **severity** of the exposure. If a percutaneous exposure is **less severe** (e.g., solid needle, superficial scratch), the **EC** is **2.** If a percutaneous exposure is **more severe** (e.g., large-bore hollow needle, deep puncture, visible blood on device, or needle used in source patient's artery or vein[14] the **EC** is **3.**

2. Determining the HIV Status Code (HIV SC)

If the **exposure source** is **HIV negative**[15], **no PEP** is **needed** (HIV SC is 0)[16].

If the **exposure source** is **unknown,** or has an **unknown HIV status,** the **HIV SC** is **unknown.**

If the **exposure source is HIV positive**[17], the **HIV SC** is based on an estimated **titer** of the exposure. If an HIV positive exposure source has a **lower titer** (e.g., asymptomatic and high CD4 count), the **HIV SC** is **1.** If an HIV positive exposure source has a **higher titer** (e.g., advance AIDS, primary HIV infection, high or increasing viral load or low CD4 counts), the **HIV SC** is **2.**

3. Determining the HIV PEP Recommendation

HIV PEP recommendations are determined based on the combination of the EC and HIV SC for a particular exposure (see accompanying list).

---

[10]Other Potentially Infectious Materials (OPIM), includes semen or vaginal secretions; cerebrospinal, synovial, pleural, peritoneal, pericardial, or amniotic fluids, or tissue.

[11]CDC does not specifically rate EC or HIV SC as 0; however, for clarity, an EC or HIV SC of 0 will be used when no HIV PEP is needed.

[12]Contact with intact skin is not normally considered a risk for HIV transmission. However, if the exposure was to blood, and the circumstance suggests a higher volume exposure (e.g., an extensive area of skin was exposed or there was prolonged contact with blood), the risk for HIV transmission should be considered.

[13]Skin integrity is considered compromised if there is evidence of chapped skin, dermatitis, abrasion, or open wound.

[14]The combination of these severity factors (e.g., large-bore hollow needle *and* deep puncture) contribute to an elevated risk for transmission if the source person is HIV-positive.

[15]There is an exceedingly rare chance that an exposure source who tests HIV negative has had a false negative test, e.g., the exposure source may be in the "window phase" of HIV infection, during initial viremia, and before detectable levels of HIV antibody have formed.

[16]A source is considered negative for HIV infection if there is laboratory documentation of a negative HIV antibody, HIV polymerase chain reaction (PCR), or HIV p24 antigen test result from a specimen collected at or near the time of exposure and there is no clinical evidence of recent retroviral-like illness.

[17]A source is considerd infected with HIV (HIV positive) if there has been a positive laboratory result for HIV antibody, HIV PCR, or HIV p24 antigen or physician-diagnosed AIDS.

EC		HIV SC	PEP Recommendation
0	or	0	**No PEP needed**[18].
1		1	**PEP may not be warranted.** Exposure type does not pose a knownrisk for HIV transmission. Whether the risk for drug toxicity outweighs the benefit of PEP should be decided by the exposed HCW and treating clinician.
1		2	**Consider basic regimen.** Exposure type poses a negligible risk for HIV transmission. A high HIV titer in the source may justify consideration of PEP. Whether the risk for drug toxicity outweighs the benefit of PEP should be decided by the exposed HCW and treating clinician.
2		1	**Recommend basic regimen.***Most HIV exposures are in this category; no increased risk for HIV transmission has been observed but use of PEP is appropriate.
2		2	**Recommend expanded regimen.****Exposure type represents an increased HIV transmission risk.
3		1 or 2	**Recommend expanded regimen.** Exposure type represents an increased HIV transmission risk.
	Unknown		If the source or, in the case of an unknown source, the setting where the exposure occurred suggests a possible risk for HIV exposure and the EC is 2 or 3, consider PEP basic regimen.

HIV Post-Exposure Prophylaxis Regimens

***Basic Regimen:**[19]
4 weeks of **BOTH:**
Zidovudine 600 mg every day in divided doses (i.e., 300 mg twice a day, 200 mg three times a day, or 100 mg every 4 hours)
AND Lamivudine 150 mg twice a day.

****Expanded Regimen:**[20]
Basic regimen PLUS
Either Indinavir 800 mg every 8 hours
Or Nelfinavir 750 mg three times a day.
See addendum for more specific information on first-line drugs for HIV PEP.

[18]If either the EC or HIV SC is 0, no HIV PEP is indicated, e.g., if the source material, or the type of exposure, is low risk for HIV transmission, the HIV SC is irrelevant, and no PEP is indicated. If HIV SC is 0—the exposure source is HIV negative—the type of source material or exposure is irrelevant and no PEP is indicated.

[19]For occupational HIV exposures for which there is a recognized transmission risk.

[20]For occupational HIV exposures that pose an increase risk for transmission (e.g., larger volume of blood and/or higher virus titer in blood).

HIV Post-Exposure Prophylaxis Counseling

Because most occupational HIV exposures do not result in the transmission of HIV, potential toxicity must be carefully considered when prescribing PEP. When possible, HIV PEP recommendations should be implemented in consultation with persons having expertise in antiretroviral therapy and HIV transmission. If source individual information is not immediately available, PEP should be initiated, if indicated, without delay, and changes in the PEP regimen can be made later, after PEP is started, as appropriate.

While considering HIV PEP, HCWs should be informed that:

Knowledge about the efficacy and toxicity of drugs used for PEP are limited;
Only ZDV has been shown to prevent HIV transmission in humans;
There are no data to address whether adding other antiretroviral drugs provides any additional benefit for PEP, but experts recom-

mend combination drug regimens because of increased potency and concerns about drug-resistant virus;

Data regarding toxicity of antiretroviral drugs in persons without HIV infection or in pregnant women are limited for ZDV and not known regarding other antiretroviral drugs;

Any or all drugs for PEP may be declined by the HCW.

HCWs who have exposures for which HIV PEP is not recommended should be informed that the potential side effects and toxicity of taking PEP outweigh the negligible risk of transmission posed by the type of exposure.

If the exposure source is unknown, information about where and under what circumstances the exposure occurred should be assessed, including the prevalence of HIV in the population group from which the exposed material is derived (e.g., an exposure that occurs on an AIDS unit would be higher risk for transmission than an exposure that occurs in a nursing home for the elderly that has no known HIV-infected residents.)

If the source individual's HIV status in not known at the time of exposure (including when the source is HIV negative, but may have had a recent HIV exposure), consideration of PEP should be based on the type of exposure and the clinical or epidemiologic likelihood of HIV infection in the source. If source individual HIV testing is pending, and evaluation suggests a possibility of HIV transmission, it is reasonable to initiate a two-drug PEP regimen until lab results are obtained, and PEP can be modified or discontinued as appropriate.

HIV testing of needles or other sharps associated with an exposure, even if the source is unknown, is not recommended. The reliability and interpretation of findings in such circumstances are unknown.

Timing of HIV Post-Exposure Prophylaxis

PEP should be initiated as soon as possible. The interval within which PEP should be started for optimal efficacy is not known. To assure timely access to PEP, occupational exposure should be regarded as an urgent medical concern and PEP started as soon as possible after the exposure (i.e., in a few hours rather than days). The optimal duration of HIV PEP is unknown, but because 4 weeks of ZDV appeared protective to HCWs in a study[21], PEP probably should be administered for 4 weeks, if tolerated.

HIV Post-Exposure Prophylaxis Toxicity

Since PEP-related toxicity has been reported, drug-toxicity monitoring should be performed at baseline and at 2 weeks after starting PEP. Clinical judgement should be used to determine the scope of testing, which should be based on medical conditions that may exist in the HCW and toxicity associated with the drugs used as PEP. PEP toxicity monitoring should include:

Complete blood count

Renal function tests

Hepatic function tests

If a protease inhibitor (such as indinavir or nelfinavir) is used, hyperglycemia testing

If indinavir is used, testing for crystalluria, hematuria, hemolytic anemia, and hepatitis

Other testing based on the specific PEP drugs used.

If signs of toxicity are noted, modification of the PEP regimen should be considered after expert consultation, and further diagnostic studies may be indicated.

HCWs may fail to complete the regimen due to PEP-related side effects such as nausea and vomiting. Some of these symptoms may be managed without changing the regimen, by adding antimotility and antiemetic or other agents that target the specific symptoms. Modifying the doses interval (i.e., lowering

[21]Centers for Disease Control and Prevention. Case-control study of HIV seroconversion in health-care workers after percutaneous exposure to HIV-infected blood—France, United Kingdom, and United States, January 1988–August 1994. *MMWR Morb Mortal Wkly Rep* 1995;44:929–933.

the dose of drug, but administering more frequently during the day, as recommended by the manufacturer) may help HCWs adhere to the PEP regimen.

ADDENDUM

FIRST-LINE DRUGS FOR HIV POST-EXPOSURE PROPHYLAXIS[22]

Nucleoside Reverse Transcriptase Inhibitors

***Zidovudine (RETROVIR®*; ZDV, AZT)**

Dosage

600 mg every day in divided doses (e.g., 300 mg twice a day, 200 mg three times a day, or 100 mg every four hours).

Primary toxicities and/or side effects

Neutropenia, anemia, nausea, fatigue, malaise, headache, insomnia, and asthenia.

Comments

Caution should be used if co-administered with bone marrow suppressive drugs or cytotoxic therapy.

***Lamivudine (EPIVIR™*; 3TC)**

Dosage

150 mg twice a day.

Primary toxicities and/or side effects

Headache, abdominal pain, diarrhea, and in rare cases, pancreatitis. Toxicity of ZDV and 3TC when use in combination is approximately equal to that of ZDV alone.

***ZDV plus 3TC (COMBIVIR™*)**

Dosage

1 tablet twice a day, each table contains 300 mg ZDV and 150 mg 3TC.

Primary toxicities and/or side effects

See above for ZDV and 3TC.

Comments

Caution should be used if co-administered with bone marrow suppressive drugs or cytotoxic therapy.

Protease Inhibitors (PIs)[23]

***Indinavir (CRIXIVAN®*, IDV)**

Dosage

800 mg every 8 hours on an empty stomach (i.e., without food or with a light meal).

Primary toxicities and/or side effects

Nephrolithiasis, crystalluria, hematuria, nausea, headache, indirect hyperbilirubinemia, elevated liver function tests (LFTs), and hyperglycemia/diabetes.

Primary drug interactions[24]

No PI should be co-administered with terfenadine (Seldane®), astemizole (Hismanal®), cisapride (Propulsid®), triazolam, and midazolam. Rifampin should not be administered with PIs. Cyctochrome P450 metabolism inhibitor like detoconazole may increase PI plasma concentrations; dose reduction of the PI is only indicated for indinavir. Ergot alkaloid preparations should not be used in combination with PIs. If rifabutin is used concomitantly, rifabutin dose should be reduced because of inhibition of rifabutin metabolism; with concomitant indinavir or nelfinavir use, reduce the dose of ribafutin by 50%.

Serum levels of PIs may be increased when multiple PIs are used in combination.

Comments

Incidence of nephrolithiasis may be reduced by consuming large quantities of water [i.e., drinking six 8 oz. glasses of water (total 48 oz.) throughout the day].

***Nelfinavir (VIRACEPT™*)**

Dosage

750 mg three times a day (with meals or a light snack).

Primary toxicities and/or side effects

Diarrhea and hyperglycemia/diabetes.

Primary drug interactions[25]

See above for indinavir.

---

[22]Information included in these recommendations may not represent Food and Drug Administration (FDA) approval or approved labeling for the particular products or indications in question. Specifically, the terms "safe" and "effective" may not be synonymous with the FDA-defined legal standards for product approval.

[23]It is recommended that consultation with experts in the treatment of HIV infection and disease be sought when considering the inclusion of PIs or the use of alternative agents in PEP regimens.

[24]See package insert for other contraindications and possible drug interactions.

[25]See package insert for other contraindications and possible drug interactions.

Comments

Diarrhea usually can be controlled with over-the-counter antidiarrheal drugs (e.g., loperamide).

If oral contraceptives are being used, alternative or additional contraceptive measures should be used while taking nelfinavir.

Other antiviral drugs used for treatment of HIV infections that may be considered for PEP in special circumstances include[26]

Nucleoside Reverse Transcriptase Inhibitors:

Zalcitabine (HIVID®, ddC)
Didanosine (VIDEX®, ddI)
Stavudine (ZERIT™, d4T)

Protease Inhibitors (PIs):

Ritonavir (NORVIR™)
Saquinavir (INVIRASE™, hard-gel formulation) (FORTAVASE™, soft-gel formulation)

Non-nucleoside Reverse Transciptase Inhibitors:

Nevirapine (VIRAMUNE®)
Delavirdine (RESCRIPTOR®)

Appendix A

OSHA Bloodborne Pathogens Standard Regulatory Text[1]

(a) SCOPE AND APPLICATION

This section applies to all occupational exposure to blood or other potentially infectious materials as defined by paragraph (b) of this section.

[26]The use of these non-first-line drugs should be used in consultation with persons having expertise in antiretroviral therapy. Consult package insert for specific information on dosage, contraindications, and possible side effects.

[1]As published in the *Federal Register,* Friday, December 6, 1991; 29CFR, part 1910.1030.

(b) DEFINITIONS

For purposes of this section, the following shall apply:

Assistant Secretary means the Assistant Secretary of Labor for Occupational Safety and Health, or designated representative.

Blood means human blood, human blood components, and products made from human blood.

Bloodborne Pathogens means pathogenic microorganisms that are present in human blood and can cause disease in humans. These pathogens include, but are not limited to, Hepatitis B Virus [HBV] and Human Immunodeficiency Virus [HIV].

Clinical Laboratory means a workplace where diagnostic or other screening procedures are performed on blood or other potentially infectious materials.

Contaminated means the presence or the reasonably anticipated presence of blood or other potentially infectious materials on an item or surface.

Contaminated Laundry means laundry which has been soiled with blood or other potentially infectious materials or may contain sharps.

Contaminated Sharps means any contaminated object that can penetrate the skin including, but not limited to, needles, scalpels, broken glass, broken capillary tubes, and exposed ends of dental wires.

Decontamination means the use of physical or chemical means to remove, inactivate, or destroy bloodborne pathogens on a surface or item to the point where they are no longer capable of transmitting infectious particles and the surface or item is rendered safe for handling, use, or disposal.

Director means the Director of the National Institute for Occupational Safety and Health, U.S. Department of Health and Human Services, or designated representative.

Engineering Controls means controls (e.g., sharps disposal containers, self-sheathing needles) that isolate or remove the bloodborne pathogens hazard from the workplace.

Exposure Incident means a specific eye, mouth, other mucous membrane, non-intact skin, or parenteral contact with blood or other potentially infectious materials that results from the performance of an employee's duties.

Handwashing Facilities means a facility providing an adequate supply of running potable water, soap, and single use towels or hot air drying machines.

Licensed Healthcare Professional is a person whose legally permitted scope of practice allows him or her to independently perform the activities required by paragraph (f) Hepatitis B vaccination and Post-Exposure Evaluation and Follow-Up.

HBV means Hepatitis B Virus.

HIV means Human Immunodeficiency Virus.

Occupational Exposure means reasonably anticipated skin, eye, mucous membrane, or parenteral contact with blood or other potentially infectious materials that may result from the performance of an employee's duties.

Other Potentially Infectious Materials means

(1) The following human body fluids: semen, vaginal secretions, cerebrospinal fluid, synovial fluid, pleural fluid, pericardial fluid, peritoneal fluid, amniotic fluid, saliva in dental procedures, any body fluid that is visibly contaminated with blood, and all body fluids in situations where it is difficult or impossible to differentiate between body fluids;

(2) Any unfixed tissue or organ (other than intact skin) from a human (living or dead); and

(3) HIV-containing cell or tissue cultures, organ cultures, and HIV- or HBV-containing culture medium or other solutions; and blood, organs, or other tissues from experimental animals infected with HIV or HBV.

Parenteral means piercing mucous membranes or the skin barrier through such events as needlesticks, human bites, cuts, and abrasions.

Personal Protective Equipment is specialized clothing or equipment worn by an employee for protection against a hazard. General work clothes (e.g., uniforms, pants, shirts, or blouses) not intended to function as protection against a hazard are not considered to be personal protective equipment.

Production Facility means a facility engaged in industrial-scale, large-volume, or high concentration production of HIV or HBV.

Regulated Waste means liquid or semi-liquid blood or other potentially infectious materials; contaminated items that would release blood or other potentially infectious materials in a liquid or semi-liquid state if compressed; items that are caked with dried blood or other potentially infectious materials and are capable of releasing these materials during handling; contaminated sharps; and pathological and microbiological wastes containing blood or other potentially infectious materials.

Research Laboratory means a laboratory producing or using research-laboratory-scale amounts of HIV or HBV. Research laboratories may produce high concentrations of HIV or HBV but not in the volume found in production facilities.

Source Individual means any individual, living or dead, whose blood or other potentially infectious materials may be a source of occupational exposure to the employee. Examples include, but are not limited to, hospital and clinic patients; clients in institutions for the developmentally disabled; trauma victims; clients of drug and alcohol treatment facilities; residents of hospices and nursing homes; human remains; and individuals who donate or sell blood or blood components.

Sterilize means the use of a physical or chemical procedure to destroy all microbial life including highly resistant bacterial endospores.

Universal Precautions is an approach to infection control. According to the concept of Universal Precautions, all human blood and certain human body fluids are treated as if known to be infectious for HIV, HBV, and other bloodborne pathogens.

Work Practice Controls means controls that reduce the likelihood of exposure by altering the manner in which a task is performed (e.g., prohibiting recapping of needles by a two-handed technique).

(c) EXPOSURE CONTROL

(1) Exposure Control Plan

(i) Each employer having an employee(s) with occupational exposure as defined by paragraph (b) of this section shall establish a written Exposure Control Plan designed to eliminate or minimize employee exposure.

(ii) The Exposure Control Plan shall contain at least the following elements:
- (A) The exposure determination required by paragraph (c)(2);
- (B) The schedule and method of implementation for paragraphs (d) Methods of Compliance, (e) HIV and HBV Research Laboratories and Production Facilities, (f) Hepatitis B Vaccination and Post-Exposure Evaluation and Follow-Up, (g) Communication of Hazards to Employees, and (h) Recordkeeping of this standard; and
- (C) The procedure for the evaluation of circumstances surrounding exposure incidents as required by paragraph (f)(3)(i) of this standard.

(iii) Each employer shall ensure that a copy of the Exposure Control Plan is accessible to employees in accordance with 29 CFR 1910.20(e).

(iv) The Exposure Control Plan shall be reviewed and updated at least annually and whenever necessary to reflect new or modified tasks and procedures which affect occupational exposure and to reflect new or revised employee positions with occupational exposure.

(v) The Exposure Control Plan shall be made available to the Assistant Secretary and the Director upon request for examination and copying.

(2) Exposure Determination

(i) Each employer who has an employee(s) with occupational exposure as defined by paragraph (b) of this section shall prepare an exposure determination. This exposure determination shall contain the following:
- (A) A list of all job classifications in which all employees in those job classifications have occupational exposure;
- (B) A list of job classifications in which some employees have occupational exposure; and
- (C) A list of all tasks and procedures or groups of closely related task and procedures in which occupational exposures occur and that are performed by employees in job classifications listed in accordance with the provisions of paragraph (c)(2)(i)(B) of this standard.

(ii) This exposure determination shall be made without regard to the use of personal protective equipment.

(d) METHODS OF COMPLIANCE

(1) General

Universal precautions shall be observed to prevent contact with blood or other potentially infectious materials. Under circumstances in which differentiation between body fluid types is difficult or impossible, all body fluids shall be considered potentially infectious materials

(2) Engineering and Work Practice Controls

(i) Engineering and work practice controls shall be used to eliminate or minimize employee exposure. Where occupational exposure remains after institution of these controls, personal protective equipment shall also be used.

(ii) Engineering controls shall be examined and maintained or replaced on a regular schedule to ensure their effectiveness.

(iii) Employers shall provide handwashing facilities which are readily accessible to employees.

(iv) When provision of handwashing facilities is not feasible, the employer shall provide either an appropriate antiseptic hand cleanser in conjunction with clean cloth/paper towels or antiseptic towelettes. When antiseptic hand cleansers or towelettes are used, hands shall be washed with soap and running water as soon as feasible.

(v) Employers shall ensure that employees wash their hands immediately or as soon as feasible after removal of gloves or other personal protective equipment.

(vi) Employers shall ensure that employees wash hands and any other skin with soap and water, or flush mucous membranes with water immediately or as soon as feasible following contact of such body areas with blood or other potentially infectious materials.

(vii) Contaminated needles and other contaminated sharps shall not be bent, recapped, or removed except as noted in paragraphs (d)(2)(vii)(A) and (d)(2)(vii)(B) below. Shearing or breaking of contaminated needles is prohibited.

- (A) Contaminated needles and other contaminated sharps shall not be bent, recapped or removed unless the employer can demonstrate that no alternative is feasible or that such action is required by a specific medical or dental procedure.
- (B) Such bending, recapping or needle removal must be accomplished through the use of a mechanical device or a one-handed technique.

(viii) Immediately or as soon as possible after use, contaminated reusable sharps shall be placed in appropriate containers until properly reprocessed. These containers shall be:

- (A) Puncture resistant;
- (B) Labeled or color-coded in accordance with this standard;
- (C) Leakproof on the sides and bottom; and
- (D) In accordance with the requirements set forth in paragraph (d)(4)(ii)(E) for reusable sharps.

(ix) Eating, drinking, smoking, applying cosmetics or lip balm, and handling contact lenses are prohibited in work areas where there is a reasonable likelihood of occupational exposure.

(x) Food and drink shall not be kept in refrigerators, freezers, shelves, cabinets or on countertops or benchtops where blood or other potentially infectious materials are present.

(xi) All procedures involving blood or other potentially infectious materials shall be performed in such a manner as to minimize splashing, spraying, spattering, and generation of droplets of these substances.

(xii) Mouth pipetting/suctioning of blood or other potentially infectious materials is prohibited.

(xiii) Specimens of blood or other potentially infectious materials shall be placed in a container which prevents leakage during collection, handling, processing, storage, transport, or shipping.

- (A) The container for storage, transport, or shipping shall be labeled or color-coded according to paragraph (g)(1)(i) and closed prior to being stored, transported, or shipped. When a facility utilizes Universal Precautions in the handling of all specimens, the labeling/color-coding of specimens is not necessary provided containers are recognizable as containing specimens. This exemption only applies while such specimens/containers remain within the facility. Labeling or color-coding in accordance with paragraph (g)(1)(i) is required when such specimens/containers leave the facility.

(B) If outside contamination of the primary container occurs, the primary container shall be placed within a second container which prevents leakage during handling, processing, storage, transport, or shipping and is labeled or color-coded according to the requirements of this standard.

(C) If the specimen could puncture the primary container, the primary container shall be placed within a secondary container which is puncture-resistant in addition to the above characteristics.

(xiv) Equipment which may become contaminated with blood or other potentially infectious materials shall be examined prior to servicing or shipping and shall be decontaminated as necessary, unless the employer can demonstrate that decontamination of such equipment or portions of such equipment is not feasible.

(A) A readily observable label in accordance with paragraph (g)(1)(i)(H) shall be attached to the equipment stating which portions remain contaminated.

(B) The employer shall ensure that this information is conveyed to all affected employees, the servicing representative, and/or the manufacturer, as appropriate, prior to handling, servicing, or shipping so that appropriate precautions will be taken.

(3) Personal Protective Equipment

(i) Provision. When there is occupational exposure, the employer shall provide, at no cost to the employee, appropriate personal protective equipment such as, but not limited to, gloves, gowns, laboratory coats, face shields or masks and eye protection, and mouthpieces, resuscitation bags, pocket masks, or other ventilation devices. Personal protective equipment will be considered "appropriate" only if it does not permit blood or other potentially infectious materials to pass through to or reach the employee's work clothes, street clothes, undergarments, skin, eyes, mouth, or other mucous membranes under normal conditions of use and for the duration of time which the protective equipment will be used.

(ii) Use. The employer shall ensure that the employee uses appropriate personal protective equipment unless the employer shows that the employee temporarily and briefly declined to use personal protective equipment when, under rare and extraordinary circumstances, it was the employee's professional judgment that in the specific instance its use would have prevented the delivery of healthcare or public safety services or would have posed an increased hazard to the safety of the worker or co-worker. When the employee makes this judgment, the circumstances shall be investigated and documented in order to determine whether changes can be instituted to prevent such occurrences in the future.

(iii) Accessibility. The employer shall ensure that appropriate personal protective equipment in the appropriate sizes is readily accessible at the worksite or is issued to employees. Hypoallergenic gloves, glove liners, powderless gloves, or other similar alternatives shall be readily accessible to those employees who are allergic to the gloves normally provided.

(iv) Cleaning, Laundering, and Disposal. The employer shall clean, launder, and dispose of personal protective equipment required by paragraphs (d) and (e) of this standard, at no cost to the employee.

(v) Repair and Replacement. The employer shall repair or replace personal protective equipment as needed to maintain its effectiveness, at no cost to the employee.

(vi) If a garment(s) is penetrated by blood or other potentially infectious materials, the garment(s) shall be removed immediately or as soon as feasible.

(vii) All personal protective equipment shall be removed prior to leaving the work area.

(viii) When personal protective equipment is removed it shall be placed in an appropriately designated area or container for storage, washing, decontamination, or disposal.

(ix) Gloves. Gloves shall be worn when it can be reasonably anticipated that the employee may have hand contact with blood, other potentially infectious materials, mucous membranes, and non-intact skin; when performing vascular access procedures except as specified in paragraph (d)(3)(ix)(D); and when handling or touching contaminated items or surfaces.

(A) Disposable (single use) gloves such as surgical or examination gloves, shall be replaced as soon as practical when contaminated or as soon as feasible if they are torn, punctured, or when their ability to function as a barrier is compromised.

(B) Disposable (single use) gloves shall not be washed or decontaminated for re-use.

(C) Utility gloves may be decontaminated for re-use if the integrity of the glove is not compromised. However, they must be discarded if they are cracked, peeling, torn, punctured, or exhibit other signs of deterioration or when their ability to function as a barrier is compromised.

(D) If an employer in a volunteer blood donation center judges that routine gloving for all phlebotomies is not necessary then the employer shall:

(1) Periodically reevaluate this policy;

(2) Make gloves available to all employees who wish to use them for phlebotomy;

(3) Not discourage the use of gloves for phlebotomy; and

(4) Require that gloves be used for phlebotomy in the following circumstances:

(i) When the employee has cuts, scratches, or other breaks in his or her skin;

(ii) When the employee judges that hand contamination with blood may occur, for example, when performing phlebotomy on an uncooperative source individual; and

(iii) When the employee is receiving training in phlebotomy.

(x) Masks, Eye Protection, and Face Shields. Masks in combination with eye protection devices, such as goggles or glasses with solid side shields, or chin-length face shields, shall be worn whenever splashes, spray, spatter, or droplets of blood or other potentially infectious materials may be generated and eye, nose, or mouth contamination can be reasonably anticipated.

(xi) Gowns, Aprons, and Other Protective Body Clothing. Appropriate protective clothing such as, but not limited to, gowns, aprons, lab coats, clinic jackets, or similar outer garments shall be worn in occupational exposure situations. The type and characteristics will depend upon the task and degree of exposure anticipated.

(xii) Surgical caps or hoods and/or shoe covers or boots shall be worn in instances when gross contamination can reasonably be anticipated (e.g., autopsies, orthopedic surgery).

(4) Housekeeping

(i) General. Employers shall ensure that the worksite is maintained in a clean and sanitary condition. The employer shall determine and implement an appropriate written schedule for cleaning and method of decontamination based upon the location within the facility, type of surface to be cleaned, type of soil present, and tasks or procedures being performed in the area.

(ii) All equipment and environmental and working surfaces shall be cleaned and decontaminated after contact with blood or other potentially infectious materials.

(A) Contaminated work surfaces shall be decontaminated with an appropriate disinfectant after completion of procedures; immediately or as soon as feasible when surfaces are overtly contaminated or after any spill of blood or other potentially infectious materials; and at the end of the work shift if the surface may have become contaminated since the last cleaning.

(B) Protective coverings, such as plastic wrap, aluminum foil, or imperviously-backed absorbent paper used to cover equipment and environmental surfaces, shall be removed and replaced as soon as feasible when they become overtly contaminated or at the end of the workshift if they may have become contaminated during the shift.

(C) All bins, pails, cans, and similar receptacles intended for reuse which have a reasonable likelihood for becoming contaminated with blood or other potentially infectious materials shall be inspected and decontaminated on a regularly scheduled basis and cleaned and decontaminated immediately or as soon as feasible upon visible contamination.

(D) Broken glassware which may be contaminated shall not be picked up directly with the hands. It shall be cleaned up using mechanical means, such as a brush and dust pan, tongs, or forceps.

(E) Reusable sharps that are contaminated with blood or other potentially infectious materials shall not be stored or processed in a manner that requires employees to reach by hand into the containers where these sharps have been placed.

(iii) Regulated Waste.

(A) Contaminated Sharps Discarding and Containment.

(1) Contaminated sharps shall be discarded immediately or as soon as feasible in containers that are:

(i) Closable;

(ii) Puncture resistant;

(iii) Leakproof on sides and bottom; and

(iv) Labeled or color-coded in accordance with paragraph (g)(1)(i) of this standard.

(2) During use, containers for contaminated sharps shall be:

(i) Easily accessible to personnel and located as close as is feasible to the immediate area where sharps are used or can be reasonably anticipated to be found (e.g., laundries);

(ii) Maintained upright throughout use; and

(iii) Replaced routinely and not be allowed to overfill.

(3) When moving containers of contaminated sharps from the area of use, the containers shall be:

(i) Closed immediately prior to removal or replacement to prevent spillage or protrusion of contents during handling, storage, transport, or shipping;

(ii) Placed in a secondary container if leakage is possible. The second container shall be:

(A) Closable;

(B) Constructed to contain all contents and prevent leakage during handling, storage, transport, or shipping; and

(C) Labeled or color-coded according to paragraph (g)(1)(i) of this standard.

(4) Reusable containers shall not be opened, emptied, or cleaned manually or in any other manner which would expose employees to the risk of percutaneous injury.

(B) Regulated Waste Containment.

(1) Regulated waste shall be placed in containers that are:

(i) Closable;

(ii) Constructed to contain all contents and prevent leakage of fluids during handling, storage, transport, or shipping;

(iii) Labeled or color-coded in accordance with paragraph (g)(1)(i) of this standard; and

(iv) Closed prior to removal to prevent spillage or protrusion of contents during handling, storage, transport, or shipping.

(2) If outside contamination of the regulated waste container occurs, it shall be placed in a second container. The second container shall be:

(i) Closable;

(ii) Constructed to contain all contents and prevent leakage of fluids during handling, storage, transport, or shipping;

(iii) Labeled or color-coded in accordance with paragraph (g)(1)(i) of this standard; and

(iv) Closed prior to removal to prevent spillage or protrusion of contents during handling, storage, transport, or shipping.

(C) Disposal of all regulated waste shall be in accordance with applicable regulations of the United States, States and Territories, and political subdivisions of States and Territories.

(iv) Laundry.

(A) Contaminated laundry shall be handled as little as possible with a minimum of agitation.

(1) Contaminated laundry shall be bagged or containerized at the location where it was used and shall not be sorted or rinsed in the location of use.

(2) Contaminated laundry shall be placed and transported in bags or containers labeled or color-coded in accordance with paragraph (g)(1)(i) of this standard. When a facility utilizes Universal Precautions in the handling of all soiled laundry, alternative labeling or color-coding is sufficient if it permits all employees to recognize the containers as requiring compliance with Universal Precautions.

(3) Whenever contaminated laundry is wet and presents a reasonable likelihood of soak-through of or leakage from the bag or container, the laundry shall be placed and transported in bags or containers which prevent soak-through and/or leakage of fluids to the exterior.

(B) The employer shall ensure that employees who have contact with contaminated laundry wear protective gloves and other appropriate personal protective equipment.

(C) When a facility ships contaminated laundry off-site to a second facility which does not utilize Universal Precautions in the handling of all laundry, the facility generating the contaminated laundry must place such laundry in bags or containers which are labeled or color-coded in accordance with paragraph (g)(1)(i).

(e) HIV AND HBV RESEARCH LABORATORIES AND PRODUCTION FACILITIES

(1) **This paragraph applies to research laboratories and production facilities** engaged in the culture, production, concentration, experimentation, and manipulation of HIV and HBV. It does not apply to clinical or diagnostic laboratories engaged solely in the analysis of blood, tissues, or organs. These requirements apply in addition to the other requirements of the standard.

(2) **Research laboratories and production facilities shall meet the following criteria:**

(i) Standard microbiological practices. All regulated waste shall either be incinerated or decontaminated by a method such as autoclaving known to effectively destroy bloodborne pathogens.

(ii) Special practices:

(A) Laboratory doors shall be kept closed when work involving HIV or HBV is in progress.

(B) Contaminated materials that are to be decontaminated at a site away from the work area shall be placed in a durable, leakproof, labeled or color-coded container that is closed before being removed from the work area.

(C) Access to the work area shall be limited to authorized persons. Written policies and procedures shall be established whereby only persons who have been advised of the potential biohazard, who meet any specific entry requirements, and who comply with all entry and exit procedures shall be allowed to enter the work areas and animal rooms.

(D) When other potentially infectious materials or infected animals are present in the work area or containment module, a hazard warning sign incorporating the universal biohazard symbol shall be posted on all access doors. The hazard warning sign shall comply with paragraph (g)(1)(ii) of this standard.

(E) All activities involving other potentially infectious materials shall be conducted in biological safety cabinets or other physical-containment devices within the containment module. No work with these other potentially infectious materials shall be conducted on the open bench.

(F) Laboratory coats, gowns, smocks, uniforms, or other appropriate protective clothing shall be used in the work area and animal rooms. Protective clothing shall not be worn outside of the work area and shall be decontaminated before being laundered.

(G) Special care shall be taken to avoid skin contact with other potentially infectious materials. Gloves shall be worn when handling infected animals and when making hand contact with other potentially infectious materials is unavoidable.

(H) Before disposal all waste from work areas and from animal rooms shall either be incinerated or decontaminated by a method such as autoclaving known to effectively destroy bloodborne pathogens.

(I) Vacuum lines shall be protected with liquid disinfectant traps and high efficiency particulate air (HEPA) filters or filters of equivalent or superior efficiency and which are checked routinely and maintained or replaced as necessary.

(J) Hypodermic needles and syringes shall be used only for parenteral injection and aspiration of fluids from laboratory animals and diaphragm bottles. Only needle-locking syringes or disposable syringe-needle units (i.e., the needle is integral to the syringe) shall be used for the injection or aspiration of other potentially infectious materials. Extreme caution shall be used when handling needles and syringes. A needle shall not be bent, sheared, replaced in the sheath or guard, or removed from the syringe following use. The needle and syringe shall be promptly placed in a puncture-resistant container and autoclaved or decontaminated before reuse or disposal.

(K) All spills shall be immediately contained and cleaned up by appropriate professional staff or others properly trained and equipped to work with potentially concentrated infectious materials.

(L) A spill or accident that results in an exposure incident shall be immediately reported to the laboratory director or other responsible person.

(M) A biosafety manual shall be prepared or adopted and periodically reviewed and updated at least annually or more often if necessary. Personnel shall be advised of potential hazards, shall be required to read instructions on practices and procedures, and shall be required to follow them.

(iii) Containment Equipment

(A) Certified biological safety cabinets (Class I, II, or III) or other appropriate combinations of personal protection or physical containment devices, such as special protective clothing, respirators, centrifuge safety cups, sealed centrifuge rotors, and containment caging for animals, shall be used for all activities with other potentially infectious materials that pose a threat of exposure to droplets, splashes, spills, or aerosols.

(B) Biological safety cabinets shall be certified when installed, whenever they are moved, and at least annually.

(3) HIV and HBV research laboratories shall meet the following criteria:

(i) Each laboratory shall contain a facility for handwashing and an eye wash facility which is readily available within the work area.

(ii) An autoclave for decontamination of regulated waste shall be available.

(4) HIV and HBV production facilities shall meet the following criteria:

(i) The work areas shall be separated from areas that are open to unrestricted traffic flow within the building. Passage through two sets of doors shall be the basic requirement for entry into the work area from access corridors or other contiguous areas. Physical separation of the high-containment work area from access corridors or other areas or activities may also be provided by a double-doored clothes-change room (showers may be included), airlock, or other access facility that requires passing through two sets of doors before entering the work area.

(ii) The surfaces of doors, walls, floors, and ceilings in the work area shall be water resistant so that they can be easily cleaned. Penetrations in these surfaces shall be sealed or capable of being sealed to facilitate decontamination.

(iii) Each work area shall contain a sink for washing hands and readily available eye wash facility. The sink shall be foot, elbow, or automatically operated and shall be located near the exit door of the work area.

(iv) Access doors to the work area or containment module shall be self-closing.

(v) An autoclave for decontamination of regulated waste shall be available within or as near as possible to the work area.

(vi) A ducted exhaust-air ventilation system shall be provided. This system shall create directional airflow that draws air into the work area through the entry area. The exhaust air shall not be recirculated to any other area of the building, shall be discharged to the outside, and shall be dispersed away from occupied areas and air intakes. The proper direction of the airflow shall be verified (i.e., into the work area).

(5) Training Requirements. Additional training requirements for employees in HIV and HBV research laboratories and HIV and HBV production facilities are specified in paragraph (g)(2)(ix).

(f) HEPATITIS B VACCINATION AND POST-EXPOSURE EVALUATION AND FOLLOW-UP

(1) General

(i) The employer shall make available the Hepatitis B vaccine and vaccination series to all employees who have occupational exposure, and post-exposure evaluation and follow-up to all employees who have had an exposure incident.

(ii) The employer shall ensure that all medical evaluations and procedures including the Hepatitis B vaccine and vaccination series and post-exposure evaluation and follow-up, including prophylaxis, are:
- (A) Made available at no cost to the employee;
- (B) Made available to the employee at a reasonable time and place;
- (C) Performed by or under the supervision of a licensed physician or by or under the supervision of another licensed healthcare professional; and
- (D) Provided according to recommendations of the U.S. Public Health Service current at the time these evaluations and procedures take place, except as specified by this paragraph (f).

(iii) The employer shall ensure that all laboratory tests are conducted by an accredited laboratory at no cost to the employee.

(2) Hepatitis B Vaccination

(i) Hepatitis B vaccination shall be made available after the employee has received the training required in paragraph (g)(2)(vii)(I) and within 10 working days of initial assignment to all employees who have occupational exposure unless the employee has previously received the complete Hepatitis B vaccination series, antibody testing has revealed that the employee is immune, or the vaccine is contraindicated for medical reasons.

(ii) The employer shall not make participation in a prescreening program a prerequisite for receiving Hepatitis B vaccination.

(iii) If the employee initially declines Hepatitis B vaccination but at a later date while still covered under the standard decides to accept the vaccination, the employer shall make available Hepatitis B vaccination at that time.

(iv) The employer shall assure that employees who decline to accept Hepatitis B vaccination offered by the employer sign the statement in Appendix A1.

(v) If a routine booster dose(s) of Hepatitis B vaccine is recommended by the U.S. Public Health Service at a future date, such booster dose(s) shall be made available in accordance with section (f)(1)(ii).

(3) Post-Exposure Evaluation and Follow-Up

Following a report of an exposure incident, the employer shall make immediately available to the exposed employee a confidential medical evaluation and follow-up, including at least the following elements:

(i) Documentation of the route(s) of exposure, and the circumstances under which the exposure incident occurred;

(ii) Identification and documentation of the source individual, unless the employer can establish that identification is infeasible or prohibited by state or local law:
   (A) The source individual's blood shall be tested as soon as feasible and after consent is obtained in order to determine HBV and HIV infectivity. If consent is not obtained, the employer shall establish that legally required consent cannot be obtained. When the source individual's consent is not required by law the source individual's blood, if available, shall be tested and the results documented.
   (B) When the source individual is already known to be infected with HBV or HIV, testing for the source individual's known HBV or HIV status need not be repeated.
   (C) Results of the source individual's testing shall be made available to the exposed employee, and the employee shall be informed of applicable laws and regulations concerning disclosure of the identity and infectious status of the source individual.

(ii) Collection and testing of blood for HBV and HIV serological status:
   (A) The exposed employee's blood shall be collected as soon as feasible and tested after consent is obtained.
   (B) If the employee consents to baseline blood collection, but does not give consent at that time for HIV serologic testing, the sample shall be preserved for at least 90 days. If, within 90 days of the exposure incident, the employee elects to have the baseline sample tested, such testing shall be done as soon as feasible.

(iv) Post-exposure prophylaxis, when medically indicated, as recommended by the U.S. Public Health Service;
(v) Counseling; and
(vi) Evaluation of reported illnesses.

(4) Information Provided to the Healthcare Professional

(i) The employer shall ensure that the healthcare professional responsible for the employee's Hepatitis B vaccination is provided a copy of this regulation.
(ii) The employer shall ensure that the healthcare professional evaluating an employee after an exposure incident is provided the following information:
   (A) A copy of this regulation;
   (B) A description of the exposed employee's duties as they relate to the exposure incident;
   (C) Documentation of the route(s) of exposure and circumstances under which the exposure occurred;
   (D) Results of the source individual's blood testing, if available; and
   (E) All medical records relevant to the appropriate treatment of the employee including vaccination status which are the employer's responsibility to maintain.

(5) Healthcare Professional's Written Opinion

The employer shall obtain and provide the employee with a copy of the evaluating healthcare professional's written opinion within 15 days of the completion of the evaluation.

(i) The healthcare professional's written opinion for Hepatitis B vaccination shall be limited to whether Hepatitis B vaccination is indicated for an employee, and if the employee has received such vaccination.

(ii) The healthcare professional's written opinion for post-exposure evaluation and follow-up shall be limited to the following information:
  (A) That the employee has been informed of the results of the evaluation; and
  (B) That the employee has been told about any medical conditions resulting from exposure to blood or other potentially infectious materials which require further evaluation or treatment.

(iii) All other findings or diagnoses shall remain confidential and shall not be included in the written report.

(6) Medical Recordkeeping

Medical records required by this standard shall be maintained in accordance with paragraph (h)(1) of this section.

(g) COMMUNICATION OF HAZARDS TO EMPLOYEES

(1) Labels and Signs

(i) Labels
  (A) Warning labels shall be affixed to containers of regulated waste, refrigerators and freezers containing blood or other potentially infectious material; and other containers used to store, transport, or ship blood or other potentially infectious materials, except as provided in paragraph (g)(1)(i)(E), (F), and (G).
  (B) Labels required by this section shall include the BIOHAZARD legend (Fig. 3-1).

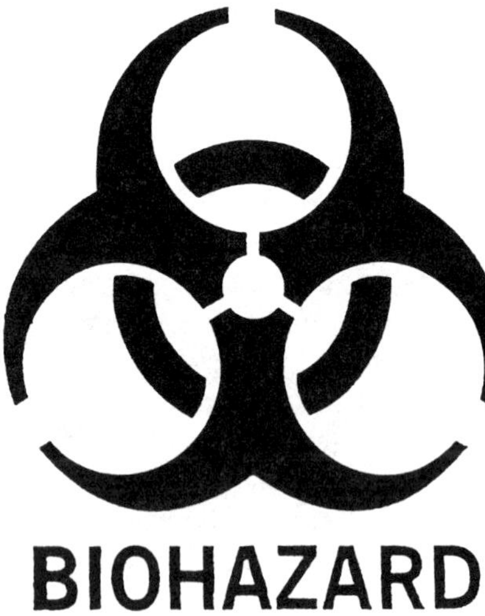

FIG. 3-1. Biohazard legend.

  (C) These labels shall be fluorescent orange or orange-red or predominantly so, with lettering or symbols in contrasting color.
  (D) Labels required be affixed as close as feasible to the container by string, wire, adhesive, or other method that prevents their loss or unintentional removal.
  (E) Red bags or red containers may be substituted for labels.
  (F) Containers of blood, blood components, or blood products that are labeled as to their contents and have been released for transfusion or other clinical use are exempted from labeling requirements of paragraph (g).
  (G) Individual containers of blood or other potentially infectious materials that are placed in a labeled container during storage, transport, shipment, or disposal are exempted from the labeling requirement.
  (H) Labels required for contaminated equipment shall be in accordance with this paragraph and shall also state which portions of the equipment remain contaminated.
  (I) Regulated waste that has been decontaminated need not be labeled or color-coded.

(ii) Signs.
  (A) The employer shall post signs at the entrance to work areas

specified in paragraph (e), HIV and HBV Research Laboratory and Production Facilities, which shall bear the following legend:

BIOHAZARD

(Name of the Infectious Agent) (Special requirements for entering the area) (Name, telephone number of the laboratory director or other responsible person)

(B) These signs shall be fluorescent orange-red or predominantly so, with lettering or symbols in a contrasting color.

(2) Information and Training

(i) Employers shall ensure that all employees with occupational exposure participate in a training program which must be provided at no cost to the employee and during working hours.

(ii) Training shall be provided as follows:
- (A) At the time of initial assignment to tasks where occupational exposure may take place;
- (B) Within 90 days after the effective date of the standard; and
- (C) At least annually thereafter.

(iii) For employees who have received training on bloodborne pathogens in the year preceding the effective date of the standard, only training with respect to the provisions of the standard which were not included need be provided.

(iv) Annual training for all employees shall be provided within one year of their previous training.

(v) Employers shall provide additional training when changes such as modification of tasks or procedures or institution of new tasks or procedures affect the employee's occupational exposure. The additional training may be limited to addressing the new exposures created.

(vi) Material appropriate in content and vocabulary to educational level, literacy, and language of employees shall be used.

(vii) The training program shall contain at a minimum the following elements:
- (A) An accessible copy of the regulatory text of this standard and an explanation of its contents;
- (B) A general explanation of the epidemiology and symptoms of bloodborne diseases;
- (C) An explanation of the modes of transmission of bloodborne pathogens;
- (D) An explanation of the employer's exposure control plan and the means by which the employee can obtain a copy of the written plan;
- (E) An explanation of the appropriate methods for recognizing tasks and other activities that may involve exposure to blood and other potentially infectious materials;
- (F) An explanation of the use and limitations of methods that will prevent or reduce exposure including appropriate engineering controls, work practices, and personal protective equipment;
- (G) Information on the types, proper use, location, removal, handling, decontamination, and disposal of personal protective equipment;
- (H) An explanation of the basis for selection of personal protective equipment;
- (I) Information on the Hepatitis B vaccine, including information on its efficacy, safety, method of administration, the benefits of being vaccinated, and that the vaccine and vaccination will be offered free of charge;
- (J) Information on the appropriate actions to take and persons to contact in an emergency involving blood or other potentially infectious materials;
- (K) An explanation of the procedure to follow if an exposure incident

occurs, including the method of reporting the incident and the medical follow-up that will be made available;

(L) Information on the post-exposure evaluation and follow-up that the employer is required to provide for the employee following an exposure incident;

(M) An explanation of the signs and labels and/or color-coding required by paragraph (g)(1); and

(N) An opportunity for interactive questions and answers with the person conducting the training session.

(viii) The person conducting the training shall be knowledgeable in the subject matter covered by the elements contained in the training program as it relates to the workplace that the training will address.

(ix) Additional Initial Training for Employees in HIV and HBV Laboratories and Production Facilities. Employees in HIV or HBV research laboratories and HIV or HBV production facilities shall receive the following initial training in addition to the above training requirements:

(A) The employer shall assure that employees demonstrate proficiency in standard microbiological practices and techniques and in the practices and operations specific to the facility before being allowed to work with HIV or HBV.

(B) The employer shall assure that employees have prior experience in the handling of human pathogens or tissue cultures before working with HIV or HBV.

(C) The employer shall provide a training program to employees who have no prior experience in handling human pathogens. Initial work activities shall not include the handling of infectious agents. A progression of work activities shall be assigned as techniques are learned and proficiency is developed. The employer shall assure that employees participate in work activities involving infectious agents only after proficiency has been demonstrated.

(h) RECORDKEEPING

(1) Medical Records

(i) The employer shall establish and maintain an accurate record for each employee with occupational exposure, in accordance with 29 CFR 1910.20.

(ii) This record shall include:

(A) The name and social security number of the employee;

(B) A copy of the employee's Hepatitis B vaccination status including the dates of all the Hepatitis B vaccinations and any medical records relative to the employee's ability to receive vaccination as required by paragraph (f)(2);

(C) A copy of all results of examinations, medical testing, and follow-up procedures as required by paragraph (f)(3);

(D) The employer's copy of the healthcare professional's written opinion as required by paragraph (f)(5); and

(E) A copy of the information provided to the healthcare professional as required by paragraphs (f)(4)(ii)(B), (C), and (D).

(iii) Confidentiality. The employer shall ensure that employee medical records required by paragraph (h)(1) are:

(A) Kept confidential; and

(B) Not disclosed or reported without the employee's express written consent to any person within or outside the workplace except as required by this section or as may be required by law.

(iv) The employer shall maintain the records required by paragraph (h) for at least the duration of employment plus 30 years in accordance with 29 CFR 1910.20.

(2) Training Records

(i) Training records shall include the following information:
- (A) The dates of the training sessions;
- (B) The contents or a summary of the training sessions;
- (C) The names and qualifications for the persons conducting the training; and
- (D) The names and job titles of all persons attending the training sessions.

(ii) Training records shall be maintained for 3 years from the date on which the training occurred.

(3) Availability

(i) The employer shall ensure that all records required to be maintained by this section shall be made available upon request to the Assistant Secretary and Director for examination and copying.

(ii) Employee training records required by this paragraph shall be provided upon request for examination and copying to employees, to employee representatives, to the Director, and to the Assistant Secretary in accordance with 29 CFR 1910.20.

(iii) Employee medical records required by this paragraph shall be provided upon request for examination and copying to the subject employee, to anyone having written consent of the subject employee, to the Director, and to the Assistant Secretary in accordance with 29 CFR 1910.20.

(4) Transfer of Records

(i) The employer shall comply with the requirements involving transfer of records set forth in 29 CFR 1910.20(h).

(ii) If the employer ceases to do business and there is no successor employer to receive and retain the records for the prescribed period, the employer shall notify the Director, at least three months prior to their disposal and transmit them to the Director, if required by the Director to do so, within that three month period.

(i) DATES

(1) Effective Date. The standard shall become effective on March 6, 1992.

(2) The Exposure Control Plan required by paragraph (c)(1) of this section shall be completed on or before May 5, 1992.

(3) Paragraph (g)(2) Information and Training and (h) Recordkeeping shall take effect on or before June 4, 1992.

(4) Paragraphs (d)(2) Engineering and Work Practice Controls, (d)(3) Personal Protective Equipment, (d)(4), Housekeeping, (e) HIV and HBV Research Laboratories and Production Facilities, (f) Hepatitis B Vaccination and Post-Exposure Evaluation and Follow-Up, and (g)(1) Labels and Signs shall take effect July 6, 1992.

APPENDIX A1 TO SECTION 1910.1030—HEPATITIS B VACCINE DECLINATION (MANDATORY)

I understand that due to my occupational exposure to blood or other potentially infectious materials I may be at risk of acquiring Hepatitis B Virus (HBV) infection. I have been given the opportunity to be vaccinated with Hepatitis B vaccine, at no charge to myself. However, I decline Hepatitis B vaccination at this time. I understand that by declining this vaccine, I continue to be at risk of acquiring Hepatitis B, a serious disease. If in the future I continue to have occupational exposure to blood or other potentially infectious materials and I want to be vaccinated with Hepatitis B vaccine, I can receive the vaccination series at no charge to me.

Appendix B

Universal Precautions for Prevention of Transmission of HIV, HBV, and Other Bloodborne Pathogens in Healthcare Settings[2]

INTRODUCTION

The purpose of this report is to clarify and supplement the CDC publication entitled "Recommendations for Prevention of HIV Transmission in Health-Care Settings" (1).

In 1983, CDC published a document entitled "Guideline for Isolation Precautions in Hospitals" (2) that contained a section entitled "Blood and Body Fluid Precautions." The recommendations in this section called for blood and body fluid precautions when a patient was known or suspected to be infected with bloodborne pathogens. In August 1987, CDC published a document entitled "Recommendations for Prevention of HIV Transmission in Health-Care Settings" (1). In contrast to the 1983 document, the 1987 document recommended that blood and body fluid precautions be consistently used for all patients regardless of their bloodborne infection status. This extension of blood and body fluid precautions to ***all*** patients is referred to as "Universal Blood and Body Fluid Precautions" or "Universal Precautions." Under universal precautions, blood and certain body fluids of all patients are considered potentially infectious for human immunodeficiency virus (HIV), hepatitis B virus (HBV), and other bloodborne pathogens.

Universal precautions are intended to prevent parenteral, mucous membrane, and nonintact skin exposures of health-care workers to bloodborne pathogens. In addition, immunization with HBV vaccine is recommended as an important adjunct to universal precautions for health-care workers who have exposures to blood (3,4).

Since the recommendations for universal precautions were published in August 1987, CDC and the Food and Drug Administration (FDA) have received requests for clarification of the following issues: 1) body fluids to which universal precautions apply, 2) use of protective barriers, 3) use of gloves for phlebotomy, 4) selection of gloves for use while observing universal precautions, and 5) need for making changes in waste management programs as a result of adopting universal precautions.

BODY FLUIDS TO WHICH UNIVERSAL PRECAUTIONS APPLY

Universal precautions apply to blood and to other body fluids containing visible blood. Occupational transmission of HIV and HBV to healthcare workers by blood is documented (4,5). **Blood is the single most important source of HIV, HBV, and other bloodborne pathogens in the occupational setting. Infection control efforts for HIV, HBV, and other bloodborne pathogens must focus on preventing exposures to blood as well as on delivery of HBV immunization.**

Universal precautions also apply to semen and vaginal secretions. Although both of these fluids have been implicated in the sexual transmission of HIV and HBV, they have not

[2] *Morbidity and Mortality Weekly Report* June 24, 1988;37 (no. 24).

been implicated in occupational transmission from patient to health-care worker. This observation is not unexpected, since exposure to semen in the usual health-care setting is limited, and the routine practice of wearing gloves for performing vaginal examinations protects health-care workers from exposure to potentially infectious vaginal secretions.

Universal precautions also apply to tissues and to the following fluids: cerebrospinal fluid (CSF), synovial fluid, pleural fluid, peritoneal fluid, pericardial fluid, and amniotic fluid. The risk of transmission of HIV and HBV from these fluids is unknown; epidemiologic studies in the health-care and community setting are currently inadequate to assess the potential risk to health-care workers from occupational exposures to them. However, HIV has been isolated from CSF, synovial, and amniotic fluid (6,8), and HBsAg has been detected in synovial fluid, amniotic fluid, and peritoneal fluid (9–11). One case of HIV transmission was reported after a percutaneous exposure to bloody pleural fluid obtained by needle aspiration (12). Whereas aseptic procedures used to obtain these fluids for diagnostic or therapeutic purposes protect health-care workers from skin exposures, they cannot prevent penetrating injuries due to contaminated needles or other sharp instruments.

BODY FLUIDS TO WHICH UNIVERSAL PRECAUTIONS DO NOT APPLY

Universal precautions do not apply to feces, nasal secretions, sputum, sweat, tears, urine, and vomitus unless they contain visible blood. The risk of transmission of HIV and HBV from these fluids and materials is extremely low or nonexistent. HIV has been isolated and HBsAg has been demonstrated in some of these fluids; however, epidemiologic studies in the health-care and community setting have not implicated these fluids or materials in the transmission of HIV and HBV infections (13,14). Some of the above fluids and excretions represent a potential source for nosocomial and community-acquired infections with other pathogens, and recommendations for preventing the transmission of nonbloodborne pathogens have been published (2).

PRECAUTIONS FOR OTHER BODY FLUIDS IN SPECIAL SETTINGS

Human breast milk has been implicated in perinatal transmission of HIV, and HBsAg has been found in the milk of mothers infected with HBV (10,13). However, occupational exposure to human breast milk has not been implicated in the transmission of HIV nor HBV infection to health-care workers. Moreover, the health-care worker will not have the same type of intensive exposure to breast milk as the nursing neonate. Whereas universal precautions do not apply to human breast milk, gloves may be worn by health-care workers in situations where exposures to breast milk might be frequent, for example, in breast milk banking.

Saliva of some persons infected with HBV has been shown to contain HBV-DNA at concentrations 1/1,000 to 1/10,000 of that found in the infected person's serum (15). HBsAg-positive saliva has been shown to be infectious when injected into experimental animals and in human bite exposures (16–18). However, HBsAg-positive saliva has not been shown to be infectious when applied to oral mucous membranes in experimental primate studies (18) or through contamination of musical instruments or cardiopulmonary resuscitation dummies used by HBV carriers (19,20). Epidemiologic studies of nonsexual household contacts of HIV-infected patients, including several small series in which HIV transmission failed to occur after bites or after percutaneous inoculation or contamination of cuts and open wounds with saliva from HIV-infected patients, suggest that the potential for salivary transmission of HIV is remote (5,13,14,21,22). One case report from Germany has suggested the possibility of transmission of HIV in a household setting from an infected child to a sibling through a human bite (23). The bite did not break the skin or result in bleeding. Since the date of seroconversion to HIV was not known for either child in this case, evidence of the role of saliva in the transmission of virus is unclear (23). Another case report suggested the possibility of transmission of HIV from husband to wife by contact with saliva during kissing (24). However, follow-up studies did not confirm HIV infection in the wife (21).

Universal precautions do not apply to saliva. General infection control practices already in existence—including the use of gloves for digital examination of mucous membranes and endotracheal suctioning, and handwashing after exposure to saliva should further minimize the minute risk, if any, for salivary transmission of HIV and HBV (1,25). Gloves need not be worn when feeding patients and when wiping saliva from skin.

Special precautions, however, are recommended for dentistry (1). Occupationally acquired infection with HBV in dental workers has been documented (4), and two possible cases of occupationally acquired HIV infection involving dentists have been reported (5,26). During dental procedures, contamination of saliva with blood is predictable, trauma to health-care workers' hands is common, and blood spattering may occur. Infection control precautions for dentistry minimize the potential for nonintact skin and mucous membrane contact of dental health-care workers to blood-contaminated saliva of patients. In addition, the use of gloves for oral examinations and treatment in the dental setting may also protect the patient's oral mucous membranes from exposures to blood, which may occur from breaks in the skin of dental workers' hands.

USE OF PROTECTIVE BARRIERS

Protective barriers reduce the risk of exposure of the health-care worker's skin or mucous membranes to potentially infective materials. For universal precautions, protective barriers reduce the risk of exposure to blood, body fluids containing visible blood, and other fluids to which universal precautions apply. Examples of protective barriers include gloves, gowns, masks, and protective eyewear. Gloves should reduce the incidence of contamination of hands, but they cannot prevent penetrating injuries due to needles or other sharp instruments. Masks and protective eyewear or face shields should reduce the incidence of contamination of mucous membranes of the mouth, nose, and eyes.

Universal precautions are intended to supplement rather than replace recommendations for routine infection control, such as handwashing and using gloves to prevent gross microbial contamination of hands (27). Because specifying the types of barriers needed for every possible clinical situation is impractical, some judgment must be exercised.

The risk of nosocomial transmission of HIV, HBV, and other bloodborne pathogens can be minimized if health-care workers use the following general guidelines:

1. Take care to prevent injuries when using needles, scalpels, and other sharp instruments or devices; when handling sharp instruments after procedures; when cleaning used instruments; and when disposing of used needles. Do not recap used needles by hand; do not remove used needles from disposable syringes by hand; and do not bend, break, or otherwise manipulate used needles by hand. Place used disposable syringes and needles, scalpel blades, and other sharp items in puncture-resistant containers for disposal. Locate the puncture-resistant containers as close to the use area as is practical.
2. Use protective barriers to prevent exposure to blood, body fluids containing visible blood, and other fluids to which universal precautions apply. The type of protective barrier(s) should be appropriate for the procedure being performed and the type exposure anticipated.
3. Immediately and thoroughly wash hands and other skin surfaces that are contami-

nated with blood, body fluids containing visible blood, or other body fluids to which universal precautions apply.

GLOVE USE FOR PHLEBOTOMY

Gloves should reduce the incidence of blood contamination of hands during phlebotomy (drawing blood samples), but they cannot prevent penetrating injuries caused by needles or other sharp instruments. The likelihood of hand contamination with blood containing HIV, HBV, or other bloodborne pathogens during phlebotomy depends on several factors: 1) the skill and technique of the health-care worker, 2) the frequency with which the health-care worker performs the procedure (other factors being equal, the cumulative risk of blood exposure is higher for a health-care worker who performs more procedures), 3) whether the procedure occurs in a routine or emergency situation (where blood contact may be more likely), and 4) the prevalence of infection with bloodborne pathogens in the patient population. The likelihood of infection after skin exposure to blood containing HIV or HBV will depend on the concentration of virus (viral concentration is much higher for hepatitis B than for HIV), the duration of contact, the presence of skin lesions on the hands of the health-care worker, and for HBV the immune status of the health-care worker. Although not accurately quantified, the risk of HIV infection following intact skin contact with infective blood is certainly much less than the 0.5% risk following percutaneous needlestick exposures (5). In universal precautions, *all* blood is assumed to be potentially infective for bloodborne pathogens, but in certain settings (e.g., volunteer blood-donation centers) the prevalence of infection with some bloodborne pathogens (e.g., HIV, HBV) is known to be very low. Some institutions have relaxed recommendations for using gloves for phlebotomy procedures by skilled phlebotomists in settings where the prevalence of bloodborne pathogens is known to be very low.

Institutions that judge that routine gloving for *all* phlebotomies is not necessary should periodically reevaluate their policy. Gloves should always be available to health-care workers who wish to use them for phlebotomy. In addition, the following general guidelines apply:

1. Use gloves for performing phlebotomy when the health-care worker has cuts, scratches, or other breaks in his/her skin.
2. Use gloves in situations where the health-care worker judges that hand contamination with blood may occur, for example, when performing phlebotomy on an uncooperative patient.
3. Use gloves for performing finger and/or heel sticks on infants and children.
4. Use gloves when persons are receiving training in phlebotomy.

SELECTION OF GLOVES

The Center for Devices and Radiological Health, FDA, has responsibility for regulating the medical glove industry. Medical gloves include those marketed as sterile surgical or nonsterile examination gloves made of vinyl or latex. General purpose utility ("rubber") gloves are also used in the health-care setting, but they are not regulated by FDA since they are not promoted for medical use. There are no reported differences in barrier effectiveness between intact latex and intact vinyl used to manufacture gloves. Thus, the type of gloves selected should be appropriate for the task being performed.

The following general guidelines are recommended:

1. Use sterile gloves for procedures involving contact with normally sterile areas of the body.
2. Use examination gloves for procedures involving contact with mucous membranes, unless otherwise indicated, and for other patient care or diagnostic procedures that do not require the use of sterile gloves.

3. Change gloves between patient contacts.
4. Do not wash or disinfect surgical or examination gloves for reuse. Washing with surfactants may cause "wicking," i.e., the enhanced penetration of liquids through undetected holes in the glove. Disinfecting agents may cause deterioration.
5. Use general-purpose utility gloves (e.g., rubber household gloves) for housekeeping chores involving potential blood contact and for instrument cleaning and decontamination procedures. Utility gloves may be decontaminated and reused but should be discarded if they are peeling, cracked, or discolored, or if they have punctures, tears, or other evidence of deterioration.

WASTE MANAGEMENT

Universal precautions are not intended to change waste management programs previously recommended by CDC for health-care settings (1). Policies for defining, collecting, storing, decontaminating, and disposing of infective waste are generally determined by institutions in accordance with state and local regulations. Information regarding waste management regulations in health-care settings may be obtained from state or local health departments or agencies responsible for waste management.

Reported by: Center for Devices and Radiological Health, Food and Drug Administration. Hospital Infections Program, AIDS Program, and Hepatitis Branch, Division of Viral Diseases, Center for Infectious Diseases, National Institute for Occupational Safety and Health, CDC.

Editorial Note: Implementation of universal precautions does not eliminate the need for other category- or disease-specific isolation precautions, such as enteric precautions for infectious diarrhea or isolation for pulmonary tuberculosis (1,2). In addition to universal precautions, detailed precautions have been developed for the following procedures and/or settings in which prolonged or intensive exposures to blood occur: invasive procedures, dentistry, autopsies or morticians' services, dialysis, and the clinical laboratory. These detailed precautions are found in the August 21, 1987, "Recommendations for Prevention of HIV Transmission in Health-Care Settings" (1). In addition, specific precautions have been developed for research laboratories (28).

REFERENCES

1. Centers for Disease Control. Recommendations for prevention of HIV transmission in health-care settings. *MMWR* 1987;369(suppl no. 2S).
2. Garner JS, Simmons BP. Guideline for isolation precautions in hospitals. *Infect Control* 1983;4:245–325.
3. Immunization Practices Advisory Committee. Recommendations for protection against viral hepatitis. *MMWR* 1985;34:313–24,329–35.
4. Department of Labor, Department of Health and Human Services. Joint advisory notice: protection against occupational exposure to hepatitis B virus (HBV) and human immunodeficiency virus (HIV). Washington, D.C.: U.S. Department of Labor, U.S. Department of Health and Human Services, 1987.
5. Centers for Disease Control. Update: Acquired immunodeficiency syndrome and human immunodeficiency virus infection among health-care workers. *MMWR* 1988;37:229–234,239.
6. Hollander H, Levy JA. Neurologic abnormalities and recovery of human immunodeficiency virus from cerebrospinal fluid. *Ann Intern Med* 1987;106:692–695.
7. Wirthrington RH, Cornes P, Harris JRW, et al. Isolation of human immunodeficiency virus from synovial fluid of a patient with reactive arthritis. *Br Med J* 1987;294:484.
8. Mundy DC, Schinazi RF, Gerber AR, Nahmias AJ, Randall HW. Human immunodeficiency virus isolated from amniotic fluid. *Lancet* 1987;2:459–460.
9. Onion DK, Crumpacker CS, Gilliland BC. Arthritis of hepatitis associated with Australia antigen. *Ann Intern Med* 1971;75:29–33.
10. Lee AKY, Ip HMH, Wong VCW. Mechanisms of maternal-fetal transmission of hepatitis B virus. *J Infect Dis* 1978;138:668–671.
11. Bond WW, Petersen NI, Gravelle CR, Favero MS. Hepatitis B virus in peritoneal dialysis fluid: a potential hazard. *Dial Transplantation* 1982;11:592–600.
12. Oskenhendler E, Harzic M, Le Roux JM, Rabian C, Clauvel JP. HIV infection with seroconversion after a superficial needlestick injury to the finger [Letter]. *N Engl J Med* 1986;315:582.
13. Lifson AR. Do alternate modes for transmission of human immunodeficiency virus exist? a review. *JAMA* 1988;259:1353–1356.
14. Friedland GH, Saltzman BR, Rogers MF, et al. Lack of transmission of HTLV-III/LAV infection to household contacts of patients with AIDS or AIDS-related complex with oral candidiasis. *N Engl J Med* 1986;314:344–349.
15. Jenison SA, Lemon SM, Baker LN, Newbold JE. Quantitative analysis of hepatitis B virus DNA in saliva and semen of chronically infected homosexual men. *J Infect Dis* 1987;156:299–306.

16. Cancio-Bello TP, de Medina M, Shorey J, Valledor MD, Schiff ER. An institutional outbreak of hepatitis B related to a human biting carrier. *J Infect Dis* 1982;146: 652–656.
17. MacQuarrie MB, Forghani B, Wolochow DA. Hepatitis B transmitted by a human bite. *JAMA* 1974;230:723–724.
18. Scott RM, Snitbhan R, Bancroft WH, Alter HJ, Tingpalapong M. Experimental transmission of hepatitis B virus by semen and saliva. *J Infect Dis* 1980;142:67–71.
19. Glaser JB, Nadler JP. Hepatitis B virus in a cardiopulmonary resuscitation training course: risk of transmission from a surface antigen-positive participant. *Arch Intern Med* 1985;145:1653–1655.
20. Osterholm MT, Bravo ER, Crosson JT, et al. Lack of transmission of viral hepatitis type B after oral exposure to HBsAg-positive saliva. *Br Med J* 1979;2:1263–1264.
21. Curran JW, Jaffe HW, Hardy AM, et al. Epidemiology of HIV infection and AIDS in the United States. *Science* 1988;239:610–616.
22. Jason JM, McDougal JS, Dixon G, et al. HTLV-III/LAV antibody and immune status of household contacts and sexual partners of persons with hemophilia. *JAMA* 1986;255:212–215.
23. Wahn V, Kramer HH, Voit T, Bruster HT, Scrampical B, Scheid A. Horizontal transmission of HIV infection between two siblings [Letter]. *Lancet* 1986;2:694.
24. Salahuddin SZ, Groopman JE, Markham PD, et al. HTLV-III in symptom-free seronegative persons. *Lancet* 1984;2:1418–1420.
25. Simmons BP, Wong ES. Guideline for prevention of nosocomial pneumonia. Atlanta: U.S. Department of Health and Human Services, Public Health Service, Centers for Disease Control, 1982.
26. Klein RS, Phelan JA, Freeman K, et al. Low occupational risk of human immunodeficiency virus infection among dental professionals. *N Engl J Med* 1988;318:86–90.
27. Garner JS, Favero MS. Guideline for handwashing and hospital environmental control; 1985. Atlanta: U.S. Department of Health and Human Services, Public Health Service, Centers for Disease Control, 1985: HHS pub. no. 99-1117.
28. Centers for Disease Control. 1988 Agent summary statement for human immunodeficiency virus and report on laboratory-acquired infection with human immunodeficiency virus. *MMWR* 7988;37(suppl no. S4:1S–22S).

Medical Center Occupational Health and Safety,
edited by Robert J. McCunney.
Lippincott Williams & Wilkins, Philadelphia © 1999.

4
Tuberculosis

Victor S. Roth and *Brian G. Forrester

University of Michigan Occupational Health Services, Ann Arbor, Michigan 48103-5827;
**Department of Occupational Medicine, Regional First Care, Athens, Georgia 30603*

Tuberculosis and a multidrug-resistant form of tuberculosis have reemerged in epidemic proportions (1). Nowhere is the increasing problem of tuberculosis more apparent than in acute care hospitals (2). High rates of tuberculosis among patients who are served by large urban hospitals mean that these institutions face the greatest risk for transmission of this disease to health care workers and patients.

Tuberculosis is more prevalent among persons with human immunodeficiency virus (HIV) infection, homeless persons, persons from countries with high rates of tuberculosis, prison inmates, residents of long-term care facilities, persons from low socioeconomic backgrounds, and users of intravenous drugs. Ambulatory (urgent) care centers and acute care hospitals are where most persons in these high-risk groups seek medical care. Therefore such institutions are at risk for encountering patients with undetected tuberculosis.

Nosocomial cases of tuberculosis have affected both health care workers and hospitalized patients, and each group has transmitted the infection to the other. Exacerbating factors are an increasing prevalence of concurrent HIV infection and multidrug-resistant tuberculosis; inadequate implementation of procedures for the recognition, isolation, and treatment of patients with tuberculosis in health care facilities; and a lack of practical engineering interventions and personal protective equipment, both of which serve to control airborne transmission of *Mycobacterium tuberculosis* (3).

The following factors make the threat of tuberculosis to health care workers of increasing concern:

- Increased incidence of the tuberculosis
- Existence of multidrug-resistant strains of tuberculosis
- The presence of HIV infection, which increases risk for tuberculosis and increases susceptibility to the multidrug-resistant form

HISTORY OF REGULATIONS FOR TUBERCULOSIS

The Centers for Disease Control and Prevention (CDC) has released reports that several health care workers have died of nosocomially acquired multidrug-resistant tuberculosis. The CDC also has found that additional health care workers have contracted the disease and are under treatment (4). Many other hospital workers have become acutely infected during nosocomial outbreaks of multidrug-resistant tuberculosis (documented with tuberculosis skin test conversion) without developing active disease (4). The CDC first published recommendations for controlling tuberculosis in hospitals in 1982 (5). In 1990, the CDC published Guidelines for Preventing the Transmission of Tuberculosis in Health Care Facilities with Special Focus on HIV-Related Issues (6). Subsequent investigations by the CDC supported these recommendations with documentation that implementation of measures contained in these guidelines considerably reduced or eliminated nosocomial transmission of tuberculosis to patients and health care workers.

In 1992, in response to outbreaks of multidrug-resistant tuberculosis, the multidrug-resistant tuberculosis task force published the National Action Plan to Combat Multidrug-Resistant Tuberculosis (7). The document called for an update and revision of the 1990 recommendations. This evolved into the CDC Draft Guidelines for Preventing the Transmission of Tuberculosis in Health-Care Facilities, second edition, which appeared in the *Federal Register* on October 12, 1993 (58 FR:52810-54). After a public comment period, the final version was released on October 24, 1994 (8). Important in the 1994 publication were revisions regarding worker education, administrative controls, specific ventilation recommendations, and clarification on the use of respiratory protection.

A tuberculosis standard is forthcoming from the Occupational Safety and Health Administration (OSHA) that will closely follow the CDC recommendations. Until such a standard is published, OSHA, through the office of health compliance assistance, will expect facilities to comply with instruction CPL 2.106, Enforcement Procedures and Scheduling for Occupational Exposure to Tuberculosis, released on February 9, 1996. This directive covers inspection procedures and guidelines for issuing citations, making use of the general duty clause and the respiratory protection standard as its foundation. OSHA's proposed standard for Occupational Exposure to Tuberculosis was published October 17, 1997, and contains basic information about occupational tuberculosis, including those populations most at risk of exposure.

RISK FOR TRANSMISSION OF TUBERCULOSIS TO HEALTH CARE WORKERS

The risk for transmission of tuberculosis to health care workers depends on the following factors:

- The institution's (a) ratio of patients with tuberculosis admitted to the number of health care workers at the facility and (b) percentage of tuberculosis cases that are multidrug resistant
- Duration of employment at the facility
- Potential for contact with tuberculosis within that institution on the basis of job duties or job title
- State of the health care worker's personal health and well-being, such as HIV status, presence of other condition of compromised immunity, or use of corticosteroid therapy
- Delay by treating physicians in diagnosis of the source of infection
- The presence of effective surveillance and preventive measures at the institution to prevent spread of infection from patients or coworkers

The Institution

In institutions with fewer than 10 annual admissions for tuberculosis or less than one admission per year per 100 workers (<1% ratio), one study determined that the risk for infection among workers was extremely low (<0.2% per year) (9) (Table 4-1). In institutions in which the annual worker to tuberculosis admission ratio was between 18 and 92, the risk for health care worker infection ranged from 1.7% to 3.9% per year (5). In hospitals with more than 200 annual admissions for tuberculosis or with a ratio of workers to tuberculosis admissions less than 10, a study showed an infection risk to workers of 1% to 10% each year (9). The larger the number of patients admitted with multidrug-resistant tuberculosis, the greater was the probability for exposure because of the prolonged period of infectivity of persons with the multidrug-resistant form of the disease. In summary, the larger the number of patients with tuberculosis treated or admitted and the larger the number of patients with multidrug-resistant tuberculosis treated or admitted to the facility, the greater is the risk for infection among medical center employees.

Duration of Employment

In one study investigators found that duration of employment in a hospital was directly

TABLE 4-1. *Categorization of tuberculosis risk in health care facilities*

Situation	Risk level
No TB patients in facility or community	*Minimal*
No patients with TB admitted as inpatients to facility during preceding year *and* plan to refer patients with confirmed or suspected TB to a collaborating facility if inpatient care is required	*Very low*
Fewer than six patients with TB admitted to the area during preceding year	*Low*
Six or more patients with TB admitted to area during preceding year	*Intermediate*
Health care worker PPD conversion rates in area or group significantly higher than rates for areas or groups in which occupational exposure to *Mycobacterium tuberculosis* is unlikely or than a previous rate in same area or group *or* Cluster of health care worker PPD conversions *or* Evidence of person-to-person transmission *and* Cause of transmission[a] not identified and consequently not corrected	*High*

[a]If cause of transmission is identified and corrected, repeat PPD tests and risk assessment at 3 months. Resume appropriate lower-risk protocol if there are no further PPD conversions or other evidence of transmission.
TB, tuberculosis; PPD, purified protein derivative (tuberculin).

proportional to the prevalence of infection and skin test conversion (10). This finding is expected because length of employment is directly proportional to probability of exposure.

Potential for Contact with Tuberculosis on the Basis of Job Duties

A review (11) of specific health care occupations and risk for *M. tuberculosis* infection among persons in those occupations came to the following conclusions.

Nurses

Nurses have the highest rate of infection and disease.

Pathologists

Prosector's wart (inoculation tuberculosis) has long been recognized as an occupational hazard for pathologists. Other risks faced by pathologists include potential spread through aerosolization during autopsies of patients who had tuberculosis and during autopsies of patients who had tuberculosis but the disease was not suspected. In one report, 8 of 55 health care workers (including several pathologists) had purified protein derivative (PPD) skin test conversions after exposure to an elderly man with progressive small-cell carcinoma of the lung and unsuspected tuberculosis. Active tuberculosis developed in two of the health care workers (12).

Laboratory Workers

The potential for infection among laboratory workers is through accidental aerosolization by means of inhalation or inadvertent inoculation.

Medical Specialists

Pulmonary medicine specialists have the highest rate of PPD skin test conversion and are followed by infectious disease specialists. The increased risk among pulmonologists is thought to be caused by time spent with patients with tuberculosis during the performance of bronchoscopy and providing care in intensive care units.

Inhalation Therapists

A study (13) found that the standardized mortality ratio (SMR) for tuberculosis among inhalation therapists was substantially elevated. These workers have intense interaction with patients who have pulmonary disease, and they may be at high risk for *M. tuberculosis* infection.

Nursing Aides, Orderlies, and Attendants

Nursing aides, orderlies, and attendants are at slightly elevated risk for active tuberculosis. This association, however, is probably confounded by the correlation between lower socioeconomic status backgrounds and tuberculosis (13).

Health Care Workers' Health and Well-Being and HIV Status

Infection with HIV and immunosuppression increase risk for tuberculosis (14). Persons with HIV infection and tuberculosis are at increased risk for active tuberculosis, and health care workers exposed to patients with multidrug-resistant tuberculosis are at risk for *M. tuberculosis* infection (15). This risk is even more of a concern when health care workers with HIV infection are assigned to high-risk areas of the hospital, such as areas where patients with HIV are treated. Working in such areas increases the likelihood of exposure to tuberculosis and the probability that the exposure is to multidrug-resistant tuberculosis.

In 1990 through 1992, the CDC investigated seven outbreaks of multidrug-resistant tuberculosis involving more than 200 persons. Most cases involved persons with HIV infection. In these outbreaks, most cases appeared to be the result of nosocomial transmission. The period from exposure to development of infectious tuberculosis was brief, and the fatality rate was high (72% to 89%). Death occurred within weeks of the onset of symptoms (16). The risk for nosocomial transmission of multidrug-resistant tuberculosis is high because conventional initial antituberculosis chemotherapy is inadequate to treat multidrug-resistant strains. As a result, patients infected with such strains may remain infectious for long periods of time (15). In addition to HIV, several other medical risk factors should be considered, such as immunocompromise caused by cancer chemotherapy or corticosteroid therapy.

Delay in Diagnosis of the Source of *M. tuberculosis* Infection

Evidence from several studies of infection rates in the preantibiotic era and reports of recent outbreaks consistently indicate that rates of nosocomial transmission are highest when the diagnosis of tuberculosis among hospitalized patients is delayed, patients do not receive adequate therapy, or there is unrecognized drug resistance (9). The delay in diagnosis may be caused by lack of awareness by physicians, atypical clinical manifestations, clinical manifestations of concurrent disease that may mask typical tuberculosis symptoms, or inadequate laboratory diagnosis. According to one report, tests for acid-fast bacilli or sputum smears were not available in 16% of U.S. hospitals caring for patients with tuberculosis (17). The same study found that routine sensitivity testing of isolates was not performed in 80% of the hospitals.

Preplacement and Periodic Surveillance for Disease among Health Care Workers

Skin Testing

Risk and Frequency

Health care workers at risk for *M. tuberculosis* infection are a specific group to screen with a tuberculin skin test. Baseline skin testing should be done for all health care workers with potential patient contact. The intradermal Mantoux test, not a multiple puncture test, should be used to determine whether infection has occurred (18). The CDC in the publication Guidelines for Preventing the Transmission of *M. tuberculosis* in Health Care Facilities bases the recommendations for periodicity of skin testing on risk categories (8). Risk categories are determined from information contained in the CDC guide (see Table 4-1). The CDC recommends the following procedures for conducting tuberculosis risk assessment in a health care facility for determining periodicity of PPD skin testing:

- Review of community tuberculosis profiles
- Review of the number of patients with tuberculosis examined as inpatients and outpatients at the facility

Once risk level is determined (see Table 4-1), the recommendations in Table 4-2 are made regarding the frequency of PPD skin testing. It is assumed that all health care workers in the facility have received at least a baseline skin test before beginning employment. Recommendations made by the American Hospital Association regarding skin testing are more inclusive (19) (Table 4-3).

TABLE 4-3. *American Hospital Association recommendations for tuberculosis skin testing*

Perform skin testing annually
Include medical staff, volunteers, temporary staff, students, and all others who may be affected
Use trained personnel to administer and read all skin tests
Enter skin test results into database and review skin test conversion rates by area and job category to assess risk and determine which groups need more frequent testing
Manage skin test converters clinically and assess possible sources of infection (hospital or community acquired)
Educate and train staff to ensure compliance

Administration of the Tuberculin Skin Test

The Mantoux test (18) is performed by means of intradermal injection of 0.1 mL PPD tuberculin containing 5 tuberculin units (TU) into either the volar or dorsal surface of the forearm. The injection should be made with a disposable tuberculin syringe and be just below the skin surface with the needle bevel facing upward to produce a discrete wheal 6 to 10 mm in diameter. Needles should not be recapped. Gloves are not necessary for this procedure. The Mantoux test should be read 48 to 72 hours after the injection. If the skin test is not read as scheduled, positive reactions may still be measured up to 1 week after testing. The reading should measure induration, not erythema.

TABLE 4-2. *Frequency of skin testing for tuberculosis according to risk category*

Risk category	Frequency of testing
Minimal	Not applicable
Very low	Variable[a]
Low	Yearly
Intermediate	Every 6–12 months
High	Every 3 months

[a]Because very-low-risk facilities do not admit patients who may have active tuberculosis to inpatient areas, most health care workers in such facilities do not need routine follow-up PPD screening after a baseline PPD test is done. However, those who are involved in the initial assessment and diagnostic evaluation of patients in the ambulatory care, emergency, and admitting departments of such facilities or in the outpatient care of patients with active tuberculosis could be exposed to a patient with active TB. These health care workers may need to receive routine periodic PPD screening. These health care workers also may need to be included in a respiratory protection program.

Classification of the Tuberculin Skin Test

Table 4-4 shows when induration of 5 mm or more is considered positive (8). Induration of 10 mm or more is classified as positive for those who do not meet the criteria in Table 4-4 but who have the risk factors in Tables 4-5 through 4-7. The recommendations regarding interpretation of PPD skin tests should be applied to health care workers but should be qualified as follows.

The prevalence of tuberculosis in the facility should determine what is considered a positive test. In minimal- risk to low-risk facilities (see Table 4-1), a positive test result is 15 mm or greater induration for health care workers with no other risk factors and work in facilities with no exposure risk. In intermediate- to high-risk facilities (see Table 4-1), a

TABLE 4-4. *Instances in which induration of 5 mm or more is classified as positive*

Person has HIV infection or risk factors for HIV infection but unknown HIV status
Person has had recent close contact with persons who have active tuberculosis
Person has fibrotic lesions on chest radiograph likely to represent old healed tuberculosis

HIV, human immunodeficiency virus.

TABLE 4-5. *Instances in which induration of 10 mm or more is classified as positive*

High-risk groups
- Injecting drug user is known to be HIV seronegative
- Person has other medical conditions that reportedly increase risk for progression from latent TB infection to active TB infection (e.g., silicosis, gastrectomy or jejunoileal bypass, ≥10% below ideal body weight, chronic renal failure with dialysis, diabetes, immunosuppressive therapy, some hematologic disorders such as leukemia or lymphoma), other malignant tumors
- Child is younger than 4 years

High-prevalence groups
- Person is born in a country in Asia, Africa, Caribbean, and Latin America that has high prevalence of TB
- Person is from a medically underserved, low-income population
- Person is a resident of a long-term-care facility (nursing home)
- Person is from a high-risk population in the community, as determined by local public health authorities

HIV, human immunodeficiency virus; TB, tuberculosis.

positive test result is 10 mm or more induration for health care workers with no other risk factors who work in facilities where tuberculosis patients receive care.

Recent skin test conversion among health care workers is considered significant if there is a 10 mm or greater increase in induration within a 2-year period in most facilities or 15 mm or greater within a 2-year period in minimal risk facilities. Because of anergy, persons with HIV infection may have suppressed reactions to the PPD. Therefore persons with HIV infection should be evaluated for anergy in conjunction with PPD testing. The tests should involve two companion antigens, such as *Candida* organisms and tetanus toxoid. Persons with more than 3 mm induration in

TABLE 4-6. *Instances in which induration of 15 mm or more is classified as positive*

Person does not meet any of the criteria in Tables 4-4 or 4-5. For example, in facilities in which there is essentially no risk for exposure to tuberculosis (minimal or very-low-risk facilities) induration of 15 mm or more may be a suitable cut point for health care workers who have no other risk factors.

TABLE 4-7. *Recent converters*[a]

- ≥ 10 mm increase within a 2-year period is classified as recent conversion for persons younger than 35 years
- ≥ 15 mm increase within a 2-year period is classified as recent conversion for persons 35 years of age or older

[a]Classified by size of induration and age of the person tested.

any one of the three skin tests are not anergic, and the result confirms the validity of a negative PPD test result for these persons.

Two-Step PPD Skin Test (Booster Phenomenon)

Background

Persons unaware of a previous infection with tuberculosis may have a gradual decrease in ability to react to a PPD skin test. Such persons, though infected with latent tuberculosis, when challenged with a PPD skin test may have a negative reaction. The same negative skin test result may increase the person's sensitivity to a subsequent PPD skin test. Future positive PPD reactions among such persons may be misinterpreted as a skin test conversion from a recently acquired tuberculosis infection. This booster phenomenon increases with the age of the person being tested.

Recommendation

In PPD skin test surveillance programs for health care workers, two-step testing can be used to reduce the likelihood of a boosted reaction that can be misinterpreted as a newly acquired infection. Two-step testing should be performed on all newly employed health care workers who have an initial negative PPD test result at the preplacement examination and do not have documentation of a negative PPD result in the prior 12 months. The second PPD test should be performed 1 to 3 weeks after the first test. If the second test result is positive, a boosted reaction is assumed. The health care worker is then classified as previously infected. If the second test result is negative, the worker is classified as uninfected.

TABLE 4-8. *Indications for chest radiograph in a tuberculosis surveillance program*

Positive PPD skin test
Symptoms suggest tuberculosis regardless of PPD results

PPD, purified protein derivative (tuberculin).

Chest Radiograph

Chest radiographs are not to be used routinely in screening for tuberculosis among health care workers. A tuberculosis surveillance program, should, however, include chest radiographs based on specific indications (Table 4-8). Typical chest radiographic findings suggestive of disease include upper lobe infiltration and patchy or nodular infiltrates in the apical or subapical posterior upper lobes or the superior segment of the lower lobes. Persons with HIV infection may have atypical findings on chest radiographs.

Bacteriologic Evaluation

A health care worker with PPD skin test conversion, symptoms compatible with tuberculosis, or a chest radiograph suggestive of disease typically is referred to his or her personal physician, a pulmonologist, or local health department for further evaluation and treatment. It would be prudent, however, to suggest that the worker undergo appropriate sputum cultures and sensitivities so that other potentially infected workers can be appropriately counseled. This would serve to establish a possible source of infection and whether drug resistance is an issue. In obtaining sputum samples, it is important to bear in mind that smears and cultures for acid-fast bacilli be performed on at least three sputum specimens, each specimen obtained on different days. Normal smears do not exclude the diagnosis of tuberculosis (in the United States only 60% of patients with positive sputum culture results for tuberculosis also have positive results of acid-fast bacilli smears).

PREVENTIVE MEASURES TO REDUCE TUBERCULOSIS EXPOSURE IN MEDICAL FACILITIES: COMPONENTS OF AN EFFECTIVE TUBERCULOSIS INFECTION CONTROL PROGRAM

Suspect Tuberculosis among Patients

Control of tuberculosis begins with awareness. A delay in diagnosis increases the likelihood of inadvertent exposure. In one investigation of a tuberculosis outbreak in a county hospital in which two separate wards had PPD skin test conversion rates of 30% and 48%, it was determined that transmission was facilitated by delays of up to $2^1/_2$ months in treatment of workers with skin test conversion or tuberculosis symptoms (20). Patients should be screened for signs or symptoms at initial presentation and at admission for persistent coughing (≥3 weeks), bloody sputum, night sweats, weight loss, anorexia, or fever. Health care workers need to increase their awareness of the foregoing symptoms. For patients with symptoms, appropriate evaluation (chest radiograph and sputum smear and culture) and appropriate treatment should be initiated.

Respiratory Protection

Until recently, only high-efficiency particulate air (HEPA) filter respirators approved by the National Institute for Occupational Safety and Health (NIOSH) consistently met or exceeded the performance criteria for protection against *M. tuberculosis.* On June 8, 1995, NIOSH published a new regulation, 42 CFR 84, which replaced dust-mist, dust-fume-mist, and HEPA certifications with new classes of particulate respirators, N, P, and R. The N series is tested against a solid submicron sodium chloride particle. A respirator classified N95 has a filtration efficiency of 95% or more against sodium chloride aerosol. The N95 respirators meet CDC performance specifications for respirators that can be used for tuberculosis exposure control, allowing them to replace HEPA respirators for this purpose. The cost of N95 respirators will likely be considerably less than that of HEPA filters. Respiratory protective devices for *M. tuberculosis* (tuberculosis droplet nuclei range in size from 1 to 5 μm) should meet the following criteria (21):

- Ability to filter 1-μm particles
- Filter efficiency of 95% or more
- Proper fit according to OSHA standards
- Availability in different sizes
- Ability to have the face piece fit checked by the wearer each time the respirator is worn

Only NIOSH-approved respirators (N95, HEPA) consistently meet or exceed the performance criteria.

Cough-inducing Procedures on Patients

Cough-inducing procedures as a means of producing sputum and aerosol treatments that induce coughing are usually performed on patients with respiratory disease. Such procedures may greatly increase risk for transmission of *M. tuberculosis*. The risk varies according to type of health care facility. Recommendations for minimizing this risk are as follows:

- Cough-inducing procedures should be performed on patients with tuberculosis only if absolutely necessary.
- Cough-inducing procedures should be performed in areas that have local exhaust ventilation devices (booths) or in a room that meets ventilation requirements for tuberculosis isolation (see later).
- At the completion of cough-inducing procedures, patients with tuberculosis should remain in the booth or room until coughing subsides.

Education and Training of Staff

In trying to reduce the incidence of tuberculosis public health officials failed to consider four factors: (a) the advent of HIV, (b) the development of multidrug-resistant tuberculosis, (c) the decline in public health services and limited access to health care for those in congregative facilities, and (d) the increase in immigration of persons from countries with a high prevalence of tuberculosis. The role of occupational health nurses and occupational medicine physicians in preventing workplace exposure to tuberculosis combines education, disease prevention, early detection, and treatment to maximize the opportunity for a healthy work environment for health care workers (22).

Bacille Calmette-Guérin Vaccine

In the United States, the use of Bacille Calmette-Guérin (BCG) vaccination as a tuberculosis prevention strategy is reserved for selected persons who meet specific criteria. The selectivity in the use of BCG is caused in part by the following: (a) the effectiveness of BCG vaccine in preventing infectious forms of tuberculosis is uncertain, and (b) PPD skin test reactivity occurs after vaccination and may interfere with the treatment of those who may be infected with *M. tuberculosis*. One study has concluded that the efficacy of BCG vaccination in preventing tuberculosis among health care workers cannot be determined quantitatively through examination of available studies. Despite these disadvantages, the BCG vaccine may be considered for use among health care workers where the likelihood of transmission of and subsequent infection with *M. tuberculosis* strains resistant to isoniazid and rifampin is high. The vaccine can be used if comprehensive tuberculosis infection control precautions have been implemented in the workplace and have not been successful. BCG should not be used by persons infected with HIV because of the potential for adverse reactions (23). As a rule, the BCG vaccine should not be included in a medical center tuberculosis control program.

Isolation Rooms and Ventilation

In hospitals and other inpatient facilities, patients who have confirmed or suspected tuberculosis should be placed in isolation rooms with appropriate ventilation (8). Following recommendations for isolation would separate patients with the potential for transmitting tuberculosis from other persons, reduce the concentration of droplet nuclei in the isolation room through engineering controls, and prevent the escape of droplet nuclei from the patient's room. The number of persons entering an isolation room should be kept to a minimum. Those who do enter the isolation room, including health care personnel and visitors, should wear appropriate respiratory protection. Visitors may need to be given general instructions on how to use the respirator before entering the room. Specific isolation room recommendations are as follows:

- Single-patient room
- Maintenance of negative pressure with doors closed
- Minimum of six air changes per hour in existing construction, 12 air changes per hour in new or renovated construction
- Air exhausted to the outside unless recirculated through HEPA filters or ultraviolet germicidal irradiation devices
- Anteroom to minimize escape of droplet nuclei
- An adequate number of isolation rooms appropriate to the risk assessment of the facility (see Table 4-1)
- Grouping of isolation rooms in one area of the facility

Ultraviolet Germicidal Irradiation

Ultraviolet radiation can be used to kill or inactivate microorganisms. One of two systems can be used. In duct irradiation ultraviolet (UV) lights are placed inside ducts that remove air from rooms to disinfect the air before it is recirculated. There is no patient exposure to UV radiation. With upper-room-air irradiation, UVGI lamps are suspended from the ceiling or mounted on the wall. The bottom of the lamp is shielded to direct radiation upward. Such lamps inactivate *M. tuberculosis* organisms in the upper parts of the room while minimizing radiation exposure to persons in the room.

Prophylactic Treatment of a Health Care Worker with a Positive PPD Skin Test or Recent PPD Skin Test Conversion

Management of active tuberculosis, including multidrug-resistant tuberculosis, is beyond the scope of this text. However, recommendations regarding health care workers with an initial positive PPD skin test result or recent conversion of a previously negative skin test result are discussed in this section. The appropriateness of preventive therapy must be based on the likelihood that the skin test reaction represents true infection with *M. tuberculosis*, the estimated risk for progression from latent to active tuberculosis, and risk for potential side effects of preventive therapy (see later).

Isoniazid is used to prevent latent infection from progressing to active tuberculosis (18). It is administered in a single daily dose of 10 mg per kilogram of body weight not to exceed 300 mg/day or in two doses per week at 15 mg/kg per dose not to exceed 900 mg per dose. Although there is some evidence that 6 months of therapy may be adequate, 12 months of therapy is recommended. Isoniazid should be used with caution by persons older than 35 years, those who drink alcoholic beverages every day, those with chronic liver disease or peripheral neuropathy, those who have previously discontinued isoniazid because of side effects, those who use other long-term medications, or those who are pregnant. Persons undergoing isoniazid therapy should be monitored for compliance, neurotoxicity (paresthesias), and hepatic effects. Baseline transaminase levels (ALT and AST) should be taken before therapy for persons with the aforementioned risk factors. If transaminase levels exceed three to five times the upper limit of normal, isoniazid therapy should be reconsidered. *Rifampin* is used in preventive therapy for persons with infection by isoniazid-resistant strains of *M. tuberculosis* (22).

In a study of acceptance of preventive therapy with isoniazid by health care workers who had recent PPD skin test conversion, investigators found that more of the physician group (74%) than the hospital employee group (48%) completed preventive therapy (24). When persons are known or presumed to be infected with bacillary strains resistant to multiple drugs, usually including both isoniazid and rifampin, the appropriate course of action is not clear. In one study (25) investigators recommended prophylaxis with 750 mg ciprofloxacin twice a day and 25 to 30 mg/kg pyrazinamide a day in three divided doses for 6 to 12 months. Conclusions were based on decision analysis of drug toxicity and disease outcome.

Health Care Workers, Tuberculosis, the Americans with Disabilities Act, and Return to the Workplace

Tuberculosis is a disorder of the respiratory system subject to the provisions of the Americans with Disabilities Act (ADA). Although this chapter does not cover management of tuberculosis, health care facilities may need to determine when an employee treated for active tuberculosis should return to work. Before allowing a health care worker under treatment of active tuberculosis to return to the workplace, one must consider the risk for transmission of disease to patients, who may be compromised by other illnesses, and the risk for infection of coworkers.

Health care workers with sputum smears positive for tuberculosis and *sensitive* organisms should be considered infectious until they have received at least 2 weeks of chemotherapy (26). Before a health care worker with tuberculosis is allowed to return to work, documentation of adequate therapy, resolution of symptoms, and three consecutive sputum smears negative for tuberculosis is essential. Once the health care worker has resumed duties at the facility and is undergoing antituberculosis therapy, periodic statements should be received from the worker's health care provider documenting effective drug therapy and negative results of sputum smears. These recommendations do not apply to health care workers receiving preventive treatment for latent tuberculosis infection. Workers in this category should not be restricted from usual work activities unless they have signs or symptoms that could be caused by tuberculosis.

Postexposure Recommendations

Exposure to active tuberculosis in the health care setting is usually caused by improper diagnosis of the illness or failure to use appropriate precautions (8). A PPD skin test should be administered as soon as possible after exposure. If the initial PPD result is negative, a second skin test should be administered 12 weeks after exposure. The assumption with these postexposure recommendations is that a baseline two-step PPD skin test was performed at the start of employment if a PPD skin test had not been done within the 12 months before the start of employment, *or* that a baseline one-step PPD skin test was performed at the start of employment if a previous PPD skin test was performed within the 12 months before the start of employment, *and* the facility has a regular (that is, annual) surveillance PPD skin test program and the exposed employee is a participant in that program. If the exposed health care worker has not had a PPD skin test within previous 12 months before exposure, a two-step PPD is performed as soon as possible after the exposure. If the two step PPD result is negative, a follow-up skin test should be administered 12 weeks after exposure.

CONCLUSION

The resurgence of tuberculosis and the emergence of drug-resistant strains coupled with a growing number of immunocompromised patients and a high proportion of susceptible health care workers has increased awareness of hospital- and medical center–acquired tuberculosis. Early in 1994, OSHA announced its intent to develop a standard for occupational exposure to tuberculosis. Until such a standard becomes a reality, protection of health care workers from tuberculosis is enforced under an OSHA compliance memorandum issued October 8, 1993. This memorandum outlines the hierarchy of controls presented in the 1990 CDC publication, Guidelines for Preventing the Transmission of

Tuberculosis in Health-Care Settings, with Special Focus on HIV-Related Issues (RR-17). The memorandum indicates that effective January 6, 1994, OSHA would issue citations and fines to health care facilities under the OSHA respiratory protection standard for failure to use appropriate respiratory protection and for failure to implement a complete respiratory protection program for exposed health care workers.

The goal of the infection control guidelines in this chapter are to prevent dissemination and inhalation of infectious particles. The guidelines include (a) early diagnosis of infection and isolation of patients with infection, (b) particular care during procedures such as bronchoscopy, airway suction, and chest physiotherapy, which are likely to increase the density of the organism in the environment, and (c) regular surveillance of the hospital staff (27). If medical centers adopt such measures (depending on the prevalence of tuberculosis in the facility and community), the prevalence tuberculosis should be reduced considerably. Although not all instances of occupational infection with *M. tuberculosis* can be prevented, an understanding of the chain of infection and how to break the links in the chain aid in reducing risk and maintaining health for all health care workers (28).

REFERENCES

1. Wolf L. A tuberculosis control plan for ambulatory care centers. *Nurse Pract* 1995;20:34–36,39–40.
2. McGowan JE. Preventing nosocomial tuberculosis: progress at last [Editorial]. *Am J Infect Control* 1995; 23:141–145.
3. McGowan JE Jr. Nosocomial tuberculosis: new progress in control and prevention. *Clin Infect Dis* 1995;21:489–505.
4. Sepkowitz KA, Raffalli J. Tuberculosis at the end of the twentieth century. *Eur J Clin Microbiol Infect Dis* 1994; 13:902–907.
5. US Department of Health and Human Services, Centers for Disease Control and Prevention guidelines for prevention of tuberculosis transmission in hospitals; 1982; CDC publication no 82-8371.
6. US Department of Health and Human Services, Centers for Disease Control and Prevention. Guidelines for preventing the transmission of tuberculosis in health-care facilities, with special focus on HIV-related issues. *MMWR Morb Mortal Wkly Rep* 1990;39:[RR-17].
7. US Department of Health and Human Services, Centers for Disease Control and Prevention. National action plan to combat multidrug-resistant tuberculosis. *MMWR Morb MortWkly Rept* 1992;41:[RR-11].
8. US Department of Health and Human Services, Centers for Disease Control and Prevention. Guidelines for preventing the transmission of *Mycobacterium tuberculosis* in health-care facilities, 1994. *MMWR Morb Mortal Wkly Rep* 1994;43:[RR-13].
9. Menzies D, Fanning A, Yuan L, Fitzgerald M. Tuberculosis among health care workers. *N Engl J Med* 1995; 332:92–98.
10. Chan J, Tabak JL. Risk of tuberculosis infection among house staff in an urban teaching hospital. *South Med J* 1985;78:1061–1064.
11. Sepkowitz KA. AIDS, tuberculosis, and the health care worker. *Clin Infect Dis* 1995;22:232–242.
12. Kantor HS, Poblete R, Pusateri SL. Nosocomial transmission of tuberculosis from unsuspected disease. *Am J Med* 1988;84:833–838.
13. McKenna MT, Hutton M, Cauthen G, Onorato IM. The association between occupation and tuberculosis: a population-based survey. *Am J Resp Crit Care Med* 1996; 154:587–593.
14. Clever LH, LeGuyader Y. Infectious risks for health care workers. *Annu Rev Public Health* 1995;16:141–164.
15. Wenger PN, Otten J, Breeden A, Orfas D, Beck-Sague CM, Jarvis WR. Control of nosocomial transmission of multidrug-resistant *Mycobacterium tuberculosis* among health care workers and HIV-infected patients. *Lancet* 1995;345:235–240.
16. Beck-Sague C, Dooley SW, Hutton MD, et al. Hospital outbreak of multidrug-resistant *Mycobacterium tuberculosis* infections. *JAMA* 1992;268:1280–1286.
17. Felia P, Rivera P, Maloney C, Randolf C, Squires KL, Sepkowitz KA. Dramatic reduction of employee PPD conversions after implementation of NYS/CDC guidelines in an urban hospital. In: Program and Abstracts of APIC 20th Annual Educational Conference and International Meeting. May 23–28, 1993; Orlando, FL (abst 126).
18. US Department of Health and Human Services. CDC Core Curriculum on Tuberculosis, 2nd ed. Washington, DC: Department of Health and Human Services, 1991.
19. AHA Technical Panel on Infections. *Tuberculosis Control In Hospitals: A Special Briefing.* AHA catalog no 094692. American Hospital Association, Chicago, Illinois 1994.
20. Zaza S, Blumberg HM, Beck-Sague C, et al. Nosocomial transmission of *Mycobacterium tuberculosis*: role of health care workers in outbreak propagation. *J Infect Dis* 1995;172:1542–1549.
21. Jarvis WR, Bolyard EA, Bozzi CJ, et al. Respirators, recommendations, and regulations: the controversy surrounding protection of health care workers from tuberculosis. *Ann Intern Med* 1995;122:142–146.
22. Doyle AJ. Tuberculosis: preventing occupational transmission to health care workers. *AAOHN J* 1995;43:475–481.
23. US Department of Health and Human Services, Centers for Disease Control and Prevention. The role of BCG vaccine in the prevention and control of tuberculosis in the United States. *MMWR Morb Mortal Wkly Rep* 1995; 45:[RR-4].

24. Camins BC, Bock N, Watkins DL, Blumberg HM. Acceptance of isoniazid preventive therapy by health care workers after tuberculin skin test conversion. *JAMA* 1996;275:1013–1015.
25. Stevens JP, Daniel TM. Chemoprophylaxis of multidrug-resistant tuberculosis infection in HIV-uninfected individuals using ciprofloxacin and pyrazinamide: a decision analysis. *Chest* 1995;106:712–717.
26. Control and prevention of tuberculosis in the United Kingdom: code of practice 1994. *Thorax* 1994;49: 1193–1200.
27. DeWit D. Hospital-acquired tuberculosis. *Med J Aust* 1995;163:428–431.
28. Jackson MM, Rymer TE. Nurses: at special risk. *J Obstet Gynecol Neonatal Nurs* 1995;24:533–540.

FURTHER INFORMATION

1. US Department of Health and Human Services, Centers for Disease Control and Prevention. guidelines for preventing the transmission of *Mycobacterium tuberculosis* in health-care facilities, 1994. *MMWR Morb Mortal Wkly Rep* 1994;43:[RR-13].

   A comprehensive compilation of recommendations for control and prevention of tuberculosis in a medical center environment.
2. Markowitz SB. Epidemiology of tuberculosis among health care workers. Occup Med 1994;9:589–608.

   A comprehensive review of current methods of evaluation, management, and prevention of tuberculosis from the viewpoint of the occupational medicine physician.
3. *Am J Infect Control* 1995; volume 23.

   A large portion of this issue is devoted to tuberculosis, the modes of transmission, and the methods of prevention in the health care setting.
4. US Department of Labor, Occupational Safety and Health Administration, Office of Health Compliance Assistance. Enforcement procedures and scheduling for occupational exposure to tuberculosis. February 9, 1996. CPL 2.106.

   This document serves as an updated supplement to the CDC guidelines published in 1994. Though the purpose of this publication is to provide uniform inspection procedures and guidelines to be followed for conducting inspections and issuing citations, by necessity it relies heavily on the CDC guidelines.

Medical Center Occupational Health and Safety,
edited by Robert J. McCunney.
Lippincott Williams & Wilkins, Philadelphia © 1999

5

Infection Control and Immunization of Health Care Workers

Carol A. Sulis

Department of Medicine, Boston University School of Medicine; Epidemiology Unit, Boston Medical Center; The Maxwell Finland Laboratory for Infectious Diseases, Boston, Massachusetts 02118-2393

In today's rapidly changing health care environment, the medical center occupational health service (OHS) is in a perfect position to take a leadership role in promoting effective infection control practices and comprehensive immunization programs for health care workers. Hospital infection control was introduced in 1847 by Ignaz Semmelweis, who showed that hand washing before examining obstetric patients decreased mortality from puerperal sepsis caused by group A β-hemolytic streptococci (1). Despite subsequent improvements in disinfection and aseptic techniques in the early 1900s and the introduction of antimicrobial agents in the 1930s, worldwide outbreaks of nosocomial infections caused by *Staphylococcus aureus* in the 1950s prompted the development of formal infection control programs in hospitals (2). As evidence of the efficacy of these programs accumulated, increased attention was focused on refining hospital infection control programs (3–5). Groups of infection control practitioners formed organizations such as the Association for Professionals in Infection Control and Epidemiology (APIC), the Society for Healthcare Epidemiology of America (SHEA), and the Centers for Disease Control and Prevention Hospital Infection Control Practices Advisory Committee (HICPAC) to address infection control issues in the hospital.

Concern about the spread of multidrug-resistant organisms and the fear of occupational transmission of blood-borne pathogens has fueled the development of increasingly stringent and complex regulations and guidelines to protect both patients and health care workers (Tables 5-1 through 5-3) (6–17). The pivotal role of the OHS has become increasingly apparent and has been the focus of several reviews (2, 13,18–25). This chapter is an overview of the management of infectious diseases and exposures in the medical center. Diseases for which specific policies and procedures should be available and the need for collaboration with other hospital departments are highlighted.

PHILOSOPHY AND GOALS OF THE OCCUPATIONAL HEALTH SERVICE INFECTION CONTROL PROGRAM

Within the medical center environment, which often serves the needs of multicultural and variably educated health care workers, the OHS should assist health care workers in maintaining an optimal level of health. Services include initial and periodic health assessments, health promotion and health education activities, and appropriate utilization of medical center and community resources. Although most OHS infection control programs focus on employees who provide direct patient care, programs must also apply to all other

TABLE 5-1. *Immunizing agents and immunization schedules for health care workers*[a]

Generic name	Primary schedule and booster(s)	Indications	Major precautions and contraindications	Special considerations
Immunizing agents strongly recommended for health care workers				
Hepatitis B recombinant vaccine	Two doses IM 4 weeks apart; third dose 5 months after second; booster doses not necessary.	Preexposure: HCW at risk for exposure to blood or body fluids Postexposure: See Table 5-3.	No known risk for adverse effects to developing fetus. Pregnancy is not considered a contraindication to vaccination. Previous anaphylactic reaction to common baker's yeast is a contraindication to vaccination.	The vaccine produces neither therapeutic nor adverse effects on HBV-infected persons. Serologic screening before vaccination is not indicated for persons being vaccinated because of occupational risk unless determined to be cost effective because of HCW demographics. HCW who have contact with patients or blood should be tested 1–2 months after vaccination to determine and document serologic response.
Hepatitis B immune globulin	0.06 mL/kg IM as soon as possible after exposure. A second dose of HBIG should be administered 1 month later if the HBV vaccine series has not been started.	Postexposure prophylaxis (see Table 5-3): For persons exposed to blood or body fluids containing HBsAg and who are not immune to HBV infection give 0.06 mL/kgIM as soon as possible (but not later than 7days after exposure).	—	—
Influenza vaccine (inactivated whole-virus and split-virus vaccines)	Annual vaccination with current vaccine. Administered IM.	HCW who have contact with patients at high risk for influenza or its complications; HCW who work in chronic care facilities; HCW with high-risk medical conditions or who are 65 years of age or older.	History of anaphylactic hypersensitivity to egg ingestion.	No known risk to mother or fetus when vaccine is administered to a pregnant woman with an underlying high-risk condition. Influenza vaccination is recommended during second and third trimesters of pregnancy because of increased risk of hospitalization.

Measles live-virus vaccine	One dose SC; second dose at least 1 month later.	HCW[b] born after 1/1/57 who do not have documentation of having received two doses of live vaccine on or after the first birthday or a history of physician-diagnosed measles or serologic evidence of immunity. Vaccination should be considered for all HCW who lack proof of immunity, including those born before 1957.	Pregnancy; immunocompromised status,[c] including HIV-infected persons who have evidence of severe immunosuppression; anaphylaxis after gelatin ingestion or administration of neomycin; recent administration of immune globulin.	MMR is the vaccine of choice if recipients are likely to be susceptible to rubella, mumps, or measles. Persons vaccinated during 1963–1967 with a killed measles vaccine alone, killed vaccine followed by live vaccine, or with a vaccine of unknown type should be revaccinated with 2 doses of live measles virus vaccine.
Mumps live-virus vaccine	One dose SC; no booster.	HCW[b] believed to be susceptible can be vaccinated. Adults born before 1957 can be considered immune.	Pregnancy; immunocompromised status[a]; history of anaphylactic reaction after gelatin ingestion or administration of neomycin.	MMR is the vaccine of choice if recipients are likely to be susceptible to measles and rubella as well as to mumps.
Rubella live-virus vaccine	One dose SC, no booster.	Indicated for HCW[b] who do not have documentation of having received live vaccine on or after their first birthday or laboratory evidence of immunity. Adults born before 1957, except women who can become pregnant, are generally considered immune.	Pregnancy; immunocompromised status[c]; history of anaphylactic reaction after administration of neomycin.	Risk for rubella vaccine-associated malformations among the offspring of women pregnant when vaccinated or who become pregnant within 3 months after vaccination is negligible. Such women should be counseled regarding the theoretical basis of concern for the fetus. MMR is the vaccine of choice if recipients are likely to be susceptible to measles, mumps, or rubella.
Varicella zoster live-virus vaccine	Two 0.5-mL doses SC 4–8 weeks apart if 13 years of age or older.	Indicated for HCW[b] who do not have either a reliable history of varicella or serologic evidence of immunity.	Pregnancy, immunocompromised status[c]; history of anaphylactic reaction following receipt of neomycin or gelatin. Avoid salicylate use for 6 weeks after vaccination.	Because 71%–93% of persons without a history of varicella are immune, serologic testing before vaccination is likely to be cost effective.

(continued)

TABLE 5-1. *Continued.*

Generic name	Primary schedule and booster(s)	Indications	Major precautions and contraindications	Special considerations
Varicella zoster immune globulin	Persons weighing <50 kg: 125 U/10 kg IM	Persons known or likely to be susceptible (particularly those at high risk for complications, such as pregnant women) who have close and prolonged exposure to a contact case or to an infectious hospital staff worker or patient.		Serologic testing may help in assessing whether to administer VZIG. If use of VZIG prevents varicella disease, patient should be vaccinated subsequently.
	Persons weighing ≥50 kg: 625 U.[d]			
Bacille Calmette-Guérin (BCG) vaccination				
BCG vaccine (tuberculosis)	One percutaneous dose of 0.3 mL; no booster dose recommended.	Should be considered only for HCW in areas where multidrug-resistant tuberculosis is prevalent, a strong likelihood of infection exists, and comprehensive infection control precautions have failed to prevent TB transmission to HCW.	Should not be administered to immunocompromised persons[c] or pregnant women.	In the United States tuberculosis control efforts are directed at early identification, treatment of patients, and preventive therapy with isoniazid.
Other immunobiologic agents that are or may be indicated for health care workers				
Immune globulin (hepatitis A)	Postexposure: one IM dose of 0.02 mL/kg administered ≤2 weeks after exposure.	Indicated for HCW exposed to feces of infectious patients.	Contraindicated in persons with IgA deficiency; do not administer within 2 weeks after MMR vaccine or 3 weeks after varicella vaccine. Delay administration of MMR vaccine for ≥3 months and varicella vaccine for ≥5 months after administration of IG.	Administer in large muscle (deltoid, gluteus).

Hepatitis A vaccine	Two doses of vaccine either 6–12 months apart (HAVRIX®) or 6 months apart (VAQTA®).	Not routinely indicated for HCW in the United States. Persons who work with HAV-infected primates or with HAV in a research laboratory setting should be vaccinated.	History of anaphylactic hypersensitivity to alum or, for HAVRIX®, the preservative 2-phenoxyethanol. The safety of the vaccine among pregnant women has not been determined; the risk associated with vaccination should be weighed against the risk for hepatitis A in women who may be at high risk for exposure to HAV.	
Meningococcal polysaccharide vaccine (tetravalent A, C, W135, and Y)	One dose in volume and by route specified by manufacturer; need for boosters unknown.	Not routinely indicated for HCW in the United States.	The safety of the vaccine among pregnant women has not been evaluated; it should not be administered during pregnancy unless risk for infection is high.	
Typhoid vaccine, IM, SC, and oral	IM vaccine: One 0.5-mL dose, booster 0.5 mL every 2 years. SC vaccine: two 0.5-mL doses, ≥4 weeks apart, booster 0.5 mL SC or 0.1 mL ID every 3 years if exposure continues. Oral vaccine: four doses on alternate days. The manufacturer recommends revaccination with the entire four-dose series every 4 years.	Workers in microbiology laboratories who frequently work with *Salmonella typhi.*	Severe local or systemic reaction to a previous dose. Ty21a (oral) vaccine should not be administered to immunocompromised persons[c] or to persons receiving antimicrobial agents.	Vaccination should not be considered an alternative to the use of proper procedures when handling specimens and cultures in the laboratory.
Vaccinia vaccine (smallpox)	One dose administered with a bifurcated needle; boosters administered every 10 years.	Laboratory workers who directly handle cultures with vaccinia, recombinant vaccinia viruses, or orthopox viruses that infect humans.	The vaccine is contraindicated in pregnancy, in persons with eczema or a history of eczema, and in immunocompromised persons[c] and their household contacts.	Vaccination may be considered for HCW who have direct contact with contaminated dressings or other infectious material from volunteers in clinical studies involving recombinant vaccinia virus.
Other vaccine-preventable diseases				
Tetanus and diphtheria (toxoids [Td])	Two IM doses 4 weeks apart; third dose 6–12 months after second dose; booster every 10 years.	All adults.	Except in the first trimester, pregnancy precaution is not necessary. History of a neurologic reaction or immediate hypersensitivity	Tetanus prophylaxis in wound management.[e]

(continued)

TABLE 5-1. *Continued.*

Generic name	Primary schedule and booster(s)	Indications	Major precautions and contraindications	Special considerations
			reaction after a previous dose. History of severe local (Arthus-type) reaction after a previous dose. Such persons should not receive further routine or emergency doses of Td for 10 years.	
Pneumococcal polysaccharide vaccine (23 valent).	One dose, 0.5 mL IM or SC; revaccination recommended for those at highest risk ≥5 years after the first dose.	Adults who are at increased risk for pneumococcal disease and its complications because of underlying health conditions; older adults, especially those 65 years of age or older who are healthy.	The safety of vaccine among pregnant women has not been evaluated. It should not be administered during pregnancy unless the risk for infection is high. Previous recipients of any type of pneumococcal polysaccharide vaccine who are at highest risk for fatal infection or antibody loss may be revaccinated ≥5 years after the first dose.	
Inactivated poliovaccine (IPV) Live oral poliovaccine (OPV)	Primary series for adults: Two doses of 0.5 mL IPV SC 4–8 weeks apart, third dose 6–12 months later.[f]	Adults who are unvaccinated and at increased risk for exposure to polio because of travel to areas where polio is endemic, work in a laboratory and handle specimens that may contain poliovirus, work with patients who may be excreting poliovirus, or reside in a household where children will be receiving OPV.	Hypersensitivity or anaphylactic reaction to IPV, OPV, or components including streptomycin, polymyxin B, or neomycin. Vaccination of pregnant women should be avoided unless the patient requires immediate protection. The risk for vaccine-associated paralytic polio is small but is greater with OPV than with IPV.	OPV can spread secondarily and should not be given to patients who are immunocompromised or who live in a household with a member with known or suspected immunodeficiency from any cause, including steroid use. The risk for transmission to an immunodeficient HCW has not been determined but should be minimized by the use of standard precautions.
	Catch up vaccination: one or two doses of 0.5 mL IPV SC *or* one or two doses of 0.5 mL OPV given orally.	Incompletely vaccinated adults with the above risk factors should be given the remaining required number of doses of either OPV or IPV regardless of the interval since the last dose or the type of vaccine that was previously received.		

Booster vaccination: one dose of 0.5 mL IPV SC *or* one dose of 0.5 mL OPV given orally.	Adults who are at increased risk for exposure to wild poliovirus and who previously completed primary immunization with OPV or IPV should receive a single dose of either IPV or OPV.

[a]Persons who provide health care to patients or work in institutions that provide patient care, such as physicians, nurses, emergency medical personnel, dental professionals and students, medical and nursing students, laboratory technicians, hospital volunteers, and administrative and support staff in health-care institutions.

[b]All HCW (medical or nonmedical paid or volunteer, full time or part time, student or nonstudent, with or without patient care responsibilities) who work in health care institutions (inpatient and outpatient, public and private) should be immune to measles, rubella, and varicella.

[c]Persons immunocompromised because of immune deficiency or diseases, HIV infection, leukemia, lymphoma or generalized malignant disease or immunosuppressed as a result of therapy with corticosteroids, alkylating drugs, antimetabolities, or radiation.

[d]Some experts recommend 125 U/10 kg regardless of total body weight.

[e]See Ref 17.

[f]Accelerated immunization schedules are available. See Ref 111.

HCW, health care worker; HBV, hepatitis B virus; HBIG, hepatitis B immune globulin; HBsAg, hepatitis B surface antigen; HIV, human immunodeficiency virus; MMR, measles, mumps, rubella vaccine; VZIG, varicella zoster immune globulin; TB, tuberculosis; HAV, hepatitis A virus.

Adapted from refs. 13 and 14.

TABLE 5-2. *Summary of suggested work restrictions for health care workers exposed to or infected with diseases of importance in health care settings, in the absence of state and local regulations*

Disease or problem	Type of restriction	Duration of restriction	Category[a]
Conjunctivitis	Restriction from direct contact with patient or patient equipment.	Until discharge resolves.	II
Cytomegalovirus infection	None		
Diarrhea			
Acute stage (diarrhea and other symptoms)	Restriction from direct contact with patient or food handling.	Until symptoms resolve.	IB
Convalescent stage (*Salmonella* Spp, not typhoid)	Restriction from care of high-risk patients.	Until symptoms resolve. Consult with local and state health authorities regarding the need for negative stool cultures.	IB
Diphtheria	Exclusion from duty.	Until antimicrobial therapy completed and two cultures obtained ≥24 hours apart are negative.	IB
Enteroviral infections	Restriction from care of infants, newborns, and immunocompromised patients.	Until symptoms resolve.	II
Hepatitis A	Restriction from direct contact with patient or food handling.	Until 7 days after onset of jaundice.	IB
Hepatitis B			
HCW with acute or chronic hepatitis B surface antigenemia who does not perform exposure-prone procedures	No restriction unless epidemiologically linked to transmission of infection. Standard precautions should be observed.		
HCW with acute or chronic hepatitis, B "e" antigenemia who performs exposure-prone procedures	Exclusion from exposure-prone invasive procedures until counsel from an expert review panel has been sought. The panel should review and recommend the procedures the worker can perform, taking into account the specific procedure as well as the skill and technique of the worker. Standard precautions should be observed.	Until HBeAg is negative.	II
Hepatitis C	No recommendation.		Unresolved issue
Herpes simplex			
Genital	No restriction.		II
Hands (herpetic whitlow)	Restrict from direct contact with patient.	Until lesions heal.	IA
Orofacial	Restrict from care of high-risk patients.	Until lesions heal.	II
Human immunodeficiency virus	Exclusion from exposure-prone invasive procedures until counsel from an expert review panel has been sought. The panel should review and recommend the procedures the worker can perform, taking into account the specific procedure as well as the skill and technique of the worker. Standard precautions should be observed.		II
Measles			
Active	Exclusion from duty.	Until 4 days after appearance of rash.	IA
Postexposure (susceptible HCW)	Exclusion from duty.	From the 5th day after the first exposure through the 21st day after the last exposure and/or until 4 days after appearance of rash.	IB

Mumps			
Active	Exclusion from duty.	Until 9 days after the onset of parotitis.	IB
Postexposure (susceptible HCW)	Exclusion from duty.	From the 12th day after the first exposure through the 26th day after the last exposure, or until 9 days after the onset of parotitis.	II
Pertussis			
Active	Exclusion from duty.	From the beginning of the catarrhal stage through the 3rd week after onset of paroxysms or until 5 days after the start of effective antimicrobial therapy.	IB
Postexposure (asymptomatic)	No restriction; prophylaxis recommended.		II
Postexposure (symptomatic)	Exclusion from duty.	Until 5 days after the start of effective antimicrobial therapy.	IB
Rubella			
Active	Exclusion from duty.	Until 5 days after appearance of rash.	IA
Postexposure (susceptible HCW)	Exclusion from duty.	From 7 days after the first exposure through the 21st day after the last exposure or until 5 days after appearance of rash.	IB
Scabies or pediculosis	Restriction from patient contact.	Until treated.	IB
Staphylococcus aureus infection			
Active, draining skin lesion	Restriction from direct contact with patients, patient equipment, or food handling.	Until lesions have resolved.	IB
Carrier state	No restriction unless HCW is epidemiologically linked to transmission of infection.		IB
Streptococcal infection, group A	Restriction from direct contact with patient and food handling.	Until 24 hours after initiation of adequate therapy.	IB
Tuberculosis	Exclusion from duty.	Until proved noninfectious.	IA
Varicella, primary (chickenpox)			
Active	Exclusion from duty.	Until all lesions are dry and crusted.	IA
Postexposure (susceptible, nonvaccinated HCW; see text for discussion of management of vaccinated HCW)	Exclusion from duty.	From the 10th day after the first exposure through the 21st day after the last exposure (or through the 28th day after the last exposure if VZIG is given); If varicella occurs, until all lesions are dry and crusted.	IA
Varicella zoster (shingles)			
Active zoster (localized in normal host)	Cover lesions; restriction from care of members of high-risk groups such as neonates, immunocompromised patients of any age, and any other patient at increased risk for complications of varicella.	Until all lesions are dry and crusted.	II
Active zoster (disseminated; localized in immunosuppressed host)	Restriction from patient contact.	Until all lesions are dry and crusted.	IB
Postexposure (susceptible HCW)	Restriction from patient contact.	From the 10th day after the first exposure through the 21st day after the last exposure (or through the 28th day after the last exposure if VZIG is given); if varicella occurs, until all lesions are dry and crusted.	IA

(continued)

TABLE 5-2. *Continued.*

Disease or problem	Type of restriction	Duration of restriction	Category[a]
Viral respiratory infection, acute febrile	Consider exclusion from the care of high-risk patients during community outbreaks of respiratory syncitial virus and influenza.	Until acute symptoms resolve.	IB

[a]Definition of CDC Recommendation categories:

Category IA. Strongly recommended for all hospitals and strongly supported by well-designed experimental or epidemiologic studies.

Category IB. Strongly recommended for all hospitals and reviewed as effective by experts in the field and a consensus of HICPAC members based on strong rationale and suggestive evidence, even though definitive scientific studies have not been done.

Category II. Suggested for implementation in many hospitals. Recommendations may be supported by suggestive clinical or epidemiologic studies, a strong theoretical rationale, or definitive studies applicable to some, but not all, hospitals.

No recommendation, Unresolved issue. Practices for which insufficient evidence or consensus regarding efficacy exists.

HCW, health care worker, VZIG, varicella zoster immunoglobulin.

Adapted from refs. 13 and 14.

TABLE 5-3. *Recommendations for hepatitis B prophylaxis after percutaneous exposure*

Exposed person	HBsAg positive	HBsAg negative	HBsAg unknown or not tested
Unvaccinated	Administer HBIG[a] ×1 and initiate hepatitis B vaccine[b]	Initiate hepatitis B vaccine[b]	Initiate hepatitis B vaccine[b]
Previously vaccinated			
Known responder	No treatment	No treatment	No treatment
Known nonresponder	HBIG ×2 *or* HBIG ×1 plus one dose of hepatitis B vaccine	No treatment	If known high-risk source, may treat as if source were HBsAg positive
Response unknown	Test exposed worker for anti-hepatitis B antibody If adequate[c]: no treatment If not adequate[c]: give HBIG ×1 plus hepatitis B vaccine booster dose	No treatment	Test exposed worker for anti-hepatitis B antibody If adequate[c]: no treatment If not adequate[c]: give HBIG ×1 plus hepatitis B vaccine booster dose

[a]Hepatitis B immune globulin 0.06 mL/kg IM.
[b]See Table 5-1.
[c]Adequate level of anti-hepatitis B antibody is ≥10 μIU/mL.
Adapted from ref. 13.

medical center employees (including administrative and support staff), outside contractors (such as emergency medical personnel and laboratory technicians), physicians, dentists, students, volunteers, and visitors. Resources to provide these services must be identified.

An effective OHS infection control program must provide care for health care workers with occupational injuries or exposures, identify work-related infection risks, and institute appropriate preventive measures, including immunization programs and policies for work restriction for infected or exposed health care workers (see Tables 5-1 through 5-3). In all cases, government regulations and local public health isolation and quarantine policies must be reviewed and incorporated into the institutional policies. This is most easily accomplished in collaboration with the medical center infection control and safety departments, who can assist by monitoring and investigating infectious exposures and outbreaks among health care workers and by developing written policies and procedures to minimize infection risks. One way to maximize this type of collaboration is to have the OHS notify the infection control department or the hospital epidemiologist whenever a health care worker has a reportable infectious disease or an exposure to a communicable infectious disease. The infectious disease specialist is available to confirm the diagnosis, and investigation and control measures can be implemented without delay. It may be particularly helpful for the OHS representative to attend infection control and safety committee meetings on a regular basis and report statistics such as the number of rubella and hepatitis B vaccinations, purified protein derivative (PPD) test results, the number and circumstances surrounding unprotected exposures to blood, tuberculosis, varicella, and meningococci, and recommendations to prevent similar exposures in the future.

The institution should have a policy that guarantees that all health care workers who seek and receive care at the OHS have the right to confidentiality of all records and communications to the extent provided by law. No information regarding the health status of the health care worker should be released without the health care worker's written permission. This is particularly important with respect to exposures to blood-borne pathogens. To facilitate compliance, health care workers must be educated about the principles of infection control with an emphasis on individual responsibility.

PREPLACEMENT PHYSICAL EXAMINATION AND HEALTH INVENTORY AND INFECTIOUS DISEASE SCREENING OF STUDENTS, VOLUNTEERS, AND HOUSE OFFICERS

Because of their potential exposure to patients or infectious material from patients, all prospective health care workers in all departments should undergo a physical examination after the offer of employment to establish that the health care worker is able to perform essential job duties and to assure that the worker is free from communicable diseases. The health care worker also should undergo screening and immunization for certain vaccine-preventable infectious diseases before beginning work (see Table 5-1) (2,13,14,26–33). Appropriate screening and immunization can decrease the likelihood of infectious disease outbreaks among hospital personnel and facilitate identification of susceptible individuals in the event of an exposure, particularly when information is maintained in a computerized medical record or tracked in a database format. Health care workers should complete a health history form to facilitate data collection before infectious disease screening and immunization. The history should establish the presence of an immunosuppressive condition or therapy, chronic infection, weeping dermatitis or open wounds, or other conditions that could predispose a worker to acquisition or transmission of an infectious disease. Prospective health care workers also should undergo a tuberculosis skin test (PPD) and any other tests, such as serologic screening for vaccine-preventable diseases as determined appropriate by the provider.

Infectious Disease Screening during the Preplacement Physical

Tuberculosis PPD Skin Test

A PPD test should be administered to all new health care workers, including those who have received Bacille Calmette-Guérin (BCG), unless they have had a positive PPD result in the past or unless they have documentation of a negative PPD result within the past 6 months (11,26–28). Persons with a history of a positive PPD result who have not completed 6 to 12 months of effective therapy should be evaluated for active tuberculosis (27). The OHS may conduct its own evaluation or may refer the patient to a clinic or physician specializing in the management of tuberculosis. Under OSHA guidelines, each institution must address the management of tuberculosis in an institutional plan for preventing the transmission of tuberculosis.

Measles, Mumps, and Rubella

All health care workers should receive a measles-mumps-rubella (MMR) vaccination unless they can produce, at the physical examination, written documentation of immunity to measles, mumps, and rubella (29–31). Acceptable written documentation includes physician-diagnosed cases of measles or mumps, adequate immunization with live measles, mumps, and rubella vaccines on or after the first birthday, or laboratory evidence of immunity. Persons born before January 1, 1957, or vaccinated after 1968 are generally considered to be immune to measles and mumps.

Tetanus and Diphtheria

Health care workers who have not had a tetanus-diphtheria toxoid booster for 10 years or more may elect to receive a booster dose at the time of the preplacement physical examination (32).

Varicella

Persons who have had chickenpox are considered immune. Persons without history of the disease should undergo screening for varicella antibody during the preplacement physical examination or at the time of exposure. Varicella vaccine is indicated for health care workers who lack a reliable history or serologic evidence of immunity (33).

Hepatitis B

Hospital health care workers with potential for exposure to blood or blood products may undergo screening for antibodies to hepatitis B. Hepatitis B vaccine must be offered free of charge to health care workers. Susceptible hospital health care workers are required to receive this vaccine or sign an informed refusal (9,34–37).

Medical Evaluations

The OHS should be easily accessible on site with flexible hours. Services should be available for employees, volunteers, students, physicians, and contracted health care workers. When resources allow, evaluation and treatment should be provided at no direct cost to health care workers to encourage reporting and expedite compliance with treatment and follow-up recommendations. Health care workers should not incur loss of seniority, job, position, or vacation time if exclusion from work is required because of exposure to a communicable infectious disease.

There should be a clear, consistent written procedure for health care workers who injure themselves when the OHS is closed. An alternative care site might be the emergency department, or the worker might be asked to call a nursing supervisor. Such a procedure would apply to health care workers who sustain needle sticks or other percutaneous or mucous membrane exposures to blood or other body fluids or who have infectious diseases that may be transmitted to other workers or patients and that must be dealt with in a timely manner.

POLICIES FOR HOSPITAL HEALTH CARE WORKERS WITH CERTAIN INFECTIOUS DISEASES

It is prudent for institutions to develop general guidelines for health care workers with certain infectious diseases. These policies apply chiefly to health care workers who have direct contact with patients or patient care equipment. Health care workers have the right to seek advice and treatment from the health care provider of their choice but must adhere to OHS guidelines for certain infectious diseases or exposures that may be a danger to patients or other health care workers. Each case should be evaluated individually, and the recommendations may vary from the general guidelines in selected cases. Institutions that routinely care for patients with unusually virulent infectious diseases (hemorrhagic fevers and plague) or that have active infectious disease or animal research units (anthrax, brucellosis, herpes B virus, Q fever, rabies) should develop policies to deal with these entities (19,38–51).

Health care workers with an infectious disease, suspected infectious disease, or exposure to certain infectious diseases (described later) should report to the OHS for evaluation (see Table 5-2) (13). When the OHS is closed, the workers should report to the emergency department or other designated alternative care site. It is crucial that managers understand the relevance of infectious disease policies and send health care workers to the OHS for evaluation. It is also crucial that workers who are aware of unprotected exposures that may have occurred at work or outside the workplace be encouraged to seek evaluation at the OHS and not be penalized or made to feel guilty if exclusion from work is recommended. The infection control department or hospital epidemiologist should be consulted in most cases of infectious disease.

Examples of Infections or Conditions That Might Require Special Precautions or Work Restrictions

Acute Upper Respiratory Disease

It is neither necessary nor feasible to remove all health care workers with acute upper respiratory disease from their jobs. Special areas such as the newborn nursery may develop policies in consultation with the OHS and the infection control department. Health care workers with documented streptococcal pharyngitis may return to work 24 to 48 hours after beginning antibiotic treatment, depending on their clinical status.

Acquired Immunodeficiency Syndrome

Health care workers with symptomatic AIDS or human immunodeficiency virus (HIV) infection should be examined by the OHS and the infection control department to determine whether they have any transmissible opportunistic infections. In the absence of such infections, the decision regarding type of work should depend on the results of the examination of the individual worker by the appropriate medical consultation service.

Conjunctivitis

Health care workers with conjunctivitis should be examined in the OHS before performing direct patient care or handling medical devices or equipment. Health care workers who have epidemic keratoconjunctivitis caused by adenovirus or purulent conjunctivitis caused by other microorganisms should be restricted from patient care for the duration of symptoms. Health care workers may be referred for further evaluation and determination of continued infectiousness if symptoms persist longer than 5 days.

Dermatitis

Health care workers with dermatitis must be examined in the OHS before performing direct patient care or handling medical devices or equipment. Health care workers who have exudative lesions or weeping dermatitis should be restricted from all direct patient care, from handling patient care equipment or food, and from handling devices used in performing invasive procedures until the condition resolves.

Diarrhea of Uncertain Causation

Diarrhea is a common illness. In most instances diarrhea begins suddenly, lasts only a day or two, and resolves without harm to the patient or contacts. Transmission usually results from contact with an infected person, consumption of contaminated food or water, or exposure to contaminated objects or environmental surfaces. Health care workers with sudden onset of diarrhea should report to the OHS for a history and examination. *Salmonella, Shigella, Campylobacter*, or *Yersinia* infection, parasite infestation, cholera, pathogenic *Escherichia coli* infection, or hepatitis A should be determined as a cause as appropriate. Time away from work should be determined by the OHS and the infection control department on an individual basis depending on culture results and clinical status. The worker usually can return to work when recovered.

An exception is made for food handlers, who must be treated according to local public health isolation and quarantine regulations. In general, food handlers who have had or are household contacts of a person with *Salmonella, Shigella, Campylobacter,* or *Yersinia* infection, parasite infestation, cholera, or hepatitis A should not be allowed to work until cleared by the OHS in consultation with the infection control department. Such workers generally are required to have two consecutive negative stool cultures collected at least 48 hours apart, beginning on the date of last exposure. If antibiotics have been given, the cultures must be taken at least 48 hours after the last dose. In identified cases of infectious diarrhea, the OHS should work in collaboration with the infection control department to uncover and treat possible sources. Use of appropriate isolation techniques and good personal hygiene, particularly hand washing by health care workers before and after all patient contacts, should minimize the risk of transmission of enteric pathogens.

Monitoring Infections among Dietary Workers

To ensure a safe environment for the handling and preparation of food, the medical center should monitor food handlers for infection or colonization with organisms that can be transmitted by foods. Supervisors should refer dietary workers with diarrhea, skin lesions, jaundice, or febrile respiratory illnesses to the OHS for evaluation. This procedure should be described in a written policy.

Hepatitis B

All persons with hepatitis B should be cleared through the OHS before returning to work.

Hepatitis A

Health care workers recovering from hepatitis A should be cleared by their own health care provider and the OHS. Food-handling health care workers must be out of work until the end of the febrile period, or until 7 days after the onset of jaundice. Food-handling health care workers who have been exposed to or are a household contact of a person with hepatitis A should be excluded from work for 28 days unless they receive a prophylactic dose of immune globulin within 2 weeks of first contact, in which case they may return to work immediately.

Varicella (Chickenpox)

Health care workers with varicella-zoster or chickenpox may return to work after all lesions have crusted. Workers should be cleared through the OHS before returning to the worksite.

Herpetic Infections

Herpes simplex is a contagious viral infection. Direct contact with lesions or infected secretions is the principal mode of transmission. Health care workers with herpes simplex, including lesions on lips (cold sores) or finger (herpetic whitlow), should be examined at the OHS to determine whether they may work. Health care workers with herpes simplex should be isolated from newborn infants (first 30 days of life), women in labor, patients with severe malnutrition, patients with extensive open lesions (burns, dermatitis, patients undergoing surgical procedures), and patients receiving immunosuppressive therapy (steroids, antineoplastic agents). Health care workers with herpes simplex may not pose a special risk to other patients if the lesions can be covered. There is no evidence that health care workers with genital infections pose high risk to patients if the worker follows good patient care practices. Health care workers with oral infections, however, can reduce the risk of infecting patients by wearing an appropriate barrier such as a mask or gauze dressing to prevent hand contact with the lesions and washing hands well before and after all patient care. Health care workers with herpetic whitlow infection should be evaluated individually but are generally excluded from all direct patient contact until the lesions have dried and crusted.

Measles

Health care workers with measles may return to work 4 days after the rash appears. Workers should be cleared by the OHS before returning to the worksite.

Mumps

Health care workers may return 9 days after parotid swelling is first noticed. Workers should be cleared by the OHS before returning to the worksite.

Pertussis

Health care workers with symptoms of pertussis (unexplained rhinitis or acute cough) after unprotected exposure should be excluded from patient care until 5 days after the start of appropriate antibiotic prophylaxis.

Rubella

Health care workers may return to work 7 days after the appearance of rubella rash depending on clinical status. Workers should be cleared by the OHS before returning to the worksite.

Tuberculosis

Health care workers with tuberculosis should be cleared by the OHS or tuberculosis specialist before returning to work. In general, workers may return after three normal sputum specimens have been obtained.

Scabies and Lice

Health care workers with scabies or lice are restricted from patient care until completion of initial therapy (13).

Staphylococcal or Streptococcal Skin Disease

Health care workers with draining or crusted skin lesions should report to the OHS for evaluation and treatment. In general, the worker should not return to direct patient care activities or food handling until cultures for the causative organism have negative results and lesions are no longer draining (13).

Referrals and Follow-up Care

A referral form should be initiated by the supervisor when a health care worker becomes ill or requests evaluation in the OHS during working hours. To expedite evaluation, no form should be required in emergency cases or if the health care worker is not on duty. The OHS provider should perform the evaluation and make a recommendation that specifies return to duty, excuse from duty, or referral to another clinic. All services provided in the OHS are confidential, and no supervisor should be given details of the nature of the illness without the written consent of the health care worker. Exceptions are made for diseases such as chickenpox or infectious pulmonary tuberculosis in which unprotected exposures may have occurred before diagnosis of the worker's disease and which may require additional contact investigation or intervention to protect patients or other health care workers. The purpose of such a policy is to ensure that supervisors are aware that the health care worker is temporarily away from the worksite and to provide a means of communicating the OHS recommendation regarding work status to the supervisor.

OHS records must be maintained in accordance with local public health and hospital licensing regulations and follow OSHA recordkeeping requirements (9,52). All health care workers seen after hours at an alternative site should make a follow-up appointment with the OHS as soon as possible to review details of the infectious disease or unprotected exposure, follow up on therapy, and receive counseling if indicated.

WORK-RELATED INJURIES AND ILLNESSES

Most institutions require that a supervisor complete an accident reporting and treatment form if a health care worker sustains a work-related injury. The worker should be sent for evaluation of the injury to the OHS during its regular hours or the designated alternative site when the OHS is closed. When possible, the accident reporting and treatment form should be sent with the worker at the time of the evaluation. However, in emergency cases, or if the health care worker is not on duty, no form should be required at the initial visit.

All evaluation and management procedures for work-related illness and injury must be conducted in accordance with hospital policy, government regulations, and applicable workers' compensation law. Specific additional conditions and restrictions for health care workers with certain infectious diseases should be addressed in disease-specific infection control policies. Benefits of work restrictions must be balanced with the risks of reducing staff in critical areas such as intensive care units or nurseries. To be most effective, restriction and return to work policies should be developed by a multidisciplinary group with representation from the clinical service involved, infection control department, administration, and unions. Well-designed policies should minimize confusion about loss of benefits while maximizing compliance with infection control procedures.

Reinstatement Evaluations: Returning to Work after a Work-Related Injury or Illness

At many institutions, health care workers who have lost time from work because of an occupational injury or illness must be examined in the OHS before returning to the worksite. The purpose of the reinstatement examination is to ascertain whether the health care worker is capable of resuming previous job duties and to evaluate current infectious disease status. Specific conditions and restrictions for health care workers with certain infectious diseases should be addressed in disease-specific infection control policies. Similar policies should apply to health care workers who have been absent more than 5 days because of illness or injury and health care workers returning from a leave of absence or layoff.

Referral to Employee Assistance Program: Counseling Services for Health Care Workers

Health care workers may experience personal problems that affect their lives and job performance. Many problems can be resolved through appropriate counseling. Many institutions offer an employee assistance program free of charge to all health care workers. An employee assistance program traditionally provides evaluation, treatment, and referral services for health care workers with substance abuse problems. However, the employee assistance program may also provide referral services to outside agencies for health care workers with marital, emotional, family, or financial problems who prefer to be treated outside the medical center. Such a program might benefit health care workers after unprotected exposure to blood. Changes in sexual practices and interactions with family may require considerable additional support services.

HEALTH CARE WORKERS WHO HAVE AIDS OR WHO ARE HIV-ANTIBODY POSITIVE

AIDS is caused by HIV. Transmission of this virus occurs through intimate or percutaneous contact with infected blood or body secretions. The results of antibody tests should remain confidential information in the OHS. The risk for transmission of HIV from infected health care workers to patients has been extensively evaluated. There are no data to suggest that health care workers who do not perform invasive procedures pose a risk to patients. In general therefore health care workers with HIV infection who have no symptoms may continue to work in patient care areas. Special precautions must be taken by health care workers to prevent the passage of blood or secretions to patients or other hospital workers. The health care worker should not perform exposure-prone invasive procedures until the practice is reviewed by a panel of experts (36,53). The panel should review and recommend specific procedures that the health care worker can perform and take into consideration the skill and technique of the worker. In all cases, standard precautions should be observed.

Health care workers with symptomatic AIDS or HIV disease should be evaluated by the OHS and the infection control department to determine whether they have any transmissible opportunistic infections. In the absence of such infections, the decision regarding acceptable job tasks should depend on results of an examination of the specific health care workers by the appropriate medical consultation service.

HEALTH CARE WORKERS WHO ARE PREGNANT

Risk for occupational infection is particularly worrisome to female health care workers of childbearing age. Infection with group A β-hemolytic streptococci or varicella may be more severe during pregnancy. Infection with cytomegalovirus, hepatitis B, or rubella is commonly associated with congenital infection of the fetus (54). In general, because of the use of standard precautions in most hospitals, pregnant health care workers are not at increased risk for occupational acquisition of infection (13). Specific risks and management of exposures for pregnant health care workers are discussed later. Health care workers should be strongly encouraged to receive immunization for vaccine-preventable illnesses before becoming pregnant.

SCREENING FOR VACCINE-PREVENTABLE ILLNESSES AND TUBERCULOSIS

Hepatitis B Screening and Immunization

Hepatitis B is a common viral infection transmitted to health care workers through contact with infected blood and body fluids. Despite emphasis on preventive measures including the use of vaccine, an estimated 1,000 to 2,000 health care workers are infected each year, 5% to 10% become chronic carriers, and 100 to 200 die of the sequelae of chronic liver disease. To comply with the 1991 blood-borne pathogen standard, an institution must identify, educate, screen, and vaccinate all health care workers who are at risk for occupationally acquired hepatitis B virus infection (see Table 5-1) (13,14,34–37,53,55–57). Prevaccination serologic testing may be cost effective for health care workers with a history of hepatitis, jaundice, or unprotected blood exposures. Hepatitis B core antibody may be the preferred serologic test to avoid unnecessary vaccination of previously infected persons. If no contraindications are present, susceptible health care workers are required to receive vaccine or sign an informed refusal (declination form).

If the vaccine series is interrupted after the first dose, the second and third doses should be separated by an interval of 3 to 5 months. Health care workers who are late for the third dose may be vaccinated at any time. Previously immunized health care workers without written documentation of postimmunization serologic testing should undergo screening with the hepatitis B surface antibody test. Although vaccine-induced antibody levels wane over time, vaccine-induced immunity appears to prevent both clinical hepatitis and viremic hepatitis B infection. Therefore, booster doses for adults with normal immune status are not routinely recommended, nor is routine serologic testing to assess antibody levels necessary for vaccine recipients. However, postvaccination testing for serologic response is advised by the CDC for health care workers whose treatment after unprotected exposures to blood or body fluid depends on knowing their immune status. Approximately 1 or 2 months after the third dose, the health care workers should be tested for susceptibility to hepatitis B with the surface antibody test, and should be given a written copy of their results.

Health care workers who do not undergo seroconversion may receive up to three additional doses of vaccine 1 month apart. Hepatitis B surface antibody test testing should be performed after each additional dose to document immunity. Revaccination of nonresponders produces adequate antibody 15% to 25% of the time after one additional dose and up to 30% of the time after three additional doses. Although boosters are not currently thought to be necessary, the need for booster doses of vaccine after long intervals (more than 12 years) should be assessed as additional information becomes available. All health care workers should be instructed to report unprotected exposures to the OHS whether or not they have completed the hepatitis B vaccine series.

Measles, Mumps, and Rubella Immunization

Despite widespread availability of vaccine, nosocomial transmission of measles, mumps, and rubella continues to be reported (13–17, 29–31,58–69). To minimize transmission of measles, mumps, and rubella to susceptible persons and decrease the likelihood of outbreaks of these potentially fatal infections, it is essential that all health care workers have documentation of immunity before beginning work (see Table 5-1) (13,14,17,70). In addition, many states require immunity for health care workers, and local public health recommendations should be reviewed and incorporated into institutional policies. Acceptable written documentation includes physician-diagnosed cases of measles or mumps, adequate immunization with two doses of live measles, mumps, and rubella vaccine on or after the first birthday, or laboratory evidence of immunity. Although health care workers who were born before January 1, 1957, or were vaccinated after 1968, are generally considered to be immune to measles and mumps, serologic studies indicate that 5% to 9% actually may not be immune (71). Therefore when resources allow evaluation, unvaccinated health care workers born before January 1, 1957, who lack a history of disease or evidence of serologic immunity should be offered MMR immunization. Serologic screening need not be performed before vaccination unless the institution considers it cost effective or the health care worker requests testing (72–74). Health care workers who are unable to provide acceptable proof of immunity should receive MMR vaccine unless it is medically contraindicated (14–16,75).

Medical contraindications include severe febrile illness, hypersensitivity to the components of the vaccine, pregnancy or the intent to become pregnant within 3 months of vaccination, recent immunoglobulin injection, and immunodeficiency. Vaccine is produced in chick embryo cell cultures, so persons with a history of immediate hypersensitivity to egg products or neomycin (hives, swelling of the mouth and throat, difficulty breathing) should not receive vaccine. Nursing mothers may receive MMR vaccine. Administration of immune globulin (immune serum globulin or hepatitis B immune globulin) or whole blood products containing antibody may interfere with the immune response to vaccine, so immunization with MMR vaccine should be deferred for at least 3 months. Conversely, if it is required before travel, immune globulin ideally should be given 2 or more weeks after vaccination. Tuberculin skin testing should be performed on the day of vaccination or delayed 4 to 6 weeks.

MMR and tetanus-diphtheria toxoid vaccines may be given simultaneously because inactivated vaccines do not interfere with the immune response. However, the immune response to one live-virus vaccine might be impaired if given within 30 days of another, and live virus vaccines not administered on the same day should be given 30 days or more apart. MMR vaccine is not generally recommended for people with immunodeficiency disease or those with other suppressed immune responses; however, certain patients may benefit from vaccination and should consult their primary care provider. Health care workers born after January 1, 1957, who cannot provide acceptable proof of immunity and who refuse to receive MMR vaccine should be required to sign an informed refusal sheet and may be restricted from direct patient care. Health care workers should be instructed to report all adverse reactions to the OHS. Receipt of MMR vaccine should be documented in the OHS record. Vaccinated health care workers should be given an immunization record with documentation of vaccinations.

If immediate protection against measles is required for persons for whom use of live measles virus vaccine is contraindicated, passive immunization with immune serum globulin may be given within 6 days after a known exposure. Mumps immune globulin has not been shown to be effective and is no longer available or licensed for use in the United States. Pregnant susceptible health care workers exposed to measles or mumps should be treated jointly by the OHS, their obstetricians, and an infectious disease specialist. Susceptible health care workers who travel abroad should be protected against measles and mumps because these diseases are endemic in many countries throughout the world.

Varicella Immunization

Nosocomial transmission of varicella-zoster virus is well described (13,14,33,76–82). To prevent varicella among susceptible patients and health care workers, a varicella history should be part of the preplacement health screening for all new health care workers. The varicella history should be recorded in the health care worker's medical record. Health care workers who have had chickenpox are considered immune. Health care workers who do not meet the criteria for immunity should have a varicella titer drawn. Although 97% to 99% of adults with a positive history have seropositive results, 71% to 93% of adults with a negative history also have seropositive results. Therefore, in health care institutions serologic screening before vaccination is likely to be cost effective. Health care workers with a negative history and negative serologic results should be considered not immune to varicella. Health care workers who are not immune to varicella and have not previously received varicella vaccine should be offered the vaccine at no cost to themselves (see Table 5-1) (13,14,33,79,83–93). This is particularly important for health care workers who will have close contact with persons at high risk for serious complications of varicella, such as pregnant women, very small babies (<28 weeks gestation, <1,000 g), or immunocompromised patients.

Varicella vaccine should be administered according to published guidelines. For adults this involves two doses of vaccine separated by 4 to 8 weeks. Women who are vaccinated should avoid becoming pregnant until 3 months after completing the vaccination series. It is prudent to require that health care workers who decline immunization sign an informed refusal. Medical contraindications to vaccination include pregnancy or intent to become pregnant within 3 months; history of anaphylactic reaction to any component of vaccine, including gelatin or neomycin; immunosuppressive therapy or primary or acquired immunodeficiency, including HIV infection; untreated active tuberculosis; or malignant neoplasms that affect bone marrow or the lymphatic system.

Approximately 5% of persons who receive varicella vaccine experience a vesicular rash either at the injection site or diffusely. These persons may transmit varicella to other susceptible persons, but the risk for serious illness from transmission of attenuated virus is believed to be extremely low. Health care workers receiving varicella vaccine should be instructed to watch for development of a rash and to contact the OHS by telephone before reporting for work if a rash develops. Health care workers who experience a vesicular rash after vaccination should be given a furlough until lesions have crusted.

The rate of serologic conversion following two doses of vaccine, based on testing that is not commercially available, is estimated to be 94% among adults. The present generation of commercially available serologic tests for varicella are not sensitive enough to allow reliable detection of immunity from varicella vaccine. Therefore varicella serologic results should not be used to determine immediate postvaccination immunity. Although immunity immediately after vaccination is high, it likely decreases over time to about 70%. Despite prior immunization, a person can be naturally infected with wild-type varicella virus. Persons who have been vaccinated and have breakthrough wild-type varicella have a highly attenuated illness but may serve as a vector for cross infection in the health care setting. For this reason, and because the level of immunity cannot be reliably assessed after vaccination, workers who have been vaccinated should continue to avoid exposure to patients with infectious chickenpox or zoster. Health care workers should be informed that varicella vaccination does not necessarily prevent infection, and the worker should continue to avoid unprotected exposure to patients with infectious varicella.

Influenza Immunization

Nosocomial transmission of influenza has been reported (13,14,94–98). Administration of influenza vaccine to health care workers (including pregnant women) before the beginning of the influenza season can reduce risk for influenza infection and prevent transmission to persons at high risk for complications. Persons at greatest risk for influenza-related complications are older than 65 years, residents of nursing homes or other chronic care facilities, or have chronic pulmonary or cardiovascular conditions or diabetes mellitus (see Table 5-1) (13,14,98–103).

Other Vaccines

Certain health care workers may benefit from immunization against hepatitis A, *Neisseria meningitidis* infection, *Salmonella typhi* infection, tuberculosis, or vaccinia (see Table

5-1) (14,28,44,103–105). Nosocomial transmission of these diseases has been reported but can be minimized by the appropriate use of isolation procedures. The decision to implement vaccine programs should be based on the needs of the medical center population (6, 14,106,107).

Nosocomial transmission of pertussis has also been described (14,108). Studies on the incidence, severity, and cost of pertussis among adolescents and adults and studies on the safety and efficacy of adult vaccination are in progress. However, no formulation of the acellular pertussis vaccine has been approved for use by adults, and booster doses are not recommended at this time (see Table 5-1) (14,109,110).

Immunization against tetanus, diphtheria, and polio should be verified and updated according to published guidelines (see Table 5-1) (14–16,32,75,111). The OHS should review the status of tetanus immunity whenever a health care worker presents with a percutaneous injury, such as needle stick or bite wound. The wound should be evaluated, cleaned, debrided, and sutured if appropriate. Administration of antibiotics and tetanus prophylaxis should be initiated promptly (Table 5-4). Management of bite wounds requires knowledge about the oral flora of the biter. Appropriate reference materials should be available in the OHS if management of such wounds is anticipated. Health care workers are not at greater risk for pneumococcal disease than the general population, and immunization should follow published guidelines (see Table 5-1) (14,112).

Tuberculosis Screening

Nosocomial transmission of *Mycobacterium tuberculosis* is well documented, but the rate is generally low in the United States. Exceptions occur in communities with a high prevalence of HIV or *M. tuberculosis* infection or with a large number of persons from countries in which *M. tuberculosis* is endemic. In some areas, the incidence and prevalence of multidrug-resistant *M. tuberculosis* also have increased (11,13,26,113–121).

In 1994, the CDC published detailed recommendations for the prevention of transmission of tuberculosis in health care settings (11). A risk assessment algorithm is used to identify the nature of tuberculosis control measures that are appropriate for each facility. A tuberculosis screening program is an integral part of a health care facility's comprehensive tuberculosis control program. Skin test conversion rates among health care workers after routine testing range from 0.1% to 10% but may be as high as 55% after unprotected exposure to a patient with tuberculosis. Health care workers who have been exposed

TABLE 5-4. *Guidelines for use of tetanus prophylaxis for adults*

Immunization status	Type of injury
Completely immunized (≥3 doses)	For minor, uncomplicated wounds give a booster dose (0.5 mL IM) only if 10 years have elapsed since last dose was given. For major and/or contaminated wounds give a single booster injection promptly on the day of injury if 5 years have elapsed since last dose was given. If the patient is allergic to Td, administer human tetanus immune globulin 250 U IM and consult with an expert about need for additional therapy.
Incompletely immunized (≤3 doses) or unknown immunization status	For minor, uncomplicated wounds give a dose of Td (0.5 mL IM) promptly on the day of injury. For major and/or contaminated wounds give a dose of Td (0.5 mL IM) promptly on the day of injury and provide passive immunization with human tetanus immune globulin 250 U IM.

Td, tetanus-diphtheria toxoid.

to tuberculosis and those who convert from negative to positive status need to be examined and treated to decrease the risk for active disease and transmission of infection to others (11,26,122–125).

All health care workers must be screened for tuberculosis at the time of preplacement examination and at least annually thereafter. Health care workers who work in areas with intermediate or high risk for *M. tuberculosis* infection must undergo screening twice or four times per year, respectively. Tuberculosis testing should be a mandatory component of annual infection control recertification for all health care workers (11,26). House officers, volunteers, temporary employees, and students should undergo testing in the OHS, or they may submit documentation of their skin test status through their clinical department. Before administration of the tuberculin test (PPD), a complete history should be obtained of the following: known exposures to *M. tuberculosis*, date and result of previous tuberculosis testing, date and result of chest radiograph after positive test reaction, dates of initiation and completion of isoniazid or other preventive therapy, allergies or contraindications to the test, or history of BCG prophylaxis. The tuberculosis specialist and the infection control department should act as resources if needed in selected cases. Prior prophylaxis with BCG is not a contraindication for undergoing a PPD test. A health care worker who has not had a positive PPD result in the past and has no contraindications should be given 5 TU (0.1 mL) PPD intradermally. The worker should return in 48 to 72 hours for a reading. The degree of induration is determined by measuring millimeters of induration across the transverse axis of the arm. Interpretation of skin test results should follow American Thoracic Society guidelines (Table 5-5) (27).

Health care workers who have not undergone a PPD test within the year should be instructed to return to the OHS within the next 1 to 3 weeks for a second (two-stage) PPD. Persons with remote sensitivity to tuberculin who have not had a recent exposure to the skin test antigen may not react to the initial test. Later, because of stimulation by the recent test, they may have a positive reaction. The two-stage test technique identifies initial false-negative results and avoids an erroneous assumption later that the person has a positive skin test reaction because of a recent *M. tuberculosis* infection (126). Health care workers who have undergone a second PPD should

TABLE 5-5. *Guidelines for interpretation of the tuberculin skin test*

5 mm or more induration is positive if
- a. HCW has had recent close contact with person with active infectious TB
- b. HCW is immunosuppressed (including HIV) or risk factors for HIV infection with unknown HIV status
- c. HCW chest radiograph consistent with previous TB (untreated)

10 mm or more induration is positive for persons who do not meet any of the above criteria but who have other risk factors for TB, including
- a. High-risk groups: users of IV drugs known to be HIV seronegative; persons with certain other medical conditions, including silicosis, gastrectomy, jejunoileal bypass operation, being 10% or more below ideal body weight, chronic renal failure, diabetes mellitus, use of high-dose corticosteroids or other immunosuppressive therapy, lymphoma, leukemia, other malignant disease; and children younger than 4 years
- b. High-prevalence groups: persons from high prevalence countries in Asia, Africa, the Caribbean, and Latin America; persons from medically underserved, low-income areas; residents of long-term care facilities, including correctional institutions and nursing homes; other persons from high-risk populations in their communities as determined by the local public health authorities

15 mm or more induration is positive for persons who do not meet any of the above criteria

Recent converters are defined on the basis of both induration and age:
- a. ≥10 mm increased induration within a 2-year period for those younger than 35 years
- b. ≥15 mm increased induration for those 35 years of age or older

HCW, health care worker; TB, tuberculosis; HIV, human immunodeficiency virus.
Adapted from ref. 27.

return in 48 to 72 hours for a reading of the second test. The results of the second test should be used as the baseline for determining subsequent conversion, treatment, and follow-up care. Tuberculosis testing is labor intensive, and compliance although mandatory is difficult to achieve. Innovative incentive programs may be used to improve testing rates, but no single method has been universally successful (127).

Health care workers with positive test reactions should undergo chest radiography and evaluation of disease status. Preventive therapy should be offered to persons with positive reactions or recent conversion unless specifically contraindicated (125). Health care workers with a documented history of a positive PPD skin test result who have documentation of completion of 6 to 12 months of prophylactic treatment with isoniazid need to repeat a chest radiograph only when they have symptoms. Health care workers who have completed a full course of isoniazid preventive therapy may be discharged from tuberculosis surveillance. Health care workers with a documented history of a positive PPD skin test result who have not completed 6 to 12 months of prophylactic treatment with isoniazid should be referred to the tuberculosis clinic for evaluation. Routine follow-up chest radiographs are not necessary. Health care workers must return to the OHS for periodic evaluation only if symptoms are present. Health care workers with documented positive reactions should be exempt from screening and should be given a written copy of the test result. The efficacy of BCG vaccination in the United States is uncertain, and immunization is not generally indicated for health care workers (28).

PROCEDURES AFTER EXPOSURES TO CERTAIN INFECTIOUS DISEASES

Overview of Isolation Guidelines for Hospitals

In 1996, the CDC Hospital Infection Control Practices Advisory Committee published revised guidelines to help hospitals maintain effective isolation practices. Recommendations were developed for acute care hospitals but may be applicable to nursing homes or chronic care facilities (6,128). Recommendations for infection control in the outpatient setting, which includes ambulatory clinics, dialysis centers, and physical therapy departments, are being developed (129). The hospital isolation guidelines supersede all prior recommendations and introduce new terminology. These guidelines and a detailed rationale for each of the isolation methods have been extensively described (6).

Standard precautions combine universal (blood and body fluid) precautions and body substance isolation. Standard precautions apply to potential exposures involving blood, all body fluids, secretions, and excretions (except sweat), nonintact skin, and mucous membranes and should be used for the care of all patients. Standard precautions rely on environmental controls (adequate housekeeping services, availability of sharp-instrument disposal systems), personal protective equipment (gowns, gloves, face mask, eye protection), and scrupulous attention to hand washing to prevent transmission of infection (6,53,130–133).

Transmission-based precautions are designed for patients with known or suspected infection or colonization with highly transmissible or epidemiologically important pathogens for which additional precautions beyond standard precautions are needed to interrupt transmission in hospitals; and are divided into three categories—airborne, droplet, and contact.

Airborne precautions are used for patients with diseases such as measles, varicella, or tuberculosis, which are transmitted by tiny, airborne droplet nuclei. Patients should be placed in a private room with negative pressure and either external air exhaust or high-efficiency particulate air (HEPA) filtration if air is recirculated. These specialized HEPA filters are capable of removing 99.97% of particles 0.03 μm or more in diameter. Health care workers should use appropriate respiratory protection.

Droplet precautions are used for patients with diseases such as *Neisseria meningitidis* infection, diphtheria, or influenza which are transmitted by large-particle droplets. Patients should be placed in a private room whenever possible. In addition to use of standard precautions, health care workers should wear a mask when working within 3 feet of the patient.

Contact precautions are used for patients with diseases such as *Clostridium difficile* infection, respiratory syncytial virus infection, pediculosis, or viral hemorrhagic fever, which are transmitted through direct contact with infectious particles. Patients should be placed in a private room whenever possible. In addition to use of standard precautions, health care workers should use appropriate personal protective equipment to maintain barrier precautions.

Although implementation of isolation precautions usually rests with the infection control department, the OHS must have sufficient familiarity with the guidelines to enable collaborative development of policies and procedures to prevent unprotected exposures. The OHS must have sufficient knowledge to educate health care workers about risk-reduction strategies and be able to provide accurate and effective evaluation and prophylaxis when unprotected exposures do occur. Despite the best efforts and intentions, unprotected exposures still occur. The following section describes some of the most common situations that occur in hospitals and outlines procedures to expedite investigation and postexposure evaluation. Examination of potentially infected health care workers should proceed with appropriate infection control precautions, a detail often neglected by busy OHS practitioners.

Blood and Body Fluid Exposure

Expedient and appropriate evaluation, counseling, and treatment of health care workers who sustain unprotected exposures to blood or bloody body fluid may greatly reduce the risk for occupationally acquired infection with blood-borne pathogens such as HIV, hepatitis B virus, and hepatitis C virus and is described in detail in Chapter 3 (134–136). In 1991, OSHA mandated that most institutions develop an exposure control plan to address these risks (9). Health care workers should be encouraged to report exposures immediately to maximize potential benefit from postexposure prophylactic therapy with combination antiretroviral agents (34,35, 37,55,56,137,138). A large proportion of health care workers report side effects associated with the use of combination antiretroviral therapy (139). The OHS must be vigilant in providing monitoring and follow-up care, especially when postexposure prophylaxis is used. Avoidance of exposure with the use of safe equipment, appropriate vaccination, and risk-reduction strategies is crucial (see Tables 5-1, 5-3) (6,37,53,140).

For hepatitis C positive or unknown exposures, the health care worker should be instructed to return for a minimum of one follow-up evaluation 6 months after exposure. No vaccine or prophylactic regimen is currently available to prevent hepatitis C infection after unprotected exposure to virus in blood or secretions (13,141–143). Health care workers who have positive serologic results for hepatitis C at baseline testing or who subsequently have seroconversion, should be referred to a gastroenterologist or their primary care providers for appropriate evaluation and counseling.

Cytomegalovirus Exposure

Health care workers are not at increased risk for occupational acquisition of cytomegalovirus infection. Risk can be minimized by means of scrupulous hand washing and adherence to standard precautions (see Table 5-2) (6,13,54,144).

Measles Exposure

Measles is an acute, highly communicable viral disease spread through respiratory droplets or direct contact with infectious nasopharyngeal secretions. Measles is one of the most readily transmissible communicable diseases, and airborne precautions should be used. Immunocompetent persons shed the virus beginning 1 to 2 days before symptoms appear (5 days before the rash) and continuing until 3 to 4 days after appearance of the rash. Immunocompromised persons may shed the virus for longer periods. To minimize transmission of measles to susceptible persons, all health care workers with measles, suspicion of measles, exposure to measles or suspicion of exposure to measles should report to the OHS for joint evaluation by the OHS and infection control department (see Table 5-2) (6,13). Susceptible health care workers should contact the OHS regardless of where the exposure occurred. When practical, susceptible exposed health care workers should be offered a blood test to document immune status. Measles vaccine may prevent or modify the course of disease if it is given within 72 hours of exposure. A single dose of measles vaccine should induce measles antibodies in at least 95% of susceptible persons. Immune globulin may prevent or modify the course of disease if given within 6 days of exposure (145). Health care workers should be out of work on days 5 to 21 after exposure whether or not they received vaccine or immunoglobulin after exposure. Health care workers who develop active disease should be relieved from direct patient contact until 4 days after the rash appears.

Meningococcal Disease Exposure

When a patient is determined to have meningococcal disease, the OHS, infection control department, and the emergency or admitting department should work in collaboration to identify and evaluate all health care workers who were in contact with the patient before the initiation of isolation and precaution measures (see Table 5-2). Antibiotic prophylaxis should be considered for health care workers who have given mouth-to-mouth resuscitation, provided direct care without a mask (intubation, suctioning, standing within 3 feet of the patient for 10 minutes or more during a cardiac arrest, or performing any procedure involving face-to-face contact for more than 10 minutes, especially if the patient is coughing), or who had direct contact with the patient's secretions (cerebrospinal fluid, vomitus, saliva, sputum). Rifampin (600 mg orally twice a day for 2 days) or ciprofloxacin (500 mg orally) are effective in eradication of nasopharyngeal carriage among 90% to 95% of patients but are not recommended for pregnant women (6,104). Ceftriaxone (250 mg IM) may be used for prophylaxis for pregnant women. The quadrivalent A,C,Y,W-135 polysaccharide vaccine has been used successfully to control community outbreaks caused by serogroup C disease but is not recommended for postexposure prophylaxis in health care settings (104). Prophylaxis should be given promptly, within 24 hours if possible. Droplet precautions should be observed until completion of 24 hours of effective therapy. Health care workers should be given an educational pamphlet that describes signs and symptoms of meningococcal disease and side effects of drugs used for prophylaxis. Persons with symptoms should be examined without delay.

Mumps Exposure

Although mumps transmission has occurred in hospitals, most cases of mumps among health care workers are community acquired (146,147). Mumps is transmitted through direct contact with infectious virus in respiratory secretions. Transmission is minimized by adherence to droplet precautions until 9 days after the onset of parotid swelling (see Table 5-2). The incubation period is 16 to 18 days, but cases may occur 12 to 26 days after exposure. Susceptible health care workers should be vaccinated and excluded from work on days 12 to 26 after exposure (see Table 5-2) (6,13,30,147).

Oxacillin- or Methicillin-Resistant *Staphylococcus aureus* Infection

Patients colonized or infected with oxacillin- or methicillin-resistant *Staphylococcus aureus* should be treated with contact precautions to minimize transmission. Health care workers are not generally screened for carriage unless they are epidemiologically linked to an outbreak. If a worker is linked to an outbreak, eradication of infection or carriage should be documented before the worker resumes direct patient care or food handling (see Table 5-2) (6,13,148–152).

Parvovirus B19

Parvovirus B19 is the cause of erythema infectiosum (fifth disease), a childhood illness characterized by upper respiratory tract symptoms and a rash. Patients with chronic hemolytic anemia, leukemia, or AIDS may experience aplastic crisis or chronic infection with prolonged viral shedding. Infection among pregnant women has been associated with increased risk for hydrops fetalis and fetal wasting (54,153). Risk for transmission generally is not increased among health care workers and can be minimized with strict adherence to droplet precautions (6,13,153–155).

Pertussis (Whooping Cough)

The incidence of pertussis is increasing because of waning immunity and a lack of natural exposure. It is estimated that more than 25% of the U.S. adult population is susceptible to infection. Administration of whole-cell pertussis vaccine is contraindicated for adults, and routine administration of acellular pertussis vaccine to health care workers is not recommended at this time. Transmission of infection is facilitated by the delay in diagnosis caused by the presence of nonspecific symptoms early in the catarrhal stage of the illness, when the patient is most infectious. Transmission may be minimized by adherence to droplet precautions until the patient has completed 5 days of effective antibiotic therapy (156,157). Health care workers with symptoms of pertussis (unexplained rhinitis or acute cough) after unprotected exposure should be excluded from patient care until 5 days after the start of appropriate antibiotic prophylaxis (see Table 5-2) (6,13,156).

Rubella Exposure (German Measles)

Rubella is an acute, highly communicable viral illness spread through contact with infectious particles in nasopharyngeal secretions. Immunocompetent persons shed virus beginning 7 days before symptoms occur and continuing until 5 to 7 days after the onset of rash. Droplet precautions should be observed to minimize risk for transmission. Infants with congenital infection may shed virus substantially longer, and use of contact precautions is advised for the first year of life (6). Infection during the first 6 months of pregnancy increases risk for congenital infection and fetal malformation (54). To minimize transmission of rubella to susceptible persons, all susceptible health care workers with rubella, suspicion of rubella, exposure to rubella, or suspicion of exposure to rubella should report immediately to the OHS for evaluation and collaborative management by the OHS, infection control, and local public health departments (see Table 5-2) (6,13).

When practical, susceptible health care workers exposed to rubella should be offered serologic screening and be immunized if appropriate. Susceptible pregnant women should avoid vaccine, be comanaged with their obstetricians, and may need to remain out of work until 21 days after the last diagnosed case of rubella in the facility has resolved (6,13,14,54). All other susceptible health care workers should be given a furlough for days 7 to 21 after exposure. Health care workers who develop active disease may return to work 5 days after appearance of the rash (see Tables 5-1, 5-2) (6,13–16,31,75).

Tuberculosis Exposure

In 1994, OSHA published revised guidelines to assist hospitals in developing effective measures to prevent the nosocomial transmission of tuberculosis (11,26). Tuberculosis is spread from person to person exclusively through airborne droplets. The probability of acquiring infection is a function of patient factors (number of acid-fast bacilli in sputum, presence of cough, duration of effective therapy), type of infection (cavitary pulmonary, tracheal, or laryngeal disease), duration of exposure, mechanical factors (mechanical ventilation, suctioning, intubation, bronchoscopy, emergency resuscitation), and the adequacy of ventilation in the area. Contact investigation gears the intensity of the search for secondary cases to the probability of transmission on the basis of the foregoing factors (see Chapter 4).

Infected patients should be treated with airborne precautions in a negative pressure room with external exhaust or HEPA filtration of air before recirculation. Health care workers must use a NIOSH-approved respirator whenever they enter the room. Exposures occur most frequently when diagnosis is delayed or not suspected or when infection control measures are not followed (113–121). Evaluation and treatment after exposures should follow American Thoracic Society guidelines (11,26, 27,125). Health care workers with *M. tuberculosis* infection (positive tuberculin skin test result) may continue to work once active disease is excluded. Health care workers with active infectious pulmonary or laryngeal tuberculosis should be excluded from work until no longer infectious. This generally requires documentation of effective therapy, resolution of cough, and demonstration that three sputum smears collected on different days are negative for acid-fast bacilli. However, the OHS must ensure that specific medical center policies comply with local health department regulations.

Varicella Exposure

Primary varicella (chickenpox) is an acute contagious disease characterized by low-grade fever, general malaise, and vesicular skin eruptions. The incubation period is 10 to 21 days after exposure. A patient with varicella is considered contagious from 48 hours before the rash appears until all lesions are crusted. Person-to-person transmission occurs primarily through direct contact with patients with varicella or zoster, occasionally through airborne (droplet) spread from respiratory secretions, and rarely through direct inoculation with vesicular fluid from zoster lesions. Varicella-zoster (shingles) represents a reactivation of the original varicella infection and usually appears as a vesicular eruption involving a single dermatome. Among immunocompromised patients zoster may appear in a disseminated form involving several dermatomes and other organ systems.

Transmission can be minimized with the use of airborne and contact precautions. Susceptible health care workers (no history of disease, negative titer, or vaccine recipient) should notify the OHS if an unprotected exposure occurs. Significant exposure includes exposure for 60 minutes or more to the ambient air of a patient with primary varicella or disseminated zoster during the contagious period, close contact for 10 minutes or more with a patient with primary varicella or disseminated zoster during the contagious period, or direct contact with vesicular lesions of a patient with either primary varicella or dermatomal zoster.

Management after exposure depends on whether the health care worker has received vaccine. Exposed, susceptible health care workers who have not been immunized should be given a furlough for days 10 through 21 after exposure. If an exposed health care worker is pregnant or immunocompromised and is susceptible to varicella, varicella immunoglobulin (VZIG) should be offered after consultation with the primary physician. Receipt or declination of VZIG should be documented in the OHS medical record. VZIG does not necessarily prevent chickenpox but may attenuate the disease. VZIG is effective only if given within 96 hours after exposure. Use of VZIG may prolong the incubation period up to 28 days. Health care workers who receive VZIG should be off duty for days 10 to 28 after exposure (see Tables 5-1, 5-2) (6,13,14,33).

A vaccinated health care worker should have a varicella titer drawn after unprotected exposure. If the titer is positive, the health care worker is considered immune, and no further action is required. If the titer is negative, the health care worker should avoid direct contact with patients who have neutropenia or leukopenia or who have recently received a solid organ or bone marrow transplant for days 10–28 following exposure. Health care workers assigned to labor and delivery, general pediatrics, any nursery, the oncology clinic, or the oncology ward should be reassigned to a different work area for days 10 to 28 after exposure. Before reporting for work health care workers should be instructed to report to the OHS any rash or systemic illness that occurs 10 to 28 days after exposure to varicella. If the illness is judged to represent possible varicella, the health care worker should be given a furlough from work. Vaccine recipients who do not have a rash may have a titer drawn 4 weeks after exposure to determine whether natural immunity to varicella has developed (see Tables 5-1, 5-2) (6, 13,14,33).

Health care workers with active varicella should be excluded from work until all lesions have dried and crusted. Health care workers with suspected herpes zoster should be examined promptly by the OHS. If herpes zoster is diagnosed, appropriate treatment and follow-up care should be planned. Because of the possibility of transmission and development of severe illness among patients at high risk, health care workers with herpes zoster should be isolated or reassigned from newborn infants (first 30 days of life), women in labor, patients with severe malnutrition, patients with extensive open lesions, burns or dermatitis, patients undergoing surgical procedures, or patients receiving immunosuppressive therapy with steroids or antineoplastic agents. Health care workers with herpes zoster may not pose a special risk to other patients if the lesions can be covered. The communicable period of varicella or zoster lasts until all lesions are crusted. Health care workers should be given clearance to return to work only by the OHS.

Exposure to Patients with Other Viral Respiratory Infections

Health care workers may be exposed to a variety of respiratory pathogens, and recommendations to prevent nosocomial pneumonia have been published (158,159). Influenza is transmitted primarily through large droplets of nasopharyngeal secretions that contain infectious particles. Incubation is 1 to 5 days, and the patient is most infectious from 1 day before onset throughout the period of peak symptoms. Therefore health care workers or patients who are incubating an infection may expose many people before diagnosis (94–99). If an influenza outbreak is recognized, it is prudent to verify health care workers' immune status and offer catch-up vaccination or amantadine prophylaxis if appropriate (see Tables 5-1, 5-2) (13,98–102,159). Patients should be treated with droplet precautions for the duration of the illness. During an outbreak, health care workers may need to be excluded from high-risk areas until they are no longer shedding virus.

Respiratory syncytial virus is a common cause of acute respiratory illness among patients of all ages. It can cause devastating outbreaks among populations at high risk (13,159–162). Respiratory syncytial virus is transmitted primarily through direct contact with infectious virus in respiratory secretions and can be minimized with adherence to contact precautions until the patient is no longer shedding virus (161–163). During an outbreak, infected or colonized health care workers may need to be excluded from the care of patients at high risk until symptoms have resolved or virus shedding has stopped (see Table 5-2) (13,159,162).

Other Exposures

In rare instances health care workers may be exposed to patients with diphtheria, polio, or rabies. Appropriate management is crucial to limit transmission and should be handled in conjunction with the infection control department and local public health departments (see Tables 5-1, 5-2) (6,13,14,32,51,111).

SUMMARY AND CONCLUSIONS

Health care workers are at risk for acquiring a large number of infectious diseases in the workplace. Establishment of an occupational health service to deal with the issues described in this chapter may seem like a daunting task. Despite the increasing complexities of medicine with its emerging infectious diseases and technologic advances, the basic tenets of infection control remain quite straightforward—educate, vaccinate, isolate. As medicine enters the next millennium, it is prudent to recall the lesson taught by Dr. Semmelweis: Wash your hands.

REFERENCES

1. Classics in infectious diseases. Childbed fever by Ignaz Philipp Semmelweis. *Rev Infect Dis* 1981;3:808–811.
2. Scheckler WE, Brimhall D, Buck AS, et al. Requirements for infrastructure and essential activities of infection control and epidemiology in hospitals: a consensus panel report. *Infect Control Hosp Epidemiol* 1998;19:114–124.
3. Haley RW, Culver DH, White J, et al. The efficacy of infection surveillance and control programs in preventing nosocomial infections in US Hospitals. *Am J Epidemiol* 1985;121:182–205.
4. Haley RW, Tenney JH, Lindsey JO, Garner JS, Bennett JV. How frequent are outbreaks of nosocomial infection in community hospitals? *Infect Control* 1985;6:233–236.
5. Haley RW, Morgan WE, Culver DH, et al. Update from the SENIC project. Hospital infection control: recent progress and opportunities under prospective payment. *Am J Infect Control* 1985;13:97–108.
6. Garner JS. Hospital Infection Control Practices Advisory Committee. Guideline for isolation precautions in hospitals. *Infect Control Hosp Epidemiol* 1996;17:53–80.
7. Preventing the spread of vancomycin resistance—a report from the Hospital Infection Control Practices Advisory Committee prepared by the Subcommittee on Prevention and Control of Antimicrobial-Resistant Microorganisms in Hospitals; comment period and public meeting. Notice. *Federal Register* 1994;59: 25758–25763.
8. Joint Commission of Accreditation of Health Care Organizations. *1997 Comprehensive Accreditation Manual for Hospitals.* Oakbrook Terrace, IL: Joint Commission of Accreditation of Health Care Organizations; 1997.
9. Department of Labor. Occupational Safety and Health Administration. Occupational exposure to bloodborne pathogens. 29 CFR Part 1910.1030. *Federal Register* 1991 Dec 6:56:64004–64182.
10. CDC. Implementation of provisions of the Ryan White Comprehensive AIDS Resources Emergency Act regarding emergency response employees. *Federal Register* 1994;59:13418–13428.
11. CDC. Guidelines for preventing the transmission of mycobacterium tuberculosis in health care facilities. *MMWR Morb Mortal Wkly Rep* 1994;43(RR-13): 1–132.
12. Rutala WA, 1994, 1995, and 1996 APIC Guidelines Committee. APIC guideline for selection and use of disinfectants. *Am J Infect Control* 1996;24:313–342.
13. Draft guideline for infection control in health care personnel, 1997: Notice. *Federal Register* 1997 Sept 8:62: 47276–47327.
14. Centers for Disease Control and Prevention. Immunization of health-care workers: recommendations of the Advisory Committee on Immunization Practices (ACIP) and the Hospital Infection Control Practices Advisory Committee (HICPAC). *MMWR Morb Mortal Wkly Rep* 1997;46(RR-18):1–44.
15. Centers for Disease Control and Prevention. Update: vaccine side effects, adverse reactions, contraindications, and precautions–recommendations of the Advisory Committee on Immunization Practices (ACIP). *MMWR Morb Mortal Wkly Rep* 1996;45(RR-12):1–35.
16. Centers for Disease Control and Prevention. Recommendations of the Advisory Committee on Immunization Practices (ACIP): use of the vaccines and immune globulins for persons with altered immunocompetence. *MMWR Morb Mortal Wkly Rep* 1993;43(RR-4):1–18.
17. Centers for Disease Control and Prevention. Update on adult immunization: recommendations of the Immunization Practices Advisory Committee (ACIP). *MMWR Morb Mortal Wkly Rep* 1991;40(RR-12):1–94.
18. Sherertz RJ, Marosok RD, Streed SA. Infection control aspects of hospital employee health. In: Wenzel RP, ed. *Prevention and control of nosocomial infections*, 2nd ed. Baltimore: Williams & Wilkins, 1993:295–332.
19. Ehrenberg RL, Frumkin H. Design and implementation of occupational health and safety programs. In: Fleming DO, Richardson JH, Tulis JJ, Vesley D, eds. *Laboratory safety: principles and practices*, 2nd ed. Washington, DC: ASM, 1995:279–288.
20. Sepkowitz KA. Occupationally acquired infections in health care workers: part I. *Ann Intern Med* 1996;125: 826–834.
21. Sepkowitz KA. Occupationally acquired infections in health care workers: part II. *Ann Intern Med* 1996;125: 917–928.
22. Doebbeling BN. Protecting the health care worker from infection and injury. In: Wenzel RP, ed. *Prevention and control of nosocomial infections*, 3rd ed. Baltimore: Williams & Wilkins, 1997:397–435.
23. Schmid MM, Miller ED. Managing exposures to infections. In: Wenzel RP, ed. *Prevention and control of nosocomial infections*, 3rd ed. Baltimore: Williams & Wilkins, 1997:437–460.
24. Diekema DJ, Doebbeling BN. Employee health and infection control. *Infect Control Hosp Epidemiol* 1995; 16:292–301.
25. Polder JA, Tablan OC, Williams WW. Personnel health services. In: Bennett JV, Brachman PS, eds. *Hospital infections*, 3rd ed. Boston: Little, Brown, and Co., 1992:31–61.
26. Department of Labor. Occupational Safety and Health Administration. Occupational exposure to tuberculosis. 29 CFR Part 1910. *Federal Register* 1997 Oct 17: 62:54160–54308.
27. American Thoracic Society/Centers for Disease Control and Prevention. Diagnostic standards and classification of tuberculosis. *Am Rev Respir Dis* 1990;142: 725–735.
28. Centers for Disease Control and Prevention. The role of BCG vaccine in the prevention and control of tuberculosis in the United States: a joint statement by the Advisory Council for the Elimination of Tuberculosis

and the Advisory Committee on Immunization Practices (ACIP). *MMWR Morb Mortal Wkly Rep* 1996; 45(RR-4):1–18.
29. Centers for Disease Control and Prevention. Measles prevention: recommendations of the Immunization Practices Advisory Committee (ACIP). *MMWR Morb Mortal Wkly Rep* 1989;38(S-9):1–18.
30. Centers for Disease Control and Prevention. Mumps prevention: recommendations of the Immunization Practices Advisory Committee (ACIP). *MMWR Morb Mortal Wkly Rep* 1989;38:388–392,397–400.
31. Centers for Disease Control and Prevention. Rubella prevention: recommendations of the Immunization Practices Advisory Committee (ACIP). *MMWR Morb Mortal Wkly Rep* 1990;39(RR-15):1–13.
32. Centers for Disease Control and Prevention. Diphtheria, tetanus, and pertussis: recommendations for vaccine use and other preventive measures—recommendations of the Immunization Practices Advisory Committee (ACIP). *MMWR Morb Mortal Wkly Rep* 1991;40(RR-10):1–28.
33. Centers for Disease Control and Prevention. Prevention of varicella: recommendations of the Advisory Committee on Immunization Practices (ACIP). *MMWR Morb Mortal Wkly Rep* 1996;45(RR-11):1–36.
34. Update: universal precautions for prevention of transmission of human immunodeficiency virus, hepatitis B virus, and other bloodborne pathogens in health-care settings. *MMWR Morb Mortal Wkly Rep* 1988;37:377–388.
35. Guidelines for prevention of transmission of human immunodeficiency virus and hepatitis B virus to health-care workers and public safety workers. *MMWR Morb Mortal Wkly Rep* 1989;38[Suppl 6]:1–37.
36. Centers for Disease Control and Prevention. Recommendations for preventing transmission of human immunodeficiency virus and hepatitis B virus to patients during exposure-prone invasive procedures. *MMWR Morb Mortal Wkly Rep* 1991;40(RR-8):1–9.
37. Hepatitis B virus: a comprehensive strategy for eliminating transmission in the United States through universal childhood vaccination—recommendations of the Immunization Practices Advisory Committee (ACIP). *MMWR Morb Mortal Wkly Rep* 1991;40(RR 13):1–25.
38. Centers for Disease Control and Prevention. Management of patients with suspected viral hemorrhagic fever. *MMWR Morb Mortal Wkly Rep* 1988;37(35):1–15.
39. Update: management of patients with suspected viral hemorrhagic fever—United States. *MMWR Morb Mortal Wkly Rep* 1995;44:475–479.
40. Plague. In: Peter G, ed. *1997 Red Book: report of the committee on infectious diseases*, 24th ed. Elk Grove Village, IL: American Academy of Pediatrics, 1997: 408–410.
41. Centers for Disease Control and Prevention. Prevention of plague: recommendations of the Advisory Committee on Immunization Practices (ACIP). *MMWR Morb Mortal Wkly Rep* 1996;45(RR-14): 1–15.
42. Richmond JY, McKinney RW, eds. *Biosafety in microbiological and biomedical laboratories*, 3rd ed. Washington, DC: US Government Printing Office, 1993.
43. National Committee for Clinical Laboratory Standards. Protection of laboratory workers from infectious disease transmitted by blood, body fluids, and tissue: tentative guideline. NCCLS Document M29-T2.Villanova, Pennsylvania, 1991;11(14):1–214.
44. Centers for Disease Control and Prevention. Vaccinia (smallpox) vaccine: recommendations of the Immunization Practices Advisory Committee (ACIP). *MMWR Morb Mortal Wkly Rep* 1991;40(RR-14):1–10.
45. Gilchrist MJR. Biosafety precautions for airborne pathogens. In: Fleming DO, Richardson JH, Tulis JJ, Vesley D, eds. *Laboratory safety: principles and practices*, 2nd ed. Washington, DC: ASM, 1995:67–76.
46. Kaufmann AF, Boyce JM. Transmission of bacterial and rickettsial zoonoses in the laboratory. In: Fleming DO, Richardson JH, Tulis JJ, Vesley D, eds. *Laboratory safety: principles and practices*, 2nd ed. Washington, DC: ASM, 1995:93–104.
47. Winkler WG, Blenden DC. Transmission and control of viral zoonoses in the laboratory. In: Fleming DO, Richardson JH, Tulis JJ, Vesley D, eds. *Laboratory safety: principles and practices*, 2nd ed. Washington, DC: ASM, 1995:105–117.
48. Holmes GP, Hilliard JK, Klontz KC, et al. B virus (herpesvirus simiae) infection in humans: epidemiologic investigation of a cluster. *Ann Intern Med* 1990; 112:833–839.
49. Guidelines for prevention of herpesvirus simiae (B virus) infection in monkey handlers. *MMWR Morb Mortal Wkly Rep* 1987;36:680–682,687–689.
50. Artenstein AW, Hicks CB, Goodwin BS, Hilliard JK. Human infection with B virus following a needlestick injury. *Rev Infect Dis* 1991;13:288–291.
51. Rabies prevention—United States, 1991: recommendations of the Immunization Practices Advisory Committee (ACIP). *MMWR Morb Mortal Wkly Rep* 1991; 40(RR-3):1–19.
52. Record keeping guidelines for occupational injuries and illnesses: the Occupational Safety and Health Act of 1970 and 29 CFR 1904. OMB publication no 120-0029. Washington, DC: US Government Printing Office, 1986;
53. Burke RA, Garvin GM, Sulis CA. Infection control and risk reduction for health care workers. In: Libman H, Witzburg RA, eds. *HIV infection: a primary care manual*. Boston: Little, Brown, and Co., 1996;561–577.
54. Sulis C. Infectious disease in pregnancy. In: Carr PL, Freund KM, Somani S, eds. *The medical care of women*. Philadelphia: WB Saunders, 1995;405–422.
55. Centers for Disease Control and Prevention. Recommended infection-control practices for dentistry. *MMWR Morb Mortal Wkly Rep* 1986;35:237–242.
56. Centers for Disease Control and Prevention. Recommended infection-control practices for dentistry, 1993. *MMWR Morb Mortal Wkly Rep* 1993;42(RR-8):1–12.
57. Gibas A, Blewett DR, Schoenfeld DA, Dienstag JL. Prevalence and incidence of viral hepatitis in health workers in the prehepatitis B vaccination era. *Am J Epidemiol* 1992;136:603–610.
58. Istre GR, KcKee PA, West GR, et al. Measles spread in medical settings: an important focus of disease transmission? *Pediatrics* 1987;79:356–358.
59. Watkins NM, Smith RP, St. Germain DL, MacKay DN. Measles (rubeola) infection in a hospital setting. *Am J Infect Control* 1987;15:201–206.
60. Atkinson WL, Markowitz LE, Adams NC, Seastrom GR. Transmission of measles in medical settings—United States, 1985–1989. *Am J Med* 1991;91[Suppl 3B]:320S–324S.
61. Sienko DG, Friedman C, McGee HB, et al. A measles outbreak at university medical settings involving

health care providers. *Am J Public Health* 1987;77: 1222–1224.
62. Poland GA, Nichol KL. Medical students as sources of rubella and measles outbreaks. *Arch Intern Med* 1990; 150:44–46.
63. Centers for Disease Control and Prevention. Mumps outbreaks on university campuses—Illinois, Wisconsin, South Dakota. *MMWR Morb Mortal Wkly Rep* 1987;36:496–498,503–505.
64. van Loon FPL, Holmes SJ, Sirotkin BI, et al. Mumps surveillance—United States, 1988–1993. *MMWR Morb Mortal Wkly Rep* 1995;44(SS-3):1–14.
65. Wharton M, Cochi SL, Hutcheson RH, Schaffner W. Mumps transmission in hospitals. *Arch Intern Med* 1990;150:47–49.
66. Hersh BS, Fine PE, Kent WK, et al. Mumps outbreak in a highly vaccinated population. *J Pediatr* 1991;119: 87–93.
67. Briss PA, Fehrs LJ, Parker RA, et al. Sustained transmission of mumps in a highly vaccinated population: assessment of primary vaccine failure and waning vaccine-induced immunity. *J Infect Dis* 1994;169:77–82.
68. Fischer PR, Brunetti C, Welch V, Christenson JC. Nosocomial mumps: report of an outbreak and its control. *Am J Infect Control* 1996;24:13–18.
69. Fliegel PE, Weinstein WM. Rubella outbreak in a prenatal clinic: management and prevention. *Am J Infect Control* 1982;10:29–33.
70. Greaves WL, Orenstein WA, Stetler HC, et al. Prevention of rubella transmission in medical facilities. *JAMA* 1982;248:861–864.
71. Braunstein H, Thomas S, Ito R. Immunity to measles in a large population of varying age: significance with respect to vaccination. *Am J Dis Child* 1990;144: 296–298.
72. Sellick JA, Longbine D, Schifeling R, Mylotte JM. Screening hospital employees for measles immunity is more cost effective than blind immunization. *Ann Intern Med* 1992;116:982–984.
73. Subbarao EK, Amin S, Kumar ML. Prevaccination serologic screening for measles in health care workers. *J Infect Dis* 1991;163:876–878.
74. Stover BH, Adams G, Kuebler CA, Cost KM, Rabalais GP. Measles-mumps-rubella immunization of susceptible hospital employees during a community measles outbreak: cost-effectiveness and protective efficacy. *Infect Control Hosp Epidemiol* 1994;15:18–21.
75. American Academy of Pediatrics. Active and passive immunization. In: Peter G, ed. *1997 Red Book: report of the committee on infectious diseases*, 24th ed. Elk Grove Village, IL: American Academy of Pediatrics, 1997:1–71.
76. Leclair JM, Zaia JA, Levine MJ, Congdon RG, Goldmann DA. Airborne transmission of chickenpox in a hospital. *N Engl J Med* 1980;302:450–453.
77. Gustafson TL, Lavely GB, Brawner ER, Hutcheson RH, Wright PF, Schaffner W. An outbreak of airborne nosocomial varicella. *Pediatrics* 1982;70:550–556.
78. Gustafson TL, Shehab Z, Brunell PA. Outbreak of varicella in a newborn intensive care nursery. *Am J Dis Child* 1984;138:548–550.
79. Weber DJ, Rutala WA, Parham C. Impact and costs of varicella prevention in a university hospital. *Am J Public Health* 1988;78:19–23.
80. Josephson A, Gombert ME. Airborne transmission of nosocomial varicella from localized zoster. *J Infect Dis* 1988;158:238–241.
81. Sawyer MH, Chamberlin CJ, Wu YN, Aintablian N, Wallace MR. Detection of varicella-zoster virus DNA in air samples from hospital rooms. *J Infect Dis* 1994; 169:91–94.
82. McKinney WP, Horowitz MM, Battiola RJ. Susceptibility of hospital-based health care personnel to varicella-zoster virus infections. *Am J Infect Control* 1989; 17:26–30.
83. Gershon AA, Steinberg SP, LaRussa P, et al. Immunization of healthy adults with live attenuated varicella vaccine. *J Infect Dis* 1988;158:132–137.
84. Hardy IR, Gershon AA. Prospects for use of a varicella vaccine in adults. *Infect Dis Clin North Am* 1990;4: 159–173.
85. Takahashi M, Baba K, Horiuchi K, Kamiya H, Asano Y. A live varicella vaccine. *Adv Exp Med Biol* 1990; 278:49–58.
86. Tsolia M, Gershon AA, Steinberg SP, Gelb L. Live attenuated varicella vaccine: evidence that the virus is attenuated and the importance of skin lesions in transmission of varicella-zoster virus. *J Pediatr* 1990;116: 184–189.
87. White CJ, Kuter BJ, Hildebrand CS, et al. Varicella vaccine (Varivax) in healthy children and adolescents: results from clinical trials, 1987 to 1989. *Pediatrics* 1991; 87:604–610.
88. Gershon AA. Human immune responses to live attenuated varicella vaccine. *Rev Infect Dis* 1991;13[Suppl 11]:S957–S959.
89. White CJ, Kuter BJ, Ngai A, et al. Modified cases of chickenpox after varicella vaccination: correlation of protection with antibody response. *Pediatr Infect Dis J* 1992;11:19–23.
90. Gershon AA, LaRussa P, Hardy I, Steinberg S, Silverstein S. Varicella vaccine: the American experience. *J Infect Dis* 1992;166[Suppl 1]:S63–S68.
91. Watson BM, Piercy SA, Plotkin SA, Starr SE. Modified chickenpox in children immunized with the Oka/Merck varicella vaccine. *Pediatrics* 1993;91:17–22.
92. Bernstein HH, Rothstein EP, Watson BM, et al. Clinical survey of natural varicella compared with breakthrough varicella after immunization with live attenuated Oka/Merck varicella vaccine. *Pediatrics* 1993;92: 833–837.
93. Gershon AA. Varicella vaccine. *Isr J Med Sci* 1994;30: 482–484.
94. Patriarca PA, Weber JA, Parker RA, et al. Risk factors for outbreaks of influenza in nursing homes: a case-control study. *Am J Epidemiol* 1986;124:114–119.
95. Suspected nosocomial influenza cases in an intensive care unit. *MMWR Morb Mortal Wkly Rep* 1988;37: 3–4,9.
96. Gross PA, Rodstein M, LaMontagne JR, et al. Epidemiology of acute respiratory illness during an influenza outbreak in a nursing home: a prospective study. *Arch Intern Med* 1988;148:559–561.
97. Outbreak of influenza A in a nursing home—New York, December, 1991–January, 1992. *MMWR Morb Mortal Wkly Rep* 1992;41:129–131.
98. Pachucki CT, Walsh Pappas SA, Fuller GF, Krause SL, Lentino JR, Schaaf DM. Influenza A among hospital personnel and patients: implications for recognition, prevention, and control. *Arch Intern Med* 1990;149:77–80.
99. Adal KA, Flowers RH, Anglim AM, et al. Prevention of nosocomial influenza. *Infect Control Hosp Epidemiol* 1996;17:641–648.

100. Nichol KL, Lind A, Margolis KL, et al. The effectiveness of vaccination against influenza in healthy, working adults. *N Engl J Med* 1995;333:889–893.
101. Nichol KL, Margolis KL, Lind A, et al. Side effects associated with influenza vaccination in healthy working adults: a randomized, placebo-controlled trial. *Arch Intern Med* 1996;156:1546–1550.
102. Prevention and control of influenza: recommendations of the Advisory Committee on Immunization Practices (ACIP). *MMWR Morb Mortal Wkly Rep* 1997;46(RR-9):1–25.
103. Prevention of hepatitis A through active or passive immunization: recommendations of the Advisory Committee on Immunization Practices (ACIP). *MMWR Morb Mortal Wkly Rep* 1996;45(RR-15):1–30.
104. Control and prevention of meningococcal disease and control and prevention of serogroup C meningococcal disease: evaluation and management of suspected outbreaks-recommendations of the Advisory Committee on Immunization Practices (ACIP). *MMWR Morb Mortal Wkly Rep* 1997;46(RR-5):1–21.
105. Centers for Disease Control and Prevention. Typhoid immunization: recommendations of the Advisory Committee on Immunization Practices (ACIP). *MMWR Morb Mortal Wkly Rep* 1994;43(RR-14):1–7.
106. Goodman RA. Nosocomial hepatitis A. *Ann Intern Med* 1985;103:452–454.
107. Papaevangelou GJ, Roumeliotou-Karayannis AJ, Contoyannis PC. The risk of nosocomial hepatitis A and B virus infections from patients under care without isolation precautions. *J Med Virol* 1981;7:143–148.
108. Christie CD, Glover AM, Willke MJ, Marx ML, Reising SF, Hutchinson NM. Containment of pertussis in the regional pediatric hospital during the greater Cincinnati epidemic of 1993. *Infect Control Hosp Epidemiol* 1995;16:556–563.
109. Edwards KM, Decker MD, Graham BS, Mezzatesta J, Scott J, Hackell J. Adult immunization with acellular pertussis vaccine. *JAMA* 1993;269:53–56.
110. Centers for Disease Control and Prevention. Pertussis vaccination: use of acellular pertussis vaccines among infants and young children-recommendations of the Advisory Committee on Immunization Practices (ACIP). *MMWR Morb Mortal Wkly Rep* 1997;46(RR-7):1–25.
111. Centers for Disease Control and Prevention. Poliomyelitis prevention in the United States: introduction of a sequential vaccination schedule of inactivated poliovirus vaccine followed by oral poliovirus vaccine—recommendations of the Advisory Committee on Immunization Practices (ACIP). *MMWR Morb Mortal Wkly Rep* 1997;46(RR-3):1–25.
112. Prevention of pneumococcal disease: recommendations of the Advisory Committee on Immunization Practices (ACIP). *MMWR Morb Mortal Wkly Rep* 1997;46(RR-8):1–24.
113. Hutton MD, Stead WW, Cauthen GM, Bloch AB, Ewing WM. Nosocomial transmission of tuberculosis associated with a draining abscess. *J Infect Dis* 1990; 161:286–295.
114. Menzies D, Fanning A, Yuan L, Fitzgerald M. Tuberculosis among health care workers. *N Engl J Med* 1995; 332:92–98.
115. Nosocomial transmission of multidrug-resistant tuberculosis among HIV-infected persons—Florida and New York, 1988–1991. *MMWR Morb Mortal Wkly Rep* 1991;40(34):585–591.
116. Edlin BR, Tokars JI, Grieco MH, et al. An outbreak of multidrug-resistant tuberculosis among hospitalized patients with the acquired immunodeficiency syndrome. *N Engl J Med* 1992;326:1514–1521.
117. Beck-Sague CM, Dooley SW, Hutton MD, et al. Hospital outbreak of multidrug-resistant Mycobacterium tuberculosis infections: factors in transmission to staff and HIV-infected patients. JAMA 1992;268:1280–1286.
118. Pearson ML, Jereb JA, Frieden TR, et al. Nosocomial transmission of multidrug-resistant Mycobacterium tuberculosis: a risk to patients and health care workers. *Ann Intern Med* 1992;117:191–196.
119. Outbreak of multidrug-resistant tuberculosis at a hospital—New York City, 1991. *MMWR Morb Mortal Wkly Rep* 1993;42(22):427,433–434.
120. Valway SE, Greifinger RB, Papania M, et al. Multidrug-resistant tuberculosis in the New York State prison system, 1990–1991. *J Infect Dis* 1994;170:151–156.
121. Multidrug-resistant tuberculosis in a hospital—Jersey City, New Jersey, 1990–1992. *MMWR Morb Mortal Wkly Rep* 1994;43(22):417–419.
122. Centers for Disease Control and Prevention. Prevention and control of tuberculosis among homeless persons. Recommendations of the Advisory Council for the Elimination of Tuberculosis. *MMWR Morb Mortal Wkly Rep* 1992;41(RR-5):13–23.
123. Centers for Disease Control and Prevention. Prevention and control of tuberculosis in correctional facilities: recommendations of the Advisory Council for the Elimination of Tuberculosis. *MMWR Morb Mortal Wkly Rep* 1996;45(RR-8):1–27.
124. Stroud LA, Tokars JI, Grieco MH, et al. Evaluation of infection control measures in preventing the nosocomial transmission of multidrug-resistant *Mycobacterium tuberculosis* in a New York City hospital. *Infect Control Hosp Epidemiol* 1995;16:141–147.
125. Bass JB, Farer LS, Hopewell PC, et al. Treatment of tuberculosis and tuberculosis infection in adults and children: American Thoracic Society and The Centers for Disease Control and Prevention. *Am J Respir Crit Care Med* 1994;149:1359–1374.
126. Snider DE, Cauthen GM. Tuberculin skin testing of hospital employees: infection, "boosting," and two step testing. *Am J Infect Control* 1984;12:305–311.
127. O'Connor D, Mason S, Nieves R, et al. On-site unit-based TB skin testing: a new approach to an old problem. *Am J Respir Crit Care Med* 1996;153: A129(abst).
128. Smith PW, Rusnak PG. Draft guideline for infection prevention and control in the long term care facility: Association for Practitioners in Infection Control. *Am J Infect Control* 1990;18:30A–36A,39A–57A.
129. Herwaldt LA, Smith SD, Carter CD. Infection control in the outpatient setting. *Infect Control Hosp Epidemiol* 1998;19:41–74.
130. Garner JS, Favero MS. Centers for Disease Control and Prevention guideline for handwashing and hospital environmental control, 1985. *Infect Control* 1986;7: 231–243.
131. Garner JS, Favero MS. Centers for Disease Control and Prevention guidelines for the prevention and control of nosocomial infections: guideline for handwashing and hospital environmental control, 1985. Supersedes

guideline for hospital environmental control published in 1981. *Am J Infect Control* 1986;14:110–129.
132. Larson EL. APIC guideline for handwashing and hand antisepsis in health care settings. *Am J Infect Control* 1995;23:251–269.
133. Larson E, Kretzer EK. Compliance with handwashing and barrier precautions. *J Hosp Infect* 1995;30[Suppl]: 88–106.
134. Gerberding JL. Risks to health care workers from occupational exposure to hepatitis B virus, human immunodeficiency virus, and cytomegalovirus. *Infect Dis Clin North Am* 1989;3:735–745.
135. Gerberding JL. Incidence and prevalence of human immunodeficiency virus, hepatitis B virus, hepatitis C virus, and cytomegalovirus among health care personnel at risk for blood exposure: final report from a longitudinal study. *J Infect Dis* 1994;170:1410–1417.
136. Cardo DM, Culver DH, Ciesielksi CA, et al. A case-control study of HIV seroconversion in health care workers after percutaneous exposure. *N Engl J Med* 1997;337:1485–1490.
137. US Public Health Service statement on management of occupational exposure to human immunodeficiency virus (HIV), including considerations regarding zidovudine post-exposure use. *MMWR Morb Mortal Wkly Rep* 1990;39(RR-1):1–14.
138. Update: provisional Public Health Service recommendations for chemoprophylaxis after occupational exposure to HIV. *MMWR Morb Mortal Wkly Rep* 1996;45: 468–480.
139. Swotinsky RB, Steger KA, Sullis C, Snyder S, Craven DE. Occupational exposure to HIV: experience at a tertiary care center. *JOEM* 1998;40:1102–1109.
140. Centers for Disease Control and Prevention. Evaluation of safety devices for preventing cutaneous injuries among health-care workers during phlebotomy procedures—Minneapolis-St. Paul, New York City, and San Francisco, 1993–1995. *MMWR Morb Mortal Wkly Rep* 1997;46:21–25.
141. Howard RJ, Fry DE, Davis JM, Wiley TE, Rice CL. Hepatitis C virus infection in health care workers: Surgical Infection Society. *J Am Coll Surg* 1997;184:540–552.
142. Lanphear BP, Linnemann CC, Cannon CG, DeRonde MM, Pendy L, Kerley LM. Hepatitis C virus infection in health care workers: risk of exposure and infection. *Infect Control Hosp Epidemiol* 1994;15:745–750.
143. Recommendations for follow-up of health-care workers after occupational exposure to hepatitis C virus. *MMWR Morb Mortal Wkly Rep* 1997;46:603–606.
144. American Academy of Pediatrics. Cytomegalovirus infection. In: Peter G, ed. *1997 Red Book: report of the committee on infectious diseases*, 24th ed. Elk Grove Village, IL: American Academy of Pediatrics, 1997:187–191.
145. American Academy of Pediatrics. Measles. In: Peter G, ed. *1997 Red Book: report of the committee on infectious diseases*, 24th ed. Elk Grove Village, IL: American Academy of Pediatrics, 1997:344–357.
146. Wharton M, Cochi SL, Hutcheson RH, Schaffner W. Mumps transmission in hospitals. *Arch Intern Med* 1990;150:47–79.
147. American Academy of Pediatrics. Mumps. In: Peter G, ed. *1997 Red Book: report of the committee on infectious diseases*, 24th ed. Elk Grove Village, IL: American Academy of Pediatrics, 1997:366–369.
148. Boyce JM. Methicillin-resistant *Staphylococcus aureus* in hospitals and long-term care facilities: microbiology, epidemiology, and preventive measures. *Infect Control Hosp Epidemiol* 1992;13:725–737.
149. Panlilio AL, Culver DH, Gaynes RP, et al. Methicillin-resistant *Staphylococcus aureus* in U.S. Hospitals, 1975–1991. *Infect Control Hosp Epidemiol* 1992;13: 582–586.
150. Mulligan ME, Murray-Leisure KA, Ribner BS, et al. Methicillin-resistant *Staphylococcus aureus:* a consensus review of the microbiology, pathogenesis, and epidemiology with implications for prevention and management. *Am J Med* 1993;94:313–328.
151. Doebbeling BN, Reagan DR, Pfaller MA, et al. Long-term efficacy of intranasal mupiricin ointment: a prospective cohort study of *Staphylococcus aureus* carriage. *Arch Intern Med* 1994;154:1505–1508.
152. Miller MA, Dascal A, Portnoy J, Mendelson J. Development of mupiricin resistance among methicillin-resistant *Staphylococcus aureus* after widespread use of nasal mupiricin ointment. *Infect Control Hosp Epidemiol* 1996;17:811–813.
153. American Academy of Pediatrics. Parvovirus B19. In: Peter G, ed. *1997 Red Book: report of the committee on infectious diseases*, 24th ed. Elk Grove Village, IL: American Academy of Pediatrics, 1997:383–387.
154. Dowell SF, Torok TJ, Thorp JA, et al. Parvovirus B19 infections in hospital workers: community or hospital acquisition. *J Infect Dis* 1995;172:1076–1079.
155. Ray SM, Erdman DD, Berschling JD, et al. Nosocomial exposure to parvovirus B19: low risk of transmission to health care workers. *Infect Control Hosp Epidemiol* 1997;18:109–114.
156. American Academy of Pediatrics. Pertussis. In: Peter G, ed. *1997 Red Book: report of the committee on infectious diseases*, 24th ed. Elk Grove Village, IL: American Academy of Pediatrics, 1997:394–407.
157. Weber DJ, Rutala WA. Management of health care workers exposed to pertussis. *Infect Control Hosp Epidemiol* 1994;15:411–415.
158. Tablan OC, Anderson LJ, Arden NH, Breiman RF, Butler JC, McNeil MM. Guideline for prevention of nosocomial pneumonia: the Hospital Infection Control Practices Advisory Committee, Centers for Disease Control and Prevention. *Infect Control Hosp Epidemiol* 1994;15:587–627.
159. Centers for Disease Control and Prevention. Guidelines for prevention of nosocomial pneumonia. *MMWR Morb Mortal Wkly Rep* 1997;46(RR-1):1–79.
160. Falsey AR, Cunningham CK, Barker WH, et al. Respiratory syncytial virus and influenza A infections in the hospitalized elderly. *J Infect Dis* 1995;172:389–394.
161. Snydman DR, Greer C, Meissner HC, McIntosh K. Prevention of nosocomial transmission of respiratory syncytial virus in a newborn nursery. *Infect Control Hosp Epidemiol* 1988;9:105–108.
162. American Academy of Pediatrics. Respiratory syncytial virus. In: Peter G, ed. *1997 Red Book: report of the committee on infectious diseases*, 24th ed. Elk Grove Village, IL: American Academy of Pediatrics, 1997:443–447.
163. Leclair JM, Freeman J, Sullivan BF, Crowley CM, Goldmann DA. Prevention of nosocomial respiratory syncytial virus infections through compliance with gown and glove isolation precautions. *N Engl J Med* 1987;317:329–334.

Medical Center Occupational Health and Safety,
edited by Robert J. McCunney.
Lippincott Williams & Wilkins, Philadelphia © 1999.

6

Research Activities Including Pathogens, Recombinant DNA, and Animal Handling

Richard W. Gilpin

Division of Occupational Medicine, Department of Medicine, School of Medicine, Biosafety Division, Department of Health, Safety, and Environment, The Johns Hopkins Institutions, Baltimore, Maryland 21205-2223

Occupational health issues have become increasingly prominent in recent years at medical research centers, and regulators have been turning their attention toward laboratory and clinical research activities. This chapter covers occupational health issues involving laboratory research with pathogens, recombinant DNA, and animals. Institutional responsibility, oversight of research, containment procedures, and equipment associated with these activities are discussed. The information is directed at occupational health professionals who formulate biosafety policies and procedures for research programs at medical centers, government agencies, industry, universities, and other research facilities.

Safety programs in research date back to the 1940s and early programs that concentrated on chemical and physical safety. Anecdotal reports of laboratory fires, explosions, and chemical exposures provided ideas that researchers used to decrease hazards in their environment. Biologic safety experience also dates back to the 1940s, when biologic warfare research became important. Occupational health issues related to biologic safety were studied with animals and human volunteers. Some of this information was published, and a number of individuals learned the rules and passed them on to their students. Much of this information appeared in publications during the 1960s and 1970s from the National Cancer Institute, the Centers for Disease Control and Prevention (CDC), and the National Institutes of Health (NIH). The American Biological Safety Association, among other biologic safety activities, has published historical articles of early biologic containment practices written by A. G. Wedum and introduced by W. E. Barkley in the *Journal of the American Biological Safety Association* (1,2).

During the 1960s, researchers formulated guidelines for laboratory animal research, a substantial component of which involved biosafety practices and procedures. The Guide for the Care and Use of Laboratory Animals (3) is the consensus standard for animal research today. During the 1970s research with recombinant DNA expanded across the research community. To decrease the risk for releasing recombinant organisms into the environment, researchers established guidelines for experiments with recombinant DNA. These guidelines were formalized in the NIH Guidelines for Research Involving Recombinant DNA Molecules (4), currently the worldwide consensus standard. During this period the NIH and CDC began to publish biosafety guidelines for research with pathogenic microorganisms with Biosafety in Microbiological and Biomedical Laboratories (5). Many of the guideline recommendations have been developed over the years from earlier publications and experiences with infectious agents, oncogenic agents, and other biologic materials (6–19).

ADMINISTRATIVE RESPONSIBILITIES

Administrative Officers

It is the responsibility of the institution and those associated with it to adhere to the intent of current guidelines and standards to reduce the hazard of research activities to employees, patients, students, visitors, and the surrounding community. The institution, through its administrative officers, must provide the resources and establish oversight mechanisms to accomplish compliance. The institutional biosafety committee (IBC) and institutional animal care and use committee (IACUC), among others, are responsible for assuring that research is performed safely. General recognition of institutional authority and responsibility properly establishes accountability for safe conduct of research.

According to NIH guidelines, "The institution must determine the necessity for health surveillance of personnel involved in connection with individual projects; and if appropriate, conduct a health surveillance program for such projects" (4). The institution should establish and maintain a health surveillance program for personnel engaged in large-scale research or production activities or in animal research involving viable organisms that require biosafety level 3 (BL3) containment in the laboratory. The publication *Laboratory Safety Monograph* (20) discusses various components of such a program, such as records of agents handled, active investigation of relevant illnesses, and maintenance of serial serum samples for monitoring serologic changes that may result from an employee's work experience. Certain medical conditions or treatments may place a laboratory worker at increased risk when infectious agents are handled. Examples cited in the monograph include gastrointestinal disorders and treatment with steroids, immunosuppressive drugs, or antibiotics. Vulnerable workers should undergo an evaluation to determine whether they should be engaged in research with potentially hazardous organisms during their treatment or illness.

Administrative responsibilities are discussed in the recently promulgated select agents regulations (21):

The transferor's

> responsible facility official means an official authorized to transfer and receive select agents covered by this part [the select agents regulation] on behalf of the transferor's and/or requestor's facility. This person should be either a safety officer, a senior management official of the facility, or both. The responsible facility official should not be an individual who actually transfers or receives an agent at the facility. Prior to transferring any agent covered by this part, the transferor's responsible facility official must verify with the requestor's responsible facility official, and as appropriate, with the registering entity: (i) That the requesting facility retains a valid, current registration; (ii) That the requestor is an employee of the requesting facility; and (iii) That the proposed use of the agent by the requestor is correctly indicated on CDC Form EA-101.

The responsible facility official at many institutions is the biosafety officer, who may have the background and experience to satisfy the requirements of the select agent registration program.

Department Chair, Chief, or Director

Responsibility for the health and safety of employees, visitors, and students rests with each department head. The department heads interpret institutional policies and recommendations and assure compliance with the provisions. Each department head is responsible for approving all research and all protocols for research.

Principal Investigator and Supervisor

Supervisors at every level are responsible for biohazard control. They are responsible for assuring appropriate training of employees on safe practices and correction of errors and defective conditions that could result in personal injury or property damage. Supervisors are situated to develop a positive attitude among employees toward biohazard safety and accident prevention.

Principal investigators and supervisors must develop specific protocols to assure safe practices and procedures for use of biologic agents. They must obtain protocol approval from the institution for their biohazardous research from the department chair and IBC. This includes registration of potentially infectious agents or materials and recombinant DNA projects. The investigators and supervisors also should register all biologic safety cabinets, clean air benches, and other high-efficiency particulate air (HEPA) filtered devices with the biosafety officer or designated institutional official. These devices should be certified at least annually.

Individual Researchers and Technicians

Employees must comply with safety rules, regulations, and procedures for each assigned task. Employees are responsible for reporting all incidents that actually or potentially result in personal injury, illness, or property damage and any action or existing condition that may result in such incidents.

REGISTRATION OF RESEARCH

Research applicants should complete an information checklist that identifies specific procedures and materials that may be hazardous when not handled properly. The checklist includes, among other things, information about research involving pathogens, recombinant DNA, animals, radionuclides, toxic chemicals, and other materials. When one of these items is checked off, there is a requirement that appropriate institutional offices be notified. Many institutions use a checklist concept for all research, not just federally funded programs. Therefore it is prudent practice for a research institution to determine whether facilities and procedures proposed by a researcher are appropriate at that institution. These evaluations must involve individuals and committees that have the expertise to properly review proposed research and maintain records of these reviews. Two of the main committees for oversight of research involving pathogens, recombinant DNA, and animals are the IBC (22) and the IACUC. IACUC functions are covered in the section on animal research.

Composition of an IBC is described in the NIH Guidelines for Research Involving Recombinant DNA Molecules (4):

> The Institutional Biosafety Committee must be comprised of no fewer than five members so selected that they collectively have experience and expertise in recombinant DNA technology and the capacity to assess the safety of recombinant DNA research and to identify any potential risk to public health or the environment. At least two members shall not be affiliated with the institution (apart from their membership on the Institutional Biosafety Committee) and who represent the interest of the surrounding community with respect to health and protection of the environment (e.g., officials of state or local public health or environmental protection agencies, members of other local governmental bodies, or persons active in medical, occupational health, or environmental concerns in the community).
>
> The Institutional Biosafety Committee shall include at least one scientist with expertise in animal containment principles when experiments utilizing Appendix Q, *Physical and Biological Containment for Recombinant DNA Research Involving Animals*, require Institutional Biosafety Committee prior approval. When the institution conducts recombinant DNA research at BL3, BL4, or large scale (greater than 10 liters), a Biological Safety Officer is mandatory and shall be a member of the Institutional Biosafety Committee.

However, many institutions conducting research at lower biosafety levels have a biosafety officer on staff to track the institution's compliance with research guidelines and regulations. The NIH guidelines (4) continue:

> In order to ensure the competence necessary to review and approve recombinant DNA activities, it is recommended that the Institutional Biosafety Committee: (i) include persons with expertise in recombinant DNA technology, biological safety, and physical containment; (ii) include or have available as consultants persons

knowledgeable in institutional commitments and policies, applicable law, standards of professional conduct and practice, community attitudes, and (iii) include at least one member representing the laboratory technical staff.

The NIH Office of Recombinant DNA Affairs (ORDA) requires that each federally funded institution submit a list of IBC members every year. The list should include each member's curriculum vitae and names of the committee chair, outside members, and biosafety officer.

Registration of Research with Pathogenic and Oncogenic Materials

During the mid-1970s, researchers such as Pike (23,24) investigated laboratory accidents and methods to reduce potential hazards associated with the use of biologic agents and materials. In response to Pike's articles, the 1988 CDC Agent Summary Statement for Human Immunodeficiency Virus and Report on Laboratory Acquired Infection with Human Immunodeficiency Virus (25) and other publications (26,27), many institutions established a central registry of biologic agents and materials. The biosafety officer or the IBC should maintain this registry and assign the degree of hazard to registered agents or materials after review of information supplied by the investigator. Agents to be registered include human and animal pathogenic or oncogenic agents. Also included are tissue cultures, tissues, blood, body fluids, and specimens and samples presumed to contain potential or suspect infectious agents and toxins.

The biosafety officer or IBC should maintain a registry of research with recombinant DNA, pathogens, sheep and goats, and nonhuman primates. The IBC also must register research with toxins with a mean lethal dose (LD_{50}) for vertebrates of less than 100 nanograms per kilogram body weight (21). Each principal investigator should furnish information for all biohazardous agents and materials in use in investigative research and all agents maintained in stock culture collections for research or teaching purposes. Each principal investigator should provide revised information for each new biologic agent or material.

The level of competence and physical containment required for work with biologic agents or materials depend on results of an evaluation of the degree of hazard associated with each research protocol. Criteria for establishing biosafety levels are not absolute. The degree of hazard depends not only on the agent but also on the risk of exposure, which may vary depending on the research procedures. Aerosol studies, passage in animals, and infection of animal vectors increase the hazard. Strict adherence to in vitro experiments or the use of attenuated agents decreases the hazard.

The purpose of research registration is to assure adequate review to determine compliance with biohazard safety guidelines and regulations regarding the safe handling, storage, and disposal of hazardous agents. Registration also provides information about possible hazards that may be encountered in the laboratory by emergency responders. Investigators planning a laboratory project or procedure involving biologic agents, oncogenic viruses, certain toxins, recombinant DNA, or potentially infectious blood-borne pathogen materials should register with the biosafety officer or IBC. Potentially infectious blood-borne materials include blood from humans or nonhuman primates, internal body fluids, tissue specimens, semen and vaginal secretions, breast milk, and tissue cultures containing any of the foregoing materials. The principal investigator should also notify the biosafety officer or IBC before concentrating large quantities of antigen, which could be immunogenic, and other potentially hazardous materials. The biosafety officer or IBC should be notified before containment equipment is altered, moved, modified, repaired, or replaced.

Researchers should submit a completed registration form to the biosafety officer or IBC. For new grants in particular it is to the advantage of the investigator to allow enough time to allow inclusion of the IBC's action on the protocol with the grant application. When the biosafety officer or IBC reviews a protocol, the institution's guidelines and policies determine whether further review will involve approval by the IBC. Review of medical microbiology evaluations (28,29) and laboratory manual references (30) can assist in the evaluation of research proposals involving biologic agents or materials. Evaluations of the degree of hazard associated with proposed research projects and development of appropriate containment procedures can also be expedited by consulting current biosafety publications (31–36). The biosafety officer should present projects requiring BL3 and above to the IBC. A report of the committee's action should be sent to administrative and research offices, such as research administration, the IACUC, institutional review board (human subjects committee if applicable), and the employee occupational health office if medical surveillance is needed.

The principal investigator or laboratory director working with moderate- or high-risk biologic agents or materials should prepare a written research protocol and send it to the biosafety officer or IBC. A potentially pathogenic or oncogenic agent or material registration form should accompany the written protocol. The registration form should identify the etiologic or oncogenic agent, its pathogenicity, and its host range. Submissions should include descriptions of the quantities of organisms used for research. The form should include techniques, facilities, and methods to ensure containment and terminal inactivation of the agent or material. The registration should include descriptions of special requirements for handling experimentally infected animals.

Standard Operating Procedure Manual for Biosafety Level 3 and Biosafety Level 4 Laboratories

The principal investigator or laboratory director should submit a standard operating procedure (SOP) manual to the biosafety officer or IBC for review. This has become a consensus standard for research conducted in BL3 and BL4 facilities. The SOP should include a table of contents, a list of personnel permitted to work in the laboratory, a hazardous chemical inventory, a laboratory floor plan, and emergency contact numbers. The SOP should include laboratory operating hours and descriptions of entrance requirements for housekeeping and maintenance personnel. The manual also should outline decontamination and waste disposal procedures. It should list the types, locations, and proposed uses of available personal protective equipment. Signature pages for each researcher to record successful completion of required laboratory-specific training should be part of the manual.

Registration of Research with Hepatitis B Virus and Human Immunodeficiency Virus

Investigators using human blood, tissue, internal body fluids, and other materials containing potential pathogens, such as hepatitis B virus (HBV), hepatitis C virus (HCV), or human immunodeficiency virus (HIV), should register with the biosafety officer or IBC. Registration includes materials such as peripheral blood leukocyte cultures, tissue cultures containing HBV, HCV, HIV, simian immunodeficiency virus (SIV), and all other known or suspected retroviruses or lentiviruses. Experimental animal studies involving these agents should not begin without approval from the biosafety officer or IBC and the IACUC. According to NIH guidelines (4)

> Activities such as the production of research-laboratory scale quantities of HIV or other bloodborne pathogens, manipulating concentrated virus preparations, or conducting procedures that may produce droplets or aerosols are performed in a BL2 facility using the additional practices and containment equipment recommended for BL3. Activities involving large scale volumes or preparations of concentrated HIV are conducted in a BL3 facility, or BL3 Large Scale if appropriate, using BL3 practices and containment equipment.

Standard Precautions for Research Laboratories

The Occupational Safety and Health Administration (OSHA) document Occupational Exposure to Bloodborne Pathogens: Final Rule (37) covers all human blood, tissue, body fluids from inside the body, and any material with visible blood. OSHA-defined universal precautions consider these materials to contain HBV, HIV, and other blood-borne pathogens. OSHA published an enforcement procedure document (38) that provides expanded descriptions of several research-related issues, such as exemption from the standard for certain immortalized human cell lines that have been in use for many years. Careful handling should minimize cutaneous, oral, or parenteral exposure of personnel (39,40).

Postexposure prophylaxis guidelines for serious HIV exposures have changed recently and should be incorporated into the institutional occupational medicine program (41). Researchers have become more aware of HCV contamination of human tissue. Therefore the institutional occupational medicine program should keep up to date on the recommendations for prevention and control of HCV (42). CDC Hospital Infection Control Practices Advisory Committee guidelines (43) recommend that universal precautions be revised to standard precautions:

> Standard Precautions synthesize the major features of Universal (Blood and Body Fluid) Precautions (designed to reduce risk of transmission of bloodborne pathogens) and Body Substance Isolation (designed to reduce the risk of transmission of pathogens from moist body substances). Standard Precautions apply to (1) blood; (2) all body fluids, secretions, and excretions except sweat, regardless of whether or not they contain visible blood; (3) non-intact skin; and, (4) mucous membranes.

Biosafety Level 2 (BL2) standards and special practices, containment equipment, and facilities are appropriate for activities involving clinical specimens, body fluids, and tissues from humans or inoculated laboratory animals.

Sputa may contain *Mycobacterium tuberculosis* organisms. Therefore work involving sputum liquefaction should follow BL3 guidelines, because of possible generation of aerosols (44).

Production of research laboratory-scale amounts of HIV, manipulating concentrated virus preparations, and conducting procedures that may produce aerosols or droplets requires at least a BL2 facility with BL3 practices and procedures. Industrial-scale, large-volume production (volumes of 10 L or more) or high concentrations or manipulations of concentrated HIV requires a BL3 facility and BL3 practices and equipment. Research with animals experimentally inoculated with HIV requires at least BL2 facilities with BL3 practices.

Medical surveillance programs should be in place in all laboratories that test specimens, perform research, or produce reagents involving HIV. Other primary and opportunistic pathogenic agents may be present in the body fluids and tissues of persons infected with HIV. Laboratory workers should follow accepted biosafety practices to assure maximum protection against inadvertent laboratory exposure to agents that may be present in clinical specimens. The laboratory director or designated laboratory supervisor is responsible for carrying out the biosafety program in the laboratory. The laboratory director or designated supervisor and the biosafety officer or IBC should establish the biosafety level for each research area. The laboratory director or designated laboratory supervisor should provide periodic training to the laboratory staff. The principal investigator or laboratory director controls laboratory access and provides entry requirements for the laboratory.

Registration of Research with Sheep, Goats, and Nonhuman Primates

Investigators register research with sheep, goats, and nonhuman primates with the biosafety officer or IBC to ensure that persons who work with the animals undergo appropriate medical surveillance. Registration also ensures that appropriate biologic containment is assigned by the IBC and the IACUC. Registration databases also provide emergency responders information about potential biologic hazards in a particular laboratory or animal facility. The registration should include an experimental protocol with details on how products of conception and excrement are discarded. Information about the room or rooms where the animals are housed and the room or rooms where animal-related biologic samples will be handled is important and should be part of the registration. Maintaining a list of all professional personnel, employees, and students who will come into contact with the animals and animal products allows appropriate medical surveillance of these persons. Medical surveillance in the past often involved employee baseline serum banking. A recent occupational health and safety publication titled *Occupational Health and Safety in the Care and Use of Research Animals* states, "Substantial issues should be considered in advance of instituting a serum-banking program" (45). Biannual tuberculin testing is suggested for employees who work with nonhuman primates.

Registration of Research with Recombinant DNA

Research involving recombinant DNA requires strict adherence to the most current NIH Guidelines for Research Involving Recombinant DNA Molecules (4) and any local, state, or federal regulation promulgated to cover activities with recombinant DNA. Several local councils or boards around the country have authority to approve projects that involve recombinant DNA and potential pathogens. Local public authorities should be contacted to obtain information about local regulations.

A principal investigator who conducts recombinant DNA research should file a recombinant DNA registration form with the biosafety officer or IBC. The biosafety officer or IBC should review all proposals to identify those covered by the NIH guidelines. IBC members who are not molecular biologists may find a general review of genetics and gene transfer procedures will help them familiarize themselves with molecular biology terms used by researchers (46). The IBC should review all nonexempt proposals. At some institutions, the biosafety officer may review and maintain a database for all proposals, including those that are exempt. Principal investigators have the opportunity to make changes to their registration during annual updates of recombinant DNA activities. The biosafety officer or IBC should establish containment conditions for the research and maintain a research database.

Registration of Research with Select Agents

According to the final rule of the CDC (21)

> Prior to transferring or receiving a select agent . . . a facility shall register with a registering entity authorized by the Secretary [Secretary of the Department of Health and Human Services or her or his designee] or be approved by the Secretary as equipped and capable of handling the covered agent at Biosafety Level (BL) 2, 3, or 4, depending on the agent. Registration will include: (i) Sufficient information provided by the responsible facility official indicating that the applicant facility, and its laboratory or laboratories, are equipped and capable of handling the agents at BL 2, 3, or 4, depending upon the agent, and the type of work being performed with the agents; (ii) Inspection of the applicant facility at the discretion of the Secretary or the registering entity in consultation with the Secretary; (iii) Issuance by the registering entity of a registration number unique to each facility; (iv) Collection of a periodic site registration fee by the registering entity or the Secretary.

The biosafety officer would be an appropriate person to represent the facility for the purposes of this statute. Inclusion of the IBC in this process would be appropriate. The IBC should review all select-agent registrations and maintain a database for these registrations.

BIOSAFETY PRACTICES, TRAINING, AND PRECAUTIONS

The physical containment objective for biohazardous materials is to reduce potential injury to laboratory workers and persons outside the laboratory. Physical containment involves use of appropriate laboratory practices and containment equipment and special laboratory design. Primary emphasis involves primary containment provided by laboratory practices and containment equipment. Special laboratory design provides secondary containment to prevent accidental release of organisms or materials outside the laboratory.

Biosafety level standards have four levels of containment outlined by the CDC publication Biosafety in Microbiological and Biomedical Laboratories (5). The NIH Guidelines for Research Involving Recombinant DNA Molecules (4) have an expanded version of biosafety level standards that include research with recombinant DNA involving animals and plants. The biosafety level standards presented in this chapter are based on those presented in the CDC publication (5) but are taken directly from the most current NIH recombinant DNA guidelines (4).

Personnel involved in experiments with biologic agents or recombinant DNA must receive instruction including, but not limited to potential biohazard risks, microbiologic aseptic technique, and techniques for decontamination. There should be strict adherence to good microbiologic practice in all experiments. All research groups must have a written emergency plan that outlines procedures to follow after an accident. Vaccination for research with selected disease agents, such as vaccinia virus, may be appropriate. Workers should report all accidents and illnesses to their occupational health or workers' compensation clinic.

The selection of an appropriate biosafety level for work with a particular agent or animal depends on a number of factors. Factors such as agent pathogenicity, biologic stability, endemicity, transmissibility, and availability of effective vaccines or therapeutic measures are considerations in the assignment of biosafety levels (33). The assignment of risk groups, quite similar to biosafety levels, is a useful exercise in decisions about biosafety levels. With a combination of increasingly stringent primary and secondary containment procedures and facilities, laboratory studies and manipulations can be safely conducted with agents that are correspondingly more hazardous. Assignment of biosafety level should cover the agent of highest virulence encountered during research in a particular laboratory.

Biosafety Containment Levels

Combinations of laboratory practices, containment equipment, and special laboratory design can be made to achieve different levels of physical containment. Four levels of physical containment, BL1 through BL4, are described. Very few BL4 laboratories exist in the United States. Therefore discussion of BL4 containment is not covered in this chapter. It should be emphasized that the descriptions and assignments of biosafety level detailed herein are based on existing approaches to containment of pathogenic organisms. The National Cancer Institute *Biological Safety Manual for Research Involving Oncogenic Viruses* (47) describes three levels for research on oncogenic viruses that roughly correspond to the BL2, BL3, and BL4 levels in the CDC guidelines (5).

Several different combinations of laboratory practices, containment equipment, and special laboratory design may be appropriate for containment of specific research activities. The NIH guidelines (4) allow alternative selections of primary containment equipment within facilities that have been designed to provide BL3 and BL4 levels of physical containment. The selection of alternative methods of primary containment depends, however, on the level of biologic containment provided by the host-vector system used in the experiment. Consideration is given by the NIH director, with the advice of the NIH Recombinant DNA Affairs Committee, to other combinations that achieve an equivalent level of containment.

Biosafety Level I Guidelines

According to the CDC guidelines (5)

> Biosafety Level 1 is suitable for work involving well-characterized agents not known to cause disease in healthy adult humans, and of minimal

potential hazard to laboratory personnel and the environment. The laboratory is not necessarily separated from the general traffic patterns in the building. Work is generally conducted on open bench tops using standard microbiologic practices. Special containment equipment or facility design is not required nor generally used. Laboratory personnel have specific training in the procedures conducted in the laboratory and are supervised by a scientist with general training in microbiology or a related science.

Biosafety Level 2 Guidelines

According to the CDC guidelines (5)

Biosafety Level 2 is similar to Level 1 and is suitable for work involving agents of moderate potential hazard to personnel and the environment. It differs in that (1) laboratory personnel have specific training in handling pathogenic agents and are directed by competent scientists; (2) access to the laboratory is limited when work is being conducted; (3) extreme precautions are taken with contaminated sharp items, and (4) certain procedures in which infectious aerosols or splashes may be created are conducted in biological safety cabinets or other physical containment equipment.

According to the NIH guidelines (4)

Spills and accidents which result in overt or potential exposures to organisms containing recombinant DNA molecules are immediately reported to the Institutional Biosafety Committee, and NIH/ORDA. When appropriate, considering the agent(s) handled, baseline serum samples for laboratory and other at-risk personnel are collected and stored. Additional serum specimens may be collected periodically depending on the agents handled or the function of the facility. A biosafety manual is prepared and adopted. Personnel are advised of special hazards and are required to read and follow instructions on practices and procedures.

Biosafety Level 3 Guidelines

According to the NIH guidelines (4)

Biosafety Level 3 is applicable to clinical, diagnostic, teaching, research, or production facilities in which work is done with indigenous or exotic agents which may cause serious or potentially lethal disease as a result of exposure by the inhalation route. Laboratory personnel have specific training in handling pathogenic and potentially lethal agents, and are supervised by competent scientists who are experienced in working with these agents. All procedures involving the manipulation of infectious materials are conducted within biological safety cabinets or other physical containment devices, or by personnel wearing appropriate personal protective clothing and equipment. The laboratory has special engineering and design features. It is recognized, however, that many existing facilities may not have all the facility safeguards recommended for Biosafety Level 3 (e.g., access zone, sealed penetrations, and directional airflow, etc.). In these circumstances, acceptable safety may be achieved for routine or repetitive operations (e.g., diagnostic procedures involving the propagation of an agent for identification, typing, and susceptibility testing) in Biosafety Level 2 facilities. However, the recommended Standard Microbiological Practices, Special Practices, and Safety Equipment for Biosafety Level 3 must be rigorously followed. The decision to implement this modification of Biosafety Level 3 recommendations should be made only by the laboratory director.

IBCs often play a major role in these decisions. The NIH guidelines (4) continue:

Spills and accidents which result in overt or potential exposures to organisms containing recombinant DNA molecules are immediately reported to the Biological Safety Officer, Institutional Biosafety Committee, and NIH/ORDA. When appropriate, considering the agent(s) handled, baseline serum samples for laboratory and other at-risk personnel are collected and stored. Additional serum specimens may be collected periodically depending on the agents handled or the function of the facility. A biosafety manual is prepared and adopted. Personnel are advised of special hazards and are required to read and follow instructions on practices and procedures.

ANIMAL CARE AND HANDLING

Animal Exposure Surveillance Programs

This section is derived from handbook *The Use of Experimental Animals at Johns Hopkins University* (48). A program should be developed for workers with direct contact with animals or their viable tissues, body fluids, wastes, or living quarters. The program should include identification and registration of persons at risk, medical baseline determinations, education, and postinjury or exposure treatment. All new employees who will work with animals should be enrolled in the program. Enrollment consists of filling out a registration form and submitting it to the IACUC and IBC. All persons currently employed in an institution who qualify for inclusion in the program should register. If an employee's animal exposure changes because of a job change or a change in research protocol, the registration information should be changed.

In addition to the routine preemployment screening examination performed by occupational health professionals, additional procedures should be instituted for persons whose proposed work involves exposure to or handling of laboratory animals or their tissues, body fluids, wastes, or living quarters. At a minimum this should include obtaining and storing a blood serum sample for reference purposes, although this requirement has been modified. The publication titled Occupational Health and Safety in the Care and Use of Research Animals (45) states

> Serum banking is the collection and frozen storage of serum samples drawn from employees who might be at risk for occupationally acquired infection. Typically, the purpose of the program is to give the institution the ability to compare serum obtained after an acute illness or exposure with serum obtained before the illness or exposure began. Although serum-banking has generally been regarded as a standard component of occupational health programs, it should be conducted only when there is a clear reason for obtaining the specimens and there is a plan to analyze the data as part of a risk-assessment strategy. CDC and NIH recommend serum-banking and serologic surveillance when a substantial risk of occupational illness is associated with an agent under study and methods are available to measure immunologic response to the agent. Substantial issues should be considered in advance of instituting a serum-banking program, including chain of custody, confidentiality, identification and handling of samples, retention, potential deterioration of sample quality over time, and cost. The program should include informed consent of employees and allow them to decline to participate. The collection and storage of employee serum should not be performed in the absence of a functioning occupational health and safety program.

The joint committee on health, safety and environment at Johns Hopkins University recently voted to terminate the general serum-banking program. The samples were not part of an ongoing research program, and there were concerns about sample handling and potential deterioration after several freezer breakdowns over the past 24 years.

Descriptive pamphlets should be given to registered workers that provide information regarding potential risks involved in working with animals and what to do in the case of injury or illness associated with animal exposure. If an on-the-job animal-associated injury or illness occurs, the worker should receive an evaluation, assistance, and treatment as necessary. Instructions should clearly indicate where injured or ill persons should go and whom should be contacted

Animal Zoonoses

Zoonotic diseases are those that may be transmitted between animals and humans. A number of zoonotic diseases are potential hazards in animal research. Such diseases are rare among rodents, rabbits, cats, and dogs raised specifically for laboratory research. Although rare, zoonotic diseases are more prevalent among random-source (procured from a variety of sources) cats, dogs, farm animals, such as sheep and goats, and nonhuman primates and among animals obtained from the wild, such as wild rats, prairie dogs, and rabbits.

Humans may become infected with agents that have been purposely introduced into animals for research purposes. All such biohazardous research should be registered with the biosafety officer or IBC, and workers must be instructed in how to handle infected animals. In case of injury or unexplained illness associated with such animal use, workers should be sure that the medical personnel handling their cases are informed of the possibility of infection with the agent that has been put into the animals.

Bites and Scratches

Animals are capable of inflicting bites and scratches. Small animals, such as mice, gerbils, hamsters, rats, guinea pigs, and rabbits, deliver relatively minor wounds. Larger animals such as cats, dogs, and nonhuman primates can cause severe wounds. Bite and scratch wounds can become infected because of the normal bacterial flora of the animal's mouth or toenails or from the bacterial flora of the worker's skin. Wounds may also cause scarring and disfigurement (48). In the research laboratory or animal holding facility the most important preventive measure is to learn the proper methods of handling the species used for the research. Protective garments such as gloves and long-sleeved laboratory coats reduce hand and arm injuries. Leather or chain mail gloves provide additional protection. Appropriate restraining devices, such as squeeze cages, can be purchased to reduce the risk for bites and scratches.

A bite or scratch wound should be washed with plenty of soap and water as soon as possible. A bleeding wound should be covered with sterile gauze, nonsterile gauze, facial tissue, or a paper towel. The occupational health office should be contacted. The animal service office needs to be notified if an individual is bitten by a cat, dog, nonhuman primate, or wild animal so that a clinical veterinarian can examine the animal and institute appropriate follow-up measures.

Allergies

According to the Johns Hopkins manual (48)

> Laboratory animal allergy is estimated to occur in between 10%–30% of people who are exposed to animals as part of their daily work activities. The animals to which people most commonly become allergic are small rodents (mice and rats), guinea pigs and cats. Studies indicate that proteins in excreted urine, and possibly saliva, on bedding and hair are the likely source of allergens. The symptoms of laboratory animal allergy are similar to those caused by other allergens such as grass or tree pollen: sneezing, stuffy nose, itching eyes, wheezing, asthma, and topical reactions such as reddening and itching following contact with an animal. Symptoms usually develop after exposure to animals and their bedding. Procedures such as handling or clipping hair can cause allergens to spread about.

Use of protective devices such as face masks and gloves while handling animals helps prevent the development of allergies to laboratory animals. Workers with signs of job-related animal allergies should contact the occupational health office.

Toxoplasmosis

Toxoplasmosis is a disease caused by the parasite *Toxoplasma gondii*. Although many animals, including humans, can be infected with this organism, the cat is the definitive host because the protozoan parasite can complete its life cycle only in a cat. The potentially infective form (oocyst) of the parasite can be found in the feces of infested cats. However, when initially passed, the oocyst is not capable of infestation. It takes 2 to 5 days after the feces are passed for the oocyst to become capable of infestation. Drying of the feces is detrimental to the parasite, therefore the use of cat litter inhibits the viability of the oocysts (48).

Workers who come into contact with cat feces may be exposed to *Toxoplasma* oocysts. Symptoms of infestation resemble those of influenza or infectious mononucleosis. They include a slight fever, lethargy, and swollen lymph glands. Congenital disease transmission of the infestation from a pregnant mother to her fetus sometimes causes birth defects. The general recommendations to prevent laboratory acquired toxoplasmosis involve washing hands after handling raw meat, feeding indoor cats only dry, canned, or boiled food, scalding litter pans daily or incinerating disposable litter trays daily, and wearing gloves when handling litter pans and contaminated soil. If pregnant, a woman should probably not change cat litter pans.

Rabies

According to the Johns Hopkins manual (48)

Rabies is a viral disease usually transmitted from infected animals to humans through bite wounds. Rarely, infection may occur if a scratch or abrasion is contaminated with saliva from an infected animal without an actual bite occurring. Even less likely is infection by inhalation of virus in a poorly ventilated space in which active rabies infection is present. Contact with bedding, cages or feed and water bowls does not constitute an exposure. Human cases of rabies in the United States are extremely rare. All mammals are capable of being infected with the rabies virus. Wild animals, such as skunks, raccoons, foxes and bats, account for the majority of the cases of animal rabies in this country. Infection in wild rodents (mice, rats, chipmunks) or rabbits is very rare. The most frequent source of infection for humans is through exposure to rabid cats or dogs. Some research animals are raised indoors by commercial suppliers. These animals are not a risk for transmitting rabies because they are never exposed to infected wild animals, and are usually vaccinated against rabies. Other animals, however, are obtained from licensed dealers who receive them from a variety of sources. These are referred to as random source animals—and these have the potential for being infected with rabies. Random source animals, that are "conditioned" or "pre-conditioned," are vaccinated by the dealers; those that are "acute" may not be. The background of these random source animals is unknown, and they may have been exposed to rabid animals prior to purchase. The clinical signs shown by animals infected with rabies are variable but usually have some components of personality change—a friendly animal may appear to have become shy; or it may be restless, excitable, "hyper," or aggressive. Depraved appetite—animal eats strange objects. Change in vocalization, inability to eat or drink, and excessive saliva production—caused by paralysis of the throat and voice box. Incoordination and convulsions. One way in which animal bites are classified is by intent, i.e., "provoked" or "unprovoked." That is, did the animal bite for a good reason, or completely by surprise? In most cases, persons bitten while working with dogs or cats in the research laboratory or animal holding facility would fall into the "provoked" category."

Provocation may occur when a worker tries to handle or restrain an animal or give it an injection. Some animals become aggressive when they see persons dressed in laboratory coats. Although the risk for rabies is low, all biting animals are treated as though they may have rabies.

A bitten worker should follow the standard procedures for bites and scratches. The animal service office should be notified so that the animal may be examined. Many institutions have a rabies prophylactic vaccination program available to anyone who works with potentially infected animals. A human diploid cell line vaccine administered three times in 0.1-mL doses is used. This vaccine usually produces high protective titers. Booster vaccinations are given every 2 years (48). Guidelines are available for postexposure prophylaxis with immune globulin and other management issues (49).

Q Fever

Q fever is a zoonosis caused by the rickettsial bacterium *Coxiella burnettii*. Domestic ungulates such as sheep, cattle, and goats serve as the reservoir of infection for humans and shed the desiccation-resistant organism in urine, feces, milk, and especially in birth products. Among humans, the illness is generally mild. However, Q-fever hepatitis is often seen, and Q-fever endocarditis is an uncommon but frequently fatal complication. Q fever is an occupational hazard among persons who work with these species of animals or animal products and in laboratories working with *Coxiella* organisms. Outbreaks of Q fever have occurred in medical research facilities using sheep as research animals. Skin testing is the method of choice to assess immune status in surveys of personnel at risk. Employees and students who come into direct contact with sheep and goats or products of conception from sheep and goats should be included in a medical surveillance program.

Tuberculosis

Tuberculosis is a chronic disease caused by *Mycobacterium tuberculosis*. The most common form of the disease is pulmonary tuberculosis. Human to human transmission is the common mode of transmission in the United

States. Nonhuman primates (monkeys) are highly susceptible to tuberculosis. The disease is highly infectious in a nonhuman primate colony. The most common source of infection for monkeys is infected humans or other monkeys. Many monkeys used in research are caught in the wild and may become infected from exposure to humans with tuberculosis. According to the Johns Hopkins manual (48)

> All monkeys coming into an institution should be quarantined for a minimum of 42 days to allow for at least three tuberculin tests at two week intervals. After the quarantine period, all monkeys are periodically tuberculin tested, usually at three month intervals. In order to protect the humans who come into contact with non-human primates, and to protect the monkeys who come into contact with humans, each is tuberculin tested on a routine basis. At six month intervals all persons who work with non-human primates should be tuberculin tested. The simplest preventive measure is to wear a face mask and gloves when handling or working with monkeys.

Amebic Dysentery and Bacterial Diarrhea Associated with Nonhuman Primates

Nonhuman primates are potential sources of microorganisms that can cause diarrhea among humans. Many of the monkeys used for research have been obtained from the wild. Wild animals may become infected with microorganisms that cause human disease when they are in proximity to humans. Although most of the organisms also cause illness in the monkeys, some animals may carry these microorganisms without any clinical signs of disease. The most common diarrhea-producing microorganisms among nonhuman primates are *Entamoeba histolytica* (the cause of amebic dysentery), *Shigella* (the cause of bacillary dysentery), and *Campylobacter*. Disease caused by these microorganisms may be severe with diarrhea that contains blood, mucus and pus. Less severe disease occurs with varying degrees of fever, abdominal cramps, and loose stools. The risk for acquisition of these infections is reduced when workers wear protective gloves and face masks whenever they are in contact with nonhuman primates. Other prudent practices involve frequent hand washing and not eating or drinking or applying cosmetics when working with nonhuman primates. Workers who have diarrhea that contains blood, mucus, or pus should seek an occupational health evaluation. The occupational health office should be informed that the infected person works with nonhuman primates so that further investigation may be conducted.

B Virus in Macaque Monkeys

Macaque monkeys are potential carriers of cercopithecine herpesvirus 1, also called B virus. According to the Johns Hopkins manual (48)

> In most institutions, the two macaque species commonly used are rhesus monkeys (*Macaca mulatta*) and cynomolgus monkeys (*Macaca fasicularis*). This virus is not found in non-macaque species of monkeys such as the African green, squirrel, or baboon. Herpesvirus simplex is a human virus that commonly causes oral cold-sores in people. B virus acts the same in the monkey; it sometimes causes a cold-sore lesion but generally causes no obvious physical problem in the monkey. The problem arises when a human becomes infected with the macaque virus.

Although human infection is very rare, the unfortunate consequence of such an infection usually is death or severe and lasting neurologic disease (50). Humans become infected with B virus by receiving a bite or a scratch from an infected monkey who is shedding virus, from contact with fluids or tissues from an infected monkey, or by injury from a cage or similar item that has been contaminated with material from an infected monkey. Monkeys are often tested for the presence of antibody to B virus. However, animals with negative titers are still capable of being infected and shedding virus. The wisest thing to do is to treat all macaques as though they are infected with this virus. The best way to prevent infection with this agent is to use common sense when working with monkeys and to use protective devices. Workers should always wear eye protection, face masks, long-sleeved laboratory coats or other clothing, and rubber gloves when working with monkeys. Unless absolutely necessary, one should never handle an awake macaque. A squeeze cage and a restraint drug such as ketamine should be used (48). If work must be performed with an awake animal, care should be taken near the animal's head or when one is close enough to be grabbed by the monkey.

Workers who receive a bite or scratch wound from a monkey or from a piece of equipment with which the animal or animal tissue has had contact should stop work, return the monkey to its cage, and begin first aid treatment immediately. Each primate housing area and laboratory should be equipped with a monkey injury kit that is specifically designed to provide first aid after a monkey bite or scratch. Exposed workers should report the incident to the occupational health office and the animal services office so that further investigation can be conducted (51).

Animal Research Regulations and Guidelines

Federal Regulations

Scientists and the institutions in which they conduct research or teaching with small animals fall under the Animal Welfare Act (Public Law 89544, 1966, and subsequent amendments including Public Laws 91-579, 94-279, 99-198, and 101-624). The act covers nonhuman primates, dogs, cats, rabbits, guinea pigs, hamsters, gerbils, and aquatic mammals and any other animal used for biomedical research. Mice, rats, and birds are exempted at present, although there are moves to include them in the regulated category. In essence, the act mandates unannounced inspections to ensure compliance with respect to humane care of animals used in research, their housing, and medical care including "the appropriate use of anesthetic, analgesic, or tranquilizing drugs, when such use would be proper in the opinion of the attending veterinarian at the research facility." Annual reports are required, which the animal research office should prepare on behalf of the institution.

Enabling regulations reflecting the 1985 legislation are for the most part congruent with the Public Health Service (PHS) policy outlined later. However, they also mandate annual review of all research by the IACUC and semiannual inspections of facilities by the committee. In addition, procedures that may cause more than momentary or slight pain or distress to an animal requires a written narrative description of the methods and sources (e.g., the Animal Welfare Information Center of the National Agricultural Library) used to determine that alternatives are not available. There must be written assurance that the activities do not unnecessarily duplicate previous experiments. The protocol must also describe the qualifications and training of the personnel involved in the performance of the protocol. These points should be addressed in the instructions that accompany the IACUC protocol forms. Enforcement of federal law is carried out by veterinary inspectors of the U.S. Department of Agriculture, who usually make semiannual, unannounced site visits. Reports filed by these inspectors are available to the public under the Freedom of Information Act.

A revised PHS Policy on Humane Care and Use of Laboratory Animals by Awardee Institutions was promulgated in 1985 and revised in September 1986. The policy requires that each institution receiving PHS funds for research involving animals submit detailed information in an animal welfare assurance statement regarding the institution's program for the care and use of animals. Awardee institutions are required to identify an institutional official who is ultimately responsible for the institution's program for the care and use of animals, and a veterinarian qualified in laboratory animal medicine who will participate in the program. Institutions are also required to designate clear lines of authority and responsibility for those involved in animal care and use in PHS-supported activities. The policy defines the role and responsibilities of IACUCs and enhances the involvement of such committees in all aspects of PHS-supported research at those institutions. The policy requires that IACUCs include an individual unaffiliated with the institution, a veterinarian who has program responsibilities and who has training or experience in laboratory animal science and medicine, a practicing scientist experienced in research involving animals, and a member whose concerns are in nonscientific areas.

The PHS policy requires that the IACUC review and approve sections of applications for PHS funds that relate to the care and use of animals (vertebrate animals section) before PHS funds may be awarded. Institutions that are not accredited by the Association for Assessment and Accreditation of Laboratory Animal Care International are required to conduct a self-assessment of the institution's program based on the Guide for the Care and Use of Laboratory Animals (3). Deficiencies in the institution's program must be identified, and the institution must adhere to an approved plan and schedule for correction of the deficiencies.

Animal Research Associations

Institutions should consider membership in the American Association for Laboratory Animal Science, which among other activities publishes the journal *Laboratory Animal Science*. Institutions also may choose to belong to the National Association for Biomedical Research, the Foundation for Biomedical Research, and the Scientists Center for Animal Welfare. These organizations support the biomedical research community and provide education in the use of animals in research and teaching. Several animal research publications are referenced as sources of information for occupational medicine professionals. These references provide details on subjects such as animal care (52,53), animal diseases (54), animal isolation (55,56), animal models (57–62), and alternatives to animal use in research (63).

Animal Research Involving Recombinant DNA

The NIH recombinant DNA guidelines (4) describe

> containment for animals that have been modified by stable introduction of recombinant DNA, or DNA derived therefrom, into the germ line (transgenic animals) and experiments involving viable recombinant DNA-modified microorganisms and is designed to eliminate the possibility of sexual transmission of the modified genome or transmission of recombinant DNA derived viruses known to be transmitted from animal parent to offspring only by sexual reproduction.

This applies to animal research activities (4)

> when research animals are of a size or have growth requirements that preclude the use of containment for laboratory animals. Some animals may require other types of containment. The animals covered here are those species normally categorized as animals including but not limited to cattle, swine, sheep, goats, horses, and poultry. The Institutional Biosafety Committee shall include at least one scientist with expertise in animal containment principles when experiments require Institutional Biosafety Committee prior approval. The institution shall establish and maintain a health surveillance program for personnel engaged in animal research involving viable recombinant DNA containing microorganisms that require Biosafety Level 3 (BL3) or greater containment in the laboratory. The containment levels required for research involving recombinant DNA associated with or in animals is based on classification of experiments. For the purpose of animal research, four levels of containment are established. These are referred to as BL1-Animals (N), BL2-N, BL3-N, and BL4-N.

BL4-N is not covered in this chapter because few institutions are equipped to perform research at this level of containment. Descriptions in this chapter include standard practices for physical and biologic containment and animal facilities that are of direct relevance to occupational health professionals.

Biosafety Level 2-Animals

According to the NIH guidelines (4)

> Any incident involving spills and accidents that result in environmental release or exposures of animals or laboratory workers to organisms containing recombinant DNA molecules shall be reported immediately to the Animal Facility

Director, Institutional Biosafety Committee, NIH Office of Recombinant DNA Affairs (ORDA), and other appropriate authorities (if applicable). Medical evaluation, surveillance, and treatment shall be provided as appropriate and written records maintained. If necessary, the area shall be appropriately decontaminated. When appropriate and giving consideration to the agent handled, baseline serum samples shall be collected and stored for animal care and other at-risk personnel. Additional serum specimens may be collected periodically depending on the agent handled and the function of the animal facility.

Biosafety Level 3-Animals

According to the NIH guidelines (4)

Documents regarding experimental animal use and disposal shall be maintained in a permanent record book. Any incident involving spills and accidents that result in environmental release or exposure of animals or laboratory workers to organisms containing recombinant DNA shall be reported immediately to the Biological Safety Office, Animal Facility Director, Institutional Biosafety Committee, NIH Office of Recombinant DNA Affairs (ORDA), and other appropriate authorities (if applicable). Medical evaluation, surveillance, and treatment shall be provided as appropriate and written records maintained. If necessary, the area shall be appropriately decontaminated. When appropriate and giving consideration to the agent handled, baseline serum samples shall be collected and stored for animal care and other at-risk personnel. Additional serum specimens may be collected periodically depending on the agent handled or the function of the facility.

BIOHAZARD CONTAINMENT EQUIPMENT

Types of Containment Equipment

Control of microbiologic containment in the laboratory involves proper use of containment equipment. Laboratory containment equipment is either partial barrier or absolute barrier. Partial-barrier equipment depends on negative air pressure and direction of airflow toward the most biohazardous laboratory areas to achieve containment. Absolute barrier equipment provides a separated negative-pressure working environment. Types of containment equipment include the following:

- *Partial barrier*
  - Filter-top animal cage
  - Class I open-face safety cabinet
  - Class II biological safety cabinet
- *Absolute barrier*
  - Class III gas-tight cabinet
  - Class III cage system
  - Germ-free animal chamber
  - Gas-tight centrifuge chamber
  - Gas-tight blender unit

Each of these examples offers specific solutions to biological containment. The equipment used depends on the nature of the experiment and the risk involved to laboratory personnel.

Use of Containment Equipment

A HEPA filtered biological safety cabinet is recommended for all procedures with biohazardous materials that may produce aerosols of potentially infectious or injurious materials. Examples of procedures that generate aerosols are opening test tubes, flasks, and bottles, performing dissections, using pipettes, making dilutions, performing inoculation or autopsy of animals, grinding tissue, suspending cultures, opening lyophile tubes, centrifugation, vortex mixing, and operating ultrasonic disintegrators. Placing a HEPA filtered cabinet around culture-shaking equipment and centrifuges decreases risk for aerosol escape into the laboratory. Use of safety centrifuge cups with o-ring seals reduces the possibility of aerosol escape by keeping fluids inside the cups during centrifugation.

Control of microbiologic containment in the laboratory involves proper selection and use of HEPA filtered containment equipment (64). Control of potentially hazardous materials at the source protects personnel, product, and the environment. The most elementary HEPA filtered cabinet, sometimes incorrectly called a tissue culture hood, can be described as a metal box 4 or 6 feet long and 4 to 6 feet high. Biological safety cabinets are fastened to a stand or special base cabinet. The cabinet has a waist-high work surface about 3 feet deep. The user sits at the open front of the biological safety cabinet, which has an electric blower that pulls laboratory air into the front opening of the cabinet. Some HEPA filtered cabinets require a physical connection to the building exhaust or other ancillary system. Most HEPA filtered cabinets exhaust air back into the laboratory or are thimble connected to the building exhaust system.

The heart of a HEPA filtered biological safety cabinet is the HEPA filter. The HEPA filter removes particulate material, such as dust, fungal spores, bacteria, and viruses from the internal cabinet air. HEPA filtered air flows through an exhaust HEPA filter into the laboratory (worker protection) and through a supply HEPA filter to the work surface (product protection). Biological safety cabinets have HEPA filters made of disposable, pleated filter medium encased in a rigid wood or metal frame. These HEPA filters allow passage of large volumes of air and are designed to trap 99.97% of thermally generated monodisperse dioctylphthalate smoke particles 0.3 μm in diameter. This is the size that HEPA filters capture with the least efficiency. HEPA filters trap particles both larger and smaller than 0.3 μm more efficiently than they do the 0.3 μm particles used to test the efficiency of HEPA filters.

Over the years, HEPA filtered cabinet technology has advanced to more than a simple box on a stand. Manufacturers have produced sophisticated designs with special protective safety features. Some HEPA filtered cabinets protect only personnel, not the work product or environment. Other HEPA filtered cabinets provide personnel and product protection but no protection for the environment. Hence there are many variations to HEPA filtered cabinet designs. Before choosing a cabinet, the principal investigator on advice from the biosafety officer or designated facility official should evaluate the level of safety protection needed for each work application and special needs of the research. Inexperienced workers may mistake a chemical fume hood or clean air bench for a biological safety cabinet. Chemical fume hoods allow work with potentially hazardous chemicals, although work with biohazardous material is possible in a fume hood only when contamination of the work material is not important. Clean air benches provide a clean work area for assembling sterile materials and electronic components but provide no worker protection.

Partial-barrier biological safety cabinets are open to the atmosphere on one side. They depend on constant directional negative airflow to provide containment. When a biological safety cabinet blower motor is off, there is no containment of hazardous material. Absolute barrier biological safety cabinets are enclosed on all sides and physically separate hazardous material from the environment. They provide a negative-air-pressure working environment, and manipulations involve use of arm-length rubber gloves. Introduction or removal of materials through an absolute-barrier biological safety cabinet is managed through special dunk tanks and isolation chambers with gasketed doors. Air entering and leaving an absolute barrier biological safety cabinet is HEPA filtered.

Class I: Open-face Biological Safety Cabinet

A class I biological safety cabinet is a partial-barrier biological safety cabinet with unfiltered, nonrecirculated inward airflow away from the operator and over the work surface. Class I biological safety cabinets provide worker and environmental protection only. Class I biological safety cabinets do not provide product protection. Class I biological safety cabinets are suitable for manipulations at BL1 through BL3 if there is no requirement for experiment (product) protection from laboratory air contamination. To provide environmental protection, Class I biological safety cabinet exhaust air passes through a HEPA filter before being discharged to the laboratory or outside the building.

Class II Biological Safety Cabinet

There are four types of Class II biological safety cabinets with specific performance characteristics. Type A, type B1, type B2, and

Type B3 biological safety cabinets are tested for safety, construction, and containment performance by the National Sanitation Foundation (NSF). Manufacturers of biological safety cabinets send new models of each class II biological safety cabinet to the NSF for testing. If it passes, a cabinet is listed in the *NSF Listings for Biohazard Cabinetry* (65). Class II biological safety cabinets are partial-barrier HEPA filtered cabinets. The type of biological safety cabinet dictates the configuration of the cabinet. The configuration determines what percentage of internal cabinet air is recirculated within the cabinet and what percentage of air exhausts from the cabinet. Air flows into Class II biological safety cabinets through the front work-access opening and away from the operator. This provides personnel protection. Class II biological safety cabinets usually contain supply and exhaust HEPA filters within the cabinet.

Type A biological safety cabinets are partial-containment cabinets. They provide personnel, environmental, and product protection. Type A biological safety cabinets are suitable for work with low- to moderate-risk biologic agents in the absence of volatile toxic chemicals or volatile radionuclides. They usually discharge HEPA filtered air into the laboratory or through a thimble-duct connection to the building exhaust system.

Type B1 biological safety cabinets are partial containment cabinets. They provide personnel, environmental, and product protection. Type B1 biological safety cabinets are suitable for work with low- to moderate-risk biologic agents treated with small quantities of toxic chemicals or trace amounts of radionuclides. Type B1 cabinets are not common because of difficulties associated with certification and maintenance. These cabinets must be hard ducted to the building exhaust system.

Type B2 biological safety cabinets are suitable for work with low- to moderate-risk biologic agents. Toxicology laboratories may use them when high levels of chemical vapors are present. They are useful for work with biologic agents treated with toxic chemicals and radionuclides. They typically have one internal-supply-air HEPA filter. Class II, Type B2 exhaust air is typically HEPA filtered through an ancillary HEPA filter installed upstream in a dedicated building exhaust system. The supply HEPA filter provides particle-free vertical laminar airflow over the work surface, which protects the product from contamination. The exhaust HEPA filter provides particle-free exhaust air. This prevents potentially biohazardous material in the biological safety cabinet from escaping into the environment. Type B2 biological safety cabinets are not common because of the expense associated with a dedicated HEPA filtered building exhaust system, which often is located on the building roof.

Type B3 biological safety cabinets are most commonly recommended for biologic research. They are partial-containment biological safety cabinets. These biological safety cabinets provide personnel, product, and environmental protection. Type B3 biological safety cabinets are thimble connected to the building exhaust system at Johns Hopkins University. Type B3 biological safety cabinets are suitable for work with low- to moderate-risk biologic agents treated with minute quantities of toxic chemicals and trace quantities of radionuclides. Thimble exhaust connections often are recommended over a hard exhaust connection for most biomedical research applications, because biological safety cabinet containment is less affected by airflow problems with building exhaust systems when they are thimble connected. Hard-connected Type B3 biological safety cabinets may lose their airflow containment properties because of inadequate airflow when the building exhaust system is not functioning properly.

Class III biological safety cabinets provide absolute barrier protection. They have HEPA filtered, nonrecirculated air. The air inside the cabinet does not come into contact with the operator or the environment. A physical barrier, such as glass or rubber gloves, separates the operator from biohazardous material within the cabinet. This equipment provides the highest containment reliability. Procedures in Class III biological safety cabinets involve work with high-risk biohazards often requiring BL4 containment.

Clean Air Benches

Clear air benches are not biological safety cabinets. They are not safe for work with chemical, radioactive, or biohazardous materials because they offer no protection to the operator or laboratory environment. Clean air benches look very much like Class I biological safety cabinets in size and shape but provide only product protection, not personnel or environmental protection. The hallmark characteristic of a clean air bench is direction of airflow. Unlike the airflow of Class I, II, or III biological safety cabinets, which is into the front work opening, clean air bench airflow moves in the opposite direction, toward the operator. The clean air bench blower motor pulls in air from the laboratory and forces it through a supply HEPA filter. The HEPA filtered air in horizontal clean air benches moves from the back of the work area and across the product on the work surface. Thus the HEPA filtered clean air provides the product with protection from unwanted particulate materials. Once it contacts the product, air may become contaminated. The contaminated air continues to flow out of the clean air bench and into the operator's face. Thus aerosols generated by a material, product, or process within the clean air bench are carried directly to the operator. Some clean air benches pull in air from the laboratory through the front opening and force it toward the rear of the cabinet, where it enters a HEPA filter. These reverse-flow, horizontal clean air benches are useful for administration of aerosolized drugs, such as pentamidine, to patients with acquired immunodeficiency syndrome in an environment that will not contaminate the room and health care workers during aerosol administration. These reverse-flow clean air benches also are used for sputum induction for patients being evaluated for tuberculosis to ensure that the health care workers in the room are not exposed to a potential aerosol containing tuberculosis bacteria.

Vertical clean air benches also are not biological safety cabinets. They blow HEPA filtered air down to the work surface and then out the front of the front sash into the room. They provide no worker protection. Clean air benches originally were designed to provide a clean air environment for sterile procedures in the pharmaceutical and electronics industries. Clean air benches are not recommended for biology or chemistry laboratories in which cell cultures and viable agents are handled, because unknowing operators may mistake them for biological safety cabinets. Clean air benches have limited applications in quality-control laboratories, aseptic assembly of sterile materials, and specialized microscopic micromanipulation procedures.

Chemical Fume Hoods

The hallmark characteristic of chemical fume hoods is their lack of HEPA filtration. Chemical fume hoods have externally mounted gas, vacuum, air, and sometimes water control knobs. They are built in or integrated with laboratory cabinetry. Chemical fume hoods usually are 5 feet wide; biological safety cabinets are 4 or 6 feet wide. Chemical fume hoods are connected to the building exhaust system with solid ducting. Typical chemical fume hoods do not have their own internal motor or blower system. Chemical fume hoods pull dirty air from the laboratory into the work zone. Dirty air flows over the work zone toward the back of the chemical fume hood, where it enters a plenum connected to the building exhaust system. The exhausted air mixes with other building exhaust air and is discharged to the outside. Sometimes special iodination chemical fume hoods are exhausted through rooftop charcoal filters and HEPA filters. The charcoal filters trap radioactive iodine vapors and the HEPA filters remove carbon particles escaping from the carbon filter before the air is discharged to the outside.

Operation of Biological Safety Cabinets

The principal investigator or laboratory director, with advice from the biosafety officer or IBC, is responsible for assuring proper personnel safety and use of HEPA filtered cabinets in the laboratory. At times there may be requirements for special cabinets to protect workers from airborne transmission of biohazardous agents or materials. Before use, biological safety cabinets must be performance tested (certified) by qualified personnel. The certification standard used by most institutions is the NSF Standard Number 49 Class II (Laminar Flow) Biohazard Cabinetry (66).

The effectiveness of a biological safety cabinet is a function of directional airflow, inward and downward, through a HEPA filter. Anything that disrupts the airflow pattern reduces cabinet effectiveness. Disruption can occur when workers rapidly move their arms in and out of a biological safety cabinet. People walking across the front of a biological safety cabinet, down drafts from ventilation systems, even drafts from opening and closing laboratory doors may disturb biological safety cabinet airflow patterns. Wearing a gown with knitted cuffs and gloves while working in a biological safety cabinet increases worker safety and helps reduce potential contamination of research materials. Some laboratory safety publications recommend washing hands with alcohol and not gloving while doing tissue culture work. However, alcohol can dry a worker's skin. Epithelial cells, with all associated skin-flora microorganisms, can fall off a researcher's hands and cause contamination inside the biological safety cabinet by being blown into materials on the work surface.

All HEPA filtered cabinets should be performance tested or certified in accordance with manufacturer or NSF 49 specifications (66) at least once a year. Cabinets used in pharmacy operations often require certification twice a year. Clean air benches are certified according to Federal Standard 209E specifications (67). Qualified technicians with appropriate training should conduct these performance tests and certify safe operation of HEPA filtered equipment. HEPA filtered cabinet installations that are part of new construction or renovation projects should have bid specifications that include a statement that after installation each HEPA filtered cabinet must be performance tested to the appropriate performance standard and be certified to the manufacturer's design performance specifications. Performance testing with certification is appropriate before initial use, after moving a biological safety cabinet or clean air bench from one location to another, after replacement of HEPA filters, and after repairs on the internal cabinet.

REFERENCES

1. Wedum AG. The Detrick experience as a guide to the probable efficacy of P4 microbiological containment facilities for studies of microbial recombinant DNA molecules. *J Am Biol Safety Assoc* 1996;1:7–25.
2. Wedum AG. History and epidemiology of laboratory-acquired infections (in relation to the Center Research Program). *J Am Biol Safety Assoc* 1997;2:12–29.
3. *Guide for the care and use of laboratory animals.* Washington, DC: National Academy Press, 1996.
4. Department of Health and Human Services, National Institutes of Health. Guidelines for research involving recombinant DNA molecules; 1998. Available at: http://www.nih.gov/od/orda/.
5. Centers for Disease Control and Prevention, National Institutes of Health. *Biosafety in microbiological and biomedical laboratories*, 3rd ed. HHS publication no (CDC)93-8395, May 1993.
6. Biosafety in the laboratory: prudent practices for handling and disposal of infectious materials. Washington, DC: National Academy Press, 1989.
7. Bodily JL. General administration of the laboratory. In: Bodily HL, Updyke EL, Mason JO, eds. *Diagnostic procedures for bacterial, mycotic, and parasitic infections.* New York: American Public Health Association, 1970;11–28.
8. Chatigny MA. Protection against infection in the microbiological laboratory: devices and procedures. *Adv Appl Microbiol* 1961;3:131–192.
9. US Department of Health, Education, and Welfare, Public Health Service. *Classification of etiologic agents on the basis of hazard*, 4th ed. Atlanta: Centers for Disease Control, Office of Biosafety, 1974.
10. Collins CH. *Laboratory-acquired infections,* 2nd ed. London: Butterworths, 1988.
11. Collins CH, Hartley EG, Pilsworth R. The prevention of laboratory acquired infection. London, United Kingdom. Public Health Laboratory Service, Monograph Series, No. 6, 1974.
12. Darlow HM. Safety in the microbiological laboratory. In: Norris JR, Robbins DW, eds. *Methods in microbiology*. New York: Academic Press, 1969;169–204.
13. Hellman A, Oxman MN, Pollack R, eds. *Biohazards in biological research.* Cold Spring Harbor, NY: Cold Spring Harbor Laboratory, 1973.
14. Laboratory safety at the Centers for Disease Control. DHEW publication no (CDC)75-8118. Washington, DC: US Government Printing Office, September 1974.
15. Miller BM, ed. *Laboratory safety: principles and practices.* Washington, DC: ASM Press, 1986.

16. National Cancer Institute Safety Standards for Research Involving Oncogenic Viruses. DHEW publication no. (NIH)75-790. Washington, DC: US Government Printing Office, October 1974.
17. National Institutes of Health Biohazards Safety Guide. Washington, DC: US Government Printing Office, 1974. Stock no 1740-00383,
18. Runkle RS, Phillips GB, eds. *Microbial contamination control facilities*. New York. Van Nostrand Reinhold, 1969.
19. Steere NV, ed. *Handbook of laboratory safety*, 2nd ed. Cleveland, OH: Chemical Rubber Co., 1971.
20. Office of Research Safety, National Cancer Institute, and the Special Committee of Safety and Health Experts. Laboratory safety monograph: a supplement to the NIH guidelines for recombinant DNA research. Washington, DC: National Institutes of Health, 1979.
21. Centers for Disease Control and Prevention. Additional requirements for facilities transferring or receiving select agents: final rule. 42 CFR Part 72. *Federal Register* 1996 Oct 24:61:55190–55200.
22. Dutton DB, Hochheimer JL. Institutional biosafety committees and public participation: assessing an experiment. *Nature* 1982;297:58–61.
23. Pike RM. Laboratory-associated infections: summary and analysis of 3,921 cases. *Hlth Lab Sci* 1976;13:105–114.
24. Pike RM. Laboratory-associated infections: incidence, fatalities, causes, and prevention. *Ann Rev Microbiol* 1979;33:41–66.
25. 1988 agent summary statement for human immunodeficiency virus and report on laboratory acquired infection with human immunodeficiency virus. *MMWR Morb Mortal Wkly Rep* 1988;37[Suppl].
26. Public Health Service statement on management of occupational exposure to human immunodeficiency virus, including considerations regarding zidovudine postexposure use. *MMWR Morb Mortal Wkly Rep* 1990;39:[RR-1].
27. Occupational Safety and Health Branch, NIH Division of Safety. Working safely with HIV in the research laboratory, biosafety level 2/3. Bethesda, Maryland, June 1988.
28. Benenson AS, ed. *Control of communicable diseases manual*, 16th ed. Washington, DC: American Public Health Association, 1995.
29. Jawetz, E, Melnick JL, Adelberg EA, eds. *Medical microbiology*, 20th ed. Norwalk, CT: Appleton & Lange, 1995.
30. Murray PR, Baron EJ, Pfaller MA, Tenover FC, Yolken RH, eds. *Manual of clinical microbiology*, 6th ed. Washington, DC: ASM Press, 1995.
31. Fleming D, Richardson JH, Tulis JJ, Vesley D. *Laboratory safety principles and practices*, 2nd ed. Washington, DC: ASM Press, 1995.
32. *Laboratory biosafety guidelines*, 2nd ed. Laboratory Centre for Disease Control, Ontario, Canada 1996. no MR21-1/1996-E,
33. *Laboratory biosafety manual*, 2nd ed. Geneva: World Health Organization, 1993.
34. Liberman DF. *Biohazards management handbook*, 2nd ed. New York: Marcel Dekker, 1995.
35. Rayburn SR. *The foundations of laboratory safety*. New York: Springer-Verlag, 1990.
36. Sewell DL. Laboratory-associated infections and biosafety. *Clin Microbiol Rev* 1995;8:389–405.
37. Occupational Safety and Health Administration. Occupational exposure to bloodborne pathogens: final rule. 29 CFR Part 1910.1030. *Federal Register* 1991 Dec 6:56:64175–64182.
38. Enforcement procedures for the occupational exposure to bloodborne pathogens standard, 29 CFR 1910.1030. OSHA Instruction CPL 2-2.44C, March 6, 1992.
39. Guidelines for prevention of transmission of human immunodeficiency virus and hepatitis B virus to health-care and public-safety workers. *MMWR Morb Mortal Wkly Rep* 1989;38:[S-6].
40. Guidelines for protecting the safety and health of health care workers. DHHS publication no (NIOSH)88-119, September 1988.
41. Public Health Service guidelines for the management of health-care worker exposures to HIV and recommendations for postexposure prophylaxis. *MMWR Morb Mortal Wkly Rep* 1998;47:[RR-7].
42. Recommendations for prevention and control of hepatitis C virus (HCV) infection and HCV-related chronic disease. *MMWR Morb Mortal Wkly Rep* 1998;47:[RR-19].
43. Garner JS. Guideline for isolation precautions in hospitals. *Infect Control Hosp Epidemiol* 1996;17:53–80.
44. Richmond JY, Knudsen RC, Good RC. Biosafety in the clinical mycobacteriology laboratory. *Clin Lab Med* 1996;16:527–550.
45. *Occupational health and safety in the care and use of research animals.* Washington, DC: National Academy Press, 1997.
46. Watson JD, Gilman M, Witkowski J, Zoller M. *Recombinant DNA,* 2nd ed. New York: WH Freeman, 1992.
47. Biological safety manual for research involving oncogenic viruses: Part II. Bethesda, MD: Biological Safety Monographs, National Cancer Institute, 1974.
48. The use of experimental animals at Johns Hopkins University. Baltimore, MD: Division of Comparative Medicine, School of Medicine, Johns Hopkins University, 1996.
49. Rabies Prevention–United States, 1991. Recommendations of the Immunization Practices Advisory Committee (ACIP). Morb Mortal Wkly Rep 1991;40:[RR-3].
50. Palevitz BA, Lewis R. Death raises safety issues for primate handlers. *The Scientist* 1998;12:1.
51. Holmes GP, Chapman LE, Stewart JA, et al. Guidelines for the prevention and treatment of B-virus infections in exposed persons. *Clin Infect Dis* 1995;20:421–439.
52. Melby EC, Altman NH, eds. *Handbook of laboratory animal science.* Cleveland: CRC Press, 1974.
53. National Symposium on Imperatives in Research Animal Use: Scientific Needs and Animal Welfare. Washington, DC: HHS publication no (NIH)85-2746, 1984.
54. Benirschke K, Garner FM, Jones TC, eds. *Pathology of laboratory animals*. New York: Springer-Verlag, 1978.
55. Barbeito MS. Recommended biocontainment features for research and diagnostic facilities where animal pathogens are used. *Rev Sci Tech* 1995;873–887.
56. Horsfall FL Jr, Baner JH. Individual isolation of infected animals in a single room. *J Bacteriol* 1940;40:569–580.
57. Altman PL, Katz DD, eds. *Inbred and genetically defined strains of laboratory animals.* Bethesda, MD: Federation of American Societies for Experimental Biology, 1979.
58. Andrews EJ, Ward BC, Altman NN, eds. *Spontaneous animal models of human disease.* New York: Academic Press, 1979.

59. *The biomedical investigator's handbook for researchers using animal models*, 2nd ed. Washington, DC: Foundation for Biomedical Research, 1987.
60. Foster HC, Small JD, Fox JG, eds. *The mouse in biomedical research*. Vols. 1–4. New York: Academic Press, 1982.
61. Gay WI. *Methods of animal experimentation*. Vols. I–VII. New York: Academic Press, 1965–1981.
62. Swindle MM, Adams RJ, eds. Experimental surgery and physiology: induced animal models of human disease. Baltimore: Williams & Wilkins, 1988.
63. Office of Technology Assessment. Alternatives to animal use in research, testing and education. Washington, DC: US Government Printing Office, February, 1986. OTA-BA-273.
64. Richmond JY, McKinney RW, eds. Primary containment for biohazards: selection, installation and use of biological safety cabinets. Washington, DC: US Department of Health and Human Services, Public Health Service, Centers for Disease Control and Prevention, National Institutes of Health, September 1995.
65. National Sanitation Foundation. Biohazard cabinetry, class II cabinet certification, field certifier accreditation. Ann Arbor, MI: National Sanitation Foundation, 1998.
66. National Sanitation Foundation. Standard no 49: class II (laminar flow) biohazard cabinetry. Ann Arbor, MI: National Sanitation Foundation. 1992.
67. Airborne particulate cleanliness classes in cleanrooms and clean zones: federal standard 209E. Mount Prospect, IL: Institute of Environmental Sciences, 1992.

Medical Center Occupational Health and Safety,
edited by Robert J. McCunney.
Lippincott Williams & Wilkins, Philadelphia © 1999.

7
Infectious Waste Disposal

Linda B. Wolfe

Department of Environmental Health and Safety, Whitehead Institute for Biomedical Research, Cambridge, Massachusetts 02142

In recent years, health care facility waste disposal costs have skyrocketed as cradle-to-grave and beyond liability has forced facility managers to question the adequacy of waste procedures and to find funds to improve or extend existing programs. Many types of facilities are involved. Medical centers, clinics, physicians' offices, and associated research centers generate biologically contaminated and sharp-instrument wastes. Nearly all biologically contaminated patient care and biologic research wastes are regulated. Reasons for regulating waste transport, treatment, and disposal include (a) contamination with pathogenic or potentially infectious materials, (b) potential to cause physical injury, (c) requirements to restrict distribution, as for syringes, needles, and discarded pharmaceuticals, and (d) aesthetic concerns.

When observing universal precautions (1) one assumes the presence of infectious agents in human specimens, even in the absence of symptoms. Recombinant DNA regulations (2) require decontamination of all associated biologic wastes to eliminate release into the environment and thus maintain containment. Sharp instruments and sharp laboratory wastes often are included in these rules whether they are contaminated or not. The Medical Waste Tracking Act (MWTA) (3) was driven by the high incidence of sharp-instrument injuries among waste workers and community concern over syringes and other medical paraphernalia in publicly accessible landfills and beaches. In some cases regulated biologic wastes are mixed with hazardous chemicals or radioactive materials, thus creating dual, and in some cases conflicting, regulatory responsibilities.

The goal of this chapter is to provide infectious waste generators with a regulatory perspective and the background needed to develop or evaluate a responsible infectious waste management plan. To accomplish this task, recognition, evaluation, and control of many interactive components are necessary, including (a) defining regulated waste streams and packaging, transporting, labeling, appropriately treating, and disposing of each type of waste, (b) ensuring employee safety (physical, chemical, radiation and infectious agent protection), (c) maintaining written procedures and records and providing facility and engineering controls, (d) containing costs, (e) understanding the legal liability and environmental impact of final disposal, and (f) staying abreast of evolving regulatory and permitting responsibilities.

REGULATORY CONSIDERATIONS

Environmental Protection Agency

The Resource Conservation and Recovery Act (RCRA) (4) of 1976 established the authority of the EPA to regulate hazardous wastes with the following characteristics: infectiousness, flammability, toxicity, corrosivity, and reactivity. The EPA (5) issued a draft manual for infectious waste management in

1978, updated it in 1982, and reissued it in 1986. This manual contains recommendations for treatment and disposal methods for infectious wastes.

The Comprehensive Environmental Response Compensation and Liability Act (CERCLA) (6) of 1980, also known as Superfund, has the potential to designate infectious waste as a remediable waste at hazardous waste sites. CERCLA stipulates that financial liability for remediation remains with the generator of the waste indefinitely and that this liability is retroactive. Even though many states have taken the lead in regulating medical or infectious wastes, there is currently no EPA regulation governing infectious waste treatment and disposal. If the EPA were to designate infectious waste RCRA and CERCLA waste, extensive liabilities would incur for previous disposals of infectious and medical waste in landfills.

Medical Waste Tracking Act

Public concern over the highly publicized washing-up of medical waste on beaches in 1987 and 1988 prompted Congress to pass the MWTA (3) of 1988. It was a 2-year demonstration program to track medical waste disposal and related injuries and illnesses in states where medical waste misappropriation had occurred. Other states or territories were allowed to join the effort, and the Great Lakes states and Pennsylvania opted out of the program. Final participants included New York, New Jersey, Connecticut, Rhode Island, and Puerto Rico. The program included all generators of more than 50 pounds of medical waste per month. It required packaging and manifesting of waste to track its journey to the final disposal location. Information on number of injuries, misappropriations, and infections was collected and assessed by the Agency for Toxic Substances and Disease Registry.

The public health implications of medical waste disposal were compiled in a 1990 report to Congress (7). Among the 16 conclusions was that medical waste had little adverse affect on the general public. Home health care and intravenous drug use contributed more than expected to the problem of medical waste coming into contact with the general public. Janitors, laundry workers, nurses, emergency medical workers, and refuse workers had the highest risk for injury from contaminated or uncontaminated sharps. Municipal refuse workers' risk for infection was expected to increase with the increase in home health care. It was thought, however, that once the Occupational Safety and Health Administration blood-borne pathogen rule went into effect, it would decrease employees' workplace risk for infection.

At the time of the report to Congress only one documented case of waste worker infection had been reported in the medical literature (8). A hospital housekeeper had endocarditis as a result of a stick with a discarded needle. In the 1990 Agency for Toxic Substances and Disease Registry report, statistical projections for probable numbers of infections caused by sharp objects waste handling injuries were 162 to 321 cases out of an annual 300,000 cases of hepatitis B (0.05% to 0.1% of the total number of cases of hepatitis B) and fewer than 1 to 4 cases of human immunodeficiency virus (HIV) infection out of a total of 117,781 cases of HIV infection (less than 0.003% to 0.01% of cases of HIV infection). These calculations were based on the limited data available to the Centers for Disease Control and Prevention (CDC) (9) on injuries and illnesses in 1989 and predate the 1991 OSHA blood-borne pathogen standard, which requires that hepatitis B vaccine be offered free of charge to workers at risk. Additional information is needed to better assess risk to workers.

The report to Congress (7) found environmental ramifications were insufficient to prompt the EPA to reissue or extend the MWTA. At this point states have taken the lead in issuing landfill restrictions and prescribing packaging, labeling, decontamination, transport, final disposal, and documentation. The report recommended that waste categories include cultures and stocks, pathologic wastes, blood and blood products, used sharp instruments, animal waste, selected isolation waste, and unused, discarded sharp instruments.

TABLE 7-1. *Regulated biologic and associated waste*

Material	Specific considerations
Human specimens and pathologic remains, blood, tissue, body fluids	Universal precautions required, considered potentially infectious regardless of source individual or test results
Animal specimens and pathologic remains	Usually regulated as infectious if contaminated with a known infectious agent or animal is recombinant or transgenic
Animal bleeding	Usually regulated as infectious if actually infected with a known infectious agent
Cultures of infectious agents	All biosafety levels included
All recombinant (transgenic) organisms: plant, animal, and microorganism	All biosafety levels included
Syringes with and without needles	Unused and used; restricted distribution, physically hazardous, or contaminated.
Laboratory sharps, glass slides, Pasteur pipettes, plastic pipettes, etc.	Physically hazardous and or contaminated
Surgical knives, needles, staples, cannula, etc.	Physically hazardous and or contaminated

Characterization of Regulated Waste

Infectious waste, medical waste, and biohazard waste are commonly used terms. To design a waste management program, however, it is important to determine how much of the waste stream is regulated. Because the federal government has not extended the MWTA, state and local regulations determine which wastes are regulated. Slight variations in the definition of regulated medical or biologic waste will exert modification pressures on the management system. The term *regulated biologic and associated wastes* is inclusive and allows local variation on what is and is not included. Table 7-1 shows some of the commonly generated regulated biologic and associated wastes and the rationale used for inclusion or exclusion from these regulations.

STATE AND LOCAL REGULATION

State or local regulation is the place to start when determining the restrictions on infectious waste treatment and disposal. The local board of health and or state department of environmental protection and the local municipal waste water treatment authority can provide compliance information. An excellent, annually updated handbook *The Medical Waste Handbook: Federal and State Regulation,* edited by David S. Freeman and Gregory H. Siskind (10), is highly recommended.

REGULATION OF RESEARCH WASTE

The CDC monographs, Biosafety in Microbiological and Biomedical Laboratories (11) and the National Institutes of Health (NIH) Guidelines for Research Involving Recombinant DNA Molecules (2) are the leading documents prescribing microbiologic laboratory waste decontamination and disposal. Although it is not law, the CDC monograph is considered generally acceptable practice. The NIH guidelines draw on the experience of the CDC with unengineered microbiologic systems. The NIH guidelines affect medical centers where recombinant DNA techniques and research or human gene therapy are performed. The NIH guidelines are enforceable at all institutions receiving federal funds. The NIH guidelines often are adopted or referenced by local or state laws to cover institutions using recombinant DNA regardless of funding source.

With respect to waste disposal, the CDC recommends that all cultures, stocks, and other regulated wastes be decontaminated before disposal by means of an approved decontamination method such as autoclaving.

TABLE 7-2. *CDC biosafety levels and NIH risk-group criteria*

CDC Biosafety level (BL)	NIH Risk group (RG) criteria	Examples
BL 1 is suitable for work involving well-characterized agents not known to cause disease in healthy adult humans and of minimal potential hazard to laboratory personnel and environment.	RG1 agents are not associated with disease in healthy adult humans.	*Bacillus subtilis, Escherichia coli* (K12), *Saccharomyces cerevisiae*
BL 2 is suitable for work with agents of moderate potential hazard to personnel and the environment. Medical surveillance may be required.	RG2 agents are associated with human disease that is rarely serious and for which prevent-ive or therapeutic interventions-often are available.	Enteropathogenic, enterotoxic, and enteroinvasive strains of *E. coli,* polio viruses, *Legionella* organisms
BL 3 is applicable to clinical, diagnostic, teaching, research, or production facilities in which work is done with indigenous or exotic agents that may cause serious or potentially lethal disease as a result of exposure by the inhalation route. Medical surveillance required.	RG 3 agents are associated with serious or lethal human disease for which preventive or therapeutic interventions may be available (high individual risk, low community risk).	*Mycobacterium tuberculosis, Yersinia pestis,* Japanese encephalitis virus, Vesicular stomatitis virus, HIV 1 and 2, HTLV 1 and 2, SIV, prions
BL 4 is required for work with dangerous and exotic agents that pose high individual risk for aerosol-transmitted laboratory infections and life-threatening disease. Medical surveillance required.	RG 4 agents are likely to cause serious or lethal human disease for which preventive or therapeutic interventions are not usually available (high individual risk and high community risk).	Lassa fever virus, Ebola virus, Marburg virus, Herpes simiae in production culture or concentrates

HIV, human immunodeficiency virus; HTLV, human T-lymphotrophic virus.
Adapted from refs. 2 and 10.

The NIH guidelines state that all liquid or solid wastes (microbiologic, animal, and plant) that contain recombinant DNA should be decontaminated before disposal. These guidelines apply to all biosafety levels. The higher the containment level, the higher is the risk of exposure to the infectious agent to the general public and the closer the decontamination treatment step should be to the point of the waste generation. Pass-through autoclaves or gas decontamination airlocks are used in high-containment areas to prevent any possible public exposure. Table 7-2 shows CDC biosafety levels and NIH guidelines risk-group criteria and typical agents in each category.

Animals used in research usually are disposed of by means of incineration (12). However, treatment of transgenic or recombinant animals with biologic agents, hazardous chemicals, or radioactive materials creates a mixed waste scenario. Mixed waste requires preplanning to ensure all relevant regulatory and safety issues are addressed.

REGULATION OF MIXED HAZARD WASTE

Treatment and disposal of mixed wastes generated in medical and laboratory operations, either hazardous chemical and infectious or radioactive and infectious, must comply with EPA hazardous chemical disposal requirements (13) or Nuclear Regulatory Commission (14) or state nuclear management boards requirements as appropriate. In mixed waste situations, the method of choice is to first decontaminate the biologic agent and then package, manifest, and ship the chemical residue as chemical waste. Care must be taken in choosing the disinfection method so as not to generate a more toxic or unstable chemical compound. The advice of a chemist or industrial hygienist often is necessary to evaluate chemical decontamination methods for mixed infectious and hazardous chemical wastes. Likewise, radionuclide-contaminated biologic materials should be treated initially with disinfectants or autoclaved in charcoal filtered containers before being stored for radionuclide decay or shipping as radioactive waste to a permitted burial site (see Chapters 11 and 13).

WORKER SAFETY

The MWTA study found that the general public is not likely to be put at risk through the improper disposal of biologic waste. On the other hand, medical staff generating the waste, medical and research center custodians, housekeepers, and other waste handlers are at risk because they routinely handle contaminated sharps. Also at risk are hazardous waste workers and hazardous materials emergency response teams. OSHA requires employers to assess and control infectious and related sharp-objects hazards in the workplace, whether it be a hospital, landfill, or highway.

Occupational Safety and Health Administration

The OSHA bloodborne pathogen standard (1) addresses the transmission of human bloodborne diseases. The standard covers all employees with reasonably anticipated skin, eye, mucous membrane, or parenteral contact with blood or other potentially infectious materials that may result from the performance of their work duties. Employers are required to perform a risk assessment to determine who is at risk and the work activities involved. Compliance with this standard requires documented training, use of personal protective equipment, engineering controls, a written exposure control plan, free hepatitis B vaccine, and medical evaluation in the event of an exposure.

In 1993, the EPA (15) incorporated the OSHA bloodborne pathogen standard to protect hazardous waste operators and hazardous materials teams in three situations, as follows: (a) cleanup of a hazardous waste site containing infectious waste, especially employees with collateral first-aid responder duties [operations covered by 29 CFR 1910.120 (b)-(o)]; (b) operation of an RCRA-permitted incinerator that burns infectious waste [operations covered by 1910.120 (p)]; and (c) response to an infectious waste spill, such as a transportation accident [operations covered by 1910.120 (q)]. When overlap or conflict over requirements occurs in the field a qualified health and safety professional should determine which provision is more appropriate. In most situations, the most protective provision applies.

Other OSHA standards (16) apply depending on the physical hazards to the transport and treatment operations. For example, incinerator operations present a full range of employee health and safety protection issues. Ergonomics, heat exposure, potential exposure to acid gas scrubbing chemicals (strong base), confined space, lockout or tagout, and hearing and respiratory protection are some of the issues that may need consideration in a comprehensive employee protection plan.

Joint Commission on Accreditation of Healthcare Organizations

The 1996 Joint Commission on Accreditation of Healthcare Organizations (JCAHO) Comprehensive Accreditation Manual for Hospitals (17) states that the intent of a waste management plan is to implement a management process that includes all materials and wastes that require special handling and to address identified occupational and environmental hazards. Infectious waste and medical waste fall into the special handling category because there are recognized occupational exposure issues that must be dealt with properly. The JCAHO requires that written waste programs be designed and operated in accordance with applicable law and regulation to safely control hazardous materials and wastes. It specifically provides for selecting, handling, storing, using, and disposing of hazardous materials and wastes from receipt or generation through use to final disposal.

The medical facility must identify, evaluate, and inventory hazardous materials, including regulated medical and infectious wastes and sharp objects. The plan must provide for appropriate, adequate space and equipment for safe handling and storage of hazardous materials and wastes. Reporting and investigating of all spills, exposures and other incidents are required. The plan must address an education program that covers precautions, emergency procedures, health hazards, and reporting procedures. The plan also needs to address how performance will be evaluated at many levels, including staff knowledge and skills, level of participation, monitoring, inspections and corrective action, equipment testing and preventive maintenance, routine procedures with specifics of when and to whom to report emergencies and incidents, and an annual review of the objectives, scope, performance, and effectiveness of the waste management plan. The periodic JCAHO inspection covers a health care facility's waste management plan and involves interviews with staff, review of the management plan, and evaluation of performance criteria.

PRACTICAL WASTE MANAGEMENT CONSIDERATIONS

Waste Survey

In designing, evaluating, or optimizing a waste management plan it is important to determine the resources available. Consider the following points. Does the facility have an incinerator, autoclave facility, hauling, treatment and disposal contracts, locked refrigerated holding rooms, trained personnel, procedures, and files devoted to waste management? In a large, complex organization, a facility-wide waste management survey may be necessary to identify these resources, waste handling needs, costs, and the departments and individuals involved. A survey can help assess whether personnel, users, and waste workers understand how the existing waste management system works or fails to meet the needs of the users. A carefully crafted survey can serve as a vehicle for identifying training needs or changes needed to improve the system. Interviewing personnel critical to the smooth operation of the existing system is a valuable technique. Observation of a waste worker's day, particularly in problem areas, can clarify difficulties and help identify solutions. Compare existing written procedures with inspection findings. Are procedures being followed or have they been unofficially modified? Determine the reason for any changes and document them. Can each waste container generated be tracked through the entire process from cradle-to-grave? Are wastes packaged, labeled, transported, treated, and disposed of appropriately within the current system design, time allotment, and equipment available? Is a waste minimization program in place?

Waste Sources, Composition, and Volumes

It is important to determine the types and volumes of waste generated. What percentage of the waste is paper, plastic, sharp instruments, pathologic specimens, and research animals and bedding? Are logs of waste type and volume being maintained? Where is the bulk of the waste generated? Is there a critical time frame of waste generation that needs to be considered? For example, the emergency department, operating rooms, and research laboratories may need special collections for unpredictable high-volume periods, various projects, weekends, or nights. Is the system flexible enough to meet these needs? If no service elevator or corridor is available, transport of waste through public areas should take place during times of low occupancy.

Segregation into Final Treatment and Disposal Container as Generated

To evaluate the adequacy of collection and storage containers, final disposal must be considered. Is waste discarded into the final disposal container with treatment, transport, and final disposal in mind? Sorting waste exposes workers to unknown and unnecessary risks. Separate containers should be made available for various types of waste. The OSHA bloodborne pathogen standard (1) requires that sharp waste be collected immediately into puncture-resistant, labeled containers. Sharps containers are available and in some cases are provided by treatment and disposal contractors. Some states (18) may require incineration or decontamination and mechanical grinding so that no infectious or physical hazard exists before final disposal of sharps into a disposal facility or landfill. Containers for nonsharp wastes must be leakproof, labeled, and closeable. Autoclavable, biohazard labeled, red or orange bags supported in an easily cleaned, leakproof secondary container, are often used.

State regulations may dictate additional criteria for waste containers. Massachusetts regulation (18) requires that storage containers be leakproof, rodent proof, and fly tight. There must be no discharge or release of waste, and no odor or other nuisance may be created. This regulation requires that bags be 3 mil thick, red, and labeled with the international biohazard symbol. Generator identification and treatment labels are affixed to each waste bag or container before removal from the site of generation. In case of an accident, the waste can be traced to its generator and a determination made as to the nature of the hazard and the appropriate emergency response.

Routing and Transport

Waste should always be secured. Intramural routing and transport of waste should avoid generally accessible public areas. When this is difficult because of facility restraints, transport before or after normal business hours is recommended. Facility collection staff need transport carts that are labeled, covered, and easily cleaned in case of a spill. They also need hazard training, emergency procedures, and easy access to emergency spill control materials.

Storage

A secure biohazard posted holding area is needed for biologic waste storage before treatment or shipping off site. When decomposition odors can develop, it is particularly important that the waste be refrigerated or frozen. Research animal carcasses are frozen in well-labeled, biohazard bags until removed for incineration. Waste placed into the holding area must be logged, so that the first waste in is the first out. Back-up storage must be identified in case of unusual circumstances, such as higher than normal volumes or breakdown along the treatment and disposal chain.

Treatment Options

First treatment is performed to decontaminate the waste. Then to reduce costs associated with final disposal, a volume reduction step is used. Some mechanical systems chemically decontaminate and grind waste in one operation. Incineration also is an especially efficient option because it decontaminates and reduces volume in one step. Solid waste can be decontaminated through autoclave or microwave treatment followed by grinding and landfill disposal in accordance with local laws. For liquid wastes, decontamination and disposal options involve sewer discharge of chemically decontaminated or autoclaved liquids. Municipal wastewater discharge rules apply to liquid wastes.

Treatment can take place on site, off site, or through contract services. On-site treatment offers flexibility and cost containment because operating expenses are controlled by the facility. However, a skilled maintenance staff or reliable repair vendors are needed for validation, preventive maintenance, and troubleshooting. A contingency plan is needed to provide alternatives if a shutdown occurs. On-site options need to accomplish both decontamination and volume reduction to minimize costs.

Off-site treatments and disposal by waste contractors can prove convenient, particularly if many small-volume waste streams with diverse characteristics are involved. If untreated, infectious waste is transported off site for treatment and disposal, US Department of Transportation (19) dictates packaging requirements, container tests, labeling, and truck placarding.

Contract service can prove expensive if volumes are poorly estimated, because contracts often require a minimum payment per period regardless of waste volume collected. Legal review for vendor compliance with federal, state, and local regulation is important before one signs a service contract. The due diligence review should minimally include evaluation of all operations permits, licenses, and compliance programs, including employee training, emergency response, and transport, treatment and disposal facilities.

Training

All persons involved in waste generation, handling, and treatment need training. The waste generators need to know how to safely segregate and package wastes. The transporters, treatment, and disposal workers need to understand standard operating procedures for handling the waste. They need to be aware of the physical, chemical, radioactive, and biologic hazards present and how to protect themselves. Training and signs should be in languages and educational levels understood by the workers.

The OSHA bloodborne pathogen standard (1) requires documented training for all employees with workplace exposure to potentially infectious materials. Training must be provided during the normal workday at the time of initial assignment, at least annually, and whenever procedures or new tasks change exposure risks and controls. A written exposure control plan addressing work activities in which exposure might occur must be in place and available to employees. The exposure control plan details engineering and work practice controls, housekeeping, signs and labels, selection, use and disposal of personal protective equipment, hepatitis B vaccine, emergency spill and injury response plan, and post-exposure follow-up procedures. The exposure control plan and contents of the OSHA standard are reviewed during training, as are symptoms, modes of transmission, and epidemiologic aspects of HIV infection and hepatitis B. Hepatitis B vaccine must be offered after training and within 10 days of initial assignment to covered tasks. The vaccine, personal protective equipment, and postexposure medical evaluation and treatment are made available free of charge to the employee. There are additional requirements for HIV and hepatitis B virus research laboratories and production facilities (see Chapter 3).

Additional OSHA required training (16) for ergonomics and lifting, confined space entry, lockout and tagout procedures, work involving heat stress and noise, and respirator use may be required depending on the technology employed and hazards involved.

Medical Surveillance and Fitness

Medical surveillance for waste handlers varies depending on the operations and technology used. It may include a fitness assessment for physical exertion, heat tolerance, audiometric evaluation, and respirator fitness. Susceptibility to infection, immune suppression, allergies to therapeutic antibiotics should be evaluated and discussed with the patient. The examining physician may recommend additional studies depending on specific risks.

Waste workers sustain many strains, sprains, and back problems. Needle sticks and sharps injuries are common. Anecdotal reports indicate that sharps injuries and resulting infections are most likely underreported by waste handlers. Until recently, there was only one documented waste worker case report in the literature (8). A hospital housekeeper contracted endocarditis as a result of a stick with a discarded needle. In December 1997 the Washington State Department of Health investigated transmission of tuberculosis to waste-processing workers in a Morton, Washington, waste-processing plant that used a grinder-type disposal unit (20). Two cases involving independent strains of tuberculosis were confirmed and were apparently caused by waste processing equipment. A third case was being investigated as a possible worker to worker transmission. Fifteen other workers in the same facility had evidence of exposure.

Hepatitis B is clearly a risk. Hepatitis B virus has a documented survival period (21) in the environment of up to 6 days. Hepatitis

C is also a concern. Medical evaluation and follow-up for exposure incidents should include vaccine status review, immediate postexposure prophylaxis, serum sample to hold or test if consent is given, antibiotic treatment as needed, counseling about the types of symptoms to report and behaviors to avoid, and a follow-up visit to determine whether an adverse medical consequence or illness results from the incident. The environmental instability of many infectious agents, including HIV, accounts at least in part for the discrepancy between injury and infection rates.

Record Keeping

The MWTA required waste tracking from the point of generation to the final disposal site. Many states have adopted similar manifesting requirements for the collection, shipment, treatment, and disposal of regulated biologic and sharps wastes. Even if not required by state agencies, identification of the waste source and the date the container was removed is an advantage to waste handlers and emergency response personnel. This information aids in assessment of the hazard and appropriate response in case of an injury or spill during handling. OSHA bloodborne pathogen training records are maintained for 3 years. OSHA medical records are maintained for the duration of employment plus 30 years in accordance with 29 CFR 1910.20 (15).

TREATMENT TECHNOLOGIES

Steam Autoclaves

Steam autoclaves are versatile. They decontaminate loosely packed waste such as gloves, gowns, laboratory glassware, and sharps containers. They also are used for sterilizing instruments and media. Autoclaves use steam under pressure to sterilize. Steam must penetrate the load. It is the combination of moisture and heat that kills microorganisms. Autoclave pressure must be adequate to drive the steam into the center of the container. Exposure or run time must be adequate for steam penetration and heat transfer to take place given the small opening allowed for bagged infectious or sharp wastes. Practically speaking, the temperature setting is limited by the melting point of the plastic packaging materials.

Autoclaves come in a variety of sizes and have various features. A steam source requires special plumbing. Individual electric steam generators are available for some models. Canopy exhaust hoods are recommended for venting hot waste fumes and odors. Cycle flexibility is a factor. Machines are available with drying cycles for wrapped dry goods, slow exhaust to minimize boilover of liquids, and fast exhaust for high throughput. For solid waste processing the fast exhaust or drying cycles are used. The mode of steam entry into the chamber is an option to consider. Steam pulsing or mixing baffles are recommended to distribute the steam evenly and prevent heat stratification over the cold starting air. Another mixing feature that is offered but is not recommended for wastes is a prevacuum cycle, which has the potential for contaminating the vacuum pump and rupturing containers of waste. High-containment research facilities (BL4 and BL4) should consider treating effluent condensate from the autoclave depending on the agents in use and the likelihood of liquid spills and autoclave failure during the cycle. The autoclave manufacturer should provide racks to allow even spacing of wastes in the chamber. Waste bags should be placed into shallow, heat conductive, leakproof trays to prevent overflow spillage into the chamber exhaust valve on the floor of the autoclave. Many state regulations specify the paperwork required for each run and for periodic validations. For this reason, before purchasing, one should determine the temperature and pressure recording abilities and validation-calibration ports or mechanisms.

To validate that the center of the load is killed, an ampule of *Bacillus stearothermophilus* is inserted into the center of a standard waste load, and the autoclave is run under standard conditions. The temperature is charted. Chamber pressure is recorded at intervals for evaluation in case of failure. After the run, the ampule is removed and incubated according to the manufacturer's directions. The thermal death curve of this heat-loving bacterium has been well studied. For a given concentration of culture, a predictable time at 121°C is required to reduce the viable population by a power of ten. This procedure allows determination of whether the center of the load reached an appropriate temperature for an adequate duration to kill the *B. stearothermophilus* organisms and the presumably less thermostable waste contaminants.

Another type of validation is performed with thermocouples. They are placed at various locations within the empty chamber. Continuous recordings are taken. This is often done in pharmaceutical quality assurance applications or as a diagnostic to identify cold spots in an ailing machine. Specialized equipment is needed. Not all autoclaves have access ports for this procedure.

The biologic indicator is often specified by the agencies overseeing waste validation record keeping. It is considered the acid-test of the waste system. It provides a biologic challenge within the load parameters of density, insulation, steam penetration, time, pressure, and temperature.

Incineration

Incineration is the treatment method of choice for rendering waste unidentifiable and not physically hazardous in addition to eliminating infectiousness. Incineration is appropriate for gross pathologic specimens, research animal carcasses, and sharps. Specially licensed commercial incinerators with multiple high-temperature burn chambers are needed to treat mixed hazardous chemical-contaminated infectious wastes, such as intravenous fluid bags and blood tubes contaminated with chemotherapeutic chemicals, animals used for testing toxic substances, or research mutagenicity experiment mixtures.

Medical pathologic waste incinerators can efficiently accomplish both decontamination and waste volume reduction. Depending on the materials incinerated, ash analysis may be required to identify trace contaminants and determine whether ash is subject to RCRA disposal requirements. Licensing of medical pathologic waste incinerators is increasingly difficult given required emission controls and siting requirements (see later, Proposed Regulations).

Other Technologies

Technologies are available and approved by local authorities for solid waste treatment in some areas of the United States. One method involves a conveyor belt that delivers packaged solid wastes to a decontamination bath, usually hypochlorite, and then grinds and shreds the decontaminated materials. The effluent is either discharged to the sewer or dried and the residue sent to a landfill, if allowed. Equipment of this type is large, often the size of a large truck and requires electricity, water, and a sewer hookup. All biologically contaminated waste, including gross pathologic specimens and sharp objects, can be handled with this equipment. Concerns are response in the event of a cycle failure and aerosolization of high risk agents such as *Mycobacterium tuberculosis* (see earlier, Medical Surveillance and Fitness).

Microwave-operated steam decontamination units are available in a variety of sizes. They can handle a variety of wastes, but treatment of metals and pathologic specimens is limited or not recommended depending on the unit. An advantage is that a small unit in a hospital isolation room can process waste close to the generation source with minimum utility installation requirements.

Plasma fusion is a new technology (22,23) with the potential for treating mixed wastes, infectious, hazardous chemical, and radioactive wastes. The end point is a relatively small disk of vitreous material that does not leach. This technology achieves volume reduction and a stable end product that can be stored for radioactive decay or sent to a hazardous waste landfill. Emissions are gaseous. Monitors and scrubbers are being designed to continuously monitor and minimize release to the air. Electricity is the main utility required. Units are large and require highly trained operators. Controlled pyrolysis plasma generators are available for in-house treatment. The Army Environmental Command in Newington, Virginia, is installing a controlled pyrolysis plasma unit for medical and hazardous waste processing (23).

COST CONTAINMENT

Cost containment is critical. Results from a waste management survey can be helpful in finding ways to economize. Where are the largest volumes generated? Can waste minimization be implemented? Are special wastes generated that are difficult to treat and therefore require special arrangements with outside vendors? Can some treatments be performed in house? Have the costs of potential liabilities been considered?

Choice of Reusable versus Disposable Materials

Disposable materials are a convenient choice. In some cases, however, reusable items can work well and not compromise infection control practices. For example, where a hospital laundry exists, cloth gowns and linens can be used rather than paper. The expense of purchasing and laundering has to be compared with the costs of purchasing, storage, delivery, treatment, and disposal of the paper products. Safe reuse of certain laboratory items is possible. Disposable pipette trays can be reloaded with fresh, bagged, inexpensive pipette tips, wrapped, and sterilized. Reusable glass pipettes can be used in some laboratories. Mechanical glassware and pipette washers have improved cleanliness and turnaround time. Substituting reusable items for disposable when possible reduces waste volume.

Volume and Size Reduction

Microchemistry was touted a few years ago as a great boon to chemical laboratory safety and chemical waste reduction, especially in teaching laboratories. Before purchasing clinical laboratory equipment, evaluate the waste streams generated. The cost of waste management and disposal must be factored in to cost comparisons. This requires working with the facilities and safety departments. This approach can achieve waste volume reduction and decrease disposal expenses for microbiologic research laboratories as well. Companies that develop and sell clinical and research laboratory equipment search for desirable marketing features. Waste stream minimization should be emphasized when talking with manufacturer representatives. Use their expertise in achieving waste stream minimization for present and future models.

Recycling

Commercial recycling of laboratory plastics and glass can create substantial liability because of trace contamination with potentially hazardous materials. Recyclers are unwilling to accept liability for possible contamination in a load of materials, because the current recycling process is not designed to detect or eliminate contamination. Medical center liability may occur even if contamination enters the batch of recycled materials through another facility on the pick-up circuit. Recyclers face a variable market for their product so are reluctant to commit to a particular use for the materials. Highway dividers are preferred over pacifiers and children's plastic toys because highways dividers involve minimal consumer contact and legal exposure. Wise medical center policy should discourage recycling of laboratory ware unless the recycling technology and market allow for definite end uses of the materials and provide for a clear transfer of recycled product liability.

FUTURE ISSUES

New Technology

New waste treatment technologies are constantly under development and are engineered to be in compliance with current EPA release regulations. Plasma fusion treatment for mixed waste appears to be commercially viable, particularly for mixed hazardous wastes, for which disposal options are highly regulated, limited, and therefore expensive. The high price of new technologies will come into line as additional regulatory restrictions are imposed on traditional treatment technologies, and current disposal options are eliminated.

Proposed Regulations

Air emissions control is an important topic to watch as the EPA (24) struggles with regulation of new and existing medical waste incinerators. Maximum achievable [emissions] control technology (MACT), the jargon used in the proposed regulation, will be difficult for existing incinerators to accomplish. MACT changes as technology develops and becomes a moving target. Unless medical and research centers become actively involved in rule making, it is possible that commercial incinerators alone will have the resources to maintain compliance standards. Medical facilities that currently use commercial vendors should ensure that there are protections or review triggers in the contract should regulatory changes affect the appropriateness of the contractor's waste treatment and disposal technology.

SUMMARY

Twenty years ago, medical waste did not rank as a leading concern or expense among medical centers. Medical waste has become a considerable expense. This problem is caused in part by the increasing number of available clinical tests, use of recombinant DNA and other medical research technologies, larger numbers of patients and treatments, extensive use of disposable items, beach wash-ups of medical paraphernalia, and regulations. Medical waste management affects the reputation and sound fiscal operation of medical and research centers. It is essential that the infectious waste management system be periodically reviewed to provide appropriate waste management to control costs and reduce liabilities.

REFERENCES

1. US Department of Labor, Occupational Health and Safety Administration. Occupational exposure to bloodborne pathogens. 29 CFR 1910.1030. 1991.
2. Department of Health and Human Services, National Institutes of Health. Guidelines for research involving recombinant DNA molecules. Bethesda, MD: National Institutes of Health, 1998.
3. Medical Waste Tracking Act. 42 USC 6992 et seq. 1988.
4. Resource Conservation and Recovery Act. 42 USC 690 et seq. 1976.
5. Environmental Protection Agency Guide for Infectious Waste Management. EPA Document No. 530-SW-86-014. Springfield, VA: National Technical Information Service, 1986.
6. Comprehensive Environmental Response, Compensation and Liability Act (CERCLA) 42 USC 9601 et seq. 1980.
7. The public health implications of medical waste: a report to congress. Atlanta: Agency for Toxic Substances and Disease Registry, U.S. Department of Health and Human Services, Public Health Service, September 1990.
8. Jacobson T, Burke JP, Conti MT. Injuries of hospital employees from needles and sharp objects. *Infect Control* 1983;4:100–102.
9. Centers for Disease Control. Guidelines for prevention of transmission of human immunodeficiency virus and hepatitis B virus to health-care and public-safety workers. *MMWR Morb Mortal Wkly Rep* 1989;38[S-6].
10. Freeman D, Siskind G. *Medical waste handbook: federal and state regulation.* New York: Clark, Boardman, and Callaghan, 1996.
11. US Department of Health and Human Services, Public Health Service, Centers for Disease Control/National Institute of Health. *Biosafety in microbiological and biomedical laboratories,* 3rd ed. Atlanta: Centers for Disease Control and Prevention, 1993.
12. National Research Council. Institute of Laboratory Animal Resources Commission on Life Sciences. *Guide for the care and use of laboratory animals.* Washington, DC: National Academy Press, 1996.
13. US Environmental Protection Agency. Resource conservation and recovery act regulations. 40 CFR Chapter 1, 1994.
14. US Nuclear Regulatory Commission. 10 CFR Part 20, 61, 1992.
15. The effect of OSHA's bloodborne pathogen standard on hazardous waste clean-up activities: quick reference sheet. Department of Labor publication no. 9360.0-31/FS. August 1993.
16. US Department of Labor. Occupational Health and Safety Administration regulations. 29 CFR 1910. July 1991.
17. Joint Commission on Accreditation of Healthcare Organizations. *Accreditation manual for hospitals.* Oakbrook Terrace, IL: Joint Commission on Accreditation of Healthcare Organizations, 1996.
18. State of Massachusetts, Department of Public Health, Storage and disposal of infectious or physically dangerous medical microbiological waste: State Sanitary Code, Chapter VIII, 105 CMR 480.000, 1989.
19. Department of Transportation. Research and Special Programs Administration. 49 CFR Parts 171, 172, 173, 178. 1994.

20. Medical Waste News. Silver Spring, MD: Business Publishers, March 1998.
21. Bond WW, Favero NS, Petersen NJ, Gravelle CR, Ebert JW, Maynard JE. Survival of hepatitis B virus after drying and storage for one week. *Lancet* 1981;1:550–551.
22. Cohen D. Plasma Technology for Treatment of Waste. Paper presented at: International Conference on High Power Particle Beams; June 10–14, 1996; Prague, Czech Republic,
23. www.peat.com/project/vri.html. 1998.
24. Environmental Protection Agency. Proposed standards of performance for new stationary sources and emission guidelines for existing sources: medical waste incinerators. 40 CFR Part 60 et seq. 1995.

Medical Center Occupational Health and Safety,
edited by Robert J. McCunney.
Lippincott Williams & Wilkins, Philadelphia © 1999.

8

Health Implications of Exposure to Pharmaceuticals

Alain J. Couturier

St. Joseph Mishawaka Health Services, Corporate Health Services, Mishawaka, Indiana 46545

HISTORICAL PERSPECTIVE

In modern times, our concerns over the dangers of therapeutic agents began to resonate strongly with the advent of alkylating agents, which first came into use after World War II. It became immediately evident that in addition to their antitumor efficacy, these pharmaceutical agents posed a toxic risk to the patient. A logical extension of these findings—but one that did not come to light until decades later—was the realization that health care workers who administered some of these pharmaceutical agents were not immune to their cytotoxic effects (1). Several well-known studies used markers such as sister chromatid exchanges, chromosomal abnormalities, and urine mutagenecity to detect abnormalities among workers exposed to cytotoxic pharmaceutical agents (2–7). Particularly vivid among these studies was one that showed the teratogenic effects of cytotoxic pharmaceutical agents in a population of nurses exposed to cytotoxic agents in the first trimester of pregnancy (8–11).

One of the more rational responses to these revelations was the establishment of the 1982 National Study Commission on Cytotoxic Exposure. It was composed of professionals well versed in the use of cytotoxic drugs. It drew up a set of definitive documents that set forth guidelines on the safe and responsible use of cytotoxic drugs (12).

In spite of compelling evidence, reform was slow in coming. Even during the 1980s there was a decided lack of uniformity in regulatory oversight of medical centers and their employees who handled cytotoxic pharmaceutical agents. Use of laminar flow hoods and personal protective equipment was almost unknown (13). In this vacuum of regulation, the Occupational Safety and Health Administration (OSHA) in 1986 issued guidelines covering personnel in contact with antineoplastic pharmaceutical agents (14). A summary of the OSHA provisions is contained in Table 8-1.

The American Society of Hospital Pharmacists produced a technical assistance bulletin that set forth the five characteristics of hazardous pharmaceutical agents: carcinogenicity, teratogenicity, genotoxicity, infertility, and organ impairment at low doses, shown in animal studies (15).

CLASSES OF HAZARDOUS PHARMACEUTICAL AGENTS

Since the publication of the OSHA guidelines in 1986, an explosion of pharmaceutical agents that can been classified as hazardous has emerged. A partial list is contained in Table 8-2. In general four categories of pharmaceutical agents are considered to exert potentially adverse or toxic ef-

TABLE 8-1. *Summary or Occupational Safety and Health Administration (OSHA) guidelines for handling cytotoxic drugs*

Protective measures	Activities	Rationale
Gloves		
Surgical latex gloves changed hourly or immediately if torn or contaminated	Drug preparation and administration Care of the patient Cleanup spills	Prevents contamination by absorption or ingestion: less permeable than polyvinylchloride gloves
Gowns		
Disposable gown made of lint-free, low-permeability fabric with a closed front, long sleeves, and elastic or knit-closed cuffs with cuffs tucked under the gloves	Drug preparation and administration Care of the patient Cleanup of spills	Prevents contamination caused by absorption; less permeable than cloth gown
Face protection		
Plastic face shield or splash goggles	Drug preparation and administration Cleanup of spills	Prevents contamination caused by absorption or inhalation: surgical masks do not provide adequate protection
Respirator masks	Cleanup of spills	Prevents contamination caused by inhalation
Other equipment		
Class II biologic safety cabinet	Drug preparation	Prevents contamination caused by inhalation
Plastic-backed absorbent mat	Drug preparation and administration	Prevents contamination caused by absorption
Syringes and IV sets with Luer-Lok connections (syringes should never be more than three-fourths full)	Drug preparation and administration	Prevents contamination caused by absorption or inhalation: decreases potential of spill.
IV administration sets should be attached and primed with diluent within the biologic safety cabinet before addition of the cytotoxic drugs	Drug preparation and administration	Prevents contamination caused by absorption or inhalation during priming of the infusion set ensures that the infusion set is primed in a controlled environment and that any initial fluid leackage contains no cytotoxic drug
4-mL sealable plastic or wire-tie bag with a warning label; bag large enough for transportation and waste disposal of administration equipment	Drug preparation and administration Cleanup of spills	Prevents contamination caused by absorption, inhalation, or ingestion: label properly identifies presence of cytotoxic drug
Puncture-resistant, closable, shatter-proof containers in all areas where drugs are prepared or administered	Drug preparation and administration Cleanup of spills	Prevents contamination caused by absorption of inhalation: prevents accidental spills or needle sticks

Based on ref. 28.

fects on workers who receive threshold exposures to them. These agent include antiviral drugs, antineoplastic agents, pharmaceutical agents used in anesthesia, and sex steroids.

Antineoplastic Agents

Antineoplastic agents act on rapidly dividing cells during mitosis, protein synthesis, and DNA replication. These agents traditionally are classified into five chemically discrete subtypes that manifest their own mechanisms of action. These five subtypes include alkylating agents, antibiotics, antimetabolites, mitotic inhibitors, and miscellaneous pharmaceutical agents that may include certain experimental drugs (16). The last category of pharmaceutical agents is not discussed herein.

Many antineoplastic agents are carcinogens and teratogens that affect bone marrow, hair follicles, nasopharyngeal, gastrointestinal, and genitourinary mucosa, and developing embryos (8). Potential consequences of exposure to this class of pharmaceutical

TABLE 8-2. *Drugs categorized as hazardous*

Altretamine	Etoposide	Pacitaxel
Aminothiadiazole[a]	Fazarabine[a]	Pegaspargase[a]
Amonafide[a]	Finasteride	Pentostatin
Amsacrine[a]	Floxuridine	Perfosfamide[a]
Asparaginase	Fludarabine phosphate	Pipobroman
Azaticine[a]	Fluorouracil	Piroxantrone hydrochloride[a]
Azathiopine	Flutamide	Plicamycin
Bleomycin sulfate	Ganciclovir sodium	Procargazine hydrochloride
Brequinar sodium[a]	Hydroxyurea	Pyrazcicacridine[a]
Busulfan	Idarubicin hydrochloride	Ribavirin
BV-araU[a]	Ifostamide	Ro 24-7429[a]
Carboplatin	Interferon alfa	Streptozocin
Carmustine	Interleukin-3[a]	Tamoxifen citrate
Cechalotaxine[a]	Ipomeanol[a]	Teniposide
Chlorambucil	Iproplatin[a]	Testolactone
C1-958[a]	Irinotecan hydrochloride trihydrate[a]	Thalidomide[a]
Cisplatin	Isotretinoin	Thioguanine
Cyclophosphamide	Leuprolide acetate	Thiotepa
Cytarabine	Levamiscle hydrochloide	Tocotecan hydrochloride[a]
Dacarbazine	Lomustine	Trimetrexate[a]
Dactinomycin	Mechlorethamine hydrochloride	7U85 mesylate[a]
Daunorubicin hydrochloride	Megestrol acetate	Uracil mustard
Deoxycoformycin[a]	Melphalan	Vidarabine
Diaziquone[a]	Mercaptopurine	Vinblastine sulfate
Doxorubicin hydrochloride	Methotrexate	Vincristine sulfate
Echinomycin[a]	Mitomycin	Vincrelbine tartrate[a]
Epirubicin hydrochloride[a]	Mitotane	Xcmazyme[a]
Erwinia L-asparaginase[a]	Mitoxantrone hydrochloride	Zicovudine
Etanidazole[a]	Nafarelin acetate	

[a]Investigational new drug.

agent include chromosomal abnormalities, decreased white blood cell count, liver damage, and spontaneous abortion. Less ominous physical symptoms may be headache, nausea, dermal or mucous membrane allergies and reactions, dizziness, lightheadedness, nausea, and cough. One study found that as many as 60% of oncology nursing staff at one institution had positive test results for one of the several pharmaceutical markers used to detect exposure to antineoplastic pharmaceutical agents (17).

Alkylating agents interrupt DNA replication within a cell by binding to the DNA molecule. Antibiotics, on the other hand, interfere with protein synthesis by causing misinterpretation of the DNA code. Antimetabolites disturb the process of cellular protein synthesis by halting the production of such protein precursors as folic acid, purines, and pyrimidines. Mitotic inhibitors prevent normal cell division and mitosis as they act on cell spindles (18).

Sex Steroids

It is during manufacture of synthetic estrogen by the pharmaceutical industry that maximal occupational exposure occurs. Estrogens are known to affect the breast, female reproductive organs, hypothalamus, and pituitary gland. Action on these estrogen-sensitive structures takes place in the nucleus and influences DNA synthesis (19).

Antiviral Agents

Health care workers are at particular risk for exposure to two often-used antiviral agents—ribavirin and pentamidine. These aerosolized chemicals produce their toxic effects by interfering with cellular protein synthesis (5,20). Pentamidine in particular binds to cellular molecules such as DNA, therefore this drug is implicated in potential mutagenesis or carcinogenesis. This suggestion should be sufficient to warrant all necessary preventive measures for persons working with this drug (21,22). Specific strategies are discussed in the section titled Engineering Plan.

Anesthetic Agents

The problem of escaping anesthetic gases is unique to the medical center. This issue calls for vigilance, especially because the dangers of fugitive anesthetic gas have not been clearly established. Researchers have proposed possible carcinogenic and teratogenic effects of these agents. Multiple studies, however, leave these matters unsettled (23,24). Although anesthetic equipment is designed to be a closed system, gases sometimes have the opportunity to escape during initial hookup or when a patient's mask is poorly fitted. Recovery room personnel can be exposed to gases in the exhaled breath of postoperative patients. The solution to these problems is a scavenging system, which is a vacuum device placed in areas of probable exposure such as operating rooms, recovery rooms, and labor and delivery areas (25).

The dangers of combustion and explosion that marked anesthetic gases in the past have been replaced by possible systemic effects in the newer halogenated anesthetic agents. In any case, there is no debate that waste gases can produce symptoms such as fatigue, nausea, drowsiness, headache, and irritability among health care workers exposed to them. That alone is sufficient to arouse concerns regarding employee well-being and job performance. The solution is relatively simple—an efficient and well-maintained scavenging system and periodic monitoring for fugitive gases in areas notorious for escaping anesthetic agents (26,27).

TOXICOLOGIC ASPECTS OF HAZARDOUS PHARMACEUTICAL AGENTS

Health care workers are vulnerable to toxic pharmaceutical agents in the work environment through several mechanisms. Inhalation of hazardous pharmaceutical agents in their aerosolized or powdered forms is a primary means of contamination. Absorption through skin contact is also common and can lead to secondary ingestion when workers do not take precautions such as frequent hand washing, use of personal protective equipment, and use of biologic safety cabinets. Situations that commonly give rise to workplace exposures include contact with equipment used to administer intravenous (IV) fluids and contact with body fluids from patients receiving antineoplastic or antiviral agents. Exposures to these agents may occur at any point in administration, from opening the vial to infusion.

Absorption

One of the primary determinants of how efficiently a toxic substance affects an exposed worker is the quantity, rate, and route of absorption. Absorption most commonly occurs through the skin, gastrointestinal tract, and lungs. Although the *skin* normally poses a formidable barrier to absorption of chemicals on contact, several factors affect the variability of this process. Any abrasion or break in the skin provides an opportunity for absorption through the skin. The thickness of the skin, the stratum corneum in particular, varies according to location on the body. Palmar and plantar surfaces are normally quite resistant to absorption of chemicals. This does not imply, however, that health care workers should ignore such common-sense precautions as glove use and wearing thick-soled shoes when working with hazardous chemicals. For health care workers, absorption of dangerous chemicals through the *gastrointestinal tract* most commonly occurs when good hand-washing techniques are not observed after handling materials. Eating and smoking with contaminated hands are the most likely route of access to the gastrointestinal tract.

The *lungs* are most vulnerable to absorption of gases and fine mists. Because absorption takes place at the alveolar level, particle size determines the efficiency of absorption; the smaller the particle (<1 μm), the more efficient is absorption. Other variables include gas solubility in the blood and subsequent lipid solubility once the chemical enters the blood, depth and rate of respiration, and concentration of gas or mist in the environment. Countermeasures to the hazards of inhaled chemicals should include use of well-vented biologic safety cabinets, scavenging systems where anesthetics pose a risk of leakage, and in extreme cases use of personal respirators (28,29).

Biotransformation and Excretion

Biotransformation and excretion of ingested chemicals are the metabolic processes that convert and eliminate ingested compounds through enzymatic reactions, principally in the liver, kidneys, and intestine. The rate of this process is controlled by the age, sex, nutritional status, and health state of the organism. Appropriate biologic monitoring and laboratory testing help detect end-organ disease among workers who are routinely exposed to hazardous chemicals. Organs and systems most vulnerable to adverse effects are the liver, kidney, and skin and the lymphatic, hematopoietic, cardiovascular, respiratory, and reproductive systems. Monitoring should be tailored to specific exposures and the organ systems they target.

HAZARDOUS PHARMACEUTICAL PROGRAM: ADMINISTRATIVE AND ENGINEERING CONTROLS

Most medical centers assume the responsibility of protecting their employees by limiting or eliminating exposure to hazardous pharmaceutical agents. Accepted techniques for meeting this goal include employee education, industrial hygiene, minimizing casual exposure to toxic chemicals, use of personal protective equipment, and effective removal and cleanup practices.

Administrative Plan

A formal written hazardous pharmaceutical safety and health plan is a practical necessity for institutions that use hazardous pharmaceutical agents (30,31). Minimal technical content to be included in such plans is outlined in the American Society of Hospital Pharmacists technical assistance bulletin (19). Any employee or contractor on site should have easy access to the written plan. This document represents the foundation of any employee educational program (32). Table 8-3 summarizes some of the basic ingredients of a sound health and safety plan. The document should be flexible and dynamic in the sense that departments with potentially exposed personnel, such as medical, nursing, housekeeping, and maintenance, can modify the plan according to the changing formulary and risk for exposure. The content, format, and distribution of the written plan should be presided over by a hazardous pharmaceuticals officer or a committee composed of affected workers (33–36).

A critical feature of the exposure control plan should address the issue of pregnant workers or those contemplating pregnancy. This portion of the plan should clearly outline

TABLE 8-3. *Components of a hazardous pharmaceutical program*

Safety measure	Method
Engineering: preventive measures	Biologic safety cabinets for pharmaceutical preparation
	Isolation rooms for aerosolized pharmaceutical administration
Administrative	Written hazardous pharmaceutical plan
	Reproductive toxicity policy
	Recordkeeping
Work practices	Cleanup of spills
	Pharmaceutical preparation in designated areas
	Safe handling techniques
Personal protective equipment	Gowns, gloves, masks, eye protection, and respirators

the teratogenic risks inherent in contact with cytotoxic pharmaceutical agents and offer and encourage the option of avoiding such contact by performing alternative duties during reproductively vulnerable times (9,10,37).

At a minimum, any hazardous pharmaceutical plan and prevention policy statement should include the following:

- Labeling of syringes and IV bags containing hazardous pharmaceutical agents
- Use of Luer-lock fittings on syringes and IV sets
- Use of large-bore needles to avoid high pressure within syringes
- Preparation of syringes and IV sets within a biologic safety cabinet
- Use of sufficiently large syringes to avoid overfilling
- Special care in working with powdered substances
- Wiping clean of IV bags
- Transport of pharmaceutical setups in sealed bags and special containers to avoid spills

Training Plan

An essential component of the administrative plan is a training plan whereby all health care workers who may come in contact with hazardous agents are given training on the possible adverse effects of toxic exposures. Training is designed to be specific to the actual circumstances of the individual work site and work assignment. Particular attention is paid to preventive techniques. Such training should take place at the beginning of employment and at regular intervals thereafter. Records of training sessions identify who was in attendance, material covered, qualifications of trainers, and dates. By law these records are maintained for 3 years (38). Table 8-4 outlines the knowledge and skills imparted by a well-constructed hazardous pharmaceutical training plan.

Engineering Plan

The objective of any rational engineering strategy is to separate the health care worker from toxic substances that of necessity are part of the work environment. Specific methods to achieve this aim include use of biologic safety cabinets and personal protective equipment. Among the more common-sense and less technologically intensive measures that individual workers are encouraged to observe in areas of potential contamination are avoidance of eating, drinking, chewing gum, and application of cosmetics.

Biologic Safety Cabinets

Biologic safety cabinets take on particular importance when the health care worker is called on to handle and administer pharmaceutical agents in their aerosolized forms. Hazardous pharmaceutical agents should be mixed and otherwise prepared in a class II or class III biologic safety cabinet that adheres to the safety specifications outlined in Table 8-5.

Cabinet intake and exhaust vents should be widely separated to avoid contaminating intake air with hazardous fumes. Workers using the cabinet should ensure that the exhaust fan remains on during operation. Biologic safety cabinets should not be confused with clean air workstations, which blow exhaust air in the direction of the worker.

Powered, air-circulating respirators with effective filters are occasionally used as an adjunct to or temporary substitute for a biologic safety cabinet. Surgical masks are not in compliance with OSHA standards for respiratory protection and do not provide a satisfactory substitute for the respirator, which has airtight integrity (28,29).

Two cytotoxic pharmaceutical agents commonly administered in aerosolized form are pentamidine and ribavirin. Ribavirin is used in pediatrics to treat severe cases of respiratory syncytial virus in its early stages, although occasionally it can be replaced with the less toxic respiratory syncytial virus immune globulin. The mode of delivery is typically a mist tent, oxygen hood, or face mask. Pentamidine, used prophylactically to manage recurrent *Pneumocystis carinii* pneumonia among the immunocompromised population, is administered in much the same way as rib-

TABLE 8-4. *Knowledge and skills required for work with hazardous drugs*

Employee's right to know
- List reasons for precautions
- List dangers associated with hazardous substances
- Attend safety lecture

Identification of hazardous drugs
- List drugs designated antineoplastic agents by the American Hospital Formulary Service
- Identity resources available to determine whether a drug is hazardous

Storage of hazardous drugs
- Describe secure packaging
- Describe what should be done with damaged packages
- Explain why separate storage areas are necessary
- Describe how the storage area should be labeled

Protective apparel
- Show the proper way to wear
  - Gowns
  - Gloves
  - Goggles
- Explain the rationale for each type of protective apparel

Preparation of hazardous drugs
- List relevant policies and procedures
- Demonstrate proper manipulative techniques to avoid contamination when
  - Reconstituting products
  - Handling needles
  - Withdrawing solution from vials and ampules
  - Breaking ampules
  - Using chemotherapy dispensing pins
- Describe the purpose of
  - Absorbent mats
  - Alcohol wipes
- Describe the requirements for proper labeling
- List the drugs that require use of a vesicant warning label
- Demonstrate how to prime the IV tubing for use with pumps
- Perform regular IV setups

Use of biosafety cabinets
- Name and types of cabinets
- Describe methods for venting cabinets
- Describe and demonstrate procedure for cleaning and decontaminating a cabinet
- State how often inspection and maintenance should be performed

Disposal of hazardous substances
- Demonstrate proper use of
  - Used-needle containers
  - Hazardous waste box
  - Caution tape
  - Hazardous waste box liners
- Describe proper identification of hazardous waste

Accidental spills or breakage
- Describe and demonstrate
  - How to contain a spill
  - How to clean up a spill
  - How to use the spill kit
- Explain when housekeeping department should be called

Accidental contact or exposure
- Describe how to decontaminate an exposed area
- List proper reagents for decontamination
- Locate the eye flush apparatus
- Describe circumstances when an employee should go to the
  - Medical advisor
  - Emergency department

Antineoplastic surveillance program
- Describe the purpose of this program

TABLE 8-5. *Biologic safety cabinet specifications*

Cabinet class	Specifications
II	Downward airflow with high-efficiency particulate air (HEPA) filters. Class II B cabinets vent to the outside.
III	Completely enclosed under negative pressure, allowing procedures to be performed through attached gloves. Vent to the outside.

avirin. In either case, precautions to safeguard health care workers include use of a negative-pressure isolation room with separate air-circulating systems equipped with high-efficiency particulate air (HEPA) filters (37). It also is considered prudent for medical and nursing staff to don gowns, shoe covers, and gloves when there is any potential for exposure to these pharmaceutical agents (39).

Personal Protective Equipment

Personal protective equipment used in concert with biologic safety cabinets is a crucial feature of the engineering plan. Basic protective equipment includes gowns, latex gloves, and splash goggles, all sufficient to provide a barrier against cytotoxic chemicals (40).

Gloves

In most cases, powder-free latex gloves are considered to be the superior product for prevention of hazardous pharmaceutical penetration. However, there may be exceptions depending on the nature of the hazardous chemical. Another criterion related to glove efficacy is thickness. Surgical gloves of maximum thickness (0.05 inch, 0.2 mm) were most resistant to penetration by a sampling of antineoplastic pharmaceutical agents over a 30 to 60 minute exposure. In addition to heavy weight, effective gloves should cover the wrist and forearm and exhibit good tensile strength. Gloves used in the preparation and administration of antineoplastic agents should meet the same U.S. Food and Drug Administration standards for permeability that surgical gloves are required to maintain (15,41).

Whatever the choice of glove material, nothing is a satisfactory substitute for thorough hand washing before and after application of gloves. Although double gloving provides increased protection from cytotoxic pharmaceutical agents, prudent health care workers change gloves hourly at a minimum. The worker must be diligent in performing regular self-assessments for latex allergy, whether it be a contact dermatitis or a more serious reaction (42).

Protective Gowns

Gowns that have proved effective against hazardous pharmaceutical contamination meet the following basic specifications: closed front, lint-free fabric, low-permeability fabric, long sleeves, and knit or elastic closed cuffs. Among the trade name gowns that meet these requirements are Tyvek products coated with various cytotoxic-resistant substances. The principle disadvantage inherent in these products is reduced airflow and consequent user discomfort. These limitations can be overcome with polyethylene-reinforced sleeves and fronts that increase user comfort without compromising safety (43).

Splash Goggles

Eye barrier and face protection goggles are appropriate in an environment where health care workers are vulnerable to hazardous pharmaceutical agents found in aerosolized or spray form. Risk for splashing also necessitates that such protection be worn. The dangers being addressed are contamination of oral, nasal, or ocular mucosa. In such an environment, eyewash equipment should be available. The secretions of patients receiving cytotoxic pharmaceutical agents are considered hazardous and must be treated with the same preventive measures as the pharmaceutical agents themselves. Vomitus, blood, feces, and urine are subject to universal precautions for blood-borne pathogens.

Cleanup and Disposal

Hazardous chemical spills and the institution's response must be part of an overall policy designed to remove guesswork in emergency situations. These contingencies should be covered in a hazardous pharmaceutical safety and health plan. Specifics for most plans might include the following:

Trained persons attired in personal protective equipment to attend to breakages and spills
Clearly labeled spill kits prominently displayed in areas where pharmaceutical agents are prepared and administered
Quarantine and localization of the spill area
Spill pads to absorb toxic liquids
Decontamination efforts from areas of lesser concentration to those of greater concentration
Barring of workers not involved in the cleanup effort from areas of contamination for their own safety and the safety of others
Detergent cleaning and rinse down of contamination sites
Removal of hazardous pharmaceutical waste in special containers designed for that purpose
Decontamination and medical evaluation of workers who have come in direct or indirect contact with hazardous chemicals

In one study investigators tested the efficacy of 10% sodium hypochlorite solution and sodium thiosulfate on spills of the antineoplastic agents doxorubicin and daunorubicin. It was found that these agents were effective when used sequentially rather than concurrently.

MEDICAL SURVEILLANCE

The purpose of a medical surveillance plan is to promptly identify any dangerous chemical exposures in the workplace and their prevalence, spread, and human biologic consequences. The net effect of such a plan is to limit human exposure to hazardous pharmaceutical agents. The tools necessary to reach such a goal cannot be emphasized forcefully enough; they include personal protective equipment, biologic safety cabinets, good worker technique, and training (19).

The surveillance plan must provide for monitoring of employees through an occupational history, physical examination, and laboratory studies. Often this becomes a matter of narrowing the focus of inquiry to precise job requirements and their potential hazards. For example, specialized evaluations may have to be made for workers handling infectious wastes versus those sterilizing instruments with ethylene chloride (44). Concerns relating to cytotoxic exposures occupy a dominant place in medical surveillance efforts (45–48).

History

A good occupational history as it pertains to health care workers in potential contact with hazardous pharmaceutical agents must include the types of agents found in the workplace, duration of exposure, and preventive measures. Questionnaires can prove to be time-saving tools for collecting this information. Certain hazardous pharmaceutical agents may be considered responsible for symptoms described among groups or subgroups of workers, depending on worksite and treatments performed (49). For example, exposure to aerosolized pharmaceutical agents may result in respiratory symptoms. The consequences of exposure to antineoplastic pharmaceutical agents may be expressed in the renal, hepatic, and reproductive systems; bone marrow and skin also may be affected.

Physical Examination

All workers contemplating employment in a health care setting should undergo a thorough physical examination designed to document their baseline health status. They also should receive appropriate immunizations. Subsequent examinations should be timed and focused according to types of exposure and individual vulnerability to harmful pharmaceutical agents identified on the preplacement examination. In interval evaluations of health care workers exposed over time to hazardous or cytotoxic chemicals, particular attention must be paid to physical examination of the following systems: cardiovascular, hepatic, respiratory, lymphatic, reproductive, and skin. Acute, identifiable exposure events should be managed on the basis of an understanding of the route of delivery and target organs with the highest probability of involvement. Physical signs often appear late in the development of disease.

Biomonitoring

Laboratory panels to measure serum levels of toxic chemicals are useful in monitoring health care workers chronically exposed to hazardous pharmaceutical agents (14). They are somewhat less effective and less practical in attempts to narrow the choices from among a wide variety of potentially culpable agents. This task is best left to specific laboratory tests when suspicion is high that a particular agent is implicated in an illness or symptoms. Examples of such tests include β2 globulins in cadmium toxicity and serum lead, mercury, and arsenic levels.

Laboratory tests most often used for monitoring purposes include a liver panel, blood urea nitrogen level, serum creatinine level, urinalysis, and complete blood count. Chest radiography and pulmonary function tests may have a place in establishing baseline function (19,49). A comprehensive evaluation often is performed when a health care worker terminates employment. As in other circumstances, the assessment includes history, physical examination, and laboratory studies geared to history and duration of exposure.

RECORDS

The OSHA hazard communication standard (30) mandates that appropriate records be maintained to include employee contacts with hazardous agents, methods and data for biologic monitoring, employee medical records, statistical summaries, and incident reports. By law, these records must be maintained for 30 years and should be accessible by the employee and other authorized personnel for that span of time.

SUMMARY

With the proliferation of cytotoxic pharmaceutical agents and their use in nontraditional settings comes the attendant responsibility to exercise all due precautions to limit exposure of workers who administer them. The team approach to prevention must include all parties to the process, that is, nurses, physicians, technicians, pharmacists, housekeeping personnel, and administrators. Only through compliance with a well-thought-out hazardous pharmaceutical safety and health plan in conjunction with a rational medical surveillance and training plan can the medical center provide employees with state-of-the-art prevention against the adverse consequences of hazardous pharmaceutical exposure.

REFERENCES

1. Hoover R, Fraumeni JF. Drug-induced cancer. *Cancer* 1981;47:1071–1080.
2. Hemminki K, Kyyronen P, Lindbohm ML. Spontaneous abortions and malformations in the offspring of nurses exposed to anaesthetic gases, cytostatic drugs, and other potential hazards in hospitals, based on registered information of outcome. *J Epidemiol Community Health* 1985;39:141–147.
3. Selevan SG, Lindbolm ML, Hornung RW, Hemminki K. A study of occupational exposure to antineoplastic drugs and fetal loss in nurses. *N Engl J Med* 1985;313: 1173–1178.
4. Stucker I, Caillard JF, Collin R, et al. Risk of spontaneous abortion among nurses handling antineoplastic drugs. *Scand J Work Environ Health* 1990;16:102–107.
5. Stucker I, Hirsch A, Dolroy T, et al. Urine mutagenecity, chromosomal abnormalities and sister chromatid exchanges in lymphocytes of nurses handling cytotoxic drugs. *Int Arch Occup Environ Health* 1986;57:195–205.
6. Newman MA, Valanis BG, Schoeny RS, Hee SQ. Urinary biological monitoring markers of anticancer drug exposure in oncology nurses. *Am J Public Health* 1994; 84:852–855.
7. Milkovic-Kraus S, Horvat D. Chromosomal abnormalities among nurses occupationally exposed to antineoplastic drugs. *Am J Ind Med* 1991;19:771–774.
8. Shortridge LA, Lemasters GK, Valanis B. Menstrual cycles in nurses handling antineoplastic drugs. *Cancer Nurs* 1995;18:439–444.
9. Fuchs J, Hengstler JG, Jung D, et al. DNA damage in nurses handling antineoplastic agents. *Mutat Res* 1995; 342:17–23.
10. Goloni-Bertollo EM, Tajara EH, Manzato AJ, Varella-Garcia M. Sister-chromatid exchanges and chromosome aberrations in lymphocytes of nurses handling antineoplastic drugs. *Int J Cancer* 1992;50:341–344.
11. Grummt T, Grummt HJ, Schott G. Chromosomal aberrations in peripheral lymphocytes of nurses and physicians handling antineoplastic drugs. *Mutat Res* 1993; 302:19–24.
12. US Department of Health and Human Services. Recommendations for the Safe Handling of Cytotoxic Drugs; NIH publication no 92-2621. Bethesda, MD: National Institutes of Health, 1992.
13. US Department of Health and Human Services. NIOSH Guidelines for Protecting the Safety and Health of Health Care Workers; NIOSH publication no 88-119. Cincinnati: National Institute for Occupational Safety and Health, 1988.

14. US Department of Labor, Occupational Safety and Health Administration. OSHA Technical Manual. OSHA Instruction TED 1.15 Washington, DC: OSHA, 1995.
15. Valanis B, Driscoll K, McNeil V. Comparison of antineoplastic drug handling policies of hospitals with OSHA guidelines: a pilot study. *Am J Public Health* 1990;80:480–481.
16. National Study Commission on Cytotoxic Exposure. Recommendations for Handling Cytotoxic Agents. Providence, RI: Rhode Island Hospital, 1987.
17. LeRoy ML, Roberts MJ, Theisen JA. Procedures for handling antineoplastic injections in comprehensive cancer centers. *Am J Hosp Pharm* 1983;40:601–603.
18. US Department of Labor, Occupational Safety and Health Administration. Work Practice Guidelines for Personnel Dealing with Cytotoxic (Antineoplastic) Drugs; OSHA publication no 8-1.1. Washington, DC: OSHA, 1986.
19. American Society of Hospital Pharmacists. ASHP technical assistance bulletin on handling cytotoxic and hazardous drugs. *Am J Hosp Pharm* 1990;47: 1033–1049.
20. Herr GE, McDiarmid MA, Testa MJ, Caldwell DJ. Health hazards to healthcare workers. In: Deeter D, Gaydos J, eds. *Occupational health: the soldier and the industrial base.* Washington, DC: TMM Publications, 1993:129–163.
21. Gilman GA, Rall TW, Nies AS, Taylor P, eds. *The pharmacological basis of therapeutics,* 8th ed. New York: Pergamon Press, 1990.
22. McDiarmid MA, Occupational exposure to pharmaceuticals: antineoplastics, anesthetic agents, sex steroid hormones. In: Paul M, ed. *Occupational and environmental reproductive hazards: a guide for physicians.* Baltimore: Williams & Wilkins, 1993:280–295.
23. Shults RA, Baron S, Decker J, et al. Health care worker exposure to aerosolized ribavirin: biological and air monitoring. *J Occup Environ Med* 1996;38:257–263.
24. Fackler JC, Flannery K, Zipkin M, McIntosh K. Precautions in the use of ribavirin at the children's hospital. *N Engl J Med* 1990;322:634.
25. Stansbury M. Reactive airway dysfunction syndrome in a nurse exposed to pentamidine [Letter]. *J Occup Environ Med* 1996;38:330–331.
26. Balmes JR, Estacio PL, Quinlan P, et al. Respiratory effects of occupational exposure to pentamidine. *J Occup Environ Med* 1995;37:145–150.
27. Yodaiken RE, Bennett D. OSHA work-practice guidelines for personnel dealing with cytotoxic (antineoplastic) drugs. *Am J Hosp Pharm* 1986;43:1193–1204.
28. McDiarmid MA, Gurley HT, Arrington D. Pharmaceuticals as hospital hazards: managing the risks. *J Occup Med* 1991;33:155–158.
29. Kacmarek RM. Ribavirin and pentamidine aerosols: caregiver beware! *Respir Care* 1990;35:1034–1036.
30. US Department of Labor, Occupational Safety and Health Administration. Access to employee and medical records standard. 29 CFR 1910.20, 1990.
31. Decker JA, Seitz TA, Shults RA, et al. Occupational exposure to aerosolized pharmaceuticals and control strategies. *Scand J Work Environ Health* 1992;18[Suppl 2]:100–102.
32. Anderson RW, Puckett WH, Dana WJ, et al. Risk of handling injectable antineoplastic agents. *Am J Hosp Pharm* 1982;39:1881–1887.
33. Symington IS. Controlling occupational exposure to anesthetic gases. *BMJ* 1994;309:968–969.
34. US Department of Labor, Occupational Safety and Health Administration. Air contaminants. *Federal Register* 1993;58:40191.
35. Lucchini R, Placidi D, Toffoletto F, Alessio L. Neurotoxicity in operating room personnel working with gaseous and nongaseous anesthesia. *Int Arch Occup Environ Health* 1996;68:188–192.
36. International Agency for Research on Cancer. IARC monographs on the evaluation of the carcinogenic risk of chemicals to humans: occupational exposure to mists and vapours from strong inorganic acids and other industrial chemicals. Vol. 54. Lyon, France: IARC, 1992.
37. Frase V, et al. Evaluation of rooms with negative pressure ventilation used for respiratory isolation in seven midwestern hospitals. *Infect Control Hosp Epidemiol* 1993;14:623–628.
38. American National Standards Institute. National standard for respiratory protection, respirator use, and physical qualification for personnel (Z88.6). New York: ANSI, 1984.
39. NIOSH Respirator Certification. 42 CFR 84, 1997.
40. Arrington DM, McDiarmid MA. Comprehensive program for handling hazardous drugs. *Am J Hosp Pharm* 1993;50:1170–1174.
41. Slevin ML, Ang LM, Johnston A, Turner P. The efficiency of protective gloves used in the handling of cytotoxic drugs. *Cancer Chemother Pharmacol* 1984;12:151–153.
42. Hunt LW, Fransway AF, Reed CE, et al. An epidemic of occupational allergy to latex involving health care workers. *J Occup Environ Med* 1995;37:1204–1209.
43. Laidlaw JL, Connor TH, Theiss JC, et al. Permeability of four disposable protective-clothing materials to seven antineoplastic drugs. *Am J Hosp Pharm* 1985;42: 2449–2454.
44. McDiarmid MA. Medical surveillance for antineoplastic-drug handlers. *Am J Hosp Pharm* 1990;47:1061–1066.
45. Lauwerys RR, Hoet P. Industrial *Chemical Exposures: Guidelines for Biological Monitoring.* Boca Raton, FL: Lewis, 1993.
46. Machado-Santelli GM, Cerqueira EM, Oliveira CT, de Braganca-Pereira CAA. Biomonitoring of nurses handling antineoplastic drugs. *Mutat Res* 1994;322:203–208.
47. De Meo MP, Merono S, De Baille AD, et al. Monitoring exposure of hospital personnel handling cytotoxic drugs and contaminated materials. *Int Arch Occup Environ Health* 1995;66:363–368.
48. Kevekordes S, Gebel TW, Hellwig M, Dames W, Dunkelberg H. Human effect monitoring in cases of occupational exposure to antineoplastic drugs: a method of comparison. *Occup Environ Med* 1998;55:145–149.
49. Schulte PA, Walker JT, Boeniger MF, et al. Molecular, cytogenic, and hematologic effects of ethylene oxide on female hospital workers. *J Occup Environ Med* 1995;37: 313–320.

Medical Center Occupational Health and Safety,
edited by Robert J. McCunney.
Lippincott Williams & Wilkins, Philadelphia © 1999.

9

Anesthetic Gases and Sterilants

Ross S. Myerson, *Lynn Stansbury, and Karin D. Myerson

Myerson Occupational and Environmental Medicine, Silver Spring, Maryland 20903;
**Occupational Medical Service, National Institutes of Health, Bethesda, Maryland 20813*

OVERVIEW OF ANESTHETIC GASES AND THEIR UTILIZATION

Hazards have long been associated with the use of anesthetic gases. At the beginning of the twentieth century, concerns centered around the flammability and explosive potential of the agents then in use. Today however, anesthetic agents present much different concerns to personnel working in the operating room environment. Current concerns include the possible effects of these agents on the liver, kidney, nervous system, and reproductive system. With the rapid expansion of outpatient and day surgery centers, concern for the control of these potential hazards exists far beyond the traditional confines of the hospital environment and dental office. Table 9-1 lists anesthetic goods, brand name, and year of introduction.

TABLE 9-1. *Anesthetic agents, brand name and year of introduction*

Generic name	Commercial name	Year of introduction
Diethyl ether	Ether	1842
Nitrous oxide	Nitrous oxide	1844
Chloroform	Chloroform	1933
Cyclopropane	Cyclopropane	1933
Trichloroethylene	Trilene	1934
Fluroxene	Fluoromar	1954
Halothane	Halothane	1956
Methoxyflurane	Penthrane	1959
Enflurane	Ethrane	1972
Isoflurane	Forane	—

Anesthetic gases in current use are generally of two classes: halogenated hydrocarbons and nitrous oxide. Halogenated anesthetic gases have been in general use for more than 50 years. Exposure to these agents is of course deliberate for the patients undergoing anesthesia. For operating room personnel, however, exposure is an undesired occupational hazard. Nitrous oxide was introduced as an anesthetic agent in 1844 by Horace Wells and has been an important adjunct in the care of patients undergoing operative and dental procedures ever since.

HALOGENATED ANESTHETICS

Liver and Renal Effects

The most widely known hazard associated with the use of halogenated agents was halothane hepatitis, a serious and potentially fatal postanesthesia complication. This condition was first described in the early 1960s after a number of case reports suggested a possible link between halothane and hepatotoxicity. This observation prompted the initiation of The American National Halothane Study, which found an association between severe postanesthesia hepatic dysfunction and the use of halothane anesthesia (1). Several subsequent studies went on to further characterize the disease and highlight the potentially fatal outcome of this entity (2–4). Bird and Williams (5) described a technique in which an enzyme-linked immunosorbent assay was used to detect antibodies to a halothane metabolite in patients with suspected halothane-associated hepatitis. Although this and other tests may help in the differential diagnosis of halothane-induced hepatitis, their practical application is limited by the short period in which the acute-phase antibodies are present.

In occupational studies, hepatic disease occurred more frequently among exposed medical or dental personnel than among a nonexposed control group (6,7). A study in Czechoslovakia in 1974 (8) showed a trend toward increasing hepatic disorders with increasing length of service. These findings were most probably associated with exposure to metabolites of trichloroethylene, which is no longer used as an anesthetic agent. There have been case reports of mild hepatitis possibly attributed to occupational exposure to anesthetics among surgeons and anesthesiologists (9). There have also been reports of adverse renal effects among persons occupationally exposed to anesthetic gases (5,6).

Neuropsychologic Effects

Anesthetic agents by design produce narcosis among those exposed to sufficient concentrations. Animal studies have demonstrated permanent learning deficits and neuronal damage among rats exposed to 12 ppm of halothane for long durations (10). There have been reports of increased incidence of headache, fatigue, irritability and sleep disturbance among exposed operating room personnel (11). Malhotra et al. in India conducted a prospective study to determine whether there were any effects from halothane on motor skills and short-term memory among anesthesiology residents. A group of 24 residents was evaluated after no exposure to any anesthetic gases, exposure to nonhalothane anesthetic gases, and exposure to halothane in operating room conditions. The study found consistent evidence of significant impairment of motor skills and decrements in short-term memory among the group exposed to halothane. The study made no mention of reversibility or recovery from these effects when exposure had ceased (12).

Immune System Effects

Effects of anesthetic agents on the immune system and hematologic values among patients undergoing anesthesia have been described (13–15). Studies also have addressed immune system effects from occupational exposure. A study in Eastern Europe showed numerous immunohematologic changes among persons occupationally exposed to halothane and nitrous oxide (16). However, a more recent controlled study demonstrated no differences in serum immunoglobulin concentrations (17). Additional studies would be useful in examining this issue.

Reproductive System Effects

Various authors have reported chromosomal effects after exposure to volatile anesthetic agents. Studies assessing sister-chromatid exchanges in operating room personnel have been contradictory. Sardas et al. (18) in Turkey reported an increased frequency of sister-chromatid exchanges in operating room personnel compared with controls; multiple previous studies did not show this effect. A 1994 study in Germany demonstrated a significantly higher rate of single-stranded DNA breaks in the peripheral lymphocytes of operating room personnel compared with matched controls (19).

Since the 1970s there has been considerable interest in the effects of nitrous oxide on fertility and spontaneous abortion. Several early studies suggested a link between spontaneous abortion and anesthetic exposure in operating rooms (20–22). More recent work has continued to find this association. A study conducted in France looked at the rates of spontaneous abortion and birth defects among female nurses working in a Paris hospital. The study found a significantly higher rate of spontaneous abortion among operating room nurses compared with nurses who worked elsewhere. There was no significant effect on birth defects (23). In a study of female dental assistants, Rowland et al. (24) found elevated risk for spontaneous abortion among women who worked with nitrous oxide 3 or more hours a week in offices without scavenging equipment. The same authors (25) also examined the issue of fertility among dental assistants. They reported that women exposed to high levels of nitrous oxide were significantly less fertile than those with lower or no exposure. These findings of decreased fertility may be related to undiagnosed pregnancies that end in early fetal loss. This hypothesis is consistent with findings discussed earlier with regard to spontaneous abortion. Findings of testicular effects of nitrous oxide among male rats are arguments for further research into the effects on men (26).

Carcinogenicity

Cohen et al. (6) found that there is a significant increase in cancer among women exposed to anesthetic gases compared with controls, an association not found among men. A large survey of operating room personnel in the United States conducted by the American Society of Anesthesiologists found a 1.3- to 2.0-fold increase in cancer incidence among women. Given the findings related to DNA breaks and sister-chromatid exchange discussed earlier, further study seems warranted (27).

Exposure Limits, Controls, and Monitoring

NIOSH has recommended an 8-hour time-weighted average exposure limit of 25 ppm for nitrous oxide (28). The American Conference of Governmental Industrial Hygienists (ACGIH) has set its threshold limit value (TLV) at 50 ppm per 8-hour time-weighted average. The best way to control exposures to volatile anesthetic agents is to have a well-functioning and efficient scavenging system. These systems require proper maintenance and should be checked for leaks with an infrared gas analyzer. Other common-sense measures include regular visual inspection of all hoses and connections, proper techniques in filling the vaporizer units of anesthetic machines, proper fit of masks on patients, and minimization of the administration of anesthetic gases before intubation. At the end of an operation, care should be taken to assure that all gas flow valves are shut off. Some practitioners suggest hyperoxygenating the patient at the end of the procedure to flush the residual gas from the patient's lungs. Some hospitals are taking steps to place scavenging systems in recovery rooms to collect gases exhaled by patients into individual face tents (29).

It has been postulated that psychomotor impairment may occur at exposures to nitrous oxide as low as 50 to 500 ppm (30), however, a study (31) has suggested that reports of symptoms do not correlate with ambient levels of nitrous oxide. Nitrous oxide dosimetry appears to be a cost efficient, accurate way to monitor human exposure in the occupational setting (31). It is possible to measure exposure through biologic monitoring of anesthetic agents in urine. A study in Italy (32) addressed the relation between ambient concentrations of nitrous oxide, halothane, enflurane, and isoflurane and urinary levels of these compounds in more than 1,500 exposed subjects. Significant correlations were found between ambient and urinary concentrations that indicated urinary anesthetic concentration can be used as an accurate method to assess dose. Specific biologic exposure indices were proposed (32).

STERILANTS AND DISINFECTANTS

Endoscopes and other delicate medical instruments are frequently used for a variety of procedures. Many of these devices cannot undergo steam sterilization or immersion in hypochlorite solutions. Increasing reliance on other means of sterilization and disinfection has led to a significant increase in use of chemical sterilants and disinfectants. *Sterilization* implies the removal of all spores, bacteria, and viruses and is generally required for rigid endoscopes and other instruments inserted into body cavities at laparoscopy, arthroscopy, or cystoscopy. *Disinfection* implies the removal of bacteria and viruses but does not ensure removal of spores; it is usually sufficient for devices involved in endoscopic examination of the gastrointestinal tract and respiratory tree.

This section reviews the occupational hazards associated with ethylene oxide and glutaraldehyde, two of the most common agents used for sterilization and disinfection in the current health care environment. Ethylene oxide, a highly reactive and penetrating alkylating agent, is used for sterilization. Glutaraldehyde, a low-molecular-weight aldehyde, also is used for disinfection and sterilization. Glutaraldehyde vaporizes sufficiently at room temperature for inhalation exposure to be a serious risk to personnel.

Glutaraldehyde

Glutaraldehyde, a five-carbon dialdehyde, is usually used in health care settings in 2% aqueous solution. At this concentration, it has a vapor pressure of 0.0012 mm Hg at 20°C and has a pungent odor detectable at 0.04 ppm, well below the Occupational Safety and Health Administration short-term exposure limit of 0.2 ppm. It is important that heath care workers using glutaraldehyde understand that they will detect the odor of this substance at levels that are considered safe. Many uses of glutaraldehyde, including its role as a disinfectant, are related to its ability to react with and cross link proteins. In addition to its use as a sterilant and disinfectant, glutaraldehyde is used as a tanning agent for leather, a preservative for cosmetics, and a tissue fixative and therapeutic agent for warts, hyperhidrosis, and dermal mycotic infections. It is also used in radiographic film processing solutions. Workers can be exposed to glutaraldehyde in a number of clinical and occupational settings. In the hospital environment, most adverse health effects are associated with sterilization or disinfection procedures.

Irritant and Pulmonary Effects

Glutaraldehyde is an irritant to the skin and mucous membranes. It has been shown to produce upper respiratory tract lesions (deciliation, squamous metaplasia, and focal cell damage with exfoliation and necrosis) in mice at concentrations as low as 0.3 ppm (33). It may produce eye irritation when aerosolized or when concentrations exceed 0.2 ppm. Because the use of glutaraldehyde has increased over the past decade, case reports linking glutaraldehyde and occupational asthma have raised concern for its potential as a respiratory tract sensitizer (34,35). Although most case reports of asthma involve workers who perform sterile processing, there also have been case reports of health care workers exposed in radiology departments (36). Workplace pre- and postshift pulmonary function testing and peak flow measurements can be useful in establishing the diagnosis of occupational asthma but should be interpreted with caution because the potential for misdiagnosis exists (37,38).

Dermatologic Effects

Glutaraldehyde is a primary dermal irritant known to cause dermal irritation among both animals and humans (39). It has been shown to cause contact dermatitis and skin sensitization (40,41). Typical clinical features include vesicular dermatitis, usually on the hands and forearms.

Genotoxicity, Carcinogenicity, and Reproductive Effects

Toxicity studies have shown that glutaraldehyde exhibits mutagenic activity through its ability to induce oxidative damage to DNA in cell cultures. No adequate long-term bioassay studies have evaluated the potential carcinogenicity of this substance. Limited animal studies have not shown significant reproductive toxicity associated with glutaraldehyde. There have been no reports of adverse reproductive effects among humans (39).

Controlling Exposure to Glutaraldehyde

In 1993, a study conducted in six hospitals in the United Kingdom assessed exposure to glutaraldehyde in sterile processing and radiology departments. The study found that routine exposures of hospital workers to airborne concentrations were well within the recommended exposure limit; however, potential for skin contact in many activities was found (42). Protective gloves are recommended when skin contact with glutaraldehyde is a risk. Permeation studies have indicated that polyethylene, latex, and vinyl gloves give acceptable protection against glutaraldehyde (43). Automated endoscopic washing machines are available and commonly used in many hospitals. They greatly reduce the exposure potential among employees. Care must be taken, however, to properly operate and maintain these machines and to assure regular changing of rinse water to avoid unexpected exposures to both hospital personnel and patients (44).

Ethylene Oxide

Ethylene oxide is used worldwide in the chemical industry. Annual production in the United States is estimated to be 3 million tons. Approximately 60% is used in the production of ethylene glycol; 12% is used to produce nonionic surfactants. The other 28% of ethylene oxide is used to synthesize glycol ethers, ethanolamines, and other chemicals. The health care industry uses a relatively small percentage of this amount for sterilization of medical equipment. Of all chemical sterilants, ethylene oxide is the most widely used. Ethylene oxide is a colorless gas with a distinctively sweet, ether-like odor. The main route of exposure is inhalation, which in hospitals most commonly occurs in sterile processing departments. Ethylene oxide is an irritant to the respiratory tract, eyes, mucous membranes, and skin.

Carcinogenicity of Ethylene Oxide

Swedish workers exposed to ethylene oxide exhibited an association between ethylene oxide exposure and the development of leukemia (45,46). Numerous investigators have continued to address this possible risk with equivocal results. Shore et al. (47) conducted a metaanalysis of 10 cohorts that included 29,800 workers and 2,540 deaths. Outcomes analyzed included leukemia, non-Hodgkin's lymphoma, stomach cancer, pancreatic cancer, and cancer of the brain and nervous system. A standardized mortality ratio (SMR) for leukemia of 1.06 (95% confidence interval [CI], 0.73–1.48) was reported. No trend in risk for leukemia with exposure intensity or frequency was found. The combined SMR for non-Hodgkin's's lymphoma was 1.35 (95% CI, 0.93–1.90), and as with leukemia, no trend was associated with intensity or frequency of exposure. The SMR for stomach cancer was 1.28 (95% CI, 0.98–1.65). SMRs for pancreatic and nervous system cancers did not show elevated risk (47). The authors concluded that the question of the relation between ethylene oxide and leukemia and non-Hodgkin's's lymphoma remained open but that the weight of evidence indicated no association between ethylene oxide and other types of cancer. On the basis of the entire body of scientific evidence, however, the International Agency for Research on Cancer has placed ethylene oxide in group 1 and considers it a carcinogen for humans.

Neurologic Effects of Ethylene Oxide

There have been reports of subacute sensory motor neuropathy among workers exposed to ethylene oxide during sterilizing activities (48, 49). Findings included abnormalities in electromyographic studies of the lower extremities accompanied by foot drop, sensory loss, and loss of deep tendon reflexes. Nerve biopsies performed on some workers demonstrated axonal degeneration.

Reproductive and Genotoxic Risk of Ethylene Oxide

A study of hospital workers exposed to ethylene oxide during sterilization procedures found an increased frequency of spontaneous abortions among pregnant women compared with a nonexposed control group (50). Animal data also support an association between ethylene oxide and adverse reproductive outcomes, including decreased fertility, reduced sperm counts and motility, and fetal loss (51). Ethylene oxide has been demonstrated to be associated with higher levels of single-stranded DNA breaks, chromosomal aberrations, and sister chromatid exchanges among humans with occupational exposures (52–54).

Controlling and Monitoring Exposure to Ethylene Oxide

Both the ACGIH threshold limit value and the OSHA permissible exposure limit for ethylene oxide are set a 1 ppm. OSHA standard 29 CFR 1910.1047 regulates exposure to ethylene oxide in the workplace and mandates medical surveillance for all persons who are or may be exposed at or above the action level of 0.5 ppm. Medical surveillance consists of a medical evaluation by or under the supervision of a physician before assignment and annually for each employee exposed at or above the action level. Medical evaluations also are required after any appreciable emergency exposure or on notification that any employee may have signs or symptoms of exposure. In addition to the history and physical examination, a complete blood cell count with differential is required. However, La Montagne et al. (55) recently analyzed their experience in providing ethylene oxide medical surveillance in a Massachusetts hospital. They found a lack of sensitivity and utility in the use of a complete blood cell count as an indicator of exposure and suggested that this test may not be useful in the routine medical surveillance of workers exposed to ethylene oxide. Other authors (56,57) have suggested that monitoring of chromosomal aberrations, hemoglobin adducts, and sister chromatid exchanges may be a more useful means of assessing exposure, but this is not a widespread practice. Control of exposure to ethylene oxide has improved greatly with automation, installation of exhausted gas cabinets, and installation of detectors and alarms in health care facility sterile processing departments.

A PRACTICAL GUIDE FOR THE OCCUPATIONAL HEALTH PROFESSIONAL

It is likely that occupational health professionals will become involved in some manner with the occupational health issues of a hospital or outpatient center through providing consultation services for an institution itself or treating people who work there. This section identifies the framework necessary to manage occupational health issues pertaining to anesthetic gases, sterilants, and disinfectants.

Health and Safety Assessment

The purpose of the health and safety assessment is to protect the health and safety of the employees, ensure a safe work environment, and ensure compliance with federal and state regulations. The health and safety assessment is the first step in maintaining an effective occupational injury and illness prevention program. Physical inspection of the medical center or outpatient facility should be performed on a regular basis. In larger facilities, the occupational health professional should be a member of a multidisciplinary team that includes safety, engineering, and industrial hygiene specialists. In smaller facilities that do not have these resources, the occupational professional may conduct the initial assessment and consult with specialists in safety, engineering, and industrial hygiene as needed. Table 9-2 provides exam-

TABLE 9-2. *Sample health and safety assessment for waste anesthetic gas, sterilants, and disinfectants*

Identification and labeling of agents in use in the facility	Comments
List agents:	
Are all agents properly labeled? If no, explain:	
Material safety data sheets (MSDS)	
Are current MSDS available for all agents listed above?	
Are MSDS sheets accessable to employees, managers and occupational health staff?	
Training	
Who provides employee training?	
Are employee training records current?	
Engineering controls	
Waste anesthetic gases	
What type of system to "scavenge" waste anesthetics is in place (central vacuum or nonrecirculating exhaust system)?	
What is the maintenance schedule and testing of waste anesthetic gases system?	
Are tubes and connections free of equipment leaks (nonleaking tubes, snug connection)?	
Sterilants and disinfectants	
Are sterilization operations centralized in the facility?	
Are the ethylene oxide chambers equipped with safety features (automatic door locking, controlled release of ethylene oxide into sterilization chamber, and effective exhaust system and alarms)?	
Observation of work practices	
Waste anesthetic gases	
Do employees turn off the anesthetic valve immediately when the breathing system is disconnected from the patient?	
Do employees check for leaks during hookup and checkout of the system?	
Sterilants and disinfectants	
Do employees operate sterilizing units as per established procedures?	
Do employees wear PPE to protect the skin and the eyes?	
Personal protective equipment (PPE)	
Is PPE to protect the skin and eyes from contact with sterilants and disinfectants readily available (face shields, goggles, and protective clothing)?	
Environmental monitoring	
Review air-monitoring data to ensure compliance with OSHA standards for ethylene oxide (permissible exposure limit 1 ppm per 8-hour time-weighted average)	

ples of areas to include in the health and safety assessment.

Hazard Communication

Anesthetic gases and sterilants are covered by the OSHA hazard communication standard (58). To meet the requirements of this standard, at minimum users must have written procedures for identification and labeling of specific agents used, regularly updated material safety data sheets, and employee information and training. Individual departments may contract hazard communication training to training vendors or rely on suppliers of anesthetic gases and sterilants to provide training programs and materials regarding their products. The standard that contains much useful guidance emphasizes the need for regular and responsive updating of information and training as new and sometimes unexpected hazards are introduced into the workplace, for example the recent use of nitric oxide, a potent explosive, in therapy for pulmonary hypertension. The standard also addresses less obvious issues, such as where information on workplace hazards should be located to optimize familiarity and how to manage a changing workforce, which may include contract employees or other multiple-employer situations. Though this kind of regulatory micromanagement has been appropriately challenged, it highlights the various factors that complicate compliance with regulations (59).

Engineering Controls

The most effective way to control hazards is to "engineer" out the potential hazard. Engineering controls include systems to scavenge waste anesthetic gases from the source.

Observation of Work Practices

Facilities need to review the written procedures for work practice designed to minimize employee exposure. Employee adherence to these procedures should be evaluated during normal work activities.

Personal Protective Equipment

Personal protective equipment should be available and should be used. This includes protective clothing, gloves, face shields, and respirators.

Environmental Monitoring

Hazard surveillance, environmental monitoring of waste anesthetic gases and sterilants, and calculation of time-weighted average exposure of workers is an industrial hygiene process. The occupational health professional must ensure that the required monitoring is performed and that exposure levels meet regulatory requirements.

Medical Surveillance

The monitoring of biologic effects on individuals is the direct responsibility of the occupational medical unit. Ethylene oxide is the only substance in this group for which medical surveillance is required. Medical surveillance requirements include an annual physical examination, occupational and exposure history, and a complete blood cell count for workers exposed above the 0.5 ppm action level. The usefulness of the complete blood cell count has been questioned, but the test is mandated. Sister-chromatid exchange has not yet been correlated sufficiently with the epidemiologic outcome of cancer among humans to be recommended for biologic monitoring outside well-designed epidemiologic studies. The records of persons occupationally exposed to ethylene oxide must be retained for 30 years beyond the date when exposure stops. No standard requires retention of the records of persons exposed to anesthetic gases or glutaraldehyde.

Quality Assurance

The basis of quality assurance is regular review and updating of standard operating procedures, including training and the generation of objective outcome data, by the persons who use them. For that reason, quality assurance for anesthetic gases and sterilants should be based in the departments using them. However, the multiple-employer–based nature of many medical centers suggests that occupational health staff may need to be alert to the process and outcome of quality assurance in these units.

Incident Response

Response to an exposure incident includes containment and cleanup, investigation, and identification and examination of exposed workers. Occupational health staff should be familiar with containment, cleanup, and investigation processes. Follow-up interviews with the persons responsible for these activities provides valuable information for appropriate response to the medical issues associated with the incident. Urgent care measures in the unlikely event of a major exposure incident include removal from exposure, administration of oxygen if inhalation has occurred, and copious flushing with water or normal saline solution if skin contact has occurred. Ethylene oxide is rarely contacted in liquid form, but such exposure can cause frostbite and severe irritation and blistering of skin. Hypersensitivity reactions can be caused by inhalation or dermal contact.

Given that workplace exposure is usually insidious or discovered during routine hazard surveillance, one of the most important aspects of a clinical visit to the occupational health clinic is counseling. Along with a focused history and physical examination, the occupational health professional should discuss the employee's concerns and provide accurate information about the health risks associated with exposure to anesthetic gases, sterilants, and disinfectants.

REFERENCES

1. National Halothane Study: summary of the National Halothane Study. *JAMA* 1966;197:121–134.
2. Imman WHW, Mushin WW. Jaundice after repeated exposure to halothane: a further analysis of reports to the committee on safety in medicines. *Br Med J* 1978;2: 1455–1456.
3. Walton B, Simpon BR, Strunin L, Doniach D, Perrin J, Appleyard AS. Unexplained hepatitis following halothane. *Br Med J* 1976;1:171–173.
4. Moult PJA, Sherlock S. Halothane related hepatitis. *Q J Med* 1975;44:99–114.
5. Bird GLA, Williams R. Detection of antibodies to a halothane metabolite hapten in sera from patients with halothane-associated hepatitis. *J Hepatol* 1989;9: 366–373.
6. Cohen EN, Brown BW Jr, et al. Occupational disease among operating room personnel: a national study. *Anesthesiology* 1974;41:321–340.
7. Cohen EN, Brown BW Jr, Bruce DL, et al. A survey of anesthetic health hazards among dentists. *J Am Dent Assoc* 1975;90:1291–1296.
8. Uhlirova A, Pokorny J. Results of questionnaire survey of the health hazards of anesthesiologists. *Rozhl Chir* 1974;53:761–770.
9. Williams R. Halothane and the liver: a medical review. In: *Halothane and the liver: the problem revisited.* Bristol, UK: Bristol Royal Infirmary, 1986.
10. Quimby KL, Aschkenase LJ, Bowman RE, Katz J, Chang LW. Enduring learning defects and cerebral synaptic malformation from exposure to 10 parts of halothane per million. *Science* 1975;185:625–627.
11. Saurel-Cubizolles MJ, Estryn-Behar M, Maillard MF, Mugnier N, Masson A, Monod G. Neuropsychological symptoms and occupational exposure to anesthetics. *Br J Ind Med* 1992;49:276–281.
12. Malhotra SK, Dhananjaya HS, Dwarka P. Effect of halothane exposure on motor skills and memory in anesthetists. *Indian J Med Res* 1993;98:218–222.
13. Erskine R, James MFM. Isoflurane but not halothane stimulates neutrophil chemotaxis. *Br J Anaesth* 1990; 64:723.
14. Lofstrom B, Schildt B. Reticuloendothelial function under general anesthesia. *Acta Anaesthesiol Scand* 1974; 18:34.
15. Descotes J. *Immunotoxicology of drugs and chemical.* Amsterdam: Elsevier, 1988.
16. Peric M, Varanes S, Marusic M. Immunological disturbances in anesthetic personnel chronically exposed to high occupational concentrations of nitrous oxide and halothane. *Anesthesia* 1991;23:531–537.
17. Karakaya A, Tuncel N, Yucesoy B, et al. The effects of volatile anesthetic agents on human immune system function via occupational exposure. *Immunopharmacol Immunotoxicol* 1992;14:251–259.
18. Sardas S, Cuhruk H, Karakaya AE, Atakurt Y. Sister chromatid exchanges in operating room personnel. *Mutat Res* 1992;279:12–21.
19. Reitz M, Coen R, Lanz E. DNA single strand breaks in peripheral lymphocytes of clinical personnel with occupational exposure to volatile inhalational anesthetics. *Envtron Res* 1994;65:12–21.
20. Cohen EN, Bellville JW, Brown BW. Anesthesia, pregnancy and miscarriage: a study of operating room nurses and anesthetists. *Anesthesiology* 1971;35: 343–347.
21. Knill-Jones RP, Moir DD, Rodriques LV, Spence AA. Anesthetic practice and pregnancy: controlled survey of women anesthetists in the United Kingdom. *Lancet* 1972;2:1326–1328.
22. Spence AA, Cohen EN, Brown BW, Knill-Jones RP, Himmelberger DU. Occupational hazards for operating room-based physicians: analysis of data from the United States and United Kingdom. *JAMA* 1977;238: 955–959.
23. Saurel-Cubizolles MJ, Hays M, Estryn-Behar M. Work in operating rooms and pregnancy outcome among nurses. *Int Arch Occup Environ Health* 1994;66: 235–241.
24. Rowland AS, Baird D, Shore D, Weinberg C, Savitz D, Wilcox A. Nitrous oxide and spontaneous abortion in female dental assistants. *Am J Epidemiol* 1995;141: 531–538.
25. Rowland AS, Baird DD, Weinberg C, Shore D, Shy C, Wilcox A. Reduced fertility among women employed as dental assistants exposed to high levels of nitrous oxide. *N Engl J Med* 1992;327:993–999.
26. Krupke BJ, Kelman AD, Shah NK, Balogh K, Handler AH. Testicular reaction to prolonged exposure to nitrous oxide. *Anesthesiology* 1976;44:104–113.
27. Bihari V, Srivastava AK, Gupta BN. Occupational health hazards among operation room personnel exposed to anesthetic gases: a review. *J Environ Pathol Toxicol* 1994;13:213–219.
28. National Institute for Occupational Safety and Health: Criteria for a recommended standard for occupational exposure to waste anesthetic gases and vapors; DHEW/NIOSH publication no 77-140. Washington, DC: US Government Printing Office, 1977.
29. Kubasiewicz MK. Controlling anaesthetic gas exposure in PACU. *Can Operating Room Nurs J* 1987;5:13–18.
30. Bruce D, Bach M. Effects of trace anasthetic gases on behavioral performance of volunteers. *Br. J Anaesth* 1976;48:871–876.
31. Tran N, Elias J, Rosenberg T, Wylie D, Gaborieau D, Yassi A. Evaluation of waste anesthetic gases, monitoring strategies, and correlations between nitrous oxide levels and health symptoms. *Am Ind Hyg Assoc J* 1994; 55:36–41.
32. Imbriani M, Ghittori S, Pezzagno G, Capodaglio E. Anesthetic in urine as biological index of exposure in operating-room personnel. *J Toxicol Environ Health* 1995;46:249–260.
33. Zissu D, Gagnaire F, Bonnet P. Nasal and pulmonary toxicity of glutaraldehyde in mice. *Toxicol Lett* 1994;71: 53–62.

34. Corrada OJ, Osman J, Davies RJ. Asthma and rhinitis after exposure to glutaraldehyde in endoscopy units. *Hum Toxicol* 1986;5:325–327.
35. Burge PS. Occupational risks of glutaraldehyde. *Br Med J* 1989;299:342.
36. Gannon PF, Bright P, Campbell M, O'Hickey SP, Burge PS. Occupational Asthma due to glutaraldehyde and formaldehyde in endoscopy and x-ray departments. *Thorax* 1995;50:156–159.
37. Chan-Yeung M, McMurren T, Catonio-Begley F, Lam S. Occupational asthma in a technologist exposed to glutaraldehyde. *J Allergy Clin Immunol* 1993;5: 974–978.
38. Stenton SC, Beach JR, Dennis JH, Keaney NP, Hendrick DJ. Glutaraldehyde, asthma, and work: a cautionary tale. *Occup Med* 1994;44:95–98.
39. Beauchamp RO, St Clair MG, Fennell TR, Clarke DO, Morgan KT. A critical review of the toxicology of glutaraldehyde. *Crit Rev Toxicol* 1992;22:143–174.
40. Goncalo S. Occupational contact dermatitis to glutaraldehyde. *Contact Dermatitis* 1984;10:183–184.
41. Hansen KS. Glutaraldehyde occupational dermatitis. *Contact Dermatitis* 1983;9:81–82.
42. Leinster P, Baum JM, Baxter PJ. An assessment of exposure to glutaraldehyde in hospitals: typical exposure levels and recommended control measures. *Br J Ind Med* 1993;50:107–111.
43. Mellstrom GA, Lindberg M, Boman A. Permeation and destructive effects of disinfectants on protective gloves. *Contact Dermatitis* 1992;26:163–170.
44. Lynch DA, Parnell P, Porter C, Axon AT. Patient and staff exposure to glutaraldehyde from Keymend Auto-Disinfector endoscope washing machine. *Endoscopy* 1994;26:359–361.
45. Hogstedt C, Rohlen O, Berndtsson B, Axelson O, Ehrenberg L. A cohort study of mortality and cancer incidence in ethylene oxide production workers. *Br J Ind Med* 1979;36:276–280.
46. Hogstedt C, Malmqvist N, Wadman B. Leukemia in workers exposed to ethylene oxide. *JAMA* 1979;241: 1132–1133.
47. Shore R, Gardner M, Pannet B. Ethylene oxide: an assessment of the epidemiological evidence on carcinogenicity. *Br J Ind Med* 1993;50:971–997.
48. Finelli PF, Morgan TF, Yarr I, et al. Ethylene oxide-induced polyneuropathy: a clinical and electrophysiologic study. *Arch Neurol* 1983;40:419–421.
49. Kuzukara S. Ethylene oxide polyneuropathy: report of 2 cases with biopsy studies of nerve and muscle. *Clin Neurol* 1982;22:707–713.
50. Hemminki K, Mutanen P, Saloniemi I, Niemi L, Vainio H. Spontaneous abortions in hospital staff engaged in sterilising instruments with chemical agents. *Br Med J* 1982;285:1461–1463.
51. Landrigan PJ, Meinhardt TJ, Gordon J, et al. Ethylene oxide: an overview of toxicology and epidemiological research. *Am J Ind Med* 1984;6:103–115.
52. Fuchs J, Wullenweber U, Hengstler JG, Bienfait HG, Hiltl G, Oesch F. Genotoxic risk for humans due to work place exposure to ethylene oxide: remarkable individual differences in susceptibility. *Arch Toxicol* 1994; 68:343–348.
53. Yager JW, Hines CJ, Spear RC. Exposure to ethylene oxide at work increases sister chromatid exchanges in human peripheral lymphocytes. *Science* 1983;219: 1221–1223.
54. Ethylene oxide: evidence of carcinogenicity. NIOSH Current Intelligence Bulletin 35. Springfield, VA: National Institute for Occupational Safety and Health, US Department of Health and Human Services, 1981.
55. LaMontagne AD, Christiani DC, Kelsey KT. Utility of the complete blood count in routine medical surveillance for ethylene oxide exposure. *Am J Ind Med* 1993; 24:191–206.
56. Ribeiro LR, Salvador DMF, Rios ACC, et al. Biological monitoring of workers occupationally exposed to ethylene oxide. *Mutat Res* 1994;313:81–87.
57. van Sittert MJ, Beulink G, van Vliet E, ver der Wall H. Monitoring occupational exposure to ethylene oxide by the determination of hemoglobin adducts. *Environ Health Perspect* 1993;99:217–220.
58. CFR 29 1920-1200. *Federal Register* 1987;52: 31877–31886.
59. Comments on draft OSHA instruction TED 1.15 CH-2 (June 3, 1996), Office of Science and Technology. Anesthetic Agents: Workplace Exposures. Sect V, Chap 2. Chicago: American Society for Healthcare Engineering, 1996.

Medical Center Occupational Health and Safety,
edited by Robert J. McCunney.
Lippincott Williams & Wilkins, Philadelphia © 1999.

10

Latex Allergy and Hand Dermatitis Among Health Care Workers

Elisha H. Atkins and James A. MacLean

Massachusetts General Hospital, Boston, Massachusetts 02114

Latex gloves provide both protection and potential problems for health care workers. The gloves reduce exposure to pathogens such as human immunodeficiency virus (HIV), hepatitis B and C viruses (HBV, HCV), and cytomegalovirus in the blood and body fluids of infected patients, and protect patients from skin bacteria on the hands of providers. Although synthetic alternatives are emerging, latex has been superior to most gloves in its resistance to tears, ability to reseal, impermeability to pathogens, low cost, comfort, and preservation of tactile sensation during use.

Hand dermatitis, both irritant and allergic, has long been recognized as a complication of latex glove use for some health care workers. Over the past decade, a different syndrome that may include contact urticaria, rhinitis, conjunctivitis, asthma, and even anaphylaxis has been increasing in prevalence and recognized as caused by allergy to natural rubber proteins in latex gloves (1,2). Exposure to these antigens and resulting sensitization and symptoms may occur after direct skin contact or respiratory mucosal contact with aerosolized latex particles. Occupational health personnel responsible for health care workers must be able to properly diagnose problems occurring with glove use; educate and accommodate sensitized workers; counsel those at particular risk for future problems; and advocate a preventive strategy to reduce latex exposure to all health care personnel while providing effective glove protection.

PROTECTIVE GLOVES IN HEALTH CARE

The famous surgeon William S. Halstead, it is thought, first introduced surgical gloves to protect the hands of his scrub nurse (later his wife) from the harsh carbolic acid used to sterilize instruments (3). Many in health care and biomedical research still need gloves for protection from chemicals. The prime purpose for others is protection of patients from skin bacteria or protection of health care workers from pathogens.

A variety of glove types are used in health care. Sterile gloves are used for surgical procedures, and single-use, nonsterile gloves are used for rectal, oral, and pelvic examinations. Clinical laboratory technicians often use gloves capable of more prolonged use while still affording protection against blood-borne pathogens. Others need chemical-resistant gloves for handling substances such as chemotherapeutic agents, formaldehyde, glutaraldehyde, solvents, and antiseptics. Most types of gloves used are made from latex, and despite the presence of latex in a wide range of health care products, from blood-pressure tubing to medication bottle stoppers, gloves are the principal source of latex exposure among health care workers.

The term *latex* applied to discussions about rubber is used to describe the milky sap of the rubber tree (*Hevea brasiliensis*), from which natural rubber is isolated. Natural rubber latex is a complex colloidal suspension that contains a wide variety of organic molecules. Natural rubber (*cis* 1,4 polyisoprene) is one of the largest components of natural rubber latex, and it is from this material that rubber products are manufactured. Natural rubber latex also contains a number of proteins. These proteins can remain present in the natural rubber during the manufacturing process and may be present in the end products. Persons exposed to these proteins may become immunologically sensitized, and the sensitization may lead to type I hypersensitivity reactions after repeated exposures.

A number of chemicals (accelerators, antioxidants, and antiozonants) are added to natural rubber during the manufacture of rubber products to improve the properties and extend the life of the end product. Many of these chemicals are capable of sensitizing users, resulting in type IV hypersensitivity reactions (4).

Powder may be applied to gloves after manufacture to facilitate donning. In the early 1980s, cornstarch was substituted for talc as a donning powder because talc had been shown to be fibrogenic. Cornstarch powder is frequently mistaken as a cause of allergic reaction, though studies suggest that immediate hypersensitivity to this agent by itself is extremely rare. Cornstarch powder, however, is an important factor in occupational glove reactions because it can act as a local irritant and cause irritant contact dermatitis and it can adsorb latex proteins and cause allergic reactions when the powder with adsorbed proteins becomes airborne and is inhaled by a susceptible person (5,6). Because the manufacturing process and the design of latex gloves may vary, different brands may have widely different concentrations of latex protein, chemicals, and powder and thus vary widely in capacity to cause health effects.

A number of synthetic materials have been developed as substitutes for natural latex. Vinyl is often used in single-use examination gloves but is too rigid for use in surgical procedures or for prolonged use. Nitrile is a useful alternative to latex for settings in which prolonged use is appropriate, such as clinical laboratories. Five-layer polyethylene gloves confer resistance to chemicals. Several synthetic elastomers have been developed with properties similar to those of latex and can be used for surgical procedures.

CLINICAL MANIFESTATIONS

The spectrum of glove-related illness is wide. Clinical manifestations can be classified as irritant contact dermatitis, allergic contact dermatitis (type IV), or local or systemic immediate hypersensitivity (type I). Most cases of hand dermatitis are caused by irritation rather than by hypersensitivity. Skin changes may range from mild erythema to chronic fissuring and hyperkeratosis. Friction from frequent hand washing, increased heat and moisture under the impermeable glove, and defatting of the skin through use of soaps and alcohol all increase irritation.

Allergic contact dermatitis is difficult to differentiate from irritant dermatitis simply on the basis of clinical presentation. Vesicles and relative sparing of the palms are common but not conclusive features. Rash due to glove chemical allergy tends to involve the dorsa of the hands, the thenar and hypothenar eminences, the wrists, and the distal forearms. Chronic allergic dermatitis may cause thickened, scaling, fissured skin. Agents that cause allergic contact dermatitis among health care workers include glove chemicals, glutaraldehyde (used as an instrument disinfectant), formaldehyde, nickel in instruments, and methyl methacrylate used in bone cement (Table 10-1). Fragrances in moisturizing creams and topical antibiotics may cause sensitization. After initial contact and sensitization, the rash does not appear for at least 5 days. With subsequent exposures, symptoms may begin after as few as 12 hours.

Contact urticaria is the most common initial presentation of type I allergy to latex.

TABLE 10-1. *Chemicals that cause allergic contact reactions in health personnel*

Chemicals used in glove manufactures
Thiuram
Mercaptobenzathiazole
Carbamates
Antiseptics
Glutaraldehyde
Chlorhexidine
Povidone-iodine
Hexachlorophene
Alcohol
Formaldehyde
Methyl methacrylate (in bone cement)
Nickel (surgical instruments)
Skin lotions (fragrances, lanolin)

Hives, usually intensely itchy, occur within minutes on areas of skin in contact with the gloves. Other type I, immunoglobulin E–mediated syndromes may include generalized urticaria, allergic rhinitis and conjunctivitis, angioedema, asthma, and anaphylaxis. A sensitized person may notice sneezing and rhinorrhea, or itchy, watery eyes after exposure to latex. Lip or tongue swelling may occur during work with latex products or during activities outside work such as blowing up rubber balloons.

Symptoms of asthma and reductions in measures of airflow may occur in several patterns. Some workers with latex-related asthma notice the onset of symptoms and have the maximum reduction in peak flow rate within the first hour after exposure. Persons with a late response do not experience the worst symptoms and ventilatory impairment till 6 to 10 hours after exposure. Because the initial symptom in this pattern may be a cough that becomes most noticeable after work hours, the association with latex may not be suspected. Chronic asthma and nonspecific increased bronchial hyperresponsiveness may persist even after removal from exposure to latex (7).

Some patients with latex allergies are at risk for severe systemic anaphylactic reactions, especially if they have substantial mucosal contact with latex-containing products. This may occur, for example, if latex gloves are used when the person undergoes a dental procedure, gynecologic examination, or surgical procedure. In addition to urticaria and bronchospasm, manifestations may include life-threatening laryngeal edema and hypotension. Because persons with latex allergies may have IgE antibodies that react with proteins in certain fruits and other foods (most commonly bananas, papayas, kiwi fruits, chestnuts, and avocados), ingestion of these foods has been reported to cause similar reactions (8).

The natural history of latex allergy is variable. Many reports describe a progression of symptoms that begins with hand dermatitis and proceeds to contact urticaria and systemic type I reactions (e.g., generalized urticaria, angioedema, anaphylaxis). It seems likely that the initial hand symptoms, even if caused by nonspecific irritation or to type IV allergy, predispose the person to type I reactions by allowing transdermal absorption and thus easier sensitization to latex protein.

Symptoms can be caused by a wide range of topical or airborne irritants and allergens besides latex. Contact urticaria is the symptom most highly predictive of type I latex allergy, particularly among patients with a history of atopy; 70% of nurses with atopy and a history of urticaria on contact with latex gloves had positive latex skin prick test results, the most sensitive and specific indicator of type I allergy (see Clinical Assessment) (9). Hand pruritus alone or rash without urticaria is less predictive of type I latex allergy. Health care workers with asthma may have multiple triggers, both irritant and allergic, and airborne latex protein is a possible contributor. When specific inhalation challenge testing with latex protein is conducted in the research setting, approximately 2% of all health care workers have a bronchoconstrictive response (10).

PATHOPHYSIOLOGY

Irritant contact dermatitis results from disruption of the normal skin barrier. The disruption may be caused by a variety of factors associated with glove use, including friction from surgical scrubbing, defatting action of soaps and alcohol, and increased exposure of skin to heat and moisture from occlusion. Allergic contact dermatitis is a manifestation of cell-mediated immunity, or type IV hypersensitivity. Chemicals, such as the accelerators used in glove production, bind with epidermal proteins to form antigenic determinants, which can induce production of specifically sensitized T cells. When they have a second encounter with the same antigen, these sensitized T cells become activated and release lymphokines, which recruit additional cells (macrophages, basophils, neutrophils, and eosinophils) and cause localized contact dermatitis.

Sensitization to latex proteins requires production of antigen-specific T lymphocytes. These cells assist in generation of antibody-secreting plasma cells that produce antigen-specific IgE. The latex-specific IgE then binds to the surface of mast cells, which on subsequent encounters with antigen release cytokines and inflammatory mediators such as histamine, which can cause both immediate and delayed symptoms of urticaria, asthma, rhinitis, conjunctivitis, asthma, and anaphylaxis.

A large number of proteins are present in crude natural rubber latex, and many of these proteins are believed to be immunologically relevant because they induce antibody responses among sensitized individuals (11). Exposure to the protein allergens in latex products may occur through both dermal and respiratory routes. Latex proteins are easily transferred to the skin of glove wearers. Cornstarch used as powder is not itself an allergen but has been shown to bind latex allergens. When it is released into the air with glove use, the powder and the adsorbed allergens may be absorbed through nasal or oral mucosa or inhaled into the lower respiratory tract.

EPIDEMIOLOGY

Irritant contact dermatitis and allergic contact dermatitis related to chemical additives have long been recognized as complications of the use of rubber gloves in health care, industry, and the home. IgE-mediated allergy to latex was not widely reported until the late 1980s. The increasing use of latex gloves as protection against exposure to HIV and other blood-borne pathogens may have been the cause of this rise, though changes in glove manufacture may have allowed higher concentrations of allergenic protein in some cases (12). For individual health care workers, key risk factors for the development of latex allergy are the use of gloves high in latex protein (i.e., highly allergenic), frequency of use, underlying atopy, and a history of hand dermatitis (12,13).

Although latex gloves have been used in health care for many decades, enactment of the Occupational Safety and Health Administration (OSHA) Bloodborne Pathogen standard in 1987 mandated use of latex gloves as a key protective measure against exposure to HIV, HBV, and other infectious agents. Many observers believe that gloves that were hastily made and had insufficient washing and leaching of natural allergens entered the market (14). However, high measurable levels of allergen continued even in the gloves of major manufacturers (15). Instances of latex allergy, initially found among children who needed frequent surgical procedures or indwelling latex catheters (such as children with spina bifida) increased among health care workers as well.

In the general population, latex allergy is rare, particularly among persons with no history of atopy or medical problems requiring frequent exposure to latex, but the prevalence may be increasing. In a study of 800 patients about to undergo surgical procedures, only one was found to have evidence of allergy (16). A more recent study of blood donors, though, found 2.3% of samples strongly positive for anti-latex IgE (17). The cause and importance of this higher figure are uncertain. Use of rubber products or inhalation of latex particles in urban air samples (probably related to use of recycled tires in asphalt production) may be sources of exposure (18).

Not all latex gloves appear to be equally allergenic. Measurable allergens may vary 3,000-fold among gloves from different manufacturers. The highest levels are more likely to cause sensitization through the dermal route, particularly among persons with hand dermatitis, or the respiratory route, particularly if the gloves are powdered. Latex adsorbed on powder is released to a worker's breathing zone as the gloves are donned or removed.

Although the latex protein content of gloves used may influence risk for type I latex hypersensitivity, this risk also increases with work requiring frequent glove use, a history of hand dermatitis, and a history of atopy. The greatest prevalence of both latex allergy and hand dermatitis occurs among persons whose work requires frequent changes of gloves, such as dental staff and surgical and intensive care unit personnel. Among these groups, as many as one-half of workers may report symptoms consistent with irritant dermatitis; considerably fewer have contact urticaria or other likely IgE-mediated symptoms. For example, among pediatric emergency department personnel, 48.4% reported symptoms of dermatitis, and 5.4% reported urticaria. Two of the five members who reported urticaria also had symptoms consistent with allergic rhinitis and conjunctivitis. Employee health staff should remember that not only clinical personnel are affected. Eight percent of hospital housekeepers in one study were found through skin test to have latex allergy (19).

Workers with hand dermatitis, whether it is caused by irritation or type IV contact allergy, are at increased risk for type I allergy to latex protein, probably because of increased absorption of protein through damaged skin (20). A history of atopy also markedly increases risk for latex allergy. Among physicians routinely using latex gloves, none of 38 with atopy but only 1 of 63 without atopy had positive skin prick test results for latex (21).

CLINICAL ASSESSMENT

History

In obtaining a history from a worker who has symptoms, the interviewer should focus on three areas. Is the worker at risk for sensitization because of a history of atopy or extensive exposure to gloves or other latex products on or off the job? Are there symptoms that suggest nonspecific irritation, allergic contact dermatitis, or type I immediate-type latex allergy? Are the symptoms of such severity that immediate job restriction is necessary?

The occupational history should focus on a description of exposures, particularly the type of gloves used by patients and coworkers, the frequency of use, and the environment in which the gloves are used. A listing of soaps and surgical scrub solutions, hand creams, and disinfectants should be obtained. Similar information should be requested about products used at home. A personal or family history of atopic illness, such as hay fever, urticaria, eczema, or asthma, is helpful in establishing the risk for immediate allergy.

The history should include a detailed description of symptoms and their time course, particularly their association with glove use or other work exposures. Skin symptoms should be described in detail to help differentiate true urticaria from erythema caused by irritation. Symptoms of rhinitis (sneezing, rhinorrhea, nasal pruritus) and conjunctivitis (tearing and itching) are the same as those caused by other aeroallergens. Because persons with atopy and latex allergy are more likely to have a history of allergic rhinitis, the timing of symptoms may be particularly important.

The medical history should focus on prior exposure to latex, such as during surgical or dental procedures, and any symptoms suggestive of anaphylaxis. Reactions previously thought to be caused by anesthetics or other medications should be suspected as latex related. A history of local swelling or itching on exposure to balloons, latex condoms, diaphragms, or household cleaning gloves should be addressed. Because persons with latex allergies often are allergic to certain foods, patients should be asked whether they experience perioral itching or urticaria when they eat certain foods, most commonly bananas, kiwi, chestnuts, avocado, or papaya.

Physical Examination

Physical examination often is unrevealing if not performed when symptoms are present. The examination should be focused on the skin, nasal passages, oropharynx, and chest. Evidence of erythema, fissuring, vesicles, and scaling found during the cutaneous examination should be recorded. Evidence of lip or tongue swelling, wheezing during the chest examination, or hypotension necessitates immediate treatment.

Diagnostic Testing

The role of confirmatory diagnostic testing for type I latex hypersensitivity is under debate. In the United States, a standardized latex skin-testing extract is not currently available. Some centers prepare their own extracts from latex gloves or crude latex; anaphylactic reactions to such testing have been reported (22). If latex skin tests are to be performed, informed consent is requested of the patient. Precautions to minimize risk include initial use of a dilute solution, use of a single-prick test, rather than multiple skin pricks or an intradermal test, and ready availability of intravenous fluids and medications such as epinephrine. These tests should be performed by personnel with experience in skin testing and the management of anaphylaxis.

Serologic testing for latex-specific IgE by means of enzyme-linked immunosorbent assay (ELISA) or radioallergosorbent test (RAST) is preferable as an initial test until a standardized skin test is available. These tests, however, generally are less sensitive and specific than skin testing. Latex contains a wide variety of potentially allergenic proteins. ELISA and RAST serologic tests measure antibodies with specificities for allergens that have been immobilized on a solid phase (paper or plastic) material. If the latex source material used in the serologic test does not have the full complement of allergens, the test may produce a false-positive result for persons with no clinical evidence of latex allergy. This result is caused by cross-reactive antibodies directed against a food or other antigen that contains structurally similar epitopes. Serologic testing is more likely to give positive results among persons with systemic symptoms (62%) than among those with contact urticaria alone (27%).

If serologic testing gives negative results but the diagnosis is suggested by a history such as contact urticaria, a use test may be helpful. A glove fingertip is cut off, moistened with water, and placed on the patient's finger for 15 minutes or until a positive result (urticaria) occurs.

Patch testing is used for patients with symptoms suggestive of allergic contact dermatitis. The panel of tests should include the main accelerators and antioxidants used in latex gloves. Information about the chemicals in an individual worker's gloves can be obtained from the manufacturer. Testing might be needed for other chemicals to which the patient is exposed, such as those in antiseptics and hand creams.

TREATMENT

It is likely that early recognition and management of hand dermatitis will lower the chance of later development of immediate latex hypersensitivity and help restore the skin barrier against exposure to blood-borne pathogens. Therapy for hand dermatitis depends on the severity of signs and symptoms. Weeping or vesicular lesions necessitate temporary restriction from work requiring glove use and use of drying compresses or soaks, such as Burrow's solution or Domeboro, four times a day. Oral antihistamines are helpful at reducing pruritus. A 10- to 14-day course of high-potency topical steroids (creams for moist areas, ointments for chronic dry lesions) often is indicated. Emollients are essential for chronic dermatitis. Water-based compounds are preferable to petroleum-based products, because the latter may affect the barrier protection of latex gloves.

All employees with evidence of immediate latex hypersensitivity (contact urticaria, rhinitis, conjunctivitis, asthma, or anaphylaxis) should use only nonlatex gloves (Table 10-2). Although low-protein latex gloves may con-

TABLE 10-2. *Examples of nonlatex gloves*

Surgical gloves
Chloroprene (Dermaprene, Neolon)
Copolymer (Allergard, Elastyren, Tactyl)
Examination gloves
Vinyl, polyvinyl chloride (Sensicare, Tru-Touch, Royal Shield)
Copolymer (Elastyren, Tactyl)
Nitrile (N-Dex)

tain less latex allergen and cause less initial sensitization, they still can cause reactions among persons those already sensitized.

A worker who has experienced allergic respiratory or anaphylactic symptoms must be protected from airborne latex. Transfer of the employee to an area where glove use is minimal may lessen symptoms, but continued use of high-allergen, powdered gloves by coworkers may generate enough airborne latex to cause reactions even though the affected employee uses nonlatex gloves. In one hospital laboratory, after the coworkers of a technician who had experienced anaphylaxis to latex changed to nonpowdered gloves, levels of airborne latex allergen were below the level of detection (23).

Workers with latex allergy should be educated about avoidance of latex both at home and at work. Balloons, condoms, and toys are among the most common household objects that provoke reactions among sensitized persons. Extensive lists of latex-containing products and suitable alternatives are available through the Spina Bifida Association (Table 10-3). Patients who need dental work and women who need gynecologic examinations may find it helpful to bring a pair of nonlatex gloves for the dentist, hygienist, physician, or nurse practitioner to use. A medical alert bracelet and education in the use of an automated injector syringe with epinephrine are recommended for persons with systemic reactions.

Careful preparation is needed for a latex-sensitive patient who needs surgical care. Complete avoidance of latex-containing medical equipment (catheters, tourniquets, and anesthesia equipment) is required. Many hospitals now designate a latex-safe operating room from which all latex-containing medical devices have been removed. Pretreatment with antihistamines and steroids has not been shown to provide additional protection, but is still used in some centers. There is no substitute for scrupulous latex avoidance.

TABLE 10-3. *Examples of latex-containing materials in health care environments*

Anesthesia bags
Blood pressure cuffs
Dressings and elastic wraps
Electrode pads
Endotracheal tubes and airways
Enema apparatus
Gloves
Intravenous access ports
Surgical masks, hats, shoe covers
Oxygen masks, cannulas
Spacers for metered dose inhalers
Suction tubing
Tourniquets

For up-to-date lists and lists of nonlatex alternatives, contact the Spina Bifida Association of America 1-800-621-3141 or access http://www.sbaa.org/html/sbaa_latex.html

Once the diagnosis has been established and counseling and job modification accomplished, employees with more severe reactions such as asthma or anaphylaxis should be carefully observed. Serial peak flow monitoring can show persistent work-related airflow limitation. Workers who continue to have problems may have to be transferred to an area with less glove use and consequent latex exposure, such as an outpatient unit. With early recognition, job accommodation, and environmental remediation, few workers should have to change career.

PREVENTION

Latex allergy and glove-related dermatitis may be to a large extent preventable, but only through a coordinated program of glove selection, training, surveillance, and accommodation. Prevention of irritant contact dermatitis is difficult, because the procedures and materials needed for infection control often place great stress on the skin. However, use of less alkaline soaps and provision of emollients is helpful. Avoidance of sensitizers such as fragrances and lanolin in skin creams and choosing gloves without chemical sensitizers such as thiuram, carbamate, and benzathiazoles will reduce risk for allergic contact dermatitis.

Although latex gloves remain superior to others in barrier protection, comfort, resistance to tears, and preservation of sensation, brands should be chosen that are lowest in allergens and are free of the powder that can adsorb allergens and become airborne. Comparing the latex protein content of different brands of gloves can be confusing because several assays are available, and published data may be out of date. The American Society for Testing and Materials has published a standard test method that allow easy comparison (24).

The Mayo Clinic convened a multidisciplinary task force to implement centralized changes in glove selection and purchasing. Selection of gloves that were powder free and low in latex proteins led to a reduction in levels of latex aeroallergens (25). At Massachusetts General Hospital, a task force selecting gloves used additional criteria of resistance to leaks, absence of or low concentrations of chemical accelerators, and acceptability to staff in clinical trials. As powderless, low-allergen gloves are introduced into clinical areas, shelves, laboratory coats, and medical equipment should be cleaned to remove accumulated powder and adsorbed latex allergen, which otherwise could become airborne when disturbed, causing reactions among highly sensitized persons. Ventilation systems should also be evaluated, particularly if staff continue to experience type I reactions despite the removal of high-allergen, powdered gloves. Systems in which air is recirculated may require high-efficiency filters, and above-ceiling plenums may require cleaning to prevent release of settled allergen during maintenance (McCarty J, Brigham and Women's Hospital, personal verbal communication 1997).

Such changes require institutional commitment, and efforts may encounter obstacles. Surgical staff attempting to maximize their protection against blood-borne pathogens by double gloving may find this difficult with the powderless, less antigenic gloves. Other gloves may have unpleasant odors or tear easily. Exceptions to the hospital-wide choices may be required, for example, for surgeons who find the choices unacceptable. However, highly sensitized staff may not be able to work in spaces where higher-antigen gloves are being used, so efforts must be made to track such use.

Future prevention requires manufacturing changes to lower allergen content and labeling requirements to allow easier comparisons of products. At the end of 1997, a U.S. Food and Drug Administration rule was implemented to require a health warning on latex products (26). Although a statement of the measured latex protein content is not required by this rule, manufacturers may include such information voluntarily. In the future, synthetic materials may replace latex gloves, but they currently cannot replicate all the desirable characteristics and low cost of latex. Until then, occupational health professionals must promote the careful selection and safe use of latex gloves and the prompt identification of employees for whom an alternative material is required.

REFERENCES

1. Sussman Gl, Beezhold DH. Allergy to latex rubber. *Ann Intern Med* 1995;122:43–46.
2. Slater JE. Latex allergy. *J Allergy Clin Immunol* 1992; 94):139–149.
3. Halstead W. Ligature and suture material. *JAMA* 1913; 15:199–225.
4. Fisher AA. Allergic contact reactions in health personnel. *J Allergy Clin Immunol* 1992;90:729–738.
5. Swanson MC, Bubak ME, Hunt LW, Warner MA, Reed CF. Quantification of occupational latex aeroallergens in a medical center. *J Allergy Clin Immunol* 1994;94: 445–451.
6. Tomazic VJ, Shampanie El, Lamanna A, Withrow TJ, Adkinson NF Jr, Hamilton RJ. Cornstarch powder on latex products is an allergen carrier. *J Allergy Clin Immunol* 1994;93:751–758.
7. Brugnami G, Marabini A, Siracusa A, Abbritti G. Work-related late asthmatic response induced by latex allergy. *J Allergy Clin Immunol* 1995;96:457–464.
8. Beezhold DH, Sussman GL, Liss GM, Chang NS. Latex allergy can induce clinical reactions to specific foods. *Clin Exp Allergy* 1996;26:416–422.

9. Lagier F, Vervloet D, Lhermet I, Poyen D, Carpin D. Prevalence of latex allergy in operating room nurses. *J Allergy Clin Immunol* 1992;90:319–322.
10. Vandenplas O. Prevalence of occupational asthma due to latex among hospital personnel. *Am J Respir Crit Care Med* 1995;151:54–60.
11. Kurup VP, Alenius H, Kelly KJ, Castillo L, Fink JN. A two dimensional electrophoretic analysis of latex peptides reacting with IgE and IgG antibodies from patients with latex allergy. *Int Arch Allergy Immunol* 1996;109: 58–67.
12. Hunt LW, Fransway AF, Reed CE, et al. An epidemic of occupational allergy to latex involving health care workers. *J Occup Environ Med* 1995;37:1204–1209.
13. Hunt LW. The epidemiology of latex allergy in health care workers. *Arch Pathol Lab Med* 1993;117:874–875.
14. Charous BL. The puzzle of latex allergy: some answers, still more questions. *Ann Allergy* 1994;72:277–281.
15. Jones RT, Scheppmann DL, Heilman DK, Yunginger JW. Prospective study of extractable latex allergen contents of disposable gloves. *Ann Allergy* 1994;72: 321–325.
16. Turjanmaa K. European medical experiences. In: *Latex protein allergy: the present position*. Proceedings of the International Conference of Rubber Consultants and the European Rubber Journal, 1993:17–19.
17. Ownby DR, Ownby HE, McCullough J, Shafer AW. The prevalence of anti-latex IgE antibodies in 1,000 volunteers blood donors. *J Allergy Clin Immunol* 1996;97: 1188–1192.
18. LeBerthon B, Glovsky MM, Miguel A, Weiss J, Cass G. Latex antibody in asthmatics and blood donors and latex allergens in paved road dust and airborne particles in Los Angeles. *J Allergy Clin Immunol* 1996;97: 324(abst).
19. Sussman Gl, Lem D, Liss G, Beezhold D. Latex allergy in housekeeping personnel. *Ann Allergy Clin Immunol* 1995;74:415–418.
20. Charous BL, Hamilton RG, Yunginger JW. Occupational latex exposure: characteristics of contact and systemic reactions in 47 workers. *J Allergy Clin Immunol* 1994;94:12–18.
21. Arellano R, Bradley J, Sussman G. Prevalence of latex sensitization among hospital physicians occupationally exposed to latex gloves. *Anesthesiology* 1992;77: 905–908.
22. Kelly KJ, Kurup VP, Reijula KE, Fink JN. The diagnosis of natural latex allergy. *J Allergy Clin Immunol* 1994;93:813–816.
23. Tarlo SM, Susman G, Contala A, Swanson MC. Control of airborne latex by use of powder-free latex gloves. *J Allergy Clin Immunol* 1994;93:985–989.
24. American Society for Testing and Materials. ASTM-D 5712-95. Analysis of protein in natural rubber and its products. National Technical Information Service, Springfield, Virginia, June, 1995.
25. Hunt LW, Boone-Orke JL, Fransway AF, et al. A medical-center-wide, multidisciplinary approach to the problem of natural rubber latex allergy. *J Occup Environ Med* 1996;38:765–770.
26. Food and Drug Administration, Center for Devices and Radiological Health. Natural Rubber-Containing Medical Devices; user labeling. *Federal Register* 1997;62(189):51021–51030.

Medical Center Occupational Health and Safety,
edited by Robert J. McCunney.
Lippincott Williams & Wilkins, Philadelphia © 1999.

11

Hazardous Wastes

Randy A. Roig

STC Consulting, Oakland, California 94609

Medical centers generate a variety of chemical wastes, many of which are regulated under federal laws and regulations for method and type of disposal. Most of these wastes are generated in three areas of the medical center—physical plant, laboratories, and pharmacy.

Physical plant operations generate wastes associated with major equipment operation and maintenance. These wastes typically consist of used oils from equipment, solvents used for cleaning, surplus paints, and waste refrigerant from chiller systems. Pollution control equipment, such as ethylene oxide scrubbers, also generates chemical wastes. These wastes typically are few in number but high in volume. Clinic operations generate wastes such as spills from broken mercury thermometers and manometers and rechargeable batteries, which are usually handled through housekeeping and the physical plant. Laboratory and pharmacy operations generate a wide variety of low-volume chemical wastes. Residues from laboratory tests, surplus chemicals and medicines, chemicals used for preparation and preservation of samples, and stains used in analysis of samples accumulate in laboratories and pharmacies.

The primary law that regulates the handling and disposal of wastes is the Resource Conservation and Recovery Act (RCRA). RCRA was passed in 1976, and regulations were developed and implemented in 1980. The act was amended again in 1984. RCRA regulations are exceedingly complex. As of 1998, the regulations composed more than 1,200 pages of the Code of Federal Regulations (CFR). Of these RCRA regulations, more than 40% might apply to medical center operations. These regulations include provisions that regulate the following:

- Waste generation
- Waste storage
- Waste treatment
- Waste disposal
- Emergency response planning
- Employee training

WASTE CLASSIFICATION AND REGULATION UNDER THE RESOURCE CONSERVATION AND RECOVERY ACT

How wastes are regulated by RCRA depends on the following factors: the type of material handled, how the material is handled, and the physical and chemical characteristics of the waste.

The generator of the waste is responsible for determining whether the waste is hazardous and if it is which specific RCRA or state waste code designations describe that waste. Because hazardous waste regulations are complex, the generator must first understand the way hazardous wastes are defined in the regulations. A hazardous waste is a solid waste that has been listed in the RCRA regulations (and is thus predefined as hazardous) or exhibits one of four hazardous characteristics—corrosivity, reactivity, ignitability, or toxicity. Some categories of materials may be hazardous wastes, including acutely hazardous wastes, mixtures containing hazardous waste, universal or special wastes, and excluded wastes, or be regulated under the RCRA as a controlled waste (e.g., used oil). These categories are discussed later (1).

States may add certain tests and stricter standards that cause additional wastes to qualify as hazardous. It is vital for a facility to differentiate federal hazardous waste from state hazardous waste, because different regulatory requirements often apply to each type.

Listed Hazardous Wastes

The Environmental Protection Agency (EPA) has listed approximately 500 specific materials that it considers hazardous to human health or the environment. Any wastes generated, including mixtures, that appear on these lists are considered a federal hazardous waste. Table 11-1 provides a summary of the RCRA listed wastes from 40 CFR 261 Subpart D.

Characteristic Hazardous Wastes

A waste is classified as hazardous if it is ignitable, corrosive, reactive, or toxic. Characteristic hazardous wastes are described with waste codes that begin with a *D*. A waste is *ignitable* (waste code D001) if it can be easily lighted or if ignited burns so vigorously that it produces a hazard. This category includes liquids such as xylene, alcohol, naphtha, or mineral spirits. *Corrosive wastes* (waste code D002) are those that are strongly acidic or basic or cause corrosion in steel. This category of waste includes aqueous wastes with a pH less than 2 or greater than 12.5. *Reactive wastes* (waste code D003) are those that are unstable or explosive. There are few reactive wastes in medical centers.

Toxic wastes (waste code DOO4-DO43) are those that can leach specified toxic constituents above a certain concentration when subjected to a specific leaching test. The list of constituents includes various metals, such as mercury, chromium, cadmium, and lead, and organic materials, such as pesticides and chlorinated solvents. To determine whether a waste exhibits the toxicity characteristic, a sample of the waste must be analyzed with the EPA toxicity characteristic leaching procedure (2). Examples of toxic wastes generated at medical center facilities include batteries and battery acids containing lead or cadmium, mercury compounds from various analytic residues or spills, and fixer solutions containing silver from photographic processing.

Some states have defined additional characteristics for determining whether a waste is hazardous. California and seven other states, for example, regulate persistent and bioaccumulative substances as a subset of toxic wastes. Washington specifically regulates wastes that exhibit carcinogenicity, persistence, and a more broadly defined toxicity. The biologic tests to evaluate carcinogenic substances include determination of acute

TABLE 11-1. *Resource Conservation and Recovery Act list of hazardous waste*

Type	Examples
F wastes	Spent nonhalogenated solvents such as xylene, acetone, and certain ethers and ketones (waste codes F003, F003, and F005). Spent halogenated solvents such as 1,1,1 trichloroethylene (waste code F001).
K wastes	Wastes from specific sources, such as wood preserving with creosote. There are no common medical center wastes in this category.
U or P wastes	Certain unused, discarded commercial chemical products, off-specification products that are listed, empty container or container liners that held the original listed material and have not been appropriately cleaned, and spill residues of a listed material. Common medical center listed materials include acetone (U003), mercury (U151), formaldehyde (U122), and ethylene oxide (U115). Several chemotherapy drugs are U or P wastes.

See 40 CFR 261 Subpart D.

oral, dermal, and inhalational mean lethal doses for defined exceeded threshold limits. Many additional wastes, including glutaraldehyde and ethylene oxide scrubber water (often a dilute ethylene glycol), are considered hazardous under these criteria.

Acutely Hazardous Waste

Acutely hazardous wastes (AHW) are a subset of hazardous wastes that are listed in the P group in appendix A of RCRA. These wastes are subject to a more stringent set of regulations. Facilities that generate 1 kilogram per month or more are subject to regulation. Some states establish similar additional categories for particularly hazardous wastes. Some states use the term *acutely hazardous waste* and others use different names, such as *dangerous wastes* or *extremely hazardous wastes.* It is unusual for a medical center to generate AHW except for the disposal of various chemotherapeutic agents that are on the P list.

Mixtures Containing Hazardous Wastes

The RCRA regulations generally provide that any mixture of hazardous waste and other materials is considered a hazardous waste. This is known as the mixture rule. Any material derived from hazardous waste, such as incinerator ash or residuals of treatment, remains a hazardous waste. This is known as the derived-from rule. Both the mixture and derived-from rules were vacated by a federal court in 1992 for procedural reasons, but the EPA has reinstated them on an interim basis while the agency continues to study the issues.

The EPA mixture rule provides that a mixture of a solid waste and a listed (F, K, U, or P code) hazardous waste usually becomes a hazardous waste from the moment of mixing. Thus the mixture of an F-listed solvent such as xylene with waste oil would be an F-listed hazardous waste even if only a pint of solvent were added to a 200-gallon waste oil tank. If, however, the hazardous waste is listed only because it exhibits one or more of the characteristics of a hazardous waste (ignitability, corrosivity, reactivity, or toxicity), the mixture is considered hazardous waste only if the mixture continues to exhibit the hazardous characteristics. Thus if an ignitable solvent (such as petroleum distillates) is mixed with oil as part of a normal cleaning operation, the resulting mixture would be hazardous only if the mixture were ignitable. Nonhazardous material cannot be added to render a hazardous waste nonhazardous or to dilute any hazardous waste as a substitute for proper treatment and disposal. For example, a facility may not purposely add a spent ignitable solvent to a waste oil tank to render it nonignitable.

The derived-from rule has many consequences for laboratory operations. Cleaning a surface with acetone (an F003 material when used in that manner) and wiping it with a tissue makes the tissue an F001 waste, even if the acetone evaporates from the tissue. By contrast, cleaning the same surface with alcohol would result in a wipe that would be hazardous only if it were ignitable or had some other hazardous residue. The listed character of an F waste carries over to the waste material that was derived from the solvent cleaning operation. Thus it is essential that a facility understand what materials used are listed as opposed to materials that may have a hazardous waste characteristic.

Used Oil

Used oils are recognized by the EPA to be a high-volume waste stream that does not have to be managed fully as a hazardous waste. Used oil has a special set of regulations that are less stringent than those for hazardous waste.

Mixed Wastes

Mixtures of hazardous, biologic or infectious, and radioactive wastes are subject to a complex mix of regulations and must be evaluated very carefully to determine which apply when. In general, radioactive standards take precedence over hazardous waste standards, which take precedence over infectious or biologic waste standards. However, there are exceptions to these rules; facilities should carefully consider the options and requirements when mixed wastes are involved.

HAZARDOUS WASTE GENERATOR CLASSIFICATION

The RCRA is fairly specific in its definition of a generator site. Under the RCRA, a generator is "any person, by site, whose acts or processes produce hazardous waste identified or listed in 40 CFR 261 or whose act first causes a hazardous waste to become subject to regulation." Medical facilities in adjacent buildings are considered to be one site as long as public roads are not traveled or crossed to get from one building to another.

A large medical center that contains intersections of public roads may not be considered a single site if access requires anything more than crossing a public road or traveling along a public thoroughfare such as a sidewalk. Hazardous waste cannot be legally moved along a public road without a manifest. This means that buildings near each other with public roads between have to be considered separate sites. Although many states and EPA regions have recognized the problems this interpretation presents and have made allowances, a strict reading of the regulations can mean that a medical center that consists of several buildings over several blocks may have to have several generator numbers. The resulting inability to consolidate effectively and the increased paperwork contribute to substantially higher waste management costs. Many states allow facilities with buildings directly across a public street from one another to transfer wastes between the sites as long as the transport involves going directly across the street without traveling more than 10 feet along the public highway. Facilities should consult with state regulators to determine how this exemption is interpreted.

Under the RCRA, hazardous waste generators are classified according to the amount of hazardous waste they generate during each calendar month. The federal regulations provide for the following three classes of generators. A *large quantity generator* (LQG) generates more than 1,000 kilograms per month of hazardous waste. Generators of more than 1 kilogram per month of AHW or more than 100 kilograms per month of soil or other material contaminated with AHW also are regulated as LQGs. A *small quantity generator* (SQG) generates 100 to 1,000 kilograms per month of hazardous waste. A *conditionally exempt small quantity generator* (CESQG) generates less than 100 kilograms per month of hazardous waste, less than 1 kilogram per month of AHW, or less than 100 kilograms per month of soil contaminated with AHW. LQGs are subject to the full range of RCRA requirements for generators. Many medical centers are SQGs that although regulated by the RCRA are allowed to follow a number of less-stringent standards.

ACCUMULATION OF HAZARDOUS WASTES

LQGs can accumulate hazardous wastes on site for up to 90 days without obtaining a hazardous waste storage permit, provided that certain container and tank requirements are followed and that all required plans and procedures are in place (see later).

The RCRA allows SQGs to accumulate hazardous wastes for up to 180 days without a storage permit. SQGs whose wastes must be shipped at least 200 miles to a treatment, storage, disposal (TSD) facility can accumulate wastes for up to 270 days. Many states do not extend the normal accumulation time beyond 90 days. The appropriate state agency should be consulted to confirm the allowable accumulation time. If the state time limit is exceeded, the state may require a facility to ship wastes more frequently or to obtain a storage permit. In any case, medical centers that are SQGs may not exceed a total accumulation amount of 6,000 kilograms of hazardous waste at any one time without obtaining a storage permit. An extension of up to 30 days for the accumulation time limit is available from the EPA or the state agency on an emergency basis for a situation in which is is impossible to remove wastes from the site in a timely manner. To obtain such an extension, a facility must apply to the hazardous waste agency before the time limit is reached.

Authorization to accumulate hazardous wastes without a storage permit applies only to the hazardous wastes generated at that facility. Facilities that accept hazardous wastes from other locations required to obtain a TSD facility permit under RCRA part B. RCRA regulations have special provisions for satellite (workplace) accumulation areas. These are areas where the facility can accumulate small amounts of waste near their point of generation and not be subject to the 90, 180, or 270 day limit. These satellite accumulation areas typically are used in laboratories or operations in which 55-gallon drums are not appropriate for storage of wastes. In such locations within medical centers, hazardous waste usually is stored in 1- or 5-gallon containers and then periodically emptied into a larger container in a central storage area. LQGs and SQGs may accumulate wastes in a satellite accumulation area provided that all of the following requirements are met; CESQGs are exempt from these requirements (6):

- A maximum of 55 gallons of each hazardous waste (or 1 quart of each AHW) is stored at a satellite accumulation area.
- The satellite accumulation area is located at or near the point where the wastes are generated and are under the control of the process operator.
- The wastes are stored in containers (not tanks). The containers must be in good condition, compatible with the wastes stored within, and labeled with the words *Hazardous Waste* or other words identifying the contents of the container. (The practice of using an empty glass jug and crossing out the old label should be discouraged. The contents of the container should be clear from the label.) (7).
- Within 3 days after the 55-gallon (1-quart) quantity limit is reached, the wastes are transported off site. A facility may move the wastes on site to a designated hazardous waste accumulation area for an additional 90, 180, or 270 days provided containers are labeled with the date the quantity limit was reached and comply with all additional requirements for accumulation of hazardous wastes (see later).

Many facilities use the satellite rule to increase the flexibility with which they can arrange convenient and cost-effective scheduling of their hazardous waste transport. This allows substantial accumulation of waste at local sites until enough waste is accumulated to reduce the per unit cost of disposal. Of course, these cost considerations must be balanced against the limited availability of space in laboratories and the need for safe working conditions.

Regulatory agency inspectors differ in their interpretation of "under the control of the process operator." The responsibility for managing the satellite accumulation area should be specifically assigned to a person or persons working in the immediate area, and the waste containers or their storage shelf should be clearly visible to that person from his or her workstation. There should be some means of locking or securing the container or otherwise preventing access by unauthorized persons when the assigned person is not present, particularly if it is not possible to locate the waste containers so that they are clearly visible from the workstation.

Some states place additional restrictions on satellite accumulation areas. California, for example, places a 1-year limit on accumulation at satellite areas and requires that the containers be dated at the time waste is first placed into the container to ensure compliance with this time limit. It is a good idea to discuss the requirements for satellite accumulation areas with the local regulatory agency to ensure a facility's practices meet their interpretation of the requirements.

Accumulation in Containers

Specific requirements apply to nonsatellite accumulation of hazardous wastes in containers (8) by LQGs and SQGs (CESQGs are exempt). A container is anything used for storage that is not an immobile object such as a tank, sump, or surface impoundment. A container can be moved when full; a tank cannot. Most "portable tanks" are containers. If there is doubt at the facility, the local inspection agency should be consulted. Containers must be in good condition and compatible with the waste being stored. Waste containers must not be handled in any manner that may rupture them or cause them to leak. A container holding hazardous wastes must always be closed during storage and transfer and opened only when necessary to add or remove waste. If an open funnel is left in a container, the container is considered to be open. Some agencies accept funnels with closed, locking lids, but other agencies do not. The inspecting agency should be consulted before such funnels are used.

Some local jurisdictions have adopted the latest version of the Uniform Fire Code, which requires the hazardous waste container area to have a containment system designed and operated in a manner to prevent hazardous waste migration. The local fire department may enforce other relevant fire code requirements on storage areas inside buildings.

Containers used for accumulation must be labeled with the words *Hazardous Waste* and the date accumulation began. If a container is being moved into the accumulation area from a satellite accumulation area, the label must contain the date the waste quantity limitation was exceeded or the container was moved to the storage area (whichever is earlier). The label must contain the specific words *Hazardous Waste*—not merely a description of the contents. There are additional labeling requirements when the container is removed from the accumulation area for transport.

Any areas where hazardous wastes are accumulated in containers (this does not apply to satellite storage areas), must be inspected. Aside from being a requirement, inspection of such areas is a good management practice. Inspections must be conducted often enough to identify and correct problems before harmful effects manifest themselves. At least once a week, a designated person should inspect the area containing the hazardous wastes and inspect the containers for signs of leakage or deterioration. To prove that inspections are conducted, the facility should maintain records of all inspections in an inspection log or similar summary document. These records should include, at a minimum, the following information: date and time of inspection, name of the inspector, notation of observations made, and date and nature of any repairs or other remedial actions.

Accumulation in Tanks

The RCRA contains specific requirements for the accumulation of hazardous wastes in tanks. Tanks are not commonly used for accumulation of wastes at medical centers.

OTHER HAZARDOUS WASTE MANAGEMENT REQUIREMENTS

Hazardous waste generators are subject to requirements for training of employees who handle hazardous waste, establishment of a contingency plan, development of a preparedness and prevention program, and management of empty containers.

Personnel Training

Personnel involved in hazardous waste management must successfully complete classroom instruction or on-the-job training that teaches them how to ensure the facility's compliance with hazardous waste regulations and to perform their duties in compliance with applicable regulations. Examples of personnel who must be trained are employees who do any of the following:

- Determine waste classifications
- Operate hazardous waste accumulation and satellite accumulation areas
- Move wastes from one part of the facility to another
- Complete manifests and prepare wastes for shipment
- Inspect accumulation areas
- Clean up spills and respond to emergencies
- Supervise other employees who perform these activities

Employees must be trained within 6 months after they are hired, assigned to the facility, or assigned to a new position that requires them to work with hazardous wastes (whichever is later). Employees cannot work unsupervised until they have been trained. An annual review of the initial training is required. Employee training must be documented. SQGs are required to ensure that employees are thoroughly familiar with proper waste handling and emergency procedures relevant to their responsibilities but are not required to implement a formal training program.

Contingency Plan and Emergency Procedures

Each LQG must have a written contingency plan that delineates appropriate procedures to respond to emergencies and releases of hazardous waste to air, soil, or surface water. The emergency procedures must identify at least one employee at the facility (or on call) who is responsible for coordinating all emergency response measures. Each facility also is required to have adequate communication systems, fire fighting equipment, spill control equipment, and decontamination equipment. SQGs are required to have emergency procedures, but a formal program is not required.

Requirements for Handling Empty Containers

When a container that once contained hazardous wastes or contained hazardous materials that if disposed of would be hazardous waste is "empty," it is exempt from the hazardous waste management requirements. The RCRA regulations set forth specific requirements for determining whether a container or inner liner removed from a container is empty. Some states have more stringent standards for management of empty containers. Containers or inner liners that are not empty according to the RCRA or state definition must be managed as hazardous wastes. Some drugs and chemicals are acutely hazardous wastes, and their containers cannot be directly discarded in the trash without triple rinsing. Most rinsates and inner liners that have been removed but not decontaminated must be managed as hazardous waste.

TRANSPORTING HAZARDOUS WASTES

Pretransport Actions

Before hazardous wastes are transported off site, each item must be properly packaged, labeled, and marked in accordance with Department of Transportation requirements. LQGs or SQGs shipping any hazardous waste container smaller than 110 gallons off site must include the following information on the label:

- The words *Hazardous Waste—Federal Law Prohibits Improper Disposal. If found, contact the nearest police or public safety authority or the U.S. Environmental Protection Agency.*
- The generator's name and address
- The manifest document number

Land Disposal Restrictions

Land Disposal Restrictions were established by EPA to eliminate the land disposal of untreated hazardous wastes and to set strict standards on how hazardous wastes must be treated before they are disposed of in or on the land. *Land disposal* includes disposal in landfills, pits, surface impoundments, injection wells, or similar facilities. Land disposal restrictions typically set concentration limits for constituents in a waste or treatment residue or specify the treatment technique that must be used to treat a particular waste before land disposal. There are alternative treatment standards for laboratory packs (several small containers of compatible wastes inside a larger container) and hazardous debris (solid materials exceeding 60 mm in particle size). The main concern of medical centers in regard to land disposal restrictions is preparing documentation for materials being transported to a TSD facility.

Medical centers that intend to ship wastes to an off-site TSD facility must analyze the wastes or use knowledge of the waste stream to determine whether the waste is restricted from land disposal. The TSD facility must be alerted to the appropriate treatment standards for the waste. The medical center must certify that the waste is not restricted from land disposal or must obtain a variance.

The medical center must provide the TSD facility receiving the waste with written notice identifying the waste, the EPA hazardous waste code for the waste, corresponding treatment standards, and the manifest number for the shipment. If the wastes can be land disposed without further treatment, certification to that effect must be provided. Copies of all notices, certifications, waste analysis data, and other documentation must be kept for 5 years from the date the waste was sent to an off-site TSD facility. If the waste does not meet treatment standards—that is, if the waste needs treatment rather than storage and disposal—the TSD must be notified of that fact. Further details of this process are discussed in the *Federal Simplified Guide* (3).

Manifests

The RCRA requires use of a hazardous waste manifest to assure uniform records for all shipments of hazardous waste. States use either the uniform hazardous waste manifest produced by the EPA or their own state manifests. For shipments within states that use their own manifests, the state manifest must be used. When shipping hazardous waste to an out-of-state facility, a generator generally uses the manifest of the receiving state. For more information on out-of-state manifests, the hazardous waste agency in the receiving state, the hazardous waste transporter, or the contracted hazardous waste facility in that state should be consulted.

Under the RCRA, a manifest must be completed in at least four copies. The generator, each transporter, and the destination TSD facility each must have a copy for its records. An additional copy is signed by the TSD facility and returned to the generator. Several states require additional copies.

The medical center is responsible for completing the *generator* and *waste* sections of the manifest and for signing it. The transporter must sign and date the manifest on acceptance of the wastes. The receiving TSD facility signs and dates the manifest on receipt of the waste, gives one copy of the signed manifest to the transporter, and must send a copy of the signed manifest back to the medical center within 30 days. LQGs that do not receive a signed copy of a manifest from the receiving TSD facility within 35 days of the date of shipment must contact the transporter or hazardous waste facility regarding the status of the wastes. If 10 more days pass (a total of 45 days) and it still has not received the signed copy of the manifest from the TSD facility, the medical center must file an exception report with the state agency.

SQGs shipping hazardous waste to a TSD facility or shipping to certain types of recyclers must use a manifest. If the signed copy of the manifest is not received within 60 days of the date the waste was accepted by the initial transporter, the SQG must submit to the EPA a legible copy of the manifest and indicate that confirmation of delivery has not been received. State agencies must be notified as required. Some states may require that exception reporting occur more quickly than is called for by the federal requirements.

The federal regulations allow CESQGs to ship hazardous waste to any authorized TSD facility, recycler, or solid waste facility without a manifest. Many states, however, place additional restrictions on the hazardous waste transportation and management activities of CESQGs.

MANAGING VOLATILE ORGANIC COMPOUNDS IN TANKS AND CONTAINERS

LQGs that store hazardous wastes containing volatile organic compounds (VOCs) in amounts greater than 100 ppm VOC by weight in hazardous waste accumulation areas (not satellite accumulation areas) are subject to regulations that came into effect in late

1996. Most alcohol and xylene wastes are subject to these requirements. In general, a *volatile organic compound* is considered to be any substance that participates in atmospheric photochemical reactions (measured by EPA test method 12, 24, 25, or 26) or any compound that contains carbon and hydrogen in combination with other elements and exhibits a vapor pressure of 77.6 mm Hg or greater under storage conditions. Any waste that evaporates quickly when exposed to air and smells like xylene or alcohol is likely to have a VOC content above the threshold limit of 100 ppm. The material safety data sheets for the raw materials that generated the waste should be reviewed to verify VOC content.

Containers

For storage of VOC hazardous wastes in containers larger than 26 gallons (0.12 cubic meters) the following requirements must be met:

- All containers must be closed except when wastes are being added, removed, or inspected.
- Container covers must not allow detectable levels of organic emissions. This can be demonstrated through testing of the containers for leaks or for containers less than 121 gallons (0.46 cubic meters) through use of a container meeting Department of Transportation requirements (49 CFR 173.2).
- Any warped or ill-fitting lids must be replaced with lids that fit properly.

For transfer of VOC wastes into containers larger than 121 gallons, including "portable tanks," more complex regulations apply. Tank storage of VOC wastes also is subject to more complex regulation.

SPENT UNIVERSAL WASTE BATTERY MANAGEMENT

Owners and operators of facilities that accumulate spent batteries (typically lead-acid or nickel-cadmium rechargeable batteries) before sending them to a reclaimer are subject to a reduced set of facility standards for universal waste handlers. Throwing these types of batteries in the trash is illegal disposal of hazardous waste for those not conditionally exempt SQGs of hazardous waste.

SPECIFIC MANAGEMENT PROGRAMS FOR MEDICAL CENTER WASTES

Mercury

Thermometers and Manometers

Mercury from broken thermometers and manometers is a common hospital waste stream. The spilled materials should be cleaned immediately because mercury that accumulates in cracks is extremely difficult to remove and may expose staff and patients to elevated levels of mercury vapor. Substantial mercury cleanups usually require special protective equipment (gloves and respirators) and if a powered suction device is used, a HEPA-filtered vacuum cleaner dedicated to this purpose. Use of a filter vacuum system without a HEPA filter can expose employees to high concentrations of mercury vapor. Employees who conduct the cleanup should be trained specifically in how to handle mercury spills. This is a requirement under the hazard communication standard and in many states under 29 CFR 1910.120(q) (the so-called Hazwoper regulations). Employees who respond to mercury spills as part of their job and are trained for such response are exempt from Hazwoper. The vacuum cleaner must be marked as a satellite accumulation area for hazardous waste and be handled appropriately. Many hospitals, because of the issues associated with mercury spill cleanups, have moved to thermometers and blood pressure gauges that do not contain mercury, replacing the mercury units as they break. We strongly recommend this practice.

Waste Generated in Laboratories

The Nature of Laboratory Wastes

Laboratory wastes generated within a medical center tend to be small in volume and large in number. Typical wastes include expired laboratory chemicals, specimen preparation residue (fixation, mounting, staining), waste specimens, and solvent and acid waste from cleaning. Simply put, nearly all hazardous waste regulations that apply to industry apply to laboratories. There are, however, some intricacies associated with waste determinations and a few exemptions that apply only to laboratories.

Unique Disposal Options for Laboratory Wastes

Although RCRA, its 1984 amendments, and the resultant regulations have rarely acknowledged the unique situation of laboratories in the development of environmental controls, there are a few situations in which exemptions apply. Perhaps the most important is the laboratory waste water exclusion—40CFR 261.3(a)(2)(iv)(E) and 40CFR 268.1(e)(5). This exemption states that toxic, corrosive, or ignitable waste contained in a laboratory waste water stream is exempt from RCRA as long as the total volume of laboratory waste water does not exceed 1% of the total waste water volume that reaches the facility's headworks. The domestic sewage discharge exemption—40CFR 261.4 (a)(1)(ii)—also may provide allowances for the discharge of hazardous wastes into a public sewer.

These exclusions allow discharge of small quantities of laboratory hazardous waste to the sewer, often without treatment. The medical laboratory, however, must still comply with any local publicly owned treatment works (POTW) discharge limits and prohibitions and federal regulations regarding waste water discharges. For example, under federal regulations (40 CFR 403.12), all facilities that discharge more than over 15 kilograms per month of hazardous waste or any amount of acutely hazardous waste must notify the EPA and the local POTW of the discharge. Furthermore, many local POTW have an absolute prohibition on the discharge of hazardous waste or require advance notification and approval for the discharge, even if the discharge is diluted by other medical center waste streams. Prohibitions and limits apply at the point of discharge, that is, at the laboratory sink. That the effluent is diluted by other medical center wastes is ignored for purposes of determining compliance with the provisions. The concern on the part of POTW is that a pollutant might be discharged that would inhibit the successful treatment of waste or pass through the plant untreated. Specific prohibitions against discharge of waste water to POTW under federal regulations (40 CFR 403.5) include the following:

- Pollutants that create the potential for a fire or explosion hazard in the POTW, including but not limited to waste streams with a closed cup flash point of less than 140°F or 60°C. This is basically all ignitable waste.
- Pollutants that might cause corrosive structural damage to the POTW, but in no case discharges with pH lower than 5.0, unless the POTW system is specifically designed to accommodate such discharges.
- Solid or viscous pollutants in amounts that will obstruct the flow in the POTW, resulting in interference.
- Any pollutant, including oxygen-demanding pollutants, released in a discharge at a flow rate or pollutant concentration that will cause interference with the POTW.
- Heat in amounts that will inhibit biologic activity in the POTW, resulting in interference, but in no case heat in such quantities that the temperature at the POTW treatment plant exceeds 40°C (104°F).
- Petroleum oil, nonbiodegradable cutting oil, or products of mineral oil origin in amounts that will cause interference or pass through.
- Pollutants that result in the presence of toxic gases, vapors, or fumes within the POTW in a quantity that may cause acute worker health and safety problems.

POTW usually also prohibit the discharge of certain toxic metals, such as mercury, and most chlorinated organics, such as trichloroethane acid and trichloroethylene). Many POTW also prohibit the discharge of untreated formaldehyde or formalin mixtures and glutaraldehyde wastes, because both have the potential to cause interference with the biologic treatment processes used at municipal treatment plants.

What can be discharged to the sewer? POTW usually accept the following types of wastes:

- Neutralized acidic and basic solutions
- Treated formalin and formaldehyde solutions
- Small amounts of alcohol-based solutions, such as acid-alcohol preparations, that have a flash point greater than 140°F
- Small amounts of stains that do not contain toxic metals

Off-Specification and Contaminated Chemicals

The requirements for quality control in laboratory operations often mean that the chemical user needs absolute certainty of the purity of a material. A similar assurance applies to certain medicines. When laboratory or pharmaceutical agents expire for their intended use or are no longer used or useful, the laboratory or pharmacy must decide one of the following:

- Can the chemical be requalified to be used for its original purpose?
- Can the chemical be used in another, less stringent, purpose, not necessarily in the same laboratory?

If the answer to both these questions is no, the chemical is considered waste and must be disposed or reused in some manner. There is no formal regulatory definition of when a chemical is no longer used or useful. The EPA and many states take the point of view that if a chemical has not been used within a year and has no certain usage within 6 months, it is no longer used or useful. Accumulation of such chemicals for potential use is considered speculative accumulation under federal waste regulations (40 CFR 260.10); 75% of these chemicals must be used within a year to remain in compliance. Many expired chemicals and drugs are listed wastes and are automatically defined as hazardous. A facility should carefully review disposal of these materials to ensure that they have been properly classified as hazardous or nonhazardous.

Experimental and Research Waste

Experimental and research laboratory wastes can theoretically include millions of compounds. Federal rules for such materials vary widely. For example, these research materials often are exempt from other types of regulations (such as the OSHA hazard communication standard, the laboratory chemical hygiene standard, and EPA Toxic Substances Control Act requirements. Unfortunately, once they become wastes these compounds almost always are subject to the RCRA and must be classified and disposed of according to the requirements listed therein.

Management Techniques for Common Laboratory Waste Streams

The primary function of many types of laboratories is to prepare microscopic slides of tissue specimens for review. Specimens usually are preserved with a formaldehyde or formalin solution before being affixed to a slide. After fixation, alcohol is used to dehydrate and decolorize the tissue before staining. Xylene solutions are used to remove the paraffin used in slide preparation. In some cases, alternative proprietary compounds composed primarily of petroleum naphtha are used as an alternative to xylene. Various methods of preparation are used, but typically the waste streams include one or more of the following: xylene, petroleum naphtha, xylene-paraffin mixtures, formaldehyde, formalin-methanol mixtures, xylene-methanol mixtures, and alcohol mixtures.

With the exception of the formaldehyde or formalin wastes, these materials are usually ignitable (D001) or in the case of xylene listed (F003) or ignitable (D001) depending on use. Although it is possible to reclaim these materials on site for reuse, the economics of such operations and the quality control needed to achieve complete reuse are challenging for the average medical center. Reclamation of spent or contaminated chemicals in the laboratory is a good idea as long as there is a use for the reclaimed product. A number of medical laboratories purchase expensive stills and commit to large solvent recovery programs only to find that the recovered product is not pure enough for the original use. For that reason, most medical centers have concentrated on other waste management techniques.

Calibrated Dispensing of Materials

Use of calibrated dispensing equipment such as pipettes or graduated cylinders has markedly reduced waste in several medical centers. By defining and using only a predetermined amount of alcohol or xylene, laboratories reduce the amount of excess material. In an examination of several medical centers in which this practice was instituted, my colleagues and I found that reduction averaged about 30% (unpublished data).

Use of Less Toxic Substitutes

A petroleum naphtha-based material can be used in place of xylene in slide preparation. Although not as effective as xylene for clearing slides in some applications, these substitutes are highly effective for other applications. Although the amount of waste generated is similar, the cost of disposal of ignitable solvents such as naphtha is much less than that of xylene.

Formalin and Formaldehyde

Formalin and formaldehyde waste streams often can be treated and disposed to the sewer. Several commercial products are available for this treatment. The local sewer treatment plant can determine whether permission is required before such disposal.

Photographic Laboratories

Photographic laboratories, such as that in radiology departments, generate waste fixer that usually contains silver in concentrations that are hazardous under federal criteria (D0011). Local waste water treatment regulations often limit such discharges without treatment. Fortunately, many commercial silver recovery units can precipitate the silver before discharge to local POTW.

Other Specialty Waste Streams

One of the more troublesome waste streams comes from parasitology laboratories. These facilities often use polyvinyl alcohol as a fixative for specimens. Polyvinyl alcohol waste usually contains mercury in quantities that qualify it as hazardous. Substitutes have been investigated but are currently not uniformly acceptable. In most cases, this waste must be disposed as hazardous at high cost.

REFERENCES

1. Crouth, Gary. *How to recognize a hazardous waste (even if it's wearing dark glasses).* Digby Books, New York, New York, 1993.
2. Hazardous waste management system: identification and listing of hazardous waste; toxicity characteristics and revisions—final rule. *Federal Register* 1990 Mar 29:55:11798.
3. Touchstone Environmental. *Federal simplified environmental compliance guide.* Specialty Technical Publishers, Vancouver, Canada, 1989 (updated quarterly).

SUGGESTED READING

ERM—West. Federal environmental audit checklists. Specialty Technical Publishers, Vancouver, Canada, 1993 (updated quarterly).

Medical Center Occupational Health and Safety,
edited by Robert J. McCunney.
Lippincott Williams & Wilkins, Philadelphia © 1999.

12
Ionizing Radiation

Frank X. Massé

Radiation Protection Programs, Massachusetts Institute of Technology, Cambridge, Massachusetts 02139-4307

Ionizing radiation includes electromagnetic radiation (x-rays or gamma rays) or particulate radiation (alpha particles, beta particles, electrons, positrons, or neutrons) capable of producing ions through direct or secondary processes in passage through human tissue. With the ever-increasing use of x-rays and radioactive materials in medicine, more medical center personnel may be exposed to ionizing radiation in the course of their work. Personnel range from highly trained radiation specialists to patient transport workers. Many of these employees have little information about the possible biologic effects of radiation, about amounts that may be significant, about the processes or procedures for minimizing unnecessary radiation exposure, or about levels below which concern may not be necessary. The purpose of this chapter is to provide basic information helpful to medical center personnel in judging the potential risks associated with ionizing radiation exposure related to their work and to guide them toward more comprehensive information.

RADIATION EXPOSURE

The medical care profession today is heavily dependent on the use of ionizing radiation. Radiation has become an integral tool in the prevention, diagnosis, and management of many different forms of illness. Small quantities of radioactive materials are routinely used in medical center research laboratories to learn more about normal body function and disease and to develop means of treating disease. Diagnostic studies such as routine radiographic procedures and nuclear medicine procedures and more sophisticated uses such as computed tomography and cardiac catheterization studies all involve the use of ionizing radiation to provide the necessary detail of both the anatomic structure and the physiologic features of disease or injury in the body. Radiation therapy utilizes the well-established cell-killing capability of ionizing radiation by focusing high levels of radiation on diseased tissue. To continue to derive the benefits of the use of ionizing radiation in medicine, we must continuously control the occupational radiation exposure of allied health personnel.

An understanding of the sources of medical radiation is important to all hospital workers so they may participate in the control effort. It also is important for people to understand the radiation exposure they receive from natural radiation sources. The practice for many years has been to describe the quantity of radiation in terms of exposure measured in roentgens. The roentgen, however, is a unit of exposure in air and does not take into account the effect of absorption in tissue or the biologic effect of the radiation involved. The terms *rad*, for radiation absorbed dose, and *rem*, for roentgen equivalent man, are more commonly used for the absorbed radiation dose in humans. A movement to adopt Système Internationale (SI) units, the gray (Gy) for rad and the sievert (Sv) for rem, has gained favor. The gray is defined as 100 rad and the sievert as 100 rem. Traditional units, rad and rem, are used in this chapter because they are common in the United States, but grays and sieverts are provided in parenthesis wherever exposure is quantified.

Natural Background

Although the amount of occupational radiation exposure varies widely among hospital personnel, all receive predictable amounts of natural background radiation exposure that is unavoidable. Natural background includes cosmic radiation from outer space, terrestrial radiation from the earth's crust, and radiation exposure from naturally occurring radionuclides in the body. Cosmic radiation is typically of very high energy and penetrates and interacts with the earth's atmosphere to generate secondary radiation particles that become sources of exposure to humans. The earth's atmosphere acts as a filter for cosmic radiation. Areas of high altitude, where the air is less dense, contain higher cosmic radiation levels than areas at sea level. Passengers traveling in aircraft at commercial flight altitudes are exposed to even higher levels than persons on the surface of the earth.

Terrestrial radiation comes from the naturally occurring long-lived radionuclides that have been present in the earth's surface since the beginning of time. The intensity of terrestrial radiation varies with location. Some locations contain deposits that may deliver dose rates 100 times higher than the average. These naturally occurring radioactive materials in the earth's crust may become incorporated into building materials, enhancing the terrestrial radiation dose delivered to humans as we surround ourselves with this potential radiation source.

The decay of very long-lived terrestrial sources in the earth's crust results in the emission of a gaseous radionuclide called *radon.* Radon is trapped in buildings and inhaled in enhanced concentrations. Among humans exposure to radon is the highest natural exposure attributable to internal radionuclides. The yearly dose to humans from natural radiation sources is approximately 27 millirem per year (0.27 mSv) due to cosmic radiation at sea level, approximately 28 millirem (0.28 mSv) due to average terrestrial radiation, and approximately 200 millirem (2.0 mSv) whole-body equivalent due to the average dose of radon to the general population in the United States.

Body tissues become a source of radiation exposure to humans because of the presence of radionuclides in the body. Certain naturally occurring radioactive atoms are taken into the body through ingestion and inhalation. They accumulate in tissue and contribute to natural exposure. The most important of these internal sources is potassium 40, a naturally occurring isotope of potassium that is present in all human tissue. These internal radionuclides in our bodies contribute approximately 50 millirem (0.50 mSv) to a person's annual radiation exposure. Natural background radiation is discussed in detail in a report by the National Council on Radiation Protection and Measurements (NCRP) (1).

Medical Worker Exposures

Some hospital employees, particularly those in the radiology, nuclear medicine, and radiation oncology departments, may be exposed to radiation above natural background because their occupation requires them to work closely with sources of ionizing radiation. Such workers are provided with special training in avoiding unnecessary radiation exposure in the course of their work, are provided with special equipment to protect them from the radiation exposure that might be present in their day-to-day activities, and are often specially monitored to measure the amount of radiation exposure they receive as a result of their activities.

Most hospital employees are not considered occupationally exposed workers but may occasionally come in contact with sources of radiation in their regular duties. For example, nurses or physicians may come in contact with nuclear medicine patients who have received and still retain radioactive materials for diagnostic purposes; operating room and intensive care personnel may be required to work close to portable radiographic equipment; and nurses and dietary personnel may be required to tend to patients who are undergoing radiation therapy with implanted radioactive sources. Maintenance workers or security personnel may have to work in areas where there may be peripheral exposure from nuclear medicine or radiographic sources. Even janitorial personnel may experience very low level exposures while cleaning the nuclear medicine department or research laboratories that use radioactive materials. All such exposures in hospitals must be carefully controlled. A method must be devised to provide controls in a reliable way. Personnel experts in radiation protection must play an active role in controlling exposures, and all personnel must be advised of any appreciable exposure they might receive.

Exposure Limits

Occupational and public exposure limits have been established by federal and state regulatory agencies. These limits apply to all exposures received by a radiation worker as a result of his or her occupation or a member of the public as a result of the operation of a facility such as a medical center. These limits do not include natural background radiation levels over which the facility has no control. They also do not include deliberate exposures delivered to a patient for diagnostic or therapeutic purposes, even when the patient is also a radiation worker. Occupationally exposed radiation workers are limited to an annual effective dose equivalent of 5 rem (50 mSv) from the workplace. The dose equivalent limits for the general public from the facility are one-tenth those for occupationally exposed persons. Partial body exposures and exposures of individual organs are controlled by establishment of weighting factors on the basis of the radiation sensitivity of the organ or body part. Current regulations restrict the annual dose to the organ most highly exposed for occupational purposes to no more than 50 rem (500 mSv). Occupational exposure to workers younger than 18 years are restricted to the limits applicable to the general public.

Occupational exposure of pregnant radiation workers is an area of special concern. Regulations prescribe specific limits for pregnant workers, restricting the dose to the fetus to no more than 500 millirem (5 mSv) in the gestation period. Pregnant radiation workers are urged to report to their employers as soon as the pregnancy is known so that special precautions can be taken to limit the fetal radiation dose. It is recommended that the dose to the fetus be delivered gradually through the gestation period so that no more than 50 mrem (0.5 mSv) is received in any 1-month period to avoid the potential for peak exposure at a time when the developing fetus is most sensitive. Special monitoring is generally provided for pregnant radiation workers. Because it is not practical to monitor the fetal dose directly, a monitoring badge usually is worn on the surface of the mother's abdomen. The measurement generally overestimates the dose to the fetus because the mother's overlying tissue provides radiation shielding for the fetus.

Occupational exposure may involve ingested or inhaled radionuclides, as in research or a nuclear medicine program. These internally deposited radionuclides contribute to the occupational dose. The total dose to the worker must be assessed with both the external dose measurable with the film badge and the internal deposition of radionuclides caused by ingestion or inhalation of radioactive materials. The total dose must be within the occupational limits indicated earlier (2,3).

Dose Minimization Philosophy

A general philosophy suggested for many years and now formally adopted requires that radiation protection programs be operated such that occupational exposures are held as low as reasonably achievable (ALARA). The regulations state that economic and social factors must be taken into account when determining what is reasonable with respect to minimizing unnecessary exposure. Radiation exposure regulatory guidance applicable to medical institutions implies that limiting occupational exposure to less than 10% of the maximum permissible exposure satisfies the ALARA requirement. The ALARA philosophy is considered a commitment on the part of a facility to take practical actions to minimize unnecessary exposure and to keep occupational doses low.

The ALARA approach to radiation exposure management requires participation by the worker. Workers are expected to review their own work responsibilities and make suggestions about reduction of unnecessary exposure. Training programs must include a review of ALARA principles and examples of worker action to reduce exposures through the ALARA program. The effectiveness of the ALARA principle in radiation protection is evidenced in a rate of occupational exposures in medicine well below 10% of the maximum permissible occupational exposure (4).

BIOLOGIC EFFECTS

Soon after ionizing radiation was first used in medical practice, approximately 100 years ago, it rapidly became known that excessive radiation exposure may cause detrimental effects to the recipient. Early radiation workers were observed to suffer detrimental effects months to years after initial exposures in which little care was taken for worker protection. Loss of hair and reddening of the skin among early radiologists and dentists using diagnostic x-rays led to efforts to begin controlling occupational radiation exposure. The radiation doses involved in those early exposures were hundreds to thousands of times those received by today's medical workers because little or no protection was provided for early workers in general practice. Gradual improvement in worker protection was seen through the beginning of World War II, and the increased emphasis on radiation applications after the war heightened emphasis on radiation safety.

Immediately after World War II, a massive study was initiated to investigate the effects of radiation on the survivors of the atomic bombings of Hiroshima and Nagasaki. These studies continue today. Hundreds of thousands of Japanese survivors are being observed for radiation effects. The studies include efforts to determine the radiation dose each of these survivors received. Other populations studied include medical populations treated with radiation for benign disease. Numerous radiobiologic studies have been conducted on animals and on cells to add to the knowledge of radiation effects.

There is little question that acute radiation received in large doses (20 rem [200 mSv] or more) represents measurable risk to the recipient. Biologic effects on atomic bomb survivors appear to correlate well with radiation doses of 20 rem or more; there is an approximately linear relation between dose and effect. At less than 20 rem the risks are smaller or at least proportional to those of smaller doses. That is, one-tenth the dose would result in at most one-tenth the effect, perhaps less. Because the risk at smaller doses is small, and because the possibility of other competing nonradiation causes may result in similar effects, it is difficult to see radiation effects at low dose levels. Radiation protection efforts are aimed at eliminating the probability of any observed effects of occupational radiation exposure.

Radiation-induced diseases are generally divided into two categories: stochastic effects and nonstochastic effects. *Stochastic* effects are those for which the probability of occurrence increases with increasing radiation dose but the severity among affected persons does not depend on the magnitude of the absorbed dose. A stochastic effect, once it occurs, is an all or nothing type of response as far as individuals are concerned. The increase in radiation dose simply increases the probability that an effect will occur. With *nonstochastic* effects the severity of the effect increases with an increase in dose. Nonstochastic effects are thought to involve the presence of a threshold below which the effect is unlikely to be observed. An example of a stochastic effect and perhaps the one with which radiation protection experts are most concerned is cancer. An example of a nonstochastic effect is eye lens opacity or cataracts, which have now been demonstrated to have at least an effective threshold. Radiation protection limits have been set such that the risk for occurrence of stochastic effects is small compared with the normal risks of everyday life. For nonstochastic effects, the limits are set such that the threshold is never crossed. The most complete current reference on biologic effects of ionizing radiation is the National Academy of Sciences BEIR V report (5).

Acute Effects

Acute radiation effects are those that appear within a short enough time after exposure to make it obvious that radiation was the cause. These were the effects observed by the very early radiation workers, the effects that led to early efforts at radiation protection. Such effects include erythema, epilation, nausea, and diarrhea. Acute affects usually are seen only after exposures that are very high typically 100 rem (1 Sv) or higher, and to the entire body. The early injuries experienced by workers attempting to control the fire at the Chernobyl power reactor are typical of acute radiation effects. The severity of such effects depends on the amount of radiation received and the percentage of the body exposed. The potential for occupational exposures that would result in acute effects generally does not exist in medical facilities.

Cancer

The most serious delayed effect of radiation is cancer. It takes years to decades for cancer to manifest after radiation exposure, thus linking the disease to the radiation exposure is difficult. As with the atomic bomb survivors, this linkage may be made only through statistical studies involving persons who have received known radiation exposures. These persons must be observed long enough to aid in differentiating the normal incidence of cancer applicable to all humans and the slight excess expected when radiation exposure is involved. It is generally agreed that the normal lifetime risk among the U.S. population for acquiring cancer is 33%. This rate increases about 1% with accumulated occupational exposure of 10 to 20 rem (100 to 200 mSv) (5). An increase in cancer incidence was found among some early radiation workers, notably radium dial painters and uranium miners. Current exposure levels are so low that there is no observable excess incidence; if any increase exists, it is statistically undetectable.

Genetic Effects

Genetic effects of radiation are those that are transmitted to the offspring of an exposed person. Radiation can affect the germ cell nucleus and break or alter molecular bonds; the damage can result in mutation or chromosomal breakage. The damage can manifest itself in malformation of offspring. The probability of radiation-induced genetic effects of occupational exposures is very low. The atomic bomb survival data indicate no detectable genetic effects for the survivors and their offspring. Although genetic effects still are listed as a radiation exposure concern, the levels to which occupational workers in the medical profession are exposed would generally place the concern for genetic effects at a negligible level.

Embryonic and Fetal Effects

Exposure of the embryo and fetus is of particular concern because of the rapidly dividing and hence more radiosensitive cells of the developing fetus. The amount and type of damage induced by radiation exposure depend on the stage of development at which the fetus is irradiated and on the absorbed dose. The limits applicable to a pregnant radiation worker are based on these considerations. The recommendation to divide the dose to the fetus evenly through the gestation period is to avoid risk for peak exposure during the more sensitive developmental stages. The risk decreases during the third trimester, when the fetus is more fully developed. Radiation exposure during pregnancy is generally held as low as can be reasonably achieved.

MEDICAL CENTER SOURCES OF OCCUPATIONAL EXPOSURE

X-Ray Machines

X-ray machines produce x-rays electronically by bombarding high currents of electrons against special targets to generate secondary x-rays of an energy desired for medical diagnosis or treatment. These x-ray sources are housed in heavily shielded, properly collimated systems such that the useful beam is directed and focused as necessary for diagnosis or treatment. The x-ray sources are equipped with filters to eliminate the low-energy portion of the spectrum that is rapidly absorbed in surface tissue and hence has no useful function in the medical application. The systems are designed with redundant safety devices to minimize the probability of accidental exposure. Their use in medicine is restricted to medical doctors and licensed or registered radiologic technologists. The equipment is designed such that x-rays are produced only when the exposure switch is engaged, and even that switch (should it become faulty) is backed up by an emergency timer to terminate the exposure. There are no residual x-rays in the room once an exposure terminates, and the patient undergoing an x-ray procedure does not become radioactive and does not represent a risk to other people simply because he or she has had a radiograph obtained. X-ray exposures to patients and hence to occupationally exposed personnel have been gradually reduced with better equipment design, use of faster film and better-enhancing screens, and use of more automated, computerized systems, which minimizes the need for repeat exposures.

Diagnostic radiographic procedures are generally performed in the radiology department by physicians who have been specially trained in radiology. In large medical centers, radiographs may be obtained by other physician specialists in operating suites, intensive care units, special care facilities, or coronary care units. The most complex of such facilities, cardiac catheterization laboratories, may use the highest levels of diagnostic radiation. Such widespread use indicates that all hospital personnel need to be familiar with radiation protection when using x-ray–producing equipment (6).

Nuclear Medicine Radiopharmaceuticals

Nuclear medicine involves the use of artificially produced radiopharmaceutical agents for the diagnosis and management of disease for patient inside and outside hospitals. Nuclear medicine has developed to the point at which special short-lived radiopharmaceutical agents are used for dozens of routine diagnostic procedures. The most notable radionuclide is technetium 99m, a gamma-emitting radionuclide with a half-life of only 6 hours. Technetium 99m is used because of its relatively short half-life, its ideal gamma-ray energy of 140 kV, and its ability to combine with a variety of molecules to target many different organs.

Most diagnostic procedures in nuclear medicine involve direct measurement of the amount or distribution of a radiopharmaceutical agent administered to a patient with a gamma camera. Gamma cameras have a very high efficiency and can function with administration of relatively small quantities of radiopharmaceutical agent to the patient. After administration of the radioactive tracer, images are obtained in the region of interest either immediately for observation of the dynamic process of pharmaceutical uptake or after enough time has elapsed for the radiopharmaceutical agent to be collected in an organ. Other nuclear medicine diagnostic techniques entail use of radioactive tracers for laboratory analysis of body fluids from patients. Such analyses generally do not involve administration of radioactive material directly to the patient. A NCRP report (7) describes choice of radionuclides and handling precautions for diagnostic radionuclides.

Radiopharmaceutical therapy conducted in leading centers involves administration of radionuclides compounded to localize in diseased tissue known to be effectively treated with radiation. The radioactive drug localized in the diseased tissue becomes an internal radiation source within the tissue. Such an arrangement ideally maximizes the radiation dose where it is most beneficial and minimizes the dose to surrounding healthy tissue. Relatively large doses of radiopharmaceutical agents are used for this therapy, and patients undergoing such therapy become a substantial source of radiation exposure to caregivers. Radiation protection considerations are extremely important in radiopharmaceutical therapy (8,9).

Accelerators

Accelerators are used for practically all external-beam radiation therapy. Accelerators produce high-energy x-rays for management of deep-seated tumors or high-energy electron-beams for tumors that are closer to the surface. Like x-ray machines, most accelerators do not emit radiation unless energized. Therefore there is minimal risk for radiation exposure to personnel or patients during positioning for treatment before the machine is turned on. Like x-ray machines, most medical accelerators do not operate at high enough energy to induce radioactivity into the materials they bombard. After the machine is shut off, there is no residual radiation field. Accelerators are operated in heavily shielded and tightly restricted treatment rooms. These rooms are carefully interlocked so the machine cannot be turned on until all necessary precautions have been taken and the patients are properly positioned for treatment. Final steps before treatment include providing interlocked assurance that no medical personnel are present in the room. Occupational exposure to those associated with the operation of treatment accelerators is comparable with that for x-ray workers (6).

Brachytherapy Sources

Some cancers are treated with sealed radioactive sources. A source capsule is placed directly in tissue, in a body cavity, or on a body surface for a brief period under controlled circumstances. The source is removed before the patient is discharged. Such treatment is called *brachytherapy,* and it is usually performed in a hospital in a sequestered area by specially trained medical personnel (10). The external radiation level from patients undergoing brachytherapy necessitates use of special precautions for both health care personnel and visitors. In most medical institutions, medical staff trained in general terms for care of brachytherapy patients also are specifically trained for each type of treatment just before a patient admission. Training includes specific precautions for the patient and type of treatment involved. The area receiving the implant is identified, and the staff is given instructions and precautions on the handling of the radiation source should it become dislodged.

The latest techniques involve high-dose-rate brachytherapy in which very-high-output sources are remotely implanted in patients for brief periods of time in a confined, shielded room such as is used for an external-beam accelerator. With high-dose-rate, remote-loading devices such as this, radiation exposure to medical care personnel is eliminated because no personnel are present in the room during the treatment.

The brachytherapy treatments requiring the least occupational radiation protection are those involving long-term, permanent sources implanted in patients in a hospital but that stay in place throughout the decay process. These sources are of such low dose rate and so nonthreatening to personnel that patients are allowed to go home with the sources in place.

Research Materials

Biomedical research programs in larger medical centers may use ionizing radiation sources of concern to medical staff. Such programs often handle large quantities of radioactive tracers in biomedical research. These tracers typically are longer lived than the radioactive materials used in nuclear medicine and require different management and programs. Ingestion or inhalation of such materials may result in much higher doses than would accumulate with similar quantities of the radionuclides used in nuclear medicine. In addition, special x-ray equipment, such as x-ray diffraction units, often is used for analytical purposes in research facilities. Larger programs may even include research cyclotrons for production of experimental radionuclides or for diagnostic or therapeutic research and development programs. Because research and development programs frequently change procedures and handling techniques, the risk for occupational radiation exposure is higher than in routine nuclear medicine programs. Workers in research programs must be diligent about ever-changing procedures, and safety must be paramount.

RADIATION PROTECTION PROGRAM

Medical centers that use radiation sources such as those described earlier are required to establish a formal radiation protection program for the ongoing management of all such radiation sources. The program must be instituted by the medical center's highest authorities, who must provide adequate support and funding to carry out the program in a responsible way. The support of management must be openly visible so that all medical center personnel recognize the importance of such a program and work closely to see that regulations are followed. Inherent in the establishment of such a program is the requirement that management maintain close contact with and vigilance over the program. A senior management official should oversee the routine operation of the program and initiate audits of program function and effectiveness at least annually.

Radiation Safety Officer

A key person in the organization of the radiation protection program is the radiation safety officer, who should be appointed by senior management. The radiation safety officer must be qualified by training and experience to provide the expertise required in a position of this nature. Several academic programs provide specialty training in radiation safety at the masters or doctorate level, and such specialty training is strongly advised for a person with this responsibility. Certification through the American Board of Health Physics or the American Board of Medical Physics is conferred on experienced radiation safety personnel who have passed an examination to establish their credentials. The radiation safety officer must be provided with sufficient management support and resources to establish the appropriate staff necessary to conduct the program in a responsible manner. Resources should include additional personnel to help with day to day management and monitoring techniques and the equipment needed for radiation measurement and monitoring (11) associated with the program.

Radiation Safety Committee

Licensing requirements in state and federal regulatory programs generally require organization of a radiation safety committee in a medical center with multiple sources of ionizing radiation. The size of the committee is dictated by the size of the program. Most membership requirements include a committee member from each department in which radiation sources are handled or used. The primary responsibility of the committee is development and maintenance of an effective radiation safety program for the medical facility. The committee defines the program that the radiation safety officer directs. The committee members must have adequate knowledge of radiation protection issues and procedures. Upper management must be represented on the committee, as should nursing. The committee should meet frequently, typically quarterly, to keep in close touch with the ongoing operation of the program and to receive timely reports of the day to day operation. Such a committee is typically chaired by a prominent member of the medical staff, who can assist the radiation safety officer as necessary in securing compliance in difficult situations.

Procedures and Regulations

Sources of ionizing radiation, both radiation-producing equipment and radioactive materials, are extensively regulated at the state and federal levels. Licensing of radioactive materials by the federal Nuclear Regulatory Commission or a comparable state authority and registration of radiation-producing equipment by state health agencies is required for all sources of potential exposure. A radiation protection program must include carefully drafted procedures to be followed by all persons who work with such materials or equipment. The radiation protection committee and radiation safety officer must work together to adopt appropriate procedures to cover all aspects of the program in the institution. All radiation workers must have knowledge of and access to all applicable procedures and regulations to assure compliance and to achieve the required level of radiation safety. All programs involving the use of ionizing radiation sources are subject to periodic audits by the licensing or registering authorities. The programs can best achieve satisfactory audits by preparing and adhering to complete and detailed procedure manuals, guidance documents, and up-to-date regulations applicable to their work. The management of the institution is responsible for full compliance with all regulations.

Training

All personnel involved in the use of sources of ionizing radiation must be adequately trained in the work they are assigned to perform. In most jurisdictions, key personnel such as radiologic technologists and nuclear medicine technologists are required to be registered or licensed to demonstrate their proficiency. Other persons who handle radiation sources must be trained in the procedures of the institution and in the applicable regulations. Training usually is required before work begins and must be refreshed at least annually. The level of training generally is commensurate with the responsibility of the individual, the amount the radioactivity he or she must handle, and the type of work assigned involving radiation-producing machines. For professionals who are specifically trained and licensed or registered in ionizing radiation procedures, refresher training generally involves a requirement for continuing education credits sponsored by or acceptable to the licensing agency or registering body. Management must provide reasonable opportunity for radiation workers to acquire the training necessary to perform their duties and maintain their professional status (12).

Records

Proper maintenance of adequate records to demonstrate all aspects of an operating program's complete compliance with all regulatory procedures is a key part of any radiation protection program. These records must be clear and concise and adequate to provide the means for thorough internal audits and must be kept in the form required by the regulatory authorities to facilitate proper access for regulatory audit. At a minimum, the records must address every regulatory requirement applicable to the program. Records maintenance involves program managers, such as the committee and the radiation safety officer, and individual users. Records to satisfy requirements such as daily and operational surveys and radioactive material security must be kept by the persons directly responsible. Management is ultimately responsible for full compliance with record-keeping requirements. The Code of Federal Regulations, Title 10, Part 20 (3) contains detailed record-keeping requirements for reactor-produced radioactive materials. State regulations must be followed for accelerator-produced radionuclides and radiation-producing equipment.

RADIATION PROTECTION PRINCIPLES

The principles of control of radiation sources are applicable to the many varieties of radiation sources in use. The following is a brief description of the most basic principles applicable to all programs.

Exposure Control

Ionizing radiation emanating from radioactive materials or radiation-producing equipment generally is controlled in a limited number of ways. The three basic principles applicable to radiation control are restricting the time of exposure, maximizing the distance from the radiation source, and use of appropriate shielding to absorb the radiation from the source. Length of time personnel are exposed to radioactive materials is controlled by minimizing the time between removal of the material from its shielded storage container and positioning. With radiation-producing equipment, the amount of time during which the machine is operated is controlled. In situations in which the radioactive materials are exposed continuously or the machine is operating continuously, the period of time in which individuals are in the presence of the source is limited.

Distance affects radiation dose rate the same way distance affects light intensity from a light bulb. The exposure rate from the source decreases by the square of the distance from the source; doubling the distance reduces the exposure rate by a factor of four. A tenfold increase in distance reduces the intensity by a factor of one hundred. The use of distance is a very important radiation protection technique.

Shielding is perhaps the most important tool for exposure control. Walls of radiology rooms always have a lead lining to prevent x-rays from extending into the corridors and surrounding rooms. Radioactive materials are always housed in lead-shielded containers to absorb the emitted radiation from the source. Therapy departments use massive shields, typically 2-foot or more thicknesses of concrete or several inches of lead to control the very high radiation levels that are involved in cancer treatment with external beam accelerators. The extensive use of shielding is required by all regulations and is heavily factored into all programs (13).

Surveying and Monitoring

One great advantage workers have in handling radiation sources is the ability to readily measure the radiation levels involved in a given procedure. Relatively inexpensive survey equipment can be used to make accurate and rapid measurements in work settings and provide workers with a sixth sense in working with radiation sources. All radiation workers must be thoroughly trained in the proper use of survey equipment. The training should emphasize the need for frequent measurement of radiation levels in all steps of a procedure involving potential exposure.

Monitoring of accumulated radiation doses to radiation workers or to areas accessible to members of the general public also can be readily accomplished. The well-recognized film badge for monitoring radiation workers is a widely accepted device that provides accurate, prompt, and inexpensive measurement of the quantity of radiation exposure a worker receives. Regulations specifically require at least minimal personnel monitoring to demonstrate that regulations are being followed and dose limitation requirements are being met. Areas accessible to the general public where the potential for radiation exposure exists may be monitored in a way that is not specific to any person. An example is the waiting room in a radiology or nuclear medicine department, where dose rates may be considerably greater than background levels but less than levels at which access control is required. To document that no individual member of the general public is receiving excessive exposure, it is a common practice to strategically place area monitoring badges. The readings from these badges can be used to provide sufficient evidence that adequate control has been achieved.

Control of Radioactive Material

Regulations of the licensing authority are specific in the requirement that all radioactive materials be controlled so that they are accessible only to the radiation workers and are properly secured to prevent unauthorized use or removal. Regulations define control as either secured in a locked area accessible only to radiation workers or under the direct surveillance of a radiation worker who can assure that no unauthorized person gains access or receives excessive exposure. Regulatory audits focus heavily on the control of radioactive materials, particularly when control depends on surveillance. Surveillance is generally interpreted as direct visual control. Users of radioactive materials generally follow a policy of locked storage of all radioactive materials not in immediate use. The locked storage rule for radiation sources is applied 24 hours a day even while the laboratory is occupied and radiation workers are present. It is generally considered easier and more reliable to unlock the storage area to gain access for the occasional removal of material that will be in active use than it is to try to maintain surveillance over multiple sources spread around the laboratory through the course of the day for uses that may or may not occur during the work shift.

Control of Radiation-producing Equipment

The most common method of controlling access to and operation of radiation-producing equipment is to restrict access to the equipment to persons registered in its use. X-ray machines are generally provided with a key lock for such control. Proper control of key access is particularly important for portable radiographic equipment. Years ago it was not uncommon to see a number of portable x-ray machines parked along the corridor of a radiology department for battery recharging, each with the operating key in the console. Enforcement has resulted in better compliance such that access to or unauthorized use of this equipment is now much better controlled. The state health authority that regulates such equipment is specific in the control of access to such equipment, and the equipment must be labeled by the manufacturer with clear instruction on the limitations and restrictions on its use.

Posting and Labeling

Just as the equipment for producing x-rays must be properly labeled by the manufacturer, regulations are specific on the labeling of radioactive materials. Radioactive materials in use or being transported through the hospital for administration to patients must be clearly labeled and properly shielded with adequate containment to protect others even if the person responsible for the materials were to become suddenly incapacitated. The labeling must be clear and concise and fully descriptive of the radioactive material present. The many different radiopharmaceutical compounds in the nuclear medicine department must be clearly and concisely labeled to avoid errors in administration of radioactive drugs. A rigid color-coding scheme frequently is adopted to provide the nuclear medicine technologist with a simple method of differentiating the many compounds used for different medical procedures.

Labeling techniques and practices must be known by all persons working in the program and must be backed up with full documentation to avoid any possible confusion. All areas or rooms in which radiation levels are elevated above background must be properly posted to warn those entering the area of the potential for an increase in radiation exposure. All rooms in which radioactive materials are in use must be properly posted to warn of the presence of such materials. Labeling and posting requirements are carefully spelled out in the regulations and are subject to internal and external audit. Full compliance is the responsibility of management. Posting and labeling requirements are fully covered in the Code of Federal Regulations, Title 10, Part 20 (3).

RADIATION PROTECTION CONCERNS BY PROFESSION

This section offers a brief summary of the principle radiation protection concerns to be considered by each specialty in the medical setting. It is not intended to provide complete instruction on how to achieve adequate radiation protection for each of these categories but to provide a summary of the issues that need to be considered.

Diagnostic Radiographic Technologists

Diagnostic radiographic technologists are required to receive extensive formal training before being allowed to perform medical diagnostic procedures on patients. They must continually refresh their training and remain up to date as radiographic procedures improve and equipment is updated. However, certain basic rules generally apply to assure radiation protection of workers and patients (7).

The first requirement is that posted equipment operating procedures be followed explicitly. Radiographic operators must be fully aware of all aspects of the equipment and must follow the manufacturers recommended procedures in the use of the equipment. Collimators must be adjusted to optimize the field of view for the diagnostic procedure to be performed. It is imperative that the field be large enough to accomplish the task without exposing areas not required. Adjustable filtration must be properly set depending on the x-ray energy involved in the diagnostic procedure. Proper filtration optimizes the radiation exposure a patient receives and eliminates low-energy photons that do not contribute to the diagnostic image. Equipment parameters must be selected to maximize the probability of achieving the diagnostic information sought in the prescribed examination. If motion is a potential problem in the area of the body being examined, techniques must be chosen to minimize exposure time and thus reduce the probability of motion artifacts. The patient and radiation source are positioned in the room so that the primary beam is directed to minimize potential exposure to the operator. The operator must be inside the control booth when the exposure is made to minimize exposure to stray radiation.

Technologists must avoid holding patients during diagnostic procedures. Proper use of restraining devices should eliminate the need to hold patients under almost all circumstances. On the rare occasion when a patient must be held, such as a pediatric examination, the preference is to ask a parent to hold the child. A parent would rarely be exposed to diagnostic radiation, eliminating the need for radiographic personnel to become repeatedly involved in this way.

Personnel monitoring must be properly worn by the technologist so that the maximum radiation dose is recorded. The monitor badge must be properly stored so that it does not receive exposure when not being worn, and it must be processed in a timely manner to maximize the value of the data obtained.

The use of mobile radiographic equipment warrants special safety procedures. Technologists using mobile equipment should wear an apron, control the equipment to optimize beam direction relative to surrounding patients or other medical personnel, avoid unnecessary exposure wherever possible, and operate the equipment as remotely as possible by extending the control cord.

The use of protective clothing such as a lead apron or thyroid shields or protective eye wear must always be considered when working close to fluoroscopy or special procedure fields, which involve relatively high potential occupational exposures.

Nuclear Medicine Technologists

Nuclear medicine technologists are highly trained and are required to maintain their proficiency with continuing education. Rules and regulations applicable to the handling and administration of radioactive materials must be carefully followed (7,12). Radiation shields around syringes and radiopharmaceutical vials must be used to minimize unnecessary exposure from these radioactive sources. Careful tracking of the handling and security of the radiopharmaceutical agents is extremely important to minimize the probability of error in dose administration. Special precautions are necessary in therapeutic procedures involving radiopharmaceutical agents, because these procedures always involve greater quantities of radioactivity than is normally involved in diagnostic studies. The potential for exposure in nuclear medicine is greater and proper use of shielding and radioisotope control must be emphasized.

Restraining patients for nuclear medicine procedures is less problematic than restraining those undergoing diagnostic radiologic studies, but it still is worthy of consideration. Nuclear medicine patients with diagnostic doses in their bodies represent a radiation source, and technologists who routinely stand close to such patients during relatively long imaging procedures have higher radiation exposures. As in diagnostic radiology, it is necessary to take advantage of holding and positioning devices to immobilize the patients during a long procedure to minimize the need for close contact for long periods of time. In some therapeutic nuclear medicine procedures it is advisable to use portable shielding to shield the patient to protect the technologist and other medical personnel. Such steps should be considered whenever therapy is involved.

Nuclear medicine technologists must be aware of proper procedures for an emergency involving radiopharmaceutical agents. Spills of radioactive material can occur in a busy medical practice, and all persons involved should be fully drilled in proper spill control procedures. Spill containment kits should be readily available in the nuclear medicine department and in off-site areas in which radiopharmaceutical agents are used, such as cardiac stress testing (19,20).

Radiation Therapy Technologists

Although they have the potential for the highest radiation exposure of all nuclear workers, radiation therapy technologists typically do not receive more than diagnostic radiology or nuclear medicine technologists. Although the dose rates involved in external beam therapy are higher than those of anything else in medical practice, procedures are rigidly established to minimize the possibility that anyone but the patient is in the room during treatment. Technologists working on therapeutic procedures need only follow the prescribed regulations to minimize their radiation exposure. Therapy technologists who regularly work with low dose rate brachytherapy procedures have considerably more risk for exposure. Patients with multiple sources implanted for 3- or 4-day treatments need a great deal of technologist involvement during insertion and removal of the sources and during care while the sources are in place. Just the routine handling of these sources in preparation for the treatment and removal and restoration of the sources to the storage inventory adds to the potential for exposure (10).

Physicians

Physicians of various specialties are at risk for radiation exposure in a variety of ways. Radiologists are at risk for exposure during interventional radiologic procedures that necessitate table-side presence for long fluoroscopic procedures and intermittent radiographic spot filming. Judicial use of personal shielding such as lead aprons, thyroid shields, and movable rigid shielding is imperative to protect radiologists, as is proper use of personnel monitoring for measurement of the resultant exposure. Cardiologists who use radiographic techniques to assist with pacemaker implants or high dose rate cardiac catheterization procedures also are at risk for radiation exposure. Cardiac catheterization specialists receive some of the highest occupational exposures. Other physicians who use radiographic techniques include orthopedic surgeons who use fluoroscopy in hip nailings and urologists and gastroenterologists who use radiography in their internal examinations. These physicians must use available shielding devices to minimize unnecessary exposure.

The general regulatory rule in hospitals is that x-ray equipment be under the primary control of the chief of radiology regardless of where it might be located in the hospital (6). All physicians using the equipment must be accredited in the proposed use by the chief of radiology. The chief of radiology is the person in the hospital most thoroughly trained in the use of x-ray equipment and is responsible for safe use of the equipment. It is important that the chief of radiology recognize this responsibility and control the use of all x-ray equipment to maximize the benefit of such equipment and to minimize the risk to both patients and workers.

Although they do not specifically use x-rays in their work, anesthesiologists must be carefully considered in terms of radiation exposure because they often are required to continue tending to a patient while portable radiographs are obtained during surgical procedures. Anesthesiologists must use leaded garments and portable shielding as appropriate to provide the necessary protection.

Nursing Personnel

Nurses because of their proximity to patients throughout their practice are frequently involved in the potential for exposure to radiation. Nurses usually do not have specific training in radiation protection, and it is important that the hospital and its radiation safety program provide nurses with training applicable to their duties. Sources of radiation to nurses include portable diagnostic radiographic equipment, often used in special procedures, intensive care areas, and in surgical recovery areas. It is important that nursing personnel take maximum advantage of personnel shielding devices such as lead aprons and mobile shields. Nurses should be discouraged from holding patients. They are likely to be tempted to hold patients and can acquire repeated exposures that would amount to a high dose in time if the practice were not discouraged. Positioning and restraining devices must be used. When holding is truly necessary, as in the care of some children, one of the patient's parents or a family member is the best choice for assistance.

In diagnostic nuclear medicine, the patients given imaging radiopharmaceuticals emit relatively low but nonetheless measurable doses of radiation soon after the procedure. Nurses must be aware of this and must minimize their potential for exposure while they provide the necessary patient care by minimizing the length of time they are close to these patients. This precaution generally is adequate to protect nurses, and personnel monitoring generally is not required.

With therapeutic procedures such as brachytherapy, whereby patients are treated for several days with temporarily implanted sources, nurses must be specially trained for the specific procedure and be fully aware of the steps to minimize unnecessary exposure to themselves and other patient care personnel. Nurses are relied on to control access to such patients by visitors and dietary and housekeeping personnel.

In the care of patients undergoing radiopharmaceutical therapy, nurses must be properly trained in emergency procedures involving the potential for radiation exposure. A patient who has received a therapeutic radiopharmaceutical orally and vomits soon afterward presents a difficult problem with respect to contamination control. Nurses must be properly trained to take the initial steps to minimize the spread of radioactive contamination until radiation protection personnel can assist in the proper decontamination. Patients with incontinence who have received therapeutic or diagnostic radiopharmaceutical agents may present difficulties in that their bedding materials may become radioactively contaminated. Risk for radiation exposure among nurses who handle contaminated bedding can be controlled with the use of universal precautions. Soiled bedding or clothing must be properly handled to allow safe storage for radioactive decay of the contamination involved. Training in such procedures is important for all nursing personnel (12).

Ultrasound Personnel

The general practice in most medical facilities is to attempt to schedule ultrasound procedures before diagnostic nuclear medicine procedures so that ultrasound technologists are not exposed unnecessarily to radiopharmaceutical agents. Sometimes the nuclear medicine procedure dictates the need for further information from a follow-up ultrasound procedure. Experience has shown that ultrasonographers do not receive substantial radiation exposures from such patients if a few relatively simple precautions are taken. Ultrasonographers should school themselves in the best techniques to minimize the time of direct contact with such patients and to maximize their distance from these patients as they perform their task. Radiation monitoring of hundreds of ultrasonographers who were occasionally exposed in this way has indicated that the accumulated radiation dose is well below that which would require classifying them as radiation workers or assigning routine personnel monitoring devices to satisfy regulatory requirements (12).

Other Hospital Personnel

Numerous other categories of hospital personnel occasionally have potential for radiation exposure. The pathology or morgue areas are frequently asked to handle patient tissues or deceased patients in whom radiopharmaceuticals might still be present. Generally such issues can be readily handled if radiation safety develops a tracking system to indicate which patients have substantial amounts of radiopharmaceutical agents in their bodies.

Dietary personnel who go into patient rooms to deliver meals and pick up trays are at risk for exposure to patients undergoing brachytherapy or radiopharmaceutical therapy. Oversight by properly trained nurses can address these issues. Janitorial and housekeeping personnel clean patient rooms where the potential for exposure exists. Other hospital personnel such as security and maintenance workers have lesser potential for exposure to medical radiation sources (12).

SUMMARY

Exposure of medical and allied health personnel to ionizing radiation is best controlled through education, training, and continuing dialogue. It is important to take full advantage of the assistance and guidance of radiation protection personnel and to seek the advice of experts whenever questions arise. This chapter should provide some assistance in judging when precautions may or may not be necessary and what may constitute suitable control. As with most potential hazards in the workplace, knowledge makes the most important contribution to worker safety.

REFERENCES

1. National Council on Radiation Protection and Measurements. Exposure of the population in the United States and Canada from natural background radiation; NCRP report no 94. Bethesda, MD: National Council on Radiation Protection and Measurements, 1987.
2. National Council on Radiation Protection and Measurements. Limitation of exposure to ionizing radiation; NCRP report no 116. Bethesda, MD: National Council on Radiation Protection and Measurements, 1993.
3. US Nuclear Regulatory Commission. Standards for protection against radiation; 10 CFR 20. Washington, DC: US Government Printing Office.
4. National Council on Radiation Protection and Measurements. Implementation of the principle of as low as reasonably achievable (ALARA) for medical and dental personnel; NCRP report no 107. Bethesda, MD: National Council on Radiation Protection and Measurements, 1990.
5. National Academy of Sciences/National Research Council. Health effects of exposure to low levels of ionizing radiation: report of the Advisory Committee on the Biological Effects of Ionizing Radiation—BEIR V. Washington, DC: National Academy Press, 1990.
6. National Council on Radiation Protection and Measurements. Medical x-ray, electron beam and gamma-ray protection for energies up to 50 MeV (equipment design, performance and use); NCRP report no 102. Bethesda, MD: National Council on Radiation Protection and Measurements, 1989.
7. National Council on Radiation Protection and Measurements. Nuclear medicine-factors influencing the choice and use of radionuclides in diagnosis and therapy; NCRP report no 70. Bethesda, MD: National Council on Radiation Protection and Measurements, 1982.
8. National Council on Radiation Protection and Measurements. Precautions in the management of patients who have received therapeutic amounts of radionuclides; NCRP report no 37. Bethesda, MD: National Council on Radiation Protection and Measurements, 1970.
9. National Council on Radiation Protection and Measurements. Sources and magnitude of occupational and public exposures from nuclear medicine procedures; NCRP report no 124. Bethesda, MD: National Council on Radiation Protection and Measurements, 1996.
10. National Council on Radiation Protection and Measurements. Protection against radiation from brachytherapy sources; NCRP report no 40. Bethesda, MD: National

Council on Radiation Protection and Measurements, 1972.

11. US Nuclear Regulatory Commission. Medical use of byproduct material, 10 CFR 35. US Government Printing Office, Washington, DC.
12. National Council on Radiation Protection and Measurements. Radiation protection for medical and allied health personnel; NCRP report no 105. Bethesda, MD: National Council on Radiation Protection and Measurements, 1989.
13. National Council on Radiation Protection and Measurements. Structural shielding design and evaluation for medical use of x rays and gamma rays of energies up to 10 MeV; NCRP report no 49. Bethesda, MD: National Council on Radiation Protection and Measurements, 1976).

Medical Center Occupational Health and Safety,
edited by Robert J. McCunney.
Lippincott Williams & Wilkins, Philadelphia © 1999

13

Management of Low Level Radioactive Wastes

Mitchell S. Galanek

Massachusetts Institute of Technology, Cambridge, Massachusetts 02139-4307

Whether mapping the human genome, searching for an AIDS vaccine, understanding cancer induction, or determining cardiac dysfunction, radioactive tracers are an invaluable tool to biomedical researchers and clinicians. Because of the ready availability of radiolabeled compounds and the sensitivity of radiation detectors, radioactive materials are used in countless biomedical experiments to study biologic pathways. A by-product of this use of radioactivity is the production of low level radioactive waste. This waste can take on many forms, from solid material contaminated during experimental procedures to patient excreta in a diagnostic or treatment procedure.

This chapter describes techniques and strategies for the effective management and disposal of low level radioactive waste streams. Radioactive waste management is a critical component of an effective radiation safety program to ensure the safe handling of licensed material (1). Because of skyrocketing costs for disposal, the everpresent uncertainty of disposal site access, and a continued negative public perception of associated risks, strategies for the minimization of radioactive waste that necessitate off-site disposal are more important than ever.

WASTE CATEGORIES

Low level radioactive waste from biomedical and hospital laboratories can be classified into the following five broad categories:

- Dry solid waste
- Liquid waste
- Liquid scintillation counting waste
- Animal carcasses and tissue waste
- Mixed waste
- Biologic material and radioactivity
- Chemical waste and radioactivity

SITE WASTE MANAGEMENT PLAN

The development of a site waste management plan is the most important step to safely minimize low level radioactive waste. A priority of the plan is effective experimental review and a worker training program. Radiation safety managers must review with the researchers the activities and experiments that will produce radioactive wastes, the anticipated types of waste and radioactivity levels, and strategies for waste elimination or volume reduction. Some regulators have set the unrealistic goal of zero waste production for licensees. Carefully planned experiments and procedures should preclude the generation of radioactive waste that cannot be safely disposed of under current disposal site criteria.

All workers who generate low level waste must be trained in the institution's waste management plan for the plan to be effective. Periodic review and retraining are necessary when waste handling criteria or disposal site requirements are modified. Quarterly audits of the waste management and processing program are necessary to preclude problems and to initiate new or corrective actions.

DRY SOLID RADIOACTIVE WASTE

The dry solid radioactive waste stream consists of solid material from laboratories that has been contaminated with radioactive material. Typical items are pipette tips, vials, tissue culture plates, bench cover paper, and gloves. This broad category can be further divided on the basis of the radiologic half-life of the radioactive material involved—long-half-life waste and short-half-life waste. The disposal and management strategies for the two categories differ greatly. Long-half-life waste is described as waste contaminated with radionuclides with half-lives greater than 120 days. Short-half-life waste is described as waste contaminated with radionuclides with half-lives less than 120 days.

Long-Half-life Waste

Long-half-life waste usually requires off-site treatment and disposal. Management strategies for this waste stream are waste segregation, minimization, substitution, and volume reduction. Minimization can be accomplished by means of substituting washable and reusable laboratory items for disposable items. A proved minimization strategy is use of washable plastic trays to contain radioactive spills and contamination, thus eliminating use of large volumes of bench cover paper. Contaminated trays are simply washed and reused. Washing and decontamination of glass and plastic experimental apparatus from laboratories has been effective in some waste management programs. Minimization strategies require an effective training program and a cooperative spirit among users of radioactive materials.

It is possible to substitute nonradioactive techniques for radioactive tracers. These techniques typically involve fluorescent, photochemical, or phosphorescent technologies. Some of these substitution techniques are suitable and are being used in laboratories. However, in most cases chemical waste is being substituted for radioactive waste as the ultimate by-product. Whether the chemical wastes are any easier to manage or dispose of is debatable.

Volume reduction techniques apply to waste that has already been contaminated. Commonly used volume reduction techniques are sorting and surveying, compaction and supercompaction, and incineration. The sorting and surveying of waste is simple, inexpensive, and can be accomplished at any facility. Only a portion of an object typically is contaminated with radioactivity. With proper radiation surveying, laboratory workers can eliminate the uncontaminated portion of the waste stream. There can be considerable fiscal return for a small effort.

Volume reduction by use of compaction of contaminated solid waste can be accomplished at the laboratory level with a conventional household trash compactor. The volume reduction ratio achieved with this method is not significant, on the order of 1.5:1. The physical area around laboratory compactors and the compactors themselves must be monitored frequently for contamination. Solid waste contaminated with volatile radioactive material should not be compacted in these units because most do not have a dedicated ventilation system. The compacted waste is typically transferred to a steel drum, which becomes the approved shipping container for final disposal.

Industrial scale compactors are used to obtain significant volume reduction ratios, typically about 4:1. This size compactor is part of a radiation safety waste management program. Contaminated solid waste collected from laboratories is compacted into steel drums, which become the shipping containers for final disposal. Contaminated solid waste should be sorted into burnable solid waste and physically hazardous or sharp-objects waste. These wastes should be segregated and compacted into separate drums.

Compactors should have a dedicated ventilation system with in-line filtration to trap any volatile components of the compacted waste. An environmental monitoring program for release of radionuclides should be established to ensure regulatory compliance with emission standards. Environmental air sampling of the workplace is recommended. Routine monitoring of workers for ingested radioactivity is recommended when known volatile products are part of the waste stream. Frequent radiation surveys of the compactor area are recommended to prevent the spread of contamination. Fully compacted drums may weigh between 200 and 300 pounds, so considerations must be made for the physical safety of the workers involved. Mechanical drum movers, drum dollies, and steel-toed safety shoes are necessary equipment for handling these heavy drums. The full drums are typically stored to await shipment for further processing by a licensed waste processor or shipment to a burial site.

Supercompaction is a technique offered by licensed waste processors to further improve the volume reduction ratio. The full steel drums are supercompacted and packaged in an overpack container. Volume reduction ratios are typically 5:1 to 10:1, depending on the density of the waste in the original drum. The supercompacted waste is forwarded to a licensed low level waste disposal repository. The states in which low level waste disposal sites are located have imposed disposal fees or surcharges above the fees charged by the disposal site contractor. These privilege fees are based on volume of waste to be disposed; thus supercompaction is a technique that has helped to offset the meteoritic rise in disposal costs over the past decade.

Solid radioactive waste can be incinerated at a licensed facility or at licensed commercial facilities. Incineration requires obtaining a license from a federal or state regulator. It also may require the approval of a local entity such as the board of health. Local approval of this controversial technique is typically a difficult process because of public opposition. Licensees must decide whether there is a real benefit to on-site incineration of radioactive waste. If on-site incineration is to be done at the licensees' facilities, strict controls and monitoring programs must be established.

Commercial incineration at licensed facilities such as the Scientific Ecology Group, SEG, in Oak Ridge, Tennessee, allow the licensee the advantage of tremendous volume reductions without obtaining and maintaining local approval (2,3). Incineration achieves a volume reduction ratio of approximately 200:1 and currently is the most fiscally advantageous method for solid waste disposal. The collected ash is sent to a licensed burial site for final disposal. It is important to sort burnable from nonburnable and physically hazardous waste; the latter two cannot be incinerated. The expense of having personnel at commercial incinerator sites sort the waste offsets the fiscal benefits of incineration over supercompaction.

There are three licensed low level radioactive waste disposal sites in operation in the United States. They are located in Barnell, South Carolina, Clive, Utah, and Richland, Washington. There are site-specific restrictions and acceptance criteria for the type of radioactive waste accepted for ultimate disposal at each of these sites.

Short-Half-life Solid Waste

Because of exponential cost increases and a lack of disposal site opportunities, segregation of waste according to half-life has enabled licensees to dramatically reduce the volume of waste that requires off-site disposal. Decay-in-storage is the technique used to manage short half life waste until they are no longer radioactive.

Solid waste is stored in steel, plastic, or fiberboard drums after collection from laboratories. The following conditions must be met in a successful decay-in-storage program:

1. The waste must be stored for a minimum of ten radiologic half lives.
2. The decay stored waste must be monitored with an appropriate radiation survey instrument. Radiation levels must be indistinguishable from background radiation levels.
3. All references to radioactive material (e.g., labels, radioactive material tape) in the waste stream must be obliterated.
4. A record of the management of the waste must be maintained for compliance in-

spections. The records must include the following:

a. The radionuclide and amount of it stored.
b. The date the container was sealed and placed in storage.
c. The projected date of retrieval from storage for disposal.
d. The results of the radiation survey, including the instrument used, its date of calibration, the measured radiation levels, and the measured background levels.
e. The date of disposal.
f. The name of the person performing the task.

After the solid waste is no longer radioactive, final disposition is based on activities in which the waste was generated. If generated in a biomedical research laboratory or a medical facility, the waste may require disposal as a biohazardous waste. During waste production, radiation workers should segregate physically hazardous sharp-object waste from waste that is not physically hazardous. After decay in storage, the physically hazardous waste must be disposed of in accordance with applicable regulations.

Obliteration of references to radioactive material should be done by the radiation workers generating the waste. It is extremely time consuming and frustrating for radiation safety personnel to be responsible for the obliteration during a survey for disposal.

Potential worker exposures to biologic material during radiation surveys of decayed waste must be considered. Waste can be in storage for up to 3 years before it is removed for disposal. Molds, fungi, or other biologic material can become airborne and a source of exposure to workers performing radiation surveys of the decayed-in-storage waste. Radiation surveys of decayed waste should be performed in a well-ventilated area. Workers should wear respiratory protection and the usual personnel protective equipment, such as laboratory coats, gloves, and safety glasses. Workers' gloves should be of a rugged nature (leather or Kevlar) to protect the worker against injury from sharp objects.

Preliminary studies of airborne biologic contaminants collected during the survey process at the Massachusetts Institute of Technology have indicated increased levels of dust, molds, and fungi in the workspace. A long-term study is being undertaken to determine accurate levels, species, and the possible time dependence of waste in decay storage (C. Micheklson, MIT Biosafety Officer, written personal communication, 1997).

LIQUID RADIOACTIVE WASTE

The liquid radioactive waste stream can be classified into two categories—aqueous liquid waste and organic liquid waste.

Aqueous Liquid Waste

Most of the radioactivity disposed of from biomedical research laboratories is in the form of aqueous liquid waste. The waste is generated during experimental procedures such as incubation of cells in labeled media, protein iodination, filter washing, and gel electrophoresis. The waste is typically collected in plastic bottles from the laboratories and sampled to determine its radionuclide content and activity. Once these parameters are known, the aqueous waste is disposed of through one of the following methods:

1. Disposal into the sanitary sewage system
2. Decay storage and disposal into sanitary sewage system
3. Absorption or solidification and shipment to a low level waste disposal site
4. Incineration by a licensed commercial facility

Disposal through the sanitary sewage system must comply with all applicable regulations. Federal and state regulations specify the concentration of the specific radionuclide to be disposed and the total annual radioactivity limit per radionuclide (1,4). It is important to segregate liquid waste by radionuclide at the laboratory level. Regulatory guidance requires aqueous waste to meet a solubility test. All aqueous waste disposed through the sanitary sewage system must be classified as soluble in the *Handbook of Chemistry & Physics*, with information received on the material safety data sheet or by means of calculation of the solubility product constant (C. Micheklson, written personal communication, 1997). Licensees must have records defending solubility of disposed waste. Before disposal, aqueous waste should be pH adjusted to 6 to 8.

When radioactivity concentrations exceed the regulatory limits, wastes may be stored for decay before disposal. Storage containers should be heavy-walled polyethylene jugs to minimize deterioration of the container and possible leakage of liquid. Stored liquid should be doubly contained to prevent the spread of radioactive liquid in the event of failure of the primary container.

A record must be maintained of all aqueous waste disposed into the sanitary sewage system. Records should be tabulated annually, results compared with regulatory levels, and results filed for compliance inspections.

It is good radiation safety practice to label disposal sink drains and plumbing with a warning sign or label to prevent unauthorized maintenance or removal, which can lead to worker exposure or contamination.

When radionuclide or radioactivity limits preclude sanitary sewage disposal or local restrictions prohibit the practice, aqueous waste may be solidified or absorbed and sent to a licensed waste disposal facility. Only site-approved solidification and absorption media can be used in this process. The licensee should review the site acceptance criteria for absorbed and solidified liquid wastes. Aqueous liquids are typically processed in 1- to 5-gallon (3.8 to 19 liters) containers. The solidified and absorbed containers are packaged in steel drums and shipped for disposal.

Ion exchange techniques have been developed to remove radioactivity from the liquid waste stream (2). Spent or used resin columns are disposed as solid radioactive wastes according to the methods described earlier. This management technique is valuable for programs that do not allow sanitary sewage disposal.

Some commercial waste processes offer incineration services for aqueous liquids. Collected liquid must be analyzed for radionuclide identification and activity concentration. If concentrations exceed waste processor limits, the waste can be diluted to acceptable levels. Wastes typically are collected in bulk containers, either 30- or 35-gallon drums (114 or 133 liters), which are the shipping containers.

Organic Liquid Waste

Liquid radioactive waste containing a chemical component listed in the Environmental Protection Agency (EPA) document Identification and Listing of Hazardous Waste (6) is not acceptable for disposal at disposal sites or for sanitary sewage disposal. The waste is classified as mixed waste and must be handled for its chemical and radioactive components. Mixed waste contaminated with short-half-life radionuclides is held for radiologic decay. When activities reach background levels, the chemical component of the waste can be disposed of through a licensed chemical waste broker. These mixed wastes must be handled with extreme care depending on the chemical properties of the waste. A facility should not combine or bulk together mixed wastes for storage unless it is certain of the chemical compatibilities. Storage facilities for mixed waste must be engineered to acceptable standards for chemical storage. Planning of experiments with emphasis on the types and amount of waste to be produced is critical in the management of mixed waste. Radioactively contaminated pump oil is generated in some biomedical research laboratories. Commercial incineration facilities can accept this waste if the radionuclide concentrations are within license limits and acceptance criteria.

LIQUID SCINTILLATION VIALS AND FLUID

The liquid scintillation waste stream is generated during the analysis of typically low-energy beta emitting radionuclides with liquid scintillation counting techniques. The scintillation fluid in which the reactions occur that are detected in the analyzer are categorized as drain disposable and non–drain disposable.

Non–drain-disposable scintillation fluids are usually toluene or xylene based. These chemicals are listed as hazardous substances by the EPA, thus they require disposal as waste chemicals. Nuclear Regulatory Commission and Agreement State regulations allow disposal of liquid scintillation fluid waste that contains tritium (^3H) and carbon 14 in concentrations of 0.05 microcuries per gram or less as waste flammable liquid. These wastes are termed deregulated and can be disposed of without regard to radioactivity content. Most laboratories dispose of these wastes through a licensed chemical waste disposal agent. These wastes usually are incinerated. Vials containing scintillation fluid are collected in steel drums that become the shipping container. Wastes that contain other radionuclides are termed *regulated* and can be disposed of through a licensed radioactive waste broker; these wastes almost always are incinerated.

At the commercial incinerator, vials containing fluid are processed with a ball mill or similar crushing device to separate the liquid from the solids. The liquid is incinerated. The solids are washed, surveyed for radioactive contamination, and, if free of contamination, sent to local landfills. Some institutions have adapted similar waste consolidation programs at their facilities. These programs are labor intensive but do allow bulking of scintillation fluid for disposal at greatly reduced costs.

Drain-disposable liquid scintillation fluid can be disposed of directly into the sanitary sewage system. Because of the chemical consistency, these fluids are not currently EPA listed as hazardous substances. Although drain disposal is allowed, most laboratories ship this waste for incineration. It is highly labor intensive to empty each vial, dispose of the scintillation fluid, wash the empty vial, and test for radioactive contamination. Drain-disposable liquid scintillation fluids are advertised as environmentally safe. Use of these products makes workers' environment safer because exposures to the noxious fumes and vapors of toluene- and xylene-based products are eliminated.

ANIMAL CARCASSES AND TISSUES

Animal carcass and tissue wastes are generated when scientists study materials under living conditions. The radioactive substance typically is injected directly into an animal, and after a prescribed period of time, the animal is killed. Body fluids and excreta, tissues, and organs of interest then are measured for radioactive content. When the experiment is over, the animal carcass and tissues must be disposed of as radioactive waste. As with the other waste streams, animal carcasses and tissue are segregated according to radiologic half-life for disposal purposes. Final disposal usually is by incineration.

The Nuclear Regulatory Commission and Agreement State regulations allow the disposal of animal carcass and tissue wastes containing tritium (^3H) and carbon 14 in concentrations of 0.05 microcuries per gram or less without regard to radioactivity. These wastes are termed *deregulated* and can be disposed of as nonradioactive. Incineration with nonradioactive animal waste is the usual method of disposal.

Some commercial waste processes offer incineration services for radioactive animal carcasses and tissues. Collected wastes must be frozen and segregated according to radionuclide and radioactivity concentration. Wastes typically are packaged in fiberboard containers, either 30- or 35-gallon (114 or 133 liters) drums, and shipped frozen to the incinerator site.

Animal carcass and tissue wastes contaminated with short-half-life radionuclides can be frozen and stored on site for a minimum of ten half-lives before disposal as normal animal waste. If storage space is a problem, commercial waste processors offer storage and incineration services for radioactive animal carcasses and tissues contaminated with short-half-life radionuclides.

MIXED WASTE

Waste classified as mixed consists of the radioactive component and either a chemical or biologic component. The chemical or biologic component of the waste stream makes the waste unacceptable for shallow land burial. Thus a strategy must be used to eliminate one of the components of the waste to make it acceptable for final disposal.

Chemical Radioactive Waste

Chemical radioactive waste is discussed earlier with organic liquid waste. Storage for decay of short-half-life waste followed by commercial incineration is the typical method of disposal. Licensed commercial incinerators can accept certain forms of this waste that contain long-half-life waste. Site waste management plans must include provisions for safe long-term storage of these wastes if not acceptable for commercial disposal. The potential of this mixed waste stream must be carefully investigated before it is produced in the laboratory because it is impossible to safely dispose of many forms of this waste. Researchers and radiation safety professionals need to work cooperatively before this waste is produced to have a clear understanding of amounts to be produced, potential alternatives, and disposal capabilities. Many times the researcher producing this waste form may be able to render the waste disposable by means of separation, chromatographic, or other standard chemical techniques.

Biologic Radioactive Waste

Biologic agents and by-products are made radioactive in many biomedical experiments. In this waste stream, the biologic or biohazardous component of the mixed waste should be rendered inactive before disposal as a radioactive waste. Typical inactivation procedures are chemical or steam sterilization techniques. Chemical disinfectants such as bleach or Wescodyne, a disinfectant, can be sprayed on potentially biohazardous solid materials to inactivate the biologic component. This procedure can be tedious for the persons dealing with all the different forms of solid waste generated in a biomedical research laboratory.

Steam sterilization (autoclaving) is the acceptable practice for most biologic wastes and can be done safely for mixed waste. Contaminated solid waste is placed in a plastic bag equipped with an autoclave indicator and a charcoal filter to trap potential airborne radioactivity. The bag system with the charcoal vent filter was designed to allow steam sterilization of materials contained in the bag while containing the radioactive materials so as not to contaminate the autoclave and surrounding area (5). Once inactivated, the waste can be managed with one of the techniques listed earlier.

RECORD KEEPING

Complete and accurate records must be maintained of all disposed or treated radioactive waste. Regulators require that such records be kept indefinitely. A copy of the waste-shipping manifest for materials disposed of at commercial treatment and disposal facilities is an appropriate record for archiving. Annual waste disposal volume and activity survey information required by most states is a good record for tracking progress in waste minimization or reduction efforts. Records of routine in-house audits of the waste handling and management program can be used as tools for training persons involved in the low level waste management program.

RADIOACTIVE WASTE SHIPMENTS

All shipments of radioactive wastes must be made in compliance with the regulations promulgated by the Nuclear Regulatory Commission and the Department of Transportation (1,7). The waste must be packaged in Department of Transportation acceptable packaging. These packages, typically 30- or 55-gallon (114 or 133 liters) steel drums, must be properly sealed, marked, labeled, and identified on a completed hazardous materials declaration bill. A 24-hour emergency telephone number must be listed on the shipping manifest. Also on the manifest should be certification that all materials are described by proper shipping name, are classified, packaged, marked, and labeled, and are in all respects in proper condition for transport. The ultimate responsibility for the waste remains with the generating institution.

CONCLUSIONS

Radiation safety organizations and the research community they serve have made tremendous strides in the management and disposal of low level radioactive wastes. Waste minimization and elimination efforts have reduced the volume of waste that requires long-term disposal. Workable strategies have been developed rather than dictatorial solutions that do not account for the science of the research involved in the waste production. Low level waste processing and management continue to be hard work and the least attractive of all the radiation safety disciplines. The goal of an effective management program is to be cost effective and compliant with all applicable regulations.

The single most important aspect of an effective waste management program is a solid worker-training program that has constant emphasis on source reduction techniques. Researchers and scientists need to be continually informed of changes in waste disposal requirements because of regulatory changes or modifications in specific disposal site acceptance criteria. The potential risk of safe disposal of the low level radioactive waste used in biomedical laboratories remains insignificant compared with the tremendous advances in medical science and the resulting benefit to humanity.

REFERENCES

1. Nuclear Regulatory Commission Rules and Regulations; 10 CFR 1. Washington, DC: US Government Printing Office.
2. Garcia RS. Commercially available low-level radioactive and mixed waste treatment technologies. Idaho National Engineering Laboratories; October 1996; DOE/LLW-240.
3. Scientific Ecology Group. Acceptance criteria for radioactive wastes. Oak Ridge, TN: Scientific Ecology Group, 1996.
4. US Nuclear Regulatory Commission. Solubility criteria for liquid effluent releases to sanitary sewerage under the revised 10 CFR 20. NRC information notice 94-07. Washington, DC: US Government Printing Office.
5. Stinson MC, Galanek, MS, Ducatman AM, et al. Model for inactivation and disposal human immunodeficiency virus and radioactive waste in a BL3 facility. *Appl Environ Microbiol* 1990;56:264–268.
6. Environmental Protection Agency. Identification and listing of hazardous waste; 40 CFR 261–261.1–35.
7. Department of Transportation. Subpart I-class 7 (radioactive materials); 49 CFR 173.401–476.

Medical Center Occupational Health and Safety,
edited by Robert J. McCunney.
Lippincott Williams & Wilkins, Philadelphia © 1999.

14

Nonionizing Radiation, Including Lasers

Donald L. Haes, Jr.

Environmental Medical Service, Massachusetts Institute of Technology, Cambridge, Massachusetts 02139-4304

Although the use of nonionizing radiation by the medical profession is not new, knowledge of its potential hazards is still expanding. In hospitals, sources of nonionizing radiation can be found in patient diagnostics and treatments and in administrative and physical plant activities. These sources are listed in Table 14-1.

NONIONIZING RADIATION IN THE MEDICAL PROFESSION

Physics of Nonionizing Radiation

Nonionizing radiation is a practical term for the frequency band of the electromagnetic spectrum that lacks the energy to break chemical or molecular bonds; thus they are unable to cause ionization, the energetic removal or addition of orbital electrons from the outer shells of atoms that leads to ion production. The several classes of nonionizing radiation are differentiated according to wavelength and hence by frequency. Nonionizing radiation consists of electromagnetic waves composed of electric and magnetic fields and mutually orthogonal to the direction of propagation. The waves move through a vacuum with the velocity of light. The mathematically inverse relation between frequency and wavelength is as follows. In free space

$$\text{Frequency } [f] = \text{Velocity of light } [C] \div \text{Wavelength } [\lambda]$$

Frequency usually is expressed in hertz (Hz). One hertz is defined as one cycle per second. Figure 14-1 shows the electromagnetic spectrum from the static fields to the very high frequencies found in cosmic rays. The elements of the electromagnetic spectrum included in this discussion are as follows: static fields, also known as direct current (DC); extremely low frequency (ELF) fields; radiofrequency (RF) fields, including microwaves; infrared (IR) radiation; visible light (VL); and ultraviolet (UV) light. Table 14-2 shows the frequency ranges and acronyms associated with these frequency bands.

A number of devices emit a portion of the electromagnetic spectrum as either the primary

TABLE 14-1. *Source of nonionizing radiation in hospital settings*

Patient diagnosis and therapy	Physical plant activities
Magnetic resonance imaging	Industrial alternating current line voltage
Pulsed electromagnetic stimulation	Handheld two-way communicators
Diathermy	Microwave ovens
Radiofrequency ablation	Cellular telephones
Infrared radiation	Visible light
Ultraviolet radiation	
Lasers (visible and invisible)	

Region	Frequency (Hertz)	Wavelength (Meters)	Function Device(s)	Band
	10^{0} - 1Hz	3 X 10^{8} -		
	10^{1} -	3 X 10^{7} -	Power (50/60Hz)	
	10^{2} -	3 X 10^{6} - 3Mm		
	10^{3} - 1kHz	3 X 10^{5} -		
	10^{4} -	3 X 10^{4} -	CRT/TV circuitry (17-31kHz)	
	10^{5} -	3 X 10^{3} - 3km	AM Radio (535-1705kHz)	RADIO FREQUENCY (RF)
	10^{6} - 1MHz	3 X 10^{2} -		RADIO FREQUENCY (RF)
	10^{7} -	3 X 10^{1} -	VHF Television (54-88MHz) FM Radio (88-108MHz)	RADIO FREQUENCY (RF)
	10^{8} -	3 X 10^{0} - 3m	VHF Television (174-216MHz) UHF Television (470-890MHz)	RADIO FREQUENCY (RF)
↑ NON-IONIZING	10^{9} - 1GHz	3 X 10^{-1} -	Microwave ovens (2.45GHz)	RADIO FREQUENCY (RF); MICROWAVE (MW)
NON-IONIZING	10^{10} -	3 X 10^{-2} - 3cm	Radar	RADIO FREQUENCY (RF); MICROWAVE (MW)
NON-IONIZING	10^{11} -	3 X 10^{-3} - 3mm		RADIO FREQUENCY (RF); MICROWAVE (MW)
NON-IONIZING	10^{12} - 1THz	3 X 10^{-4} -		INFRARED (IR)
NON-IONIZING	10^{13} -	3 X 10^{-5} -		INFRARED (IR)
NON-IONIZING	10^{14} -	3 X 10^{-6} - 3μm		INFRARED (IR)
		Visible Light		
NON-IONIZING	10^{15} - 1PHz	3 X 10^{-7} -		ULTRAVIOLET (UV)
NON-IONIZING	10^{16} -	3 X 10^{-8} -		ULTRAVIOLET (UV)
* * * * *	* * * * *	* * * * *	* * * * *	* * * * *
IONIZING	10^{17} -	3 X 10^{-9} - 3nm		ULTRAVIOLET (UV)
IONIZING	10^{18} - 1EHz	3 X 10^{-10} -		↑ X RAYS
IONIZING	10^{19} -	3 X 10^{-11} -		X RAYS; ↑ GAMMA RAYS
IONIZING	10^{20} -	3 X 10^{-12} - 3pm		X RAYS; GAMMA RAYS
IONIZING ↓	10^{21} -	3 X 10^{-13} -		X RAYS; GAMMA RAYS
	10^{22} -	3 X 10^{-14} -		X RAYS ↓; GAMMA RAYS
	10^{23} -	3 X 10^{-15} - 3fm		GAMMA RAYS
	10^{24} -	3 X 10^{-16} -		GAMMA RAYS ↓; ↑ COSMIC RAYS
	10^{25} -	3 X 10^{-17} -		COSMIC RAYS
	10^{26} -	3 X 10^{-18} - 3am		COSMIC RAYS
	10^{27} -	3 X 10^{-19} -		COSMIC RAYS
	10^{28} -	3 X 10^{-20} -		COSMIC RAYS
	10^{29} -	3 X 10^{-21} -		COSMIC RAYS ↓

FIG. 14-1. Electromagnetic spectrum.

TABLE 14-2. *Frequency bands of the electromagnetic spectrum*

Frequency ranged	Designated and acronym
0–30 Hz	Subextremely low frequency (SELF)[a]
30–300 Hz	Extremely low frequency (ELF)
0.3–3 kHz	Voice frequency (VF)
3–30 kHz	Very low frequency (VLF)
30–300 kHz	Low frequency (LF)
0.3–3 MHz	Medium frequency (MF)
3–30 MHz	High frequency (HF)
30–300 MHz	Very high frequency (VHF)
0.3–3 GHz	Ultra high frequency (UHF)
3–30 GHz	Superhigh frequency (SHF)
30–300 GHz	Extremely high frequency (EHF)
0.3–3 THz	Superextremely high frequency (SEHF)[a]

[a]No "official" acronym.

product or as a consequence of their use. Lasers (light amplification by stimulated emission of radiation) are designed to emit light and may be dangerous because of their primary function. Video display screens (e.g., televisions and video display terminals) emit visible light as a design function. These products and a mass of other equipment emit other frequencies of the electromagnetic spectrum as a consequence. The generated electromagnetic field is an unavoidable technologic consequence.

Static Fields

Any time electric current is flowing, magnetic fields exist. With alternating current (AC), a time-varying field exists. With DC, static fields exist. In hospitals, the typical sources of static fields are large magnets used for diagnosis and research. Although strong magnetic fields are present close to the magnets, the intensity of the field decreases dramatically with distance. These weaker fields are also known as *fringe fields.*

Strong magnetic fields have been postulated to produce potentially adverse biologic affects. These include increased blood pressure caused by magnetically induced enlargement of the T wave and rotation of sickleform red blood cells because the hemoglobin exhibits magnetic anisotropy, which causes torque. These effects have yet to be verified scientifically. The main concern with strong magnetic fields greater than 1 millitesla (mT; tesla is a unit of magnetic flux density, an indication of field strength) is the attraction of loose ferromagnetic objects (e.g., iron gas cylinders, surgical steel tools) that may be propelled toward the magnet at considerable velocity. The object adheres to the magnet, as does anything in its way. Surgical implants may be torqued, dislodged, or rotated, resulting in serious injury or death. Field strengths roughly above 0.5 mT may interfere with unshielded electronic equipment, such as implanted cardiac pacemakers (1). Even though field strengths may be in compliance with established pacemaker safety standards, patients must be warned that the strength of these fields may be enhanced by ferromagnetic objects in close contact to the wearer (2). Each pacemaker manufacturer has a specific warning available to the user regarding specific susceptibilities of the implant.

The two main sources of strong magnetic fields in the hospital environment are magnetic resonance imaging devices used for diagnosis and nuclear magnetic resonance imaging devices used for research (the word *nuclear* was dropped from the former for fear of patient apprehension). With both devices, a specimen is placed into a large static magnetic field produced by superconducting solenoid magnets and irradiated with time-varying fields (often called radio waves) to produce noninvasive internal images in vitro. A nuclear magnetic resonance device has a narrow-bore magnet of high field strength; the magnetic resonance imaging device has a large central-bore magnet for clinical imaging. During magnetic resonance imaging, the patient is exposed to static magnetic fields up to 2.0 T in intensity, which is about 25,000 times that of the background magnetic field of the earth. For these devices, magnetic field strength can be roughly determined with maps provided by the manufacturer. These maps have contour lines that relate field strength to distance from the center (bore) of the magnet. Demarcation of the 0.5 mT line (often called the 5 gauss line) (10,000 gauss = 1.0 T) is essential for pacemaker warning. Placement of this posting should be verified with measurements taken by a competent health physicist or similarly qualified person with a gaussmeter (a hall-effect probe or similar device). Although this value has regulatory significance with the Occupational Health and Safety Administration and other governmental agencies, it has no basis in science regarding risk to persons who wear cardiac pacemakers.

Standards for exposure to static magnetic fields have been published by the American Conference of Governmental Industrial Hygienists (ACGIH) (3). These published exposure standards are provided in Table 14-3. Additional standards for exposure to static magnetic fields have been published by the International Council on Non-Ionizing Radiation Protection (ICNIRP) (4). These published exposure standards are provided in Table 14-4.

Extremely Low Frequency and Very Low Frequency Fields

ELF waves have extremely long wavelengths (see Fig. 14-1). It is technically incorrect to refer to ELF fields as radiation. When the wavelength is extremely long, as in ELF fields, exposed objects, including people, are enveloped within a wavelength of the source. The physical characteristics of such confined fields dictate that the subsequent radiant energy effects are trivial (5). The exposed object encounters an induction field in which charges from the nearby electromagnetic source induce currents and charges (as opposed to radiation) on and within the exposed.

TABLE 14-3. *Standards for exposure to static magnetic fields published by ACGIH*

Exposure criteria	ACGIH limit
Routine whole-body occupational time-weighted average daily value	60 mT
Limbs	600 mT
Ceiling value	2 T
Pacemakers and similar devices	0.5 mT

ACGIH, American Conference of Governmental Industrial Hygienists.

TABLE 14-4. *Standards for exposure to static magnetic fields published by ICNIRP*

Exposure criterial	ICNIRP limit
Whole-body occupational averaged over a working day	200 mT
Limbs	5 T
Ceiling value	2 T
Public	40 mT (continuous)

ICNIRP, International Council on Non-Ionizing Radiation Protection.

The generation, transport, and use of common industrial and household electricity is associated with the generation of ELF fields. An ubiquitous potential source of this type of ELF exposure is power lines. Although the electric and magnetic field components are generated together, magnetic fields have been implicated in health problems. Despite persistent methodologic problems in assessing dose and exposure to ELF fields, residence near power lines and work with or around electrical power as surrogates of exposure have been associated with leukemia among children and adults (6). Wertheimer and Leeper (7) were the first to attempt to show a positive association between higher dose magnetic fields (albeit by a surrogate exposure assessment by the use of wiring codes, the thickness of wires) and leukemia. Other investigators (8) have attempted to overcome some of the deficiencies of earlier studies by measuring ELF field exposures at the workplace and taking work duration into consideration.

Unlike the epidemiologic results, short-term measurements of ELF fields with the magnetic field meters used in some of the studies provided no evidence of an association between exposure to 50 to 60 Hz and the risk for cancer among children. These studies prompted a National Academy of Science Committee to suggest that confounding by an unknown risk factor for childhood leukemia may account for the associations between childhood leukemia and residency in the vicinity of power lines (9).

Taken together, the epidemiologic results of exposure studies of residential magnetic fields and childhood cancer are not sufficiently compelling to warrant revisions in exposure standards, especially in light of the study by Linet et al. (8). Published standards allow exposures to ELF several orders of magnitude above levels reported in epidemiologic studies as associated with health problems. Standards for exposure to ELF fields have been published by ACGIH (<100 Hz electric fields, 25 kV/m; 1 to 30 kHz magnetic fields, 60,000/f μT) (3).

Operating computers may generate nonionizing radiation exposures. Most computers have video display terminals (VDTs) that contain cathode ray tubes. Both have a source of electrons (cathode) at one end and a phosphorous coating on the inside of the viewing screen (anode) at the other. The electrons, accelerated by high voltage, are focused onto the screen. They display information when the rapidly moving electron beam strikes the screen to produce visible light (the only type of nonionizing radiation emitted by design). The resultant nonionizing radiation fields are in both the ELF and the VLF range. Extensive measurements at the Massachusetts Institute of Technology yielded fields at 50 cm from the screen ranging from 1.9 to 87.5 mA/m (milliamperes per meter, a measure of the field strength) (10). Larger displays allow the operator to sit farther from the screen with correspondingly less exposure. Thus seating positions are crucial in assigning any dose retrospectively. It is questionable whether any information from measurements at fixed locations from VDTs can be useful in assigning a VDT dose.

Epidemiologic studies of reproductive outcomes among VDT users have the problem that exposures have not been quantified, a problem generic to all studies of nonionizing radiation fields. Reproductive outcomes have been compared retrospectively with findings of survey reports of VDT "use" time at the keyboard. This approach introduces two important limitations. First, both outcome and exposure are reconstructed retrospectively with an implied assumption that one will not bias the other. Second, any reproductive effects detected, although associated with VDT use are not necessarily related to electromagnetic emissions. The latest large study was conducted by the National Institute of Occupational Safety and Health with the conclusion, "The use of VDTs and exposure to the accompanying electromagnetic fields were not associated with an increased risk of spontaneous abortion in this study" (11).

Goldhaber et al. (12) were the first to report a statistically significant positive association between VDT use and spontaneous abortion among members attending three clinics of a large, prepaid group health care plan. Earlier, similarly designed studies had concluded that no reproductive hazards were associated with VDT use during pregnancy. Windham et al. (13) reviewed earlier data and reported the positive effect was limited to respondents in the initial studies who were contacted by telephone after not responding to questionnaires. Available data do not suggest an association between VDT use and other sources of ELF and adverse reproductive outcomes.

Very few standards apply to VDT exposure. A number of countries and agencies have created exposure limits that include the nonionizing radiation emission from a VDT. Table 14-5 shows the wide variations in frequencies covered and exposure intensities permitted.

Radio Frequency

RF bands generally are defined to include the frequencies 10 kHz to 300 GHz. Although a wide spectrum of frequencies is included, exposures are commonly grouped together under the collective term *RF exposures*. Ex-

TABLE. 14-5. *Various magnetic field exposure and emission standards in the frequency range <300 kHz*

Organization or country and year	Frequency range	Magnetic field (μT)[a]	Exposure duration and comments
ANSI C95.1 (1992)	3–100 kHz	205	Uncontrolled environment
ACGIH (1996–97)	4–30 kHz	2.01	Threshold values
453 CMR 5.00 (1986)	10–3,000 kHz	1.99	Occupational
MPR-III (1994)[b]	5–2,000 Hz	0.250	At 0.5 m, 3 planes: centerline,
	2–400 kHz	0.025	0.25 m above and below

[a]Most exposure limits list magnetic field intensity (H) in units of (A m^{-1}). These values have been converted to magnetic flux density (B) in units of μT (1×10^{-6} T), B = μH by assuming the permeability (μ) of free space ($4\pi \times 10^{-7}$) henry m^{-1}) is the same for tissue.

[b]This standard is a "performance" standard. It is based on video display terminal emissions achievable with current technology and not on any "safe" level of electromagnetic field emissions.

ANSI, American National Standards Institutes; ACGIH, American Conference of Governmental Industrial Hygienists; CMR, Commonwealth of Massachussets Regulations; MPR, Statens Mät och Provstyrelse, the Swedish National Board for Measurement and Testing.

posure to electric and magnetic fields that vary with time results in internal body currents and energy absorption in tissues, depending on the coupling mechanisms and the incident frequency. Table 14-6 lists the dosimetric quantities to be considered and corresponding units of measurement.

A significant difference between RF and ELF exposures is that RF exposures, especially RF exposures in the microwave band, may have thermal effects. Exposure to low-frequency electric and magnetic fields in air results in absorption of a negligible amount of energy and no measurable temperature rise in the body. Exposures greater than 1 milliwatt per centimeter squared (mW/cm^2, a unit of power density) at frequencies above about 10 MHz can lead to substantial energy absorption and temperature increases. Exposures greater than 10 mW/cm^2 may increase whole body temperature. Heating from RF sources is no different in producing thermal effects than exogenous sources of heat except that the degree and distribution of heating associated with RF are less predictable. The initial physiologic response among laboratory animals to exposure to RF is cutaneous vasodilation, which reverses rapidly if the source of RF is removed. Surface evaporation, metabolism, cell growth and division, and immune response can be altered by increasing the thermal effect from RF exposures. Humans heated from RF sources experience psychologic symptoms, intermittent hypertension, and burns, whereas laboratory rats and monkeys similarly exposed suffer decreased task performance at specific absorption rates (a measure of energy absorbed in the body) in the range of 1 to 3 watts per kilogram (W/kg). At body temperature elevations above 1°C to 2°C other biologic effects observed include increased permeability of the blood-brain barrier, ocular impairment, stress-associated effects on the immune system, decreased sperm production, teratogenic effects, and alterations in neural functions.

Thermally vulnerable organs, such as the eye, may sustain damage from high-energy

TABLE 14-6. *Dosimetric quantity for radiofrequency exposure assessment*

Frequency range	Dosimetric quantity	Units
1 Hz–10 MHz	Current density	Amperes per square meter (A/m^2)
1 Hz–100 MHz	Contact currents	Amperes (A)
100 kHz–10 GHz	Specific absorption rate	Watts per kilogram (W/kg)
300 MHz–10 GHz	Specific absorption	Joules per kilogram (J/kg)
10 GHz–300 GHz	Power density	Watts per square meter (W/m^2)

exposures. Microwave exposure to the eye may result in cataracts (at frequencies less than 2 GHz), corneal damage (at frequencies greater than 10 GHz), and retinal lesions. Microwave cataracts have been induced in experimental animals and have been reported in rare instances among humans. The present consensus is that very high-intensity (greater than 1.5 kW/m^2) exposures are required to produce detectable eye damage. With the exception of accidental exposures of the eyes to the feed horns of very powerful radar, such as during maintenance, this magnitude of exposure is highly unlikely. Auditory sensation from powerful RF fields is caused by rapid thermoelastic expansion and secondary pressure waves within the cochlea, a phenomenon known as a *microthermal effect* whereby a high local rate of tissue absorption and expansion occurs in the absence of any measurable change in temperature.

In the frequency range between 100 kHz and 110 MHz, shocks and burns can be caused by touching an ungrounded metal object that has acquired a charge in the field or by contact between a charged body and a grounded metal object. This phenomenon is especially dangerous in the case of long cables from cranes close to AM radio station antennae. Workers receive a shock when grabbing the cable, and the startle response from the shock compromises the grip on safety gear and causes a fall. Threshold currents that result in biologic effects that range from perception to pain have been measured in controlled experiments with human subjects (13b). When the current between the point of contact of the human body and the conductor exceeds 50 mA, there is risk for severe burns and irreversible tissue damage. I have experienced both shocks and burns while taking RF exposure measurements of RF heater-sealer units when I accidentally touched the metal table holding the jig holding the item being sealed.

RF is used in hospitals in varying frequency ranges and applications. In diathermy, first introduced in 1907, RF (commonly 27.12 MHz) is used to produce a therapeutic effect by stimulating blood flow to promote healing. Diathermy units operating at 2,450 MHz have been used but are not common. A specialized form of diathermy is pulsed electromagnetic stimulation, a noninvasive procedure used for the palliative management of postoperative pain and edema in soft tissue. In this procedure, RF at 27.12 MHz is pulsed for 65 microseconds (1 microsecond = 10^{-6} seconds) 80 to 600 times per second. Results of in vitro cell and animal experiments suggest that pulsed electromagnetic stimulation may hasten the healing of soft tissue injuries (14).

RF ablation is a nonsurgical procedure used to manage some types of cardiac conduction defects, such as Wolff-Parkinson-White syndrome. In this procedure, a physician guides a catheter with an electrode at its tip to the affected area of the heart muscle. RF is then transmitted to a very small area to kill the muscle cells conducting the extra impulses that cause rapid heart beats.

Cellular telephones operating in the frequency range of 800 to 900 MHz have been implicated in the causation of brain cancer. Numerous studies have addressed possible carcinogenic effects from exposure to RF in the range used by communication systems. A concise summary of laboratory research findings was published in 1996 by the ICNIRP (15). There is substantial evidence that RF is not mutagenic, and exposure to these fields is therefore unlikely to initiate carcinogenesis. A 1997 study (16), however, suggested another risk of use of cellular telephones—increased risk for accidents (to the level of driving inebriated) when the phones are used during driving. Concern has been expressed about the possible interference of cellular telephone use with cardiac pacemakers. The U.S. Food and Drug Administration concluded, "Based on these preliminary findings, cellular phones do not seem to pose a significant health problem for pacemaker wearers" (17).

RF exposures in hospitals are usually confined to patients undergoing electrosurgical treatment or diathermy. Hospital staff, however, may be unintentionally exposed to RF in the near-field region (within a few wavelengths) of portable transmitters, including portable transceivers (a device that combines both transmitter and receiver) and cellular telephones. Measurements of RF fields to determine regulatory compliance should be undertaken only by a competent health physicist or other suitably trained person. The appropriate equipment is very expensive to purchase and calibrate and is difficult to use (Fig. 14-2).

RF exposure standards, including contact and grasping limits, have been published by organizations worldwide. The American National Standards Institute (ANSI) (18), the National Council of Radiation Protection and Measurement (19), and ACGIH are but a few. The RF standard most cited, however, is that published by ANSI. Tables 14-7 and 14-8 show RF exposure limits for uncontrolled areas (those not restricted for reasons of RF exposure where personnel are exposed to RF as a consequence of employment).

Infrared Radiation, Visible Light, and Ultraviolet Light, Including Lasers

All objects with temperature above absolute zero emit IR radiation. The main hazard from IR exposure is a rise in the temperature of the absorbing tissue. IR is absorbed by tissue water and therefore is nonpenetrating; energy transfer is directly to outer surfaces. Pain is the best warning for thermal injury to the skin due to IR radiation. However, the eyelid and eye do not have ample thermal warning properties. Eyelid blisters are common after heat exposures, and the eye is at risk for injury from IR exposures. IR overexposure produces corneal burns and choroid and retinal damage.

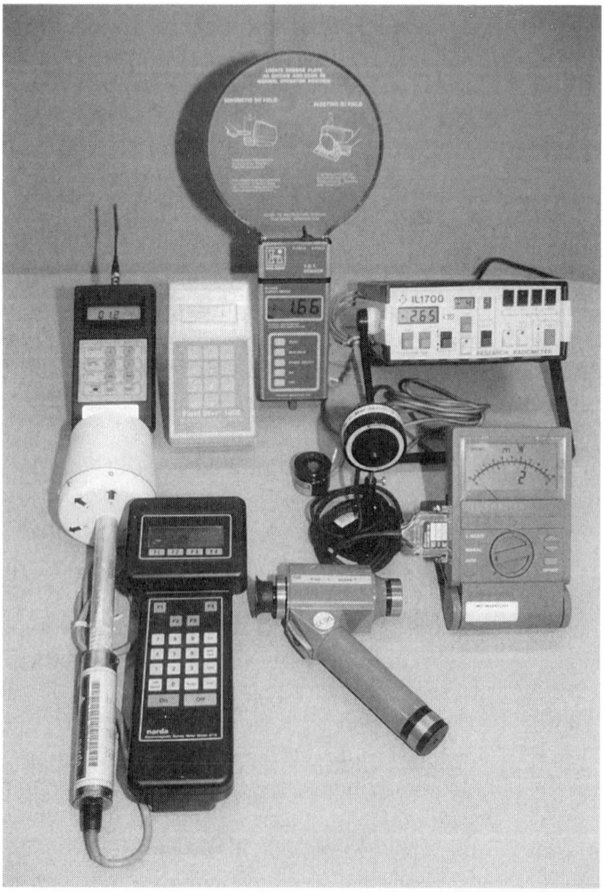

FIG. 14-2. Typical instruments used to evaluate sources of nonionizing radiation.

TABLE 14-7. *ANSI/IEEE maximum permissible exposures for uncontrolled environments*

Frequency range (MHz)	Electric field strength (E) (V/m)	Magnetic field strength (H) (A/m)	Power density (S) E field; H field (W/m^2)	Averaging time $\lvert E\rvert^2$, S, or $\lvert H\rvert^2$ (minutes)	
0.003–0.1	614	163	(1,000; 10,000,000)[a]	6	6
0.1–1.34	614	16.3/f	(1,000; 100,000/f^2)[a]	6	6
1.34–3.0	823.8/f	16.3/f	(1,800/f^2, 100,000/f^2)[a]	f^2/0.3	6
3–30	823.8/f	16.3/f	(1,800/f^2, 100,000/f^2)[a]	30	6
30–100	27.5	158/$f^{1.668}$	(2.0; 9,400,000 /$f^{3.336}$)[a]	30	0.0636/$f^{1.337}$
100–300	27.5	0.0729	2.0	30	30
300–3,000			f/150	30	
3,000–15,000			f/150	90,000/f	
15,000–300,000			100	616,000/$f^{1.22}$	

[a]Values of plane wave equivalent power densities given for comparison.
ANSI, American National Standards Institute; IEEE, Institute of Electrical and Electronics Engineers.

The human eye detects light in the narrow band between 760 nanometers (nm, 10^{-9} meters) at the red end and 380 nm at the violet end, with peak sensitivity at 555 nm. Chronic exposure to excessively bright light may lead to premature degeneration of the cones responsible for color vision (20). The retina is sensitive to excess light.

UV light extends in a narrow band between 400 and 40 nm. The harmful effects of UV light result from exposure to the range of 315 to 280 nm, also known as UV-B (20). Acute effects on the eye include photo keratitis and photo conjunctivitis. Acute eye damage may occur before a person is aware of exposure to UV light. Keratitis and conjunctivitis usually subside within several days. Burns may occur from lateral UV-B exposure to the cornea, that is, exposure that does not pass through the pupil and lens. Exposures to UV light around 297 nm induce cataract formation in a clear dose-response relation (21,22). Keratitis has been found among persons who work in biotechnology environments where UV is used for sterilization and for DNA sequencing operations. Radiation levels from germicidal UV lamps vary markedly with distance from the lamp or nearby reflecting surfaces.

A most important outcome of exposure to UV light is skin cancer. Some UV-B exposure is necessary for vitamin D_3 production if nutritional supplies are inadequate; however, UV overexposure can cause substantial pathologic changes in the skin. An alarming epidemic of skin cancer has occurred in parts of the world in association with outdoor recreation and tanning (23). The U.S. incidence of all skin cancer among white persons increases approximately 15% per degree of southern latitude. Childhood freckling and blue eyes are other consistent risk factors for the development of skin cancer.

Basal cell carcinoma, the most common skin cancer among white persons, occurs primarily on sun-exposed areas of the head and neck, and is prone to multiple lesions. There is an inverse association with ability to tan, but basal cell carcinoma is not consistently associated with cumulative UV-B exposure. Episodes of sunburn rather than cumulative UV-B exposure may be important to basal cell outcomes.

TABLE 14-8. *Maximum permissible induced and contact radiofrequency currents (ANSI/IEEE)*

	Maximum current (mA)		
Frequency range (MHz)	Through both feet	Through each foot	Contact
0.003–0.1	900f	450f	450f
0.1–100	90	45	45

Squamous cell carcinoma is caused by sun exposure, especially in outdoor occupations such as fishing and farming. Occupational links to this disease are not limited exclusively to the sun as a risk factor. Animal data show that squamous cell cancers are caused by UV exposure (24). Marked association between squamous cell carcinoma and sun exposure has been found in all well-designed epidemiologic studies.

Melanoma, the most dangerous skin cancer, is associated with fair skin and the number of benign pigmented nevi in childhood (25). It also is associated with sunlight. The relation between melanoma and sun exposure may involve age at time of exposure and degree and number of episodes of sunburning. Some studies have suggested that long-term low-level exposure may be protective but that long-term recreational exposures may be important risks.

Laser is an acronym for light amplification by stimulated emission of radiation. An energized laser beam emits intense monochromatic (one-wavelength color) visible or invisible coherent radiation (all photons of light are in phase with one another) continuously or in pulses. The most common hazard is related not to the radiation but to risk for electric shock. Fire, cryogenic, and radiation hazards are also associated with laser use. For these reasons, only appropriately qualified personnel should be involved with the design, installation, procedures, and any changes in conditions of laser use. There is a significant risk for immediate injury to the eye and skin from certain types of laser equipment. The risk depends on wavelength, intensity, and duration of exposure. Lasers may emit IR, visible, or UV light.

Infrared lasers include neodymium–yttrium-aluminum-garnet (Nd-YAG) and carbon dioxide lasers. Visible light lasers include dye lasers, argon, helium-neon lasers, and krypton lasers. The focusing ability of the eye increases the retinal hazard of any visible laser beam. UV lasers include excimer lasers and Nd-YAG lasers tripled in frequency into the UV spectrum. The excited dimers of argon fluoride or xenon chloride are used for tissue excision. Laser classification and associated hazards are described in Table 14-9.

Personal protective equipment has serious limitations as the only protective measure for use of class 4 lasers (lasers associated with permanent eye or skin injury if there is even momentary exposure to the direct beam or mirrored reflection). Eyes and skin are best kept out of the beam by use of interlock devices, which turn off the laser electronically, or use of physical barriers between personnel and the beam during operation. Not all research or medical laser activities are amenable to interlock protection. Laser surgery is a prime example. Personal protective devices are then required. Eye shielding must be selected in accordance with the wavelength used and should include side shielding. Absorptive filters are generally preferred to reflective types, because absorptive filters are reliable regardless of the incident angle of the beam. A problem with optical density markings on laser-protective eyewear has been uncertainty with the reliability of manufacturers' markings concerning transmittance. Independent checks are not truly achievable with available equipment, so it is important to pick the most reputable supplier. Another problem with eye protection is that complete protection renders otherwise visible beams invisible.

TABLE 14-9. *Laser classification*

Class	Potential danger
1	Essentially harmless
2, 2a	Dangerous to stare into the beam
3, 3a, 3b	Hazardous Direct viewing must not occur Specular reflections are dangerous Skin exposure is harmful
4	Extremely hazardous Direct viewing must not occur Specular reflections are extremely dangerous Diffuse reflections dangerous Skin exposure extremely hazardous

When class 3 and 4 lasers are fully embedded into an enclosed system that has full safety interlocks, the system may be classified as a class 1 system (per instructions of the laser safety officers).

Lasers are commonly used to manage a number of skin problems and have been used successfully in laser surgery. The three most common skin problems managed with lasers are vascular lesions, benign pigmented lesions, and unwanted tattoos. Surgical treatment with lasers includes coagulation to reduce intraoperative blood loss, prostatcctomy, lithotripsy, dacryocystorhinostomy, plastic surgical procedures, tissue welding, orthopedic operations including synovectomy, meniscectomy, and chondroplasty,.

Users of medical laser ought to assume that any laser capable of causing material surface ablation is above the safe limit for viewing diffuse reflections. Eye protection issues are outlined an ANSI standard (26). Skin protection also is important for operation of noninterlocked class 4 lasers. The American Medical Association Council on Scientific Affairs has made specific recommendations for the use of wet towels and sponges for skin protection against carbon dioxide laser burns in surgical fields (27). Carbon dioxide–nitrogen lasers emit invisible energy, so burns may be severe before the hazard is appreciated. Laser surgery or other tissue use of class 4 lasers inevitably generates heat and pressure and produces smoke and fumes, which can be malodorous. Designed ventilation is the appropriate industrial hygiene measure, but it does not adequately address the risk that the smoke plume may carry infectious organisms.

Calculations such as optical density (the protection factor for laser safety eyewear necessary to reduce a given laser hazard to the level below which permanent injury is prevented) and nominal hazard zone (the distance necessary to reduce a given laser hazard to the level below which permanent injury is avoided) are necessary in determining the safe use of any class 3 or 4 laser systems. Confirmatory measurements should be made with radiometric instruments to ensure that appropriate eye and skin protection is chosen.

Medical surveillance of surgeons who use lasers and the support staff is highly recommended to ascertain eye injury in the event of accidental exposure. Baseline eye examinations before working with the laser is essential in making this determination. Further eye examinations are needed after the incident and after employment.

SUMMARY

The three elements that must be considered in any effective safety program designed to control actual or potential occupational health hazards are recognition, evaluation, and control. After reading this chapter one should be able to recognize nonionizing radiation hazards associated with the medical profession. On recognition of each potential or actual hazard, a competent person should perform a safety evaluation. On the basis of the outcome of the evaluation, control may or may not be necessary. There is immense potential for serious injury considering all the sources of nonionizing radiation in use by the medical profession. It is imperative that a nonionizing radiation safety program be initiated and maintained in every medical facility that uses sources of nonionizing radiation. A nonionizing radiation safety program must be developed, and any actual or potential hazard must be evaluated by a person properly trained and experienced in this complex field of occupational safety. Consultants are available for such work. Qualified individuals may be found through the Health Physics Society, 1313 Dolly Madison Blvd., Suite 402, McLean, VA 22101.

REFERENCES

1. Tenforde TS. Biological effects of stationary magnetic fields. In: Grandolfo M, Michaelson S, Rindi A, eds. *Biological effects and dosimetry of static and ELF electromagnetic fields*. New York: Plenum Press, 1985:93–128.
2. Hansen DJ, Baum JW, Weilandics C, Barnhardt JF, Meninger MH. Enhancement of low-level magnetic fields by ferro-magnetic objects. *Appl Occup Environ Hyg* 1990;5:236–241.
3. American Conference of Governmental Industrial Hygienists. Threshold limit values for chemical substances and physical agents and biological indices. Cincinnati, OH: American Conference of Governmental Industrial Hygienists, 1997:123–125.
4. International Commission on Non-Ionizing Radiation Protection. Guidelines on limits of exposure to static magnetic fields. *Health Phys* 1994;66:100–106.

5. Polk C, Postow EP, eds. *Handbook of biological effects of electromagnetic fields*. Boca Raton, FL: CRC Press, 1996.
6. Savitz DA, Pearce NE, Poole C. Methodological issues in the epidemiology of electromagnetic fields and cancer. *Epidemiol Rev* 1989;11:59–77.
7. Wertheimer N, Leeper E. Electrical wiring configurations and childhood cancer. *Am J Epidemiol* 1979;109: 273–284.
8. Linet MS, Hatch EM, Kleinerman R, et al. Residential exposure to magnetic fields and acute lymphoblastic leukemia in children. *N Engl J Med* 1997;337:1–7.
9. National Academy of Science/National Research Council. Possible health effects of exposure to residential electric and magnetic *fields*. Washington, DC: National Academy of Science/National Research Council, 1996.
10. Haes DL Jr, Fitzgerald MF. VDT VLF measurements: the need for protocols in assessing VDT user "dose." *Health Phys* 1995;68:572–578.
11. Schnorr TM, Grajewski BA, Hornung RW, et al. Video display terminals and the risk of spontaneous abortion. *N Engl J Med* 1991;324:727–733.
12. Goldhaber MK, Polen MG, Hiatt PA. The risk of miscarriage and birth defects among women who use visual display terminals during pregnancy. *Am J Ind Med* 1988; 13:695–706.
13. Windham GC, Fenster L, Swan S, Neutra RR. Use of video display terminals during pregnancy and the risk of spontaneous abortion, low birthweight, or intrauterine growth retardation. *Am J Ind Med* 1990;18:675–688.
13b. Rogers SS. Radiofrequency burn hazards in the mf/hf band. In: Mitchell JC, ed. *Proceedings of a workshop on the protection of personnel against radiofrequency electro magnetic radiation*. Aeromedical Review 3-81, USAF School of Aerospace Medicine, Brooks AFB, Texas, pp. 76–89, 1981.
14. Kloth LC, Zisken MC. Diathermy and pulsed radio frequency radiation. In: Michlovitz, ed. *Thermal agents in rehabilitation.* Philadelphia: FA Davis, 1996:213–254.
15. International Commission on Non-Ionizing Radiation Protection. Heath issues related to the use of hand-held radiotelephones and base transmitters. *Health Phys* 1996; 70:587–593.
16. Redelmeier DA, Tibshirani RJ. Association between cellular telephone calls and motor vehicle collisions. *N Engl J Med* 1997;336:453–458.
17. Food and Drug Administration, Department of Health and Human Services. Update on cellular phone interference with cardiac pacemakers. Rockville, Maryland, May 3, 1995.
18. IEEE Standards Board. IEEE standard for safety levels with respect to human exposure to radio frequency electromagnetic fields, from 3 KHz to 300 GHz. New York: the Institute of Electrical and Electronic Engineers; IEEE Report 095.1-1991;1992.
19. National Council on Radiation Protection and Measurements (NCRP). Biological effects and exposure criteria for radiofrequency electromagnetic fields; NCRP report 86. Bethesda, MD: National Council on Radiation Protection and Measurements, 1986.
20. Sliney D, Wolbarsht M. *Safety with lasers and other optical sources.* New York: Plenum Press, 1985.
21. Taylor HR. The environment and the lens. *Br J Ophthalmol* 1980;64:303–310.
22. Taylor HR, West SK, Rosenthal FS, et al. Effect of ultraviolet radiation on cataract formation. *N Engl J Med* 1988;319:1429–1433.
23. Vitasa BC, Taylor HR, Strickland PT, et al. Association of nonmelanoma skin cancer and actinic keratosis with cumulative solar ultraviolet exposure in Maryland waterman. *Cancer* 1990;65:2811–2817.
24. Winklemann RK, Zollman PE, Baldes EJ. Squamous cell carcinomas produced by ultraviolet light in hairless mice. *J Invest Dermatol* 1963;40:217–240.
25. Green A, Maclennon R, Siskind V. Common acquired naevi and the risk of malignant melanoma. *Int J Cancer* 1985;35:397–400.
26. American national standard for the safe use of lasers; ANSI Z136.1-1993.: American National Standards Institute, New York, New York, 1993.
27. American Medical Association Council on Scientific Affairs. Lasers in medicine and surgery. *JAMA* 1986; 256:900–907.

Medical Center Occupational Health and Safety,
edited by Robert J. McCunney.
Lippincott Williams & Wilkins, Philadelphia © 1999.

15

Ergonomic Issues in Medical Centers

Kurt T. Hegmann and *Arun Garg

Department of Preventive Medicine, Medical College of Wisconsin, Milwaukee, Wisconsin 53226;
**Ergonomics Laboratory, Industrial and Manufacturing Engineering,*
University of Wisconsin–Milwaukee, Milwaukee, Wisconsin 53201

Ergonomics is an interdisciplinary field that has been described as fitting the task to the worker (1). Disciplines that have substantial influence on this field include industrial engineering, occupational medicine, neuromusculoskeletal epidemiology, biomechanics, industrial hygiene, physical therapy, occupational therapy, and occupational safety. Training is most often at the graduate level and most frequently follows at least baccalaureate training in one of the foregoing disciplines. Curricular composition of training programs varies from laboratory-based investigation of muscle fatigue to application of methods to assess job risks.

Certification as a certified industrial ergonomist or certified human factors professional is available through the Board of Certification in Professional Ergonomics. Candidates must fulfill education and experience requirements and pass an examination. Certification is available through the same organization for the associate ergonomics professional or associate human factors professional. The associate categories have less rigorous experience and examination requirements but the same educational requirements as full certification. The associate categories were formed to recognize persons working toward full certification who have fulfilled the 4 years' experience requirement. Approximately one half of ergonomists in the United States are certified. Most deal primarily with manufacturing settings. However, as is detailed herein, medical centers have substantial ergonomics-related issues.

Three sources of ergonomic issues in the medical center environment generate the most concerns. These are patient transfers, material handling, and keyboarding. By far, the foremost among these is back related disorders (2–15), including acute and chronic regional low-back pain and sciatica, most frequently related to patient transfers. There is also potential concern about various tasks that are common sources of back injury in medical centers, including manual materials handling in areas of laundry and shipping and receiving. Possible concerns arise with prolonged keyboarding in the area of medical transcription. This chapter focuses on the magnitude of and prevention of these disorders.

AN INDUSTRY-WIDE PERSPECTIVE

Bureau of Labor Statistics data from 1996 provide a nationwide perspective on injury and illness rates according to industry categories. Figure 15-1 shows that compared with other industry groups, health services have higher nonfatal injury rates than agriculture, transportation, and mining. These rates are only slightly lower than those for manufacturing (16). For the composite of the nation's private industries, the incidence rates of workplace injuries and illnesses in 1996 were reported as 7.4 cases per 100 equivalent full-time workers (FTE) and 9.1 cases per FTE in

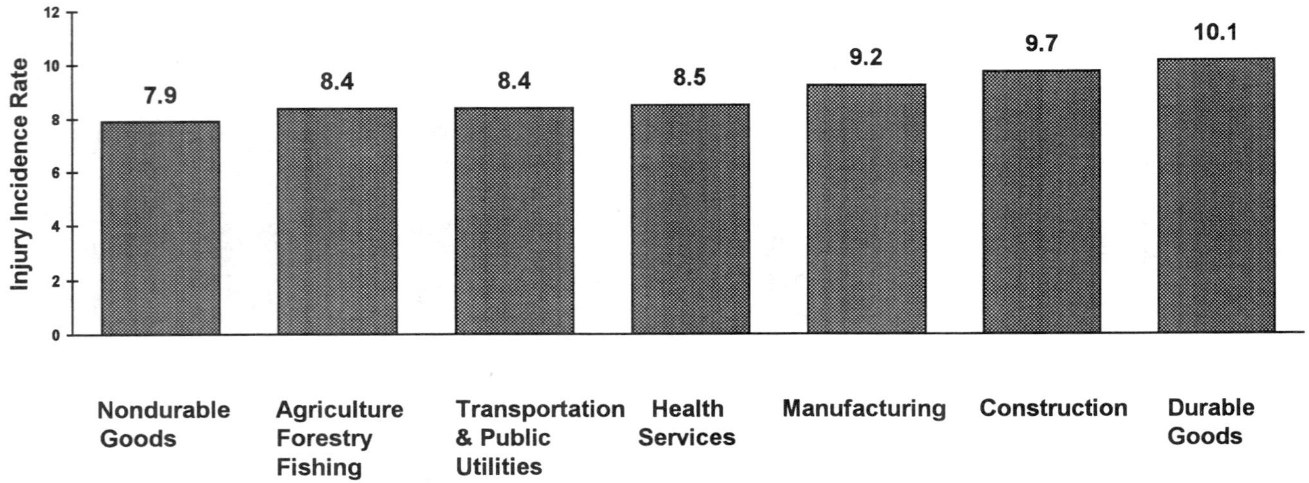

The average for all of private industry is 6.9 per 100. Other categories not represented on the graphic are, in ascending order: finance/insurance/real estate (2.1), mining (5.3), services (5.7), wholesale trade (6.5), wholesale and retail trade (6.6), and retail trade (6.7).

FIG. 15-1. Incidence of nonfatal injury (number per 100 equivalent full-time workers) by industry, 1996.

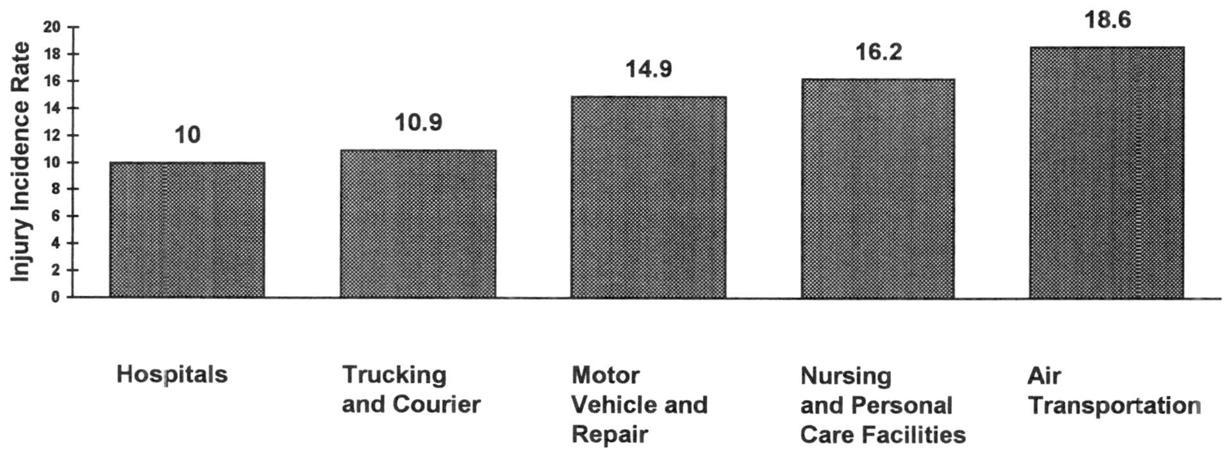

Two categories apply to the discussion in this chapter: hospitals and nursing and personal care facilities. Other categories not represented are, in ascending order: eating and drinking places (6.1), hotels and motels (8.9), grocery stores (9.7), and department stores (9.8).

FIG. 15-2. Incidence of nonfatal injury (number per 100 equivalent full-time workers in industry with 100,000 cases or more), 1996.

the health services industry (23.0% greater). Lost-workday injury and illness case rates, in which most workers' compensation costs are incurred, were also 8.8% greater (3.4 cases per FTE versus 3.7 cases per FTE) (16). Within the health services industry, hospitals and nursing and personal care facilities have been shown to have high rates of nonfatal injury (Fig. 15-2) (17).

REVIEW OF THE OCCUPATIONAL INJURY AND DISEASE DATABASE OF A LARGE MEDICAL CENTER

Because detailed analyses of medical center injuries and illnesses are infrequently reported, the experience of one urban 700-bed tertiary referral medical center is described. For an employed population of approximately 2,600 persons, data for 18 months, January 1, 1997, through June 30, 1998, were analyzed. The medical center does not have a zero lift policy (see later). A summary of this large occupational injury and illness computerized database is depicted in Fig. 15-3. A total of 1,099 cases were identified; the crude rate is approximately 28.2 instances per FTE. This rate is approximately 2.8 times higher than industry-wide reported rates, in part because it includes injuries and illnesses for which reporting is not required. Analysis of these data indicated that safety issues, such as acute accidents, toxicologic exposures, and potential infectious disease exposures encompass approximately 677 (61.6%) of cases. Nearly all of the other cases involved musculoskeletal disorders not identified as accidents. Results of an analysis of these musculoskeletal disorders (n = 400) is depicted in Fig. 15-4. Precisely half of the instances were related to regional low-back pain. Next in importance were hand and wrist, lower extremity, and rotator cuff problems. Thus back-related disorders constitute the greatest area of concern.

Although nearly all of the cases of musculoskeletal disorders are labeled as injuries, often connoting acute events, most are likely to be cases of disease and likely of potential ergonomic concern. Even in instances in which the onset of pain is acute, the pathologic findings indicate that most of these injuries are disease processes (18). However, this medical center's data are likely to contain some cases of acute injury, such as true ligamentous sprains (e.g., knee and ankle sprains), which may be safety issues rather than ergonomic concerns. This problem appears to be a systematic classification bias throughout all industry data. Most of the cases (n = 400) described herein appear to be associated with potential ergonomic concerns. Elimination from these data of injuries to other body parts in acute accidents would further magnify the back as the anatomic area of primary importance for ergonomic efforts in health care settings.

FACTORS IN HIGH RATES OF REGIONAL LOW-BACK PAIN AMONG HEALTH CARE WORKERS

Excessive rates of low-back disorders can be predicted on the basis of the typically high physical demands placed on the workers. Much lifting (Table 15-1) is excessively forceful and is believed to be hazardous to the back. The average worker cannot perform a heavy physical demand such as lifting a 100-kg patient. Because many workers performing this lifting are women, there is a great mismatch between average lifting capabilities (e.g., small average cross-sectional area of the vertebral bodies) and fixed job demands (19). This mismatch is thought to be one of the causes of the high rate of low-back disorders among health care workers (16,17). Regardless of this mismatch, high physical job demands are thought to cause high rates of low-back disorders for both sexes.

Important ergonomic reasons for the elevated risk for back disorders include the large amount of weight lifted, static exertion, long horizontal distances between the lumbosacral spine and hands when lifting, and frequency of lifts. A list of these variables is

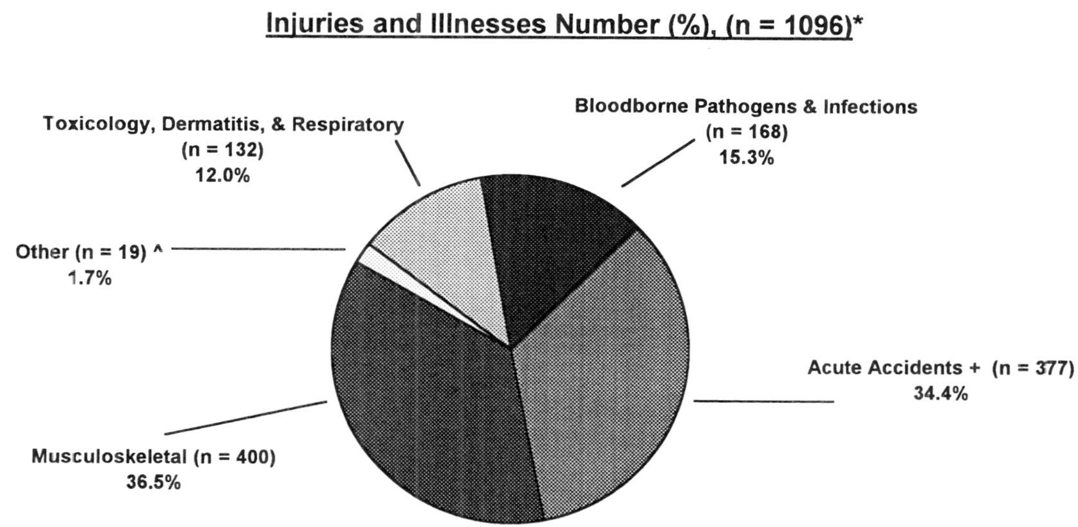

* - Unclassified "pain" cases (n = 3) are not included in the analyses
\+ - Contusions, lacerations, fractures, burns, electrical shocks, and acute injury
^ - Includes concussion, corneal abrasion and dizziness

FIG. 15-3. Injury and illness experience at a large medical center, January 1, 1997, through June 30, 1998.

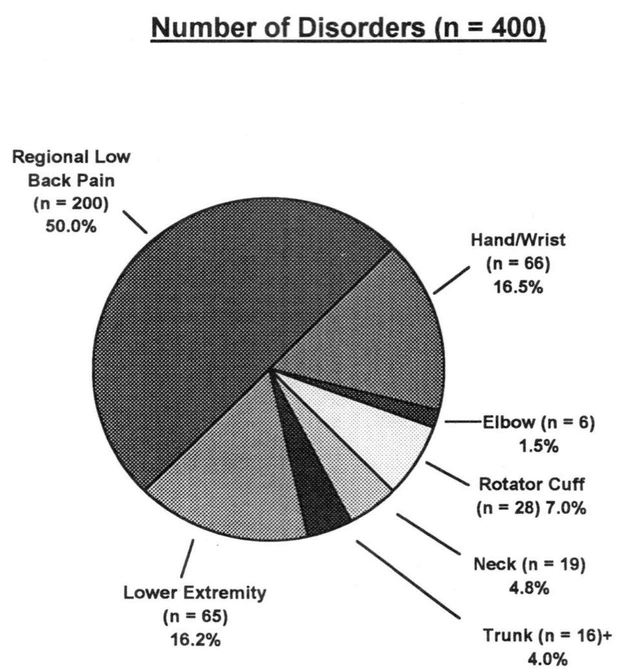

* - These data exclude what appear to be obviously acute accidents. Nevertheless, they likely include some residual acute injuries, especially of the lower extremities.

\+ - Excluding lower back. Does include thoracic spine, sternoclavicular, and groin.

FIG. 15-4. Nonacute musculoskeletal disorders among workers at a large medical center, January 1, 1997, through June 30, 1998.

TABLE 15-1. *Sources of high ergonomic demands on health care workers*

Static exertions, especially with toileting tasks
Shifting of weight and unpredictability while lifting
Sudden falls, slips, and other accidents
Patients do not have "handles" (poor coupling)
Asymmetric lifts
Long horizontal distance between the spine and the hands when lifting
Lifting over obstacles, such as the edge of bathtubs and whirlpools
Marked weights over 51 pounds, the limit considered safe for 75% of women (19)
Simultaneous lifting, flexing, and twisting
Sudden, unexpected loading
Bulky size of load
Lifting frequency
Pushing or pulling heavy loads
Lifting in confined spaces, such as bathrooms

in Table 15-1. A large number of these risk factors are unique to the health care industry; thus unique solutions are needed. Personal risk factors (Table 15-2) in addition to the physical demands of the job increase risk for low back disorders. A comprehensive program to address the entire spectrum of morbidity should address all risk factors. Despite the high rate of back injury among health care providers, studies have shown that risk for low back disorders can be markedly reduced if workers are trained and use equipment that eliminates virtually all substantial force demands associated with patient transfers—a zero lift policy.

TABLE 15-2. *Personal risk factors for back disorders*

Increasing age
Sex (female)
Obesity
Tobacco use
Prior injuries
Hypertension
Systemic arthritis
Job dissatisfaction
Other psychosocial stressors
Poor physical fitness

TABLE 15-3. *Types of patient care ergonomic transferring devices for a zero-lift policy*

Hoists, sit stand	Shower gurneys
Hoists, total	Walking belts
Repositioning devices	Weighing devices
Shower chairs	

ZERO LIFT POLICY

The term *zero lift policy* has been coined to describe an ergonomics program, usually in health services, that prohibits nearly all lifting of any consequence (20). This ergonomics program has at its core the typical occupational health program features of education, training, and equipment. Many types of ergonomically designed patient transfer devices (Table 15-3 and Figs. 15-5, 15-6) can lower physical job demands. In one comparison of equipment from different manufacturers (21), the devices were not found to be equally effective in user ratings of perceived exertion. Thus selection of the equipment appears important. Training is necessary to ensure proper use of equipment and to reduce the frequency of injuries.

Implementation of a Zero Lift Policy

The steps for implementation of a zero lift policy are given in Table 15-4. Management must be educated and committed to the project. Participation of workers and supervisors is necessary. Without this commitment, the risk for purchasing unpopular or unsuitable equipment is great. One person must be responsible for the program, and individuals may have to be responsible in each department of large medical centers. The equipment selected must match patients' and the nurses' needs. A needs assessment must include worker input. Training should include didactic and written information and practice with the equipment. After the program is implemented, periodic reassessment is needed. In-service educational retraining is needed, and new workers need extensive training as a part of their orientation. Administrative controls and discipline may be needed to resolve problems after the program is implemented. Unfortunately, without administrative controls and progressive discipline, the policy's

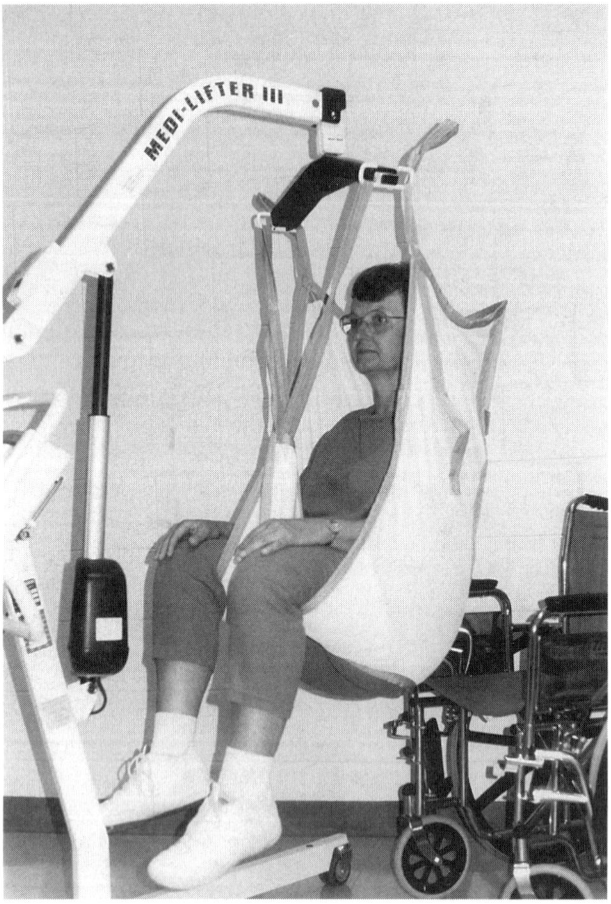

FIG. 15-5. Patient lift used to transfer patients in any seated posture to another location.

goals may be thwarted by failure to follow safe operating procedures.

Benefits of a Zero Lift Policy

A prospective interventional study was performed in three nursing homes that instituted a zero lift policy (22). Multiple benefits were documented, including an 80% decrease in lost or restricted workday injuries from patient transfers, a 62% reduction in all lost or restricted workday injuries, and an 80.6% reduction in workers' compensation costs for nursing departments. Number of lost or restricted workdays per year for nursing departments decreased 84.6% (Fig. 15-7). Total workers' compensation costs per nursing home per year decreased 75.0% (Fig. 15-8). A number of other benefits also accrued (Table 15-5), including the ability of workers less capable of forceful work demands to remain employed.

The stark magnitudes of declines in injury statistics suggest that these reductions were most likely related to the interventions. They were likely to be the result of neither shifting of causation from the occupational setting to the nonoccupational setting nor a Hawthorne effect (23,24). Because these results were obtained in nursing care facilities, which have higher rates of low-back disorders among caregivers than do hospitals (17), a zero lift policy is likely to be quite effective in the medical center environment.

Patient Transport and Dietary

Back injuries are frequent among patient transport and dietary departments. The main

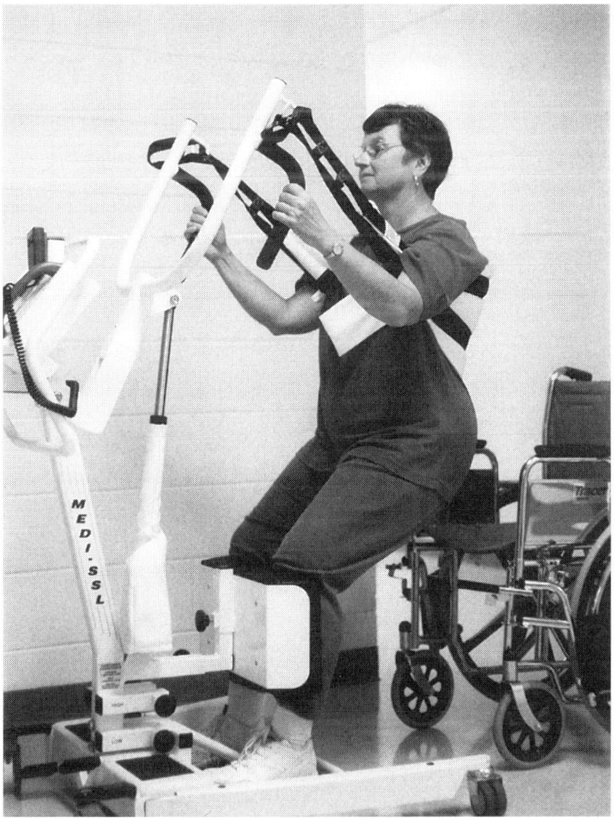

FIG. 15-6. Patient lift assist device used to transfer patients from one location to another. It is also useful for toileting tasks.

source of force that produces occupational low-back pain is pushing or pulling a patient's gurney or a cart of food trays. In both situations the common source of force is the wheel of the cart. Yet the amount of this force is relatively easily manipulated, particularly in the case of older equipment.

Irregular floor surfaces substantially increase force requirements and should be altered or repaired. Most medical centers, however, have smooth floors, so this problem is not severe. The ideal cart has large wheels. The wheels should be well lubricated and maintained. Cracking, ridging, or wearing of wheel materials necessitates repair or replacement. Equipment that tends to require lateral forces to maintain a forward direction of travel needs repair or replacement. Employee training is particularly helpful in these areas. Employees should be taught to push rather than pull whenever possible (25). Slip resis-

TABLE 15-4. *Sequencing of the key details to implement a zero-lift policy*

1. Educate management and obtain commitments.
2. Involve workers, form participatory ergonomics teams.
3. Assign overall programmatic responsibility to one person.
4. Perform needs assessments (patients' and workers').
5. Utilizing worker input, carefully select and obtain equipment (pilot before purchase).
6. Train personnel (including supervisors).
   a. Didactic
   b. Practice with each other
   c. Practice with patients
7. Assess efficacy of interventions and obtain feedback.
8. Schedule regular retraining sessions.
9. Incorporate training in new worker orientation.
10. Implement administrative discipline if there is inadequate compliance with the zero-lift policy (without substantiation).

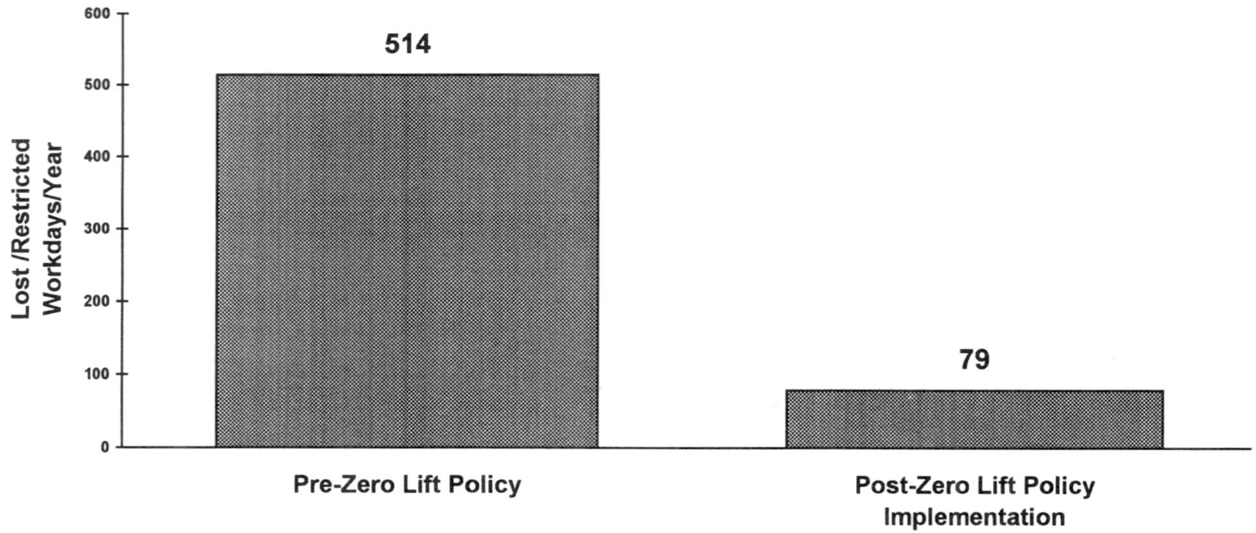

FIG. 15-7. Nursing departments' lost and restricted workdays per year.

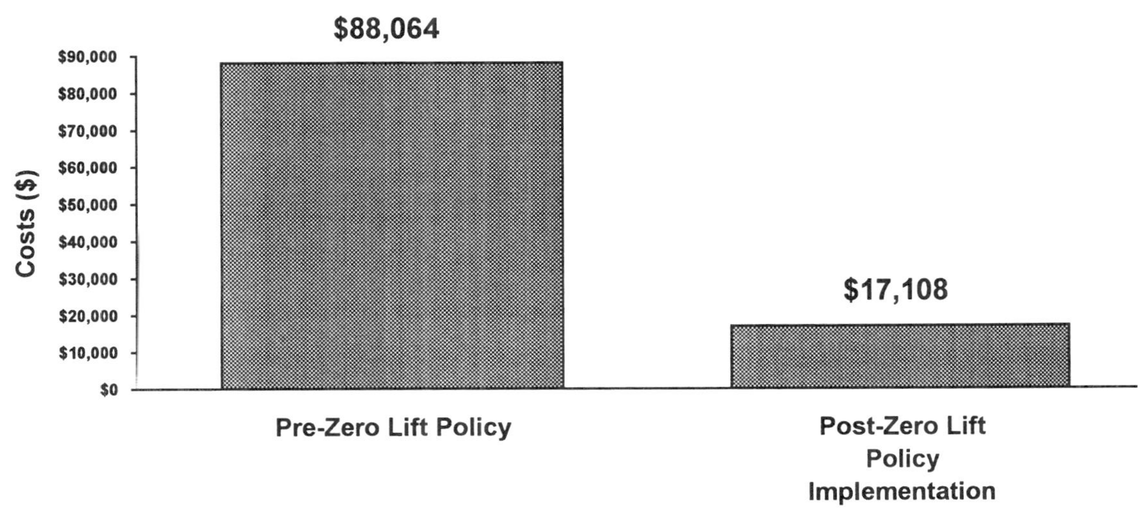

FIG. 15-8. Nursing department's workers' compensation costs per year.

TABLE 15-5. *Zero-lift policy benefits experienced in nursing homes*

Decreases	Increases
Incidence of injury and disease	Worker satisfaction
Lost-time injuries	Time a pregnant worker can give patient care
OSHA 200 recordable events	Time an older worker can work
Patient injuries (e.g., skin tears)	Morale
Worker turnover rates	
Sick days	
Costs	

TABLE 15-6. *Workstation modification to consider for potential reduction in distal upper extremity diseases among video display terminal operators*

Adjustable chair	Adjustable page holder
Adjustable back rest	Padded wrist rest
Adjustable keyboard height	Rest breaks

tant soles should be required to improve traction and decrease hazards from slipping.

Laundry

The handling of laundry is another cause of back disorders in the medical center environment. Primary causes include either repeated lumbar flexion to reach the bottoms of carts or lifting of excessively large bags of laundry. Pushing old carts with poor wheels adds unnecessary force requirements to the job. Interventions to be considered include use of spring-loaded platforms to raise the bottom of the cart as it is emptied, training to push or pull rather than lift, decreasing the size of the laundry bags, purchasing and maintaining carts with well-functioning, large wheels, and placing cart handles at a comfortable height.

OFFICE ERGONOMICS

Perhaps the single greatest area of concern about office ergonomics in medical centers involves medical transcription because high rates of key-strokes are common. Yet keyboarding is of uncertain hazard. The National Institute for Occupational Safety and Health (NIOSH) U.S. West study (26) demonstrated no dose-response relation between keystroke rates ranging from 11,304 to 22,875 per day (mean 15,950 ± 2,410) and the development of hand-wrist disorders, including carpal tunnel syndrome. The study also found no association between amount of time spent at a video display terminal station per day and hand-wrist disorders. Positive correlations were found with the occupationally related variables of high information-processing demands, uncertainty about job future, routine work that lacks decision-making opportunity, increasing work pressure, and lack of supervisor support. However, medical transcriptionists make about 80,000 per day. It is unclear whether these rates of keystroke activity are hazardous and if they are, to what extent. It is possible that this high rate of keystrokes may cause elevated risk for carpal tunnel syndrome and other hand and wrist disorders, such as flexor or extensor tenosynovitis. It is also possible that through logical extension of the U.S. West study, there is not an identifiable threshold beyond which risk for these disorders rises and that they are not related to keyboard activities.

Unfortunately, results of studies testing the foregoing hypothesis with large prospective cohorts have not yet been reported. In the absence of such studies, most recommendations rely on generic modifications of risk factors to attempt to address theoretical risks for these disorders (Table 15-6). The most important aspect of these interventions appears to be the adjustability of factors under the control of the worker. When the American National Standards Institute (ANSI) ideal job design (27) is enforced as an exact standard, there are reports of failure at reducing the incidence of disorders or at augmenting the numbers of disorders (1,28).

HOW TO CONDUCT AN ERGONOMIC ASSESSMENT

A workplace walk-through survey for physical job factors has analogies to one for chemical issues. There are differences, however, particularly if the purpose is related to concerns arising from one case. Occupational toxicologic problems, such as silicosis and benzene-induced aplastic anemia, are less likely to arise from nonoccupational exposures than are neuromusculoskeletal disorders. In addition, neuromusculoskcletal disordcrs may arise without any exposure as, for example, age-related degenerative phenomena. Thus a survey based on one case is inherently difficult for qualitative analyses. There are checklists for screening jobs for problems, but they are widely thought to be so sensitive as to be of little value, so confirmatory analyses are needed. Tools for confirmatory analyses (19, 25,29–32) require training to use and have not been completely validated.

Bccausc of the foregoing difficulties, it is recommended that an epidemiologic approach be used when practical to analyze most neuromusculoskeletal problems (Fig. 15-9). Such an

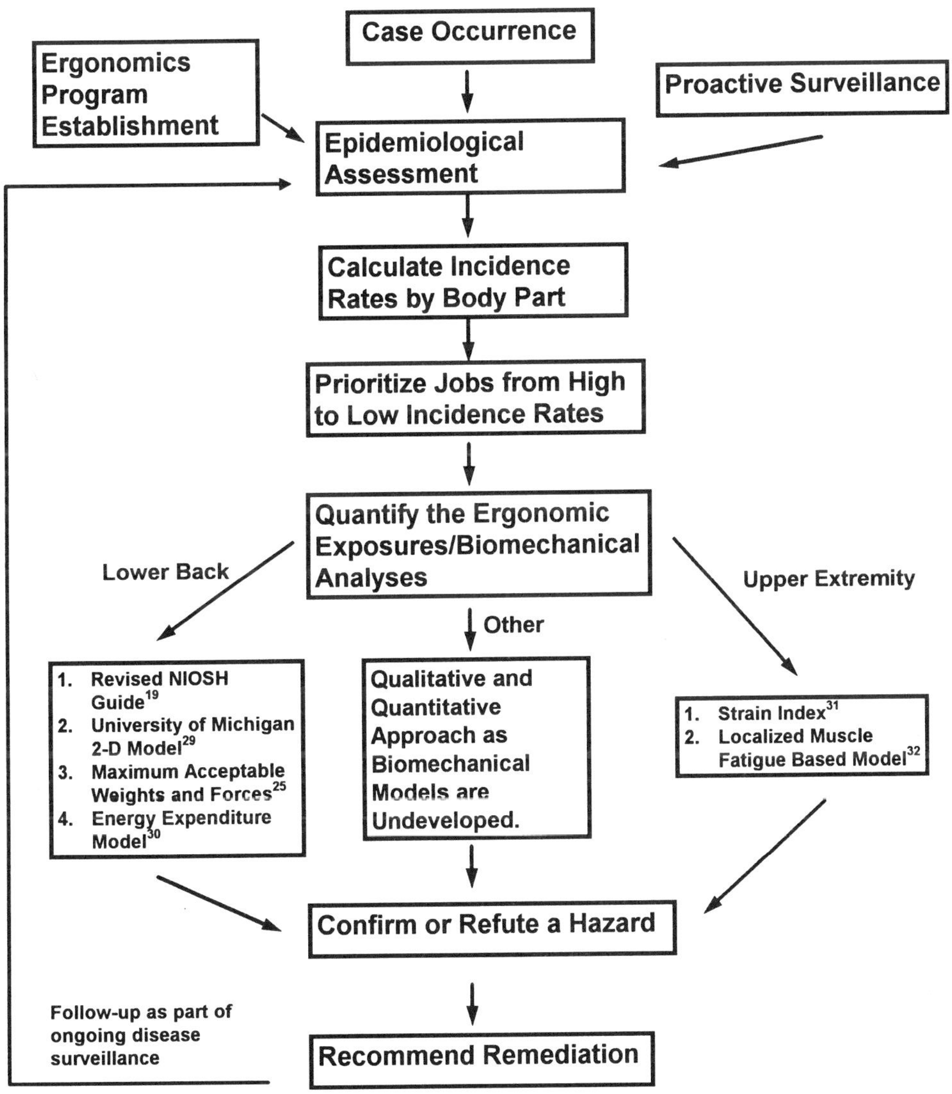

FIG. 15-9. Ergonomic surveillance by an employer based on incidence rates.

approach involves the analysis of injury and disease data to calculate incidence rates. Subsequent quantitative analyses are performed for job hazards in areas with high incidence rates. When a confirmed exposure hazard is remedied, ongoing surveillance is performed to assure the disease rate is reduced, and work begins on another issue.

ERGONOMIC REGULATIONS

National ergonomics standards may be implemented over the next few years. Currently, there is no national standard, although there has been enforcement by the Occupations Safety Health Administration (OSHA) under the general duty clause. Both OSHA and ANSI are developing such standards. Although the components of either standard have not been finalized, they may include assessment of risk, engineering and administrative controls, and training. Assessment of risk will best be accomplished with an epidemiologic approach that includes calculation of disease rates by department to ascertain the areas in greatest need of intervention.

Engineering and administrative controls will likely be epitomized in the zero lift policy. Back belts, elbow straps, and wrist braces often are considered personal protective equipment. This gear is unlikely to be specified in a standard because of pervasive opinion (33,34), including that of NIOSH regarding back belts, that these articles are not protective but might be treatment options. However, patient-lifting equipment will be necessary to fully implement a program in a medical center.

A staff education component is likely, although the scope of training is unclear. As currently drafted, for example, the scope of training is to include only occupational risk factors rather than a complete view of current knowledge of the epidemiologic features of these disorders. For example, carpal tunnel syndrome training should include teaching that elevated body mass index is a risk rather than simplistically focusing on proposed occupational risk factors. One final matter important for an ergonomics program is the maintenance of records indicating, at a minimum, prior incidence rates, hazards identified, interventions, and results of implemented changes.

Whether or not an ergonomics standard is promulgated, it appears prudent to assess risk for disease by department and intervene in those with elevated risk. Our experience has shown that implementation of a zero lift policy appears justified. A primary reason to implement a program is that, as commonly performed, many of these jobs carry high risk, and benefits are likely from an effective ergonomics program.

CONTROVERSIES IN PROPOSED ERGONOMICS STANDARDS

The following weaknesses are present in the current versions of proposed ergonomics standards:

1. Hazards are identified through complaints or single case reports rather than epidemiologically driven prioritization of jobs.
2. Job analysis methods remain largely unvalidated.
3. Cumulative trauma disorders are being defined to include virtually any injury or disease involving any tissue, rather than muscle-tendon unit disorders with or without nerve disorders.
4. The epidemiologic basis of the work relatedness of many specific diseases is weak or nonexistent (e.g., supraspinatus tendinitis or rupture, ulnar neuropathy at the wrist or elbow, radial neuropathy, cervical radiculopathy).
5. Exposures are not prioritized. Force appears to be the most important variable (i.e., it primarily drives safe versus hazardous assessments of biomechanical models), yet force is frequently considered secondary to repetition as a risk factor.
6. Unaccustomed work appears to be a substantial factor, yet it is virtually unmentioned, and controls for this factor (e.g., break-in times) are undefined.
7. There appears to be a lack of appreciation that these disorders occur frequently in

the absence of substantial occupational exposures. There is no method specified to differentiate occupational from nonoccupational causes of a disorder (35).

8. Teaching and training of employees do not include balanced information on occupational (e.g., force, percentage duration of exertion, posture, cycle time, direct compression) and nonoccupational (e.g., age, sex, obesity, lack of exercise, tobacco) risk factors to properly educate and allow for the maximum potential for reduction in disorders.
9. Psychosocial risk factors are largely ignored in the draft versions of the standards, and controls for such risk factors are currently rudimentary. Psychosocial risk factors are, however, increasingly recognized as risk factors for occupational back, shoulder, and distal upper extremity claims.

CONCLUSIONS

There are substantial ergonomic concerns in the health services industry, particularly in hospitals and nursing care facilities. Excessive risks for low-back disorders are well documented, and consequently should be the primary concern and priority for ergonomic intervention. Yet these risks appear to have been unappreciated (36). Interventions are now possible to sharply reduce the magnitudes of exertions with patient lift assist devices and implementation of a zero lift policy. These policies have been documented to result in marked reduction in injuries, illnesses, and workers' compensation costs. There are other ergonomic concerns in the medical center setting, and intervention is likely to reduce the risk of those activities.

FURTHER INFORMATION

To best address the needs of a medical center, it may be optimal if the ergonomist has experience in medical center issues. Prior employment in a medical center would be helpful, because there are many differences between the manufacturing and medical center settings. Although there is no list specific to medical centers, a list of all certified professional ergonomists is available at http://www.bcpe.org.

REFERENCES

1. Kroemer KHF, Grandjean E. *Fitting the task to the human: a textbook of occupational ergonomics,* 5th ed. London: Taylor & Francis, 1997.
2. Bell F, Dalgity ME, Fennell MJ, Aitken RCB. Hospital ward patient-lifting tasks. *Ergonomics* 1979;22: 1257–1273.
3. Biering-Sorensen F. Risk of back trouble in individual occupations in Denmark. *Ergonomics* 1985;28:51–60.
4. Cust G, Pearson JCG, Mair A. The prevalence of low back pain in nurses. *Int Nurs Rev* 1972;19:169–178.
5. Dehlin O, Hedenrud B, Horal J. Back symptoms in nursing aides in a geriatric hospital: an interview study with special reference to the incidence of low-back symptoms. *Scand J Rehabil Med* 1976;8:47–53.
6. Garg A, Owen BD, Carlson B. An ergonomic evaluation of nursing assistants' job in a nursing home. *Ergonomics* 1992;35:979–995.
7. Garg A, Owen B. Reducing back stress to nursing personnel: an ergonomic intervention in a nursing home. *Ergonomics* 1992;35:1353–1375.
8. Harber P, Billet E, Gutkowski M, Soohoo K, Lew M, Roman A. Occupational low-back pain in hospital nurses. *J Occup Med* 1985;27:518–524.
9. Jensen RC. Disabling back injuries among nursing personnel: research needs and justifications. *Res Nurs Health* 1987;10:29–38.
10. Klein BP, Jensen RC, Sanderson LM. Assessment of workers' compensation claims for back strains/sprains. *J Occup Med* 1984;26:443–448.
11. Personick ME. Nursing home aides experience increase in serious injuries. *Monthly Labor Rev* 1990;113:30–34.
12. Stubbs DA, Buckle PW, Hudson MP, Rivers PM, Worringham CJ. Back pain in the nursing profession, I: epidemiology and pilot methodology. *Ergonomics* 1983; 26:755–765.
13. Stubbs DA, Buckle PW, Hudson MP, Rivers PM. Back pain in the nursing profession, II: the effectiveness of training. *Ergonomics* 1983;26:767–779.
14. Valles-Pankratz S. What's in back of nursing home injuries? *Ohio Monitor* 1989;62:4–8.
15. Videman T, NurminenT, Tola S, Kuorinka I, Vanharanta H, Troup JD. Low-back pain in nurses and some loading factors of work. *Spine* 1984;9:400–404.
16. US Department of Labor, Bureau of Labor Statistics. Safety and Health Statistics, 1996. Available at http://stats.bls.gov/news.release/osh.t01.htm.
17. US Department of Labor, Bureau of Labor Statistics. Safety and Health Statistics, 1996. Available at http://stats.bls.gov/news.release/osh.t04.htm.
18. Hegmann KT, Moore JS. Common neuromusculoskeletal disorders. In: King P, ed. *Sourcebook of occupational rehabilitation*. New York: Plenum Press, 1998:19–41.
19. Waters TR, Putz-Anderson V, Garg A, Fine LJ. Revised NIOSH equation for the design and evaluation of manual lifting tasks. *Ergonomics* 1993;36:749–776.
20. Garg A. *Prevention of injuries to health care workers: a manual for implementing zero lift policy.* Milwaukee, WI: University of Wisconsin–Milwaukee, 1998.

21. Garg A, Owen BD. An ergonomic approach to preventing back injuries from patient lifting. *PTSM Series* 1994;2:15–22.
22. Garg A. Effectiveness of ergonomic interventions in nursing homes using participatory approach: preliminary results. In: Mital A, Krueger H, Kumar S, Menozzi M, Fernandez JE, eds. *Advances in occupational ergonomics and safety*. Vol. 1. Cincinnati: International Society for Occupational Ergonomics and Safety, 1996:164–169.
23. Mayo E. *The human problems of an industrial civilization*. New York: Macmillan, 1933.
24. Roethlisberger FJ, Dickson WJ. *Management and the worker*. Cambridge, MA: Harvard University Press, 1939.
25. Snook SH, Cirello VM. The design of manual handling tasks: revised tables of maximum acceptable weights and forces. *Ergonomics* 1991;34:1197–1213.
26. Hales T, Sauter S, Petersen M, et al. Health hazard evaluation report; HETA 89-299-2230. Phoenix: US West Communications, 1992.
27. American National Standards Institute/Human Factors Society. ANSI/HFS 100-1988. Human factors engineering of visual display terminal workstations. Santa Monica, CA: American National Standards Institute, 1988.
28. Moore JS, Garg A. A case study of an epidemic of upper extremity disorders in a corporate office. In: Mital A, Krueger H, Kumor S, Menozzi M, Fernandez JE, eds. *Advances in Occupational Ergonomics and Safety.* 1996;2:858–863.,
29. University of Michigan 2-dimensional static strength program. Ann Arbor, MI: Center for Ergonomics, 1990.
30. Garg A, Chaffin DB, Herrin GD. Prediction of metabolic rates for manual materials handling jobs. *Am Ind Hyg Assoc J* 1978;39:661.
31. Moore JS, Garg A. The strain index: a proposed method to analyze jobs for risk of distal upper extremity disorders. *Am Ind Hyg Assoc J* 1995;56:443–458.
32. Rodgers SH. A functional job analysis technique. In: Moore JS, Garg A, eds. *Ergonomics* 1992;7:679–711.
33. Van Poppel MNM, Koes BW, Van der Ploeg T, Smid T, Bouter LM. Lumbar supports and education for the prevention of low back pain in industry. *JAMA* 1998;279: 1789–1794.
34. Workplace use of back belts: review and recommendations; 1994. DHHS (NIOSH) publication no 94-1220.
35. Kusnetz S, Hutchinson MK, eds. A guide to the work-relatedness of disease—revised; 1979; DHEW (NIOSH) publication no 79-116.
36. Patterson WB, Craven DE, Schwartz DA, Nardell EA, Kasmer J, Noble J. Occupational hazards to hospital personnel. *Ann Intern Med* 1985;102:658–680.

Medical Center Occupational Health and Safety,
edited by Robert J. McCunney.
Lippincott Williams & Wilkins, Philadelphia © 1999.

16
Fire and Electrical Safety

Walter G. Diaz

Massachusetts Institute of Technology, Cambridge, Massachusetts 02139-4304

Fire safety is an important consideration for any medical center. Loss prevention experts at Factory Mutual Research and Engineering reported that in a 10-year period, hospitals and health care facilities sustained $37 million in property damage and business interruption from fire (1). More important is the loss of life and injuries sustained in medical facilities. Table 16-1 displays information that is excerpted from the National Fire Protection Association (NFPA) Web page on fire investigation abstracts. The 11 selected medical facility fires caused 41 deaths and 94 injuries. Table 16-1 shows that facilities with full and unimpaired fire protection sprinkler systems had no fatalities.

Safety awareness is essential in medical centers and nursing homes, where many occupants are often unable to leave the building in the event of an emergency. Electrical causes, the most common cause of fires in medical facilities, represented 27% of all fires and 21% of total costs (1). Smoking-related incidents, incendiary activities, cooking equipment, matches, lighters and other open flames aside from torches and heating equipment have been cited as additional causes (2). The NFPA analysis of nursing home and hospital fires suggested that smoking-related incidents rank high as a leading cause of fire (2). Electrical causes are common in hospital laboratory fires (3).

Fires can be prevented through judicious selection of equipment and proper training of personnel, including contractors. Fire safety is only one of the many disciplines needed to run a medical center. In a busy medical center encouraging people to address fire safety can be a daunting task. On the other hand, appropriate fire and disaster drills can be instrumental in ensuring that staff are properly trained and familiar with operations if a fire occurs. Many fire codes and regulations and fire insurance carrier guidelines encourage periodic drills. For example, requirements of the Joint Commission on Accreditation of Health Care Organizations (JCAHO) include fire protection, electrical safety, and evacuation and emergency planning. The Occupational Safety and Health Administration (OSHA), and other federal, state, and local governments require evacuation planning and emergency action plans. Many regulations, including building and electrical codes and environmental waste regulations, have requirements related to fire safety, such as specific types of fire alarms, fire detection and fire suppression systems, testing systems, and mandating contingency plans for hazardous waste operations.

FIRE PREVENTION

Reducing the risk for fire in a medical facility requires diligence in conducting periodic inspections of the physical plant, reviewing of policies and procedures, and training staff for fire emergency response. The most straightforward way to approach fire safety in a medical center includes fire prevention, fire planning, fire-protection evaluation, develop-

TABLE 16-1. *Selected medical facility fires abstract*

Incident no.	Date	Time	Location	Type of facility	Origin	Cause/notes	Fire protection sprinklers	No. of deaths	No. of injuries
1	10/16/96	11:16 a.m.	Hyannis, Massachusetts	Hospital	Nurses' lounge	Food tray ignited from unattended electric stove	Yes	None	9 staff 2 patients Smoke inhalation
2	12/31/94	9:00 p.m.	Petersburg, Virginia	Hospital	Patient's room	Smoking materials ignited bedding and involved air flotation mattress with foam padding and piped wall oxygen	No	5 patients	NR
3	12/1/94	3:45 a.m.	Broward County, Florida	Board and care	Resident's bedroom	NR	NR	6 residents	NR
4	9/1/93	5:42 a.m.	Brooklyn, New York	Hospital	Patient's room	Involved medical equipment; exact cause not determined	NR	3 patients	1 patient 11 firefighters
5	6/2/93	Morning	Ashland, Kentucky	Nursing home	Resident's room	NR	Yes	None	19 staff and residents
6	1/24/93	NR	Weymouth, Massachusetts	Hospital	NR	Incendiary	Yes	None	6 staff Smoke inhalation
7	10/30/92	NR	Woburn, Massachusetts	Nursing center	Gas entered building; $1.5 million loss	Natural gas released during construction caused explosion; unknown ignition source	Yes	None	21 civilians 2 firefighters
8	6/2/92	2:15 a.m.	Detroit, Michigan	Board and care	Kitchen	Probably discarded smoking materials in waste basket	No	10 occupants	NR
9	3/4/91	12:45 a.m.	Colorado Springs, Colorado	Board and care	Attic	Electric motor from ventilation fan overheated, igniting combustibles in attic; destroyed 2 of 3 wings	No	9 residents	8 residents 5 firefighters
10	9/19/90	Early morning	Bessember, Alabama	Board and care	NR	NR	Yes, but inadequate water supply and installation	4 residents	NR
11	3/13/90	NR	Dardanelle, Arkansas	Nursing home	Undetermined; cart in linen storage room	Undetermined	Yes, but partial only; in kitchen, laundry, and storage room	4 patients	10 patients
Totals								41	94

NR, not reported in the abstract.
Extracted from the National Fire Protection Association Web pages on Fire Investigations. http:www.nfpa.org.

ment of a fire-safety plan, and emergency response planning.

Preventing fires is paramount to preserving the mission of medical centers—the care and treatment of patients. Fire, essentially rapid oxidation followed by the evolution of heat and light, requires heat for ignition, fuel to burn, and air (oxygen) to support combustion. Effective fire prevention requires an extensive review of the physical environment to determine how a fire might start and be sustained once initiated.

After the facility review and evaluation of the potential for fire to initiate and propagate, fire prevention should address the containment of the fire to one particular area to prevent spread and control the sources of ignition (e.g., cooking, central heating) to designated areas within the medical center. An appreciation of the three major components of fire—fuel, oxygen, and heat—helps focus prevention efforts through the elimination of these factors. Further consideration of prevention of fires should address the following questions:

1. What can burn?
2. What can ignite it?
3. How can it be prevented from igniting?
4. How can circumstances be controlled so that ignition and fuel do not meet?

In hospitals, medical centers, and nursing homes, potential fuels include sheets, blankets, mattresses, clothing, furniture, plastic disposable items, fuel supplies, curtains, carpets, newspapers, magazines, and even food wrappers. Other combustibles include plastics, rubber, foam pillows, insulating materials, and toys, hair spray or other pressurized containers, fingernail polish remover (acetone), seasonal decorations, and table coverings.

The most likely items for starting a fire in a medical center are overloaded outlets and defective extension cords and heating appliances, such as toasters and coffee pots. Other sources are electric blankets, other appliances and diagnostic instruments, certain types of lighting, improper wiring, loose electrical connections, and improperly maintained equipment. Radiant heat from appliances such as space heaters, stove tops, and fireplaces also can be ignition sources.

Heating appliances can cause a fire from radiant or conducted heat. For example, a fire can be caused by radiant heat when an upholstered chair is too close to a fireplace or by conductive heat when a toaster is in contact with a plastic wrapper. Fires also have been started in clothes lying on top of electric space heaters. Even a hot curling iron on a cotton ball or other combustible material such as a plastic bottle of nail polish remover (acetone) can cause a fire.

Although regulations have severely limited smoking by patients and hospital staff, it is still allowable in certain areas and for designated patients, often pending physician approval. Compromised mental alertness from disease, fatigue, or medication may make a cigarette-smoking patient a fire risk. Smoking remains a major contributor to fires in medical facilities. Defective electrical wiring is another common source of fires. The heat from electrical resistance, which essentially are atoms bouncing against each other and causing friction and heat, can become an ignition source under the right conditions. For example, a short circuit can melt then ignite insulating wire and nearby materials. Once the insulation starts to melt, burn, crack, or peel away, sparking and heat can ignite nearby combustibles.

ISOLATING FIRE COMPONENTS

Oxygen cylinders should always be carefully restrained. They ideally should be stored in a noncombustible room away from ignition sources with the valve closed and protective valve caps screwed on tight. Smoking prohibition in areas where oxygen is used or stored is essential. Although oxygen is not combustible, it severely intensifies a nearby fire.

Isolating fires may involve barriers and protective coverings. Placing items behind or in a noncombustible shield (physical barrier) or using administrative hurdles such as designated smoking areas, prohibiting the use of extension cords, and fire safety inspections can serve as barriers to fire. An illustration might be storing flammable liquids in approved steel flammable liquid cabinets (Underwriters Laboratories/ Factory Mutual [UL/FM]). Storing gasoline for a snow blower, for example, in a noncombustible concrete shed or an UL/FM approved metal safety can is a barrier used to prevent fires. Placing a coffee maker on the top of a noncombustible surface is another use of a barrier. Administrative barriers and controls ensure that appropriately designated smoking areas and other policies are enforced. Keeping combustible holiday decorations to a minimum and maintaining clear exits at all times are essential. Prohibiting refueling of hot lawnmower and snow blower engines or filling fuel tanks inside a building are further illustrations of effective administrative controls.

Protective coverings, such as fire resistive mattress covers, fire retardant or resistive upholstery, gypsum wallboard, or concrete partitions can be important factors for fire protection planning. Fire-retardant materials can be applied to clothing, drapes, bed covers, seasonal decorations, and other materials. Construction or renovation efforts should consider fire retardant and resistant wall coverings, ceilings, flooring, carpet, upholstered furniture, and wooden shingles.

FIRE SAFETY TRAINING

Periodic training is essential to ensure the staff is knowledgeable about extinguishing fires, such as wastebasket fires and patients on fire, and when not to fight a fire, such as when fire is spreading up walls, across ceilings, above ceilings or other concealed spaces. Deep-seated fires in mattresses and upholstery can be tricky because reignition can occur hours after the fire was "extinguished" or when these articles are being moved from the fire area. Staff need to understand how to protect patients from ignition sources of fires and how to use routine fire emergency-preparedness techniques, such as preventing smoke migration by closing doors, calling for help immediately, using extinguishers or blankets, and quenching a fire.

Use of early-warning devices such as smoke and heat detectors is effective. Facilities greatly enhance their protection when they couple use of early-warning devices with use of a sprinkler system to automatically extinguish fires, prevent further fire spread, and quench smoke. Smoke is the killer in virtually all fires. Preparation for protecting a facility from a fire includes

- Fire protection measures for the building.
- A fire safety plan that includes an emergency action plan and emergency response procedure.

FACILITY FIRE PROTECTION

Fire protection in medical facilities may include sprinkler piping and heads. In more modern buildings, these items may not appear obvious, because sprinkler piping often is hidden above ceilings or behind walls. Sprinkler heads may be concealed above panel ceilings or hidden behind metal disks flush with the ceiling. Disks often are purchased to match the ceiling and may not be noticeable as exposed heads. The disks or sprinkler heads should not be painted in house because that will delay or prevent sprinkler operation during a fire. In addition to ceiling heads, there may be horizontal wall heads, which may be less obvious than overhead piping. If fire protection measures are not clear, consultation with someone familiar with the physical plant may be helpful. Sprinkler protection may affect the emergency evacuation plan, because a fully sprinklered building is generally safer in controlling or extinguishing fires than buildings without such a system. A fully sprinklered building with a good fire alarm and detection system often provides more options for evacuation planning.

The two most common types of fire detectors are based on either smoke or heat. A *smoke detector* can be activated by heat if there are enough airborne particles of combustion in the area. A *heat detector* is not activated by smoke unless the smoke is very hot. Smoke detectors typically give the earlier warning. Many different types of heat and smoke detectors and combination detectors have different benefits and features.

Detectors may sound a local emergency alarm, much like the battery-powered detectors used in some homes. These detectors, powered by 110-volt alternating current, are designed to sound locally and not in other parts of the building. Unless the building is supported by emergency power, a loss of electricity will cause loss of these types of smoke detectors.

Some fire detectors set off an alarm for the entire building or a part of a building. Some of these systems automatically report to a local fire department through a direct system, a proprietary system at a 24-hour operation center, or a central alarm company. Although any of these reporting systems is acceptable for most medical centers, state and community laws differ as to what signals have to go directly to a fire department. These modern systems have automatic battery emergency power in the event of a power loss. Some systems have programmable devices and self-monitoring capabilities that constantly check all devices connected to them to ensure the systems are working properly. An alert identifies the device, its location, and that it is malfunctioning.

Smoke detectors are prone to nuisance alarms, more so than heat detectors. As a result, heat detectors are used more often in kitchens, smoking rooms, bathrooms, and workshops to keep nuisance alarms to a minimum. Nuisance alarms are alarms not caused by actual fire, but by items, such as burnt toast, tobacco smoke, smoke from fireplaces, hair spray, steam from showers, or dust from woodworking machinery. Frequent and unabated nuisance alarms can annoy the workforce, who ultimately may ignore legitimate alarms that necessitate a response. Nuisance alarms also can disturb patients. To encourage the reduction of these unwanted alarms, some fire departments impose fines on facilities with repeated and avoidable nuisance alarms. It is never a good idea to delay transmission of a fire alarm (other than qualified fire alarm maintenance) to the fire department. A few minutes of lost time can make the difference between lives lost or lives saved.

Building construction is an important component to fire protection. In larger medical centers, often with a number of interconnecting buildings, containment of any fire may be a considerable challenge. Architects and engineers design buildings with the goal of preventing fires from passing from one building into another. Protection is accomplished through early fire detection and fire suppression systems, smoke evacuation systems, fire alarm evacuation systems, and fire doors that close automatically. Fire-resistant construction, which primarily refers to buildings of steel-reinforced concrete rather than with wood, is effective in protecting a building.

Older hospitals and nursing homes may have little fire protection, detection, or alarm systems or fire-resistant construction. The absence of fire protection equipment and fire resistive construction in a medical facility requires effective fire safety planning and improvement.

OSHA CONSIDERATIONS

OSHA requires an emergency action plan (subpart E, 1910.38) that addresses the elements of a written fire safety plan. OSHA fire protection requirements are outlined in 1910 subpart L, which covers fire extinguishers, fire alarms, brigades, employee training, fire detection and fire suppression systems, and maintenance. The emergency action plan includes an evacuation plan, fire prevention measures, and general emergency information. Information may include telephone numbers of persons to be notified and specific information such as how to secure narcotics and other items in the event of a fire. The emergency action plan designates responsible parties and their corresponding duties in the event of a fire. An organizational structure in the emergency action plan identifies personnel, their positions and corresponding duties, and specific roles, such as moving patients, directing visitors to evacuate using the fire stairs, closing doors, and preventing fire and smoke from spreading. During drills, personnel and patient accountability should be emphasized.

A fire plan should include a fire prevention plan, an emergency action plan, a fire and emergency equipment maintenance and testing plan, and any standard operating procedures related to fire or emergency evacuation. Points to address in developing these plans are simply who does what, when, how, and why? Consider what would happen if [insert worst-case scenarios]. What would have to be done to protect the patients and staff?

FIRE PREVENTION PLAN

A fire prevention plan lists potential fuels, combustibles, and ignition sources along with the corresponding methods to prevent fires and minimize their spread. The fire evacuation plan includes a posted floor plan that identifies the exit routes from the building and waiting and meeting areas outside to account for patients and personnel. Each area, such as a wing or suite, should have two independent ways to escape the area. In a medical facility, planning must account for the limitations of patients as a result of surgery, illness, or other physical impairments.

Fire Protection Systems and Equipment

An automatic fire sprinkler system, fire and smoke detectors, and fire alarm system to evacuate the area and notify the fire department are critical elements to the plan. Portable fire extinguishers used by trained personnel can be helpful in containing small fires. Sprinklers have an excellent record of controlling fires and saving lives and are particularly useful in medical facilities. These systems are activated only if the sprinkler head becomes hot enough to melt a fusible link. Only sprinkler heads affected by a predetermined temperature open. The others remain closed. The common temperature range for activation is 165°F to 175°F (74°C to 80°C). Smoke alone does not make these sprinklers discharge.

Sprinklers often are required by building codes and local fire department ordinances and are recommended by the JCAHO. In medical facilities, sprinklers usually are installed in combination with the fire alarm system and smoke and fire detectors. A smoke detector alarm allows enough time to remove a patient from a room before the sprinkler head discharges. After the patient has been removed, the door is closed to protect the rest of the facility and the patient.

Regular fire extinguisher training sessions are strongly recommended for staff expected to use this equipment in an emergency. Training should cover extinguishing agents, such as water, dry chemicals, foam, purple K, and carbon dioxide. Halon gas is being phased out of use because of environmental concerns.

Fire Extinguishers

Fire extinguishers often have less than a minute's worth of fire-extinguishing time. Small fires usually can be extinguished safely by a trained novice. A small fire, considered no larger than the size of an office wastebasket, a sofa cushion, or a small electrical item such as a toaster, can be contained with a fire extinguisher. Fire extinguishers must be replaced after use or sent out for replenishing.

Cautions

Medical center workers should not attempt to fight fires that are rapidly spreading or climbing walls or that involve ceilings, chemicals, or compressed gases. A worker always needs to ensure there is an exit to his or her back to avoid being trapped. In the use of fire extinguishers, the mnemonic *pass* is used in training sessions. It stands for

Pull the pin.
Aim the extinguisher nozzle at the base of the flames.
Squeeze the handle to apply the extinguishing agent in short bursts, which allows more

control and conservation of extinguishing agent.

Sweep the extinguisher nozzle back and forth to cover the base of the fire; extend 6 inches to 1 foot (15 to 30 cm) behind the edges of the base of the fire.

A blanket can be used to extinguish fire on a patient whose clothes catch on fire in bed, if the following measures are followed:

1. Call for help.
2. Ensure that the blanket is sealed to the collar bone with the rescuer's forearm closest to the patient's head. This prevents flames and smoke from being directed to the patient's head.
3. If the patient is panicking and flailing his or her arms, throw the blanket toward the collar bone with one forearm and the rest of the blanket over the flailing arms.
4. Push down the patient's arms.
5. If the patient prevents pushing down on his or her arms, use the weight of the rescuer's torso to pin down the arms, then extinguish the fire. Before lifting the blanket, make sure the fire is completely out, because reignition can occur with a fresh supply of air.
6. Wet smoldering spots after the fire only if the patient or bed is not attached to electricity.
7. Leave the room after the fire is extinguished, because there may be residual poisonous gases in the area.
8. Assess and treat patient for any injuries or complications sustained.

EMERGENCY RESPONSE PLAN

An emergency response plan can be used in fires. The acronym *aces* refers to the following elements:

Alert the staff and the people in the area. (This approach may have to be modified for areas with mentally impaired or psychiatric patients to reduce risk for panic.)

Confine the smoke or chemicals spilled by closing doors and windows and using ventilation systems to keep the fire or fumes from spreading.

Evacuate the area. Trained staff may need to defend the area by closing doors and using extinguishers, especially in situations in which patients cannot be readily moved.

Summon help while evacuating the area by pulling a fire alarm or calling an emergency number.

FIRE SAFETY SUMMARY

Organized efforts aimed at preventing fires are essential and are the best way to protect a medical facility. Planning and training, installation of automatic fire detectors, alarms, and suppression systems, and attention to building construction features are extremely important.

SELECTED FIRE PREVENTION RESOURCES

A good place to begin looking for resources is the facility's health and safety office, occupational health and safety professional, physical plant, or risk management department (sometimes called loss prevention). These offices may have applicable OSHA regulations available. If they do not, most public libraries do. The regulations also may be accessed at http://www.osha-slc.gov/OshStd_toc/OSHA_Std_toc.html or from local government book stores or OSHA offices. The Internet also offers much information on fire safety, emergency response, and planning. Other resources that may be available to assist in the development of a good fire safety program are as follows:

- Fire prevention office of the local fire department
- Medical facility's fire insurance carrier
- Local OSHA office
- Community or hospital library
- Federal Emergency Management Agency (FEMA)
- U.S. Fire Administration
- National Fire Protection Association Life Safety Code (NFPA 101)

- National Fire Protection Association, Health Care Facilities (NFPA standard 99)

ELECTRICAL SAFETY

The main concern regarding electrical safety is when electricity leaks past wire insulation. Some materials conduct electricity better than others; those that conduct electricity easily are called *conductors.* An example might be a copper wire or most metals. Some materials, however, do not conduct electricity and are considered nonconductors or insulators. Nonconductors, including wood, rubber, and glass, do not normally conduct electricity and are often used as insulators.

Electrical resistance occurs when collision between electrons produces create friction. When electron resistance is greatly increased, heat is produced. If enough heat is generated, electrical resistance can ignite combustibles and cause a fire. Electrons can escape from insulated conductors through breaks, gaps, or other openings. Table 16-2 lists the effects of electricity on the human body.

Medical center current is typically 15 to 20 amperes. Lasers, electroencephalographs, and cautery devices present an electrical source that may lead to a fire. Hospital-grade receptacles (outlets) have a green dot and are higher-quality outlets. The National Electrical Code (NEC) NFPA standard 70 provides specifications and guidance for electrical installations in medical facilities. Emergency receptacles are labeled *Emergency* and are red. Normally installed in patient areas, such as emergency departments, operating rooms, and patient rooms, emergency receptacles have specifications provided by the NEC and are designed to ensure safety and reliability of the electrical supply. NFPA standard 99 for health care facilities requires that patient care appliances have instruction manuals that are maintained and accessible. The standard also requires documentation of any associated repairs, modifications, and calibrations and a log of tests conducted. Equipment must be serviced only by qualified personnel.

Medical staff using equipment on patients should be trained to recognize the hazards associated with the equipment. Many medical facilities contract with an outside vendor who specializes in checking electrical and electronic medical equipment. The date of the last test and the maintenance performed is logged on a test form that is tagged onto the equipment itself. Equipment that is not performing properly should be taken out of service immediately, tagged as to the defect, and sent for repairs. Medical appliances and facility electrical systems should be checked regularly to ensure safety. Worn, cracked, or frayed wiring, insulation, and equipment covers should be repaired immediately or replaced. Compromised equipment, such as a ground pin cut off in an electrical plug, frayed or worn wiring, loose-fitting outlets, and loose plugs, should be removed from service.

Extension cords should not be used unless necessary, because of hazards associated with fire, electricity, and tripping. Outlets in particular should not be overloaded, and use of multiple-plug outlets should be avoided. Multioutlet surge protectors for electronic diagnostic equipment and computers are consid-

TABLE 16-2. *Effects of electricity on the human body*

Current in milliamperes	Reaction or effect on body
1	Perception level, faint
5	Slight shock felt
6–25 (women)	Painful shock, muscular
9–30 (men)	control lost. Called the "freezing current" or "let go current"
50–150	Extreme pain, respiratory
1,000–4,300	Ventricular fibrillation, severe muscular
10,000	Cardiac arrest, severe

Excerpted from OSHA publication 3075 "Controlling Electrical Hazards."

ered standard equipment by the NEC and acceptable for use with electronic and computer equipment. They are not intended for use with coffee pots or heating devices.

Bathrooms and other areas with sinks, baths, showers, or wet areas should have ground fault circuit interrupters (GFCIs) to detect minute amounts of leakage. When leakage of electricity is sensed, the GFCI disconnects the circuit to stop the flow of electricity to prevent injury. Outlets elsewhere in patient rooms may have GFCIs but others may not. Some circuits with GFCIs are easily identified and have test and reset buttons built into the outlet. Others are less obvious because they may be protected at a remote location. A licensed electrician can easily identify GFCIs for a facility.

REFERENCES

1. An Rx for hospital loss control. *Record* 1994;Winter:3–10.
2. Healthcare occupancies. In: *Fire protection handbook, 18th ed.* Quincy, Massachussets: National Fire Protection Association, 1997.
3. National Fire Protection Association. NFPA 99 standard for health care facilities, Quincy, Massachussets: National Fire Protection Association, 1999.

Medical Center Occupational Health and Safety,
edited by Robert J. McCunney.
Lippincott Williams & Wilkins, Philadelphia © 1999.

17

The Role of the Environmental Health Officer in Assuring Compliance in a Medical Center

John A. Schaefer

Department of Medicine, Division of Occupational Medicine, The Johns Hopkins University, Baltimore, Maryland 21205

The medical center environmental health officer (EHO) must comply with and coordinate the requirements of the institution imposed by the Environmental Protection Agency (EPA), Occupational Safety and Health Administration (OSHA), Joint Commission on Accreditation of Healthcare Organizations (JCAHO), and local regulators to provide a safe environment for providing quality medical care. The EHO must be able to assure that the hospital is a setting where medical procedures can be performed without interruption from environmental forces outside the institution. The EHO must be ready to assist the institution in bringing new medical treatments into the facility by being able to assure that all regulations are met. To do this, the EHO must remain knowledgeable about current regulatory requirements and changes in medical procedures and research practices.

The EHO in a medical institution should have both formal education and a solid background of practical experience in environmental procedures to assist the hospital in complying with hazardous and medical waste disposal regulations. The Clean Air Act has provisions regarding emissions and the amount and type of material released into the atmosphere. The expertise of the EHO must include the ability to understand and interpret OSHA regulations regarding worker exposure. The EHO is responsible for providing respiratory protection as required by 29 CFR 1910.134 for health care workers who must comply with Centers for Disease Control and Prevention (CDC) recommendations for tuberculosis protection. Regulatory requirements (federal, state, and local government), patient needs, and community pressure also affect the role of the EHO. The JCAHO has mandated compliance with all applicable environmental and worker safety regulations. The JCAHO inspects medical center policies and procedures for compliance with these regulations. It is therefore advisable to have policies in place that assure the institution's compliance. Policies should be reviewed annually. This chapter reviews the complex responsibilities of the medical center EHO.

ENVIRONMENTAL SAFETY

Medical center regulations fall into two categories—environmental and worker safety. The environmental issue with the most impact on a medical center is waste. Types of waste generated by a medical center include medical or infectious, chemical or toxic, radiologic, food excess, and general refuse.

Medical Waste

Medical waste includes items that are infectious or potentially infectious. Certain states have expanded their definition of medical waste to include any item that can be perceived as having been used in patient care or in a clinical laboratory. As a result, the medical center must treat many items that never come in contact with a patient or infectious material as medical waste. An example of this is any container with gradations etched into the side. Medical waste must be disposed of in a manner that assures the material is no longer infectious or recognizable. This responsibility is achieved by many institutions through incineration either on site or off site. The incinerator must meet federal and state requirements for design and emission control. Air emissions standards require that any large incinerator have a high-efficiency scrubber to remove any particulate matter and acids that may be emitted. The potential for emission of dioxin from medical waste incinerators has caused increased concern regarding medical center incinerators. Alternatives such as microwave destruction and sterilization followed by maceration are being developed and implemented in some medical centers. Medical waste disposal options have to be evaluated to fit the needs of specific medical centers.

Chemical Waste

The responsibilities of the EHO in the proper handling of controlled hazardous (chemical) wastes involves effort in educating the medical center staff about what is considered hazardous waste and what is proper disposal. Many of the substances routinely used in the treatment of patients are considered hazardous waste in regard to disposal requirements. For example, alcohol is flammable and must be disposed of as an ignitable waste under the Resource Conservation and Recovery Act (RCRA). Improper disposal can lead to citations, fines, and even criminal prosecution. More important, however, is that improper disposal can cause a fire. To dispose of hazardous waste, a medical center must be registered with the federal and local environmental regulatory agency as a generator of hazardous waste and obtain a generator identification number. This number is used to record all hazardous waste disposal and to link the medical center to the waste it generates. The collection and storage of waste material must comply with federal and possibly local regulations. Treatment, storage, and disposal facilities must have an EPA permit that specifies the activities for which the facilities are approved. The medical center is ultimately responsible for complying with all regulations concerning hazardous waste disposal and for the proper disposal of its hazardous waste. The medical center is responsible for the compliance of its contractors.

Responsibility for the disposal of hazardous waste is referred to as cradle to grave and may actually extend further. The generator of hazardous waste is held responsible by the EPA under the Comprehensive Environmental Response, Compensation, and Liability Act (CERCLA), also known as Superfund, for the mishandling of hazardous materials by permitted disposal facilities. There is no protection against future liability even by the most diligent of medical centers to prevent them from being named as a potentially responsible party in Superfund site remediation and decontamination. Being named in as a potentially responsible party in a Superfund site requires that the EHO conduct a search of all hazardous waste manifests and records to determine the amount and type of material sent to the site. It is a prudent practice to maintain files of the manifests beyond the regulatory time of 3 years. Most Superfund activities involve hazardous waste disposal that occurred much more than 3 years earlier, sometimes even before the regulations governing hazardous waste existed. Copies of the records are requested as the initial steps in determining the liability and cost associated with the cleanup. From these records and the records recovered from the waste site the medical center's liability is determined by the EPA. The first step is to determine the actual amount of the hazardous waste sent to the site from the medical center. The EHO should verify the accuracy of the information the EPA is using and be ready to document the correct amount of waste sent to the site. The amount of hazardous waste sent to the site determines the portion of the cleanup, administrative, and legal costs assigned to the medical center.

The medical center and the EHO can take action to minimize the potential for Superfund sites in the future. The first step is to take an active role in determining the facilities through which the hazardous waste is disposed of (Table 17-1). Each site chosen should be investigated by the EHO. Because changes are likely to occur within any organization, it is prudent to review annually the status of each facility used for disposal of hazardous waste.

Radiologic Waste

The use and disposal of radioactive materials is under the control of the Nuclear Regulatory Commission, which places limits on the amount of radioactive material that can be used and stored. These limits are delineated in the radioactive material license. Radioactivity is a cause of fear in many communities, and a not-in-my-backyard response confronts the medical center. One east coast city, in an attempt to protect its citizens from nuclear weapon manufacturing, declared itself a nuclear free zone. As originally written, the bill effectively would have banned the use of any radioactive material within the city limits. If passed as written, the bill would have prevented hospitals and medical centers from performing radioactive diagnostic testing. When the city council was informed, the law was quickly amended to allow medical and research use of radioactive materials. The medical center EHO needs to maintain an active role in reviewing pending legislation and providing factual information to the appropriate government agencies and community groups.

TABLE 17-1. *Review items for consideration of disposal facilities*

Permitted procedures for treatment and disposal
Closure plans
Closure funding
Environmental insurance
Internal inspection records
State inspection records
Records of accidental releases
Citations
Fines
Corrective actions

Hazardous Materials

Controls on how waste is handled must begin in the medical center with documented policies and procedures detailing responsibility and appropriate actions for the handling of wastes and a training program to inform staff of the proper disposal of hazardous wastes. Even with a comprehensive system of controlling wastes internally, problems can arise. For example, a misinformed laboratory technician given the task of disposing of an acid cleaning solution pours it down a sink drain, which causes a reaction, destruction of the drain pipe, an exposure, and an acid burn. Hazardous material if placed in the wrong disposal container can expose custodial staff as the trash is emptied. The EHO may be called in to retrieve improperly disposed material. When emergency situations like these arise in the medical center, the EHO must decide first who should respond—the fire department or a hazardous waste handler, both of whom are experts at handling large-volume hazardous spills. Most spills in a medical center are small. For example, OSHA considers a spill of chemotherapy solution greater than 5 mL a large spill. The medical center needs to decide whether to have an outside team or an in-house team respond to spills in patient care areas.

The dilution and sink disposal of controlled hazardous wastes is illegal and can lead to fines for the medical center and criminal penalties for the individual. However, there are no restrictions on this type of disposal of material not regulated under the RCRA. Although not illegal, it is not acceptable to dispose of hazardous materials by means of dilution and sink disposal. Dilution does not occur instantaneously, and contact between the discarded material and material already in the system can cause adverse interactions. Another factor that precludes sink disposal is that the amount of vapor and aerosols generated during the action of pouring material down the drain may exceed permissible exposure levels.

A pathologist monitored in a surgical pathology area exceeded the OSHA permissible exposure limit for formaldehyde. The levels routinely exceeded 4 ppm averaged over an 8-hour work day. Specimens were retrieved from the formalin by means of pouring the contents of the specimen container into a strainer held over a stream of running water. A simple change in work practices—retrieving the specimen from the formalin with forceps and placing the closed container into a bin for disposal—resulted in reducing the exposure to less than 1 ppm.

Another parameter that affects disposal of material through the drain is the restrictions placed on this activity by the local waste treatment facility. The waste treatment facility bans from sewer disposal material incompatible with the methods used to detoxify the wastes it receives (Table 17-2). Glutaraldehyde is an example of a material the disposal of which is not regulated by EPA but one that may adversely affect the functions of the treatment plant. Glutaraldehyde, a highly effective germicidal disinfectant, can in high concentrations adversely affect the bacteria colony used in the treatment plant. Many treatment plants issue guidelines for materials to be disposed of through the drain on the basis of their effect on bacteria. This is usually described as the EC_{50} (effluent concentration fatal to 50% of a colony of test bacteria) and is expressed as a percentage concentration. If EC_{50} is 10%, the material is fatal to 50% of the bacterial colony at a concentration of 10% in a diluted solution. Although an EC_{50} for glutaraldehyde has not been determined, Union Carbide, a manufacturer of glutaraldehyde, has stated that a 10 ppm solution is safe for disposal through the drain. A 2% glutaraldehyde solution would have to be diluted more than 1,000-fold to be considered safe for drain disposal. Every gallon (3.8 L) of glutaraldehyde would have to be diluted with 1,000 gallons (3,800 L) of water before flushing down the drain. This effort can be time consuming and wasteful.

TABLE 17-2. *Material restricted from disposal through the sanitary sewer*

Hazardous
Flammable
Nonmiscible with water
Colored
Creates noxious fumes
Detrimental to function of the treatment plant[a]

[a]This is listed as the EC_{50} of the material, the concentration fatal to 50% of the bacterial colony.

Alternatives to regulated disposal of hazardous waste are substitution, redistillation, and detoxification. A substitute material must be compatible with the medical center procedures and capable of assuring the same quality of results as the original material. Consideration should be given to environmental and treatment facility requirements. Redistillation necessitates knowledge of fire codes, purity, suitability with specimens, and staffing needs. Redistillation procedures should include procedures for certification of the purity of the redistilled material before use in a clinical laboratory. Detoxification procedures should be reviewed by the local EPA to assure that the procedures meet requirements and do not pose environmental hazards and to determine whether a treatment permit is needed. Records of detoxification should include letters of approval for the procedure, a log of all material detoxified, and the results of any testing to assure that the material has been completely detoxified.

General Waste Disposal

Many wastes generated by a medical center although not hazardous may pose environmental concern because of the volume of material. These materials include food, paper, and plastic wastes. The role of a medical center as protector of health requires proper disposal of all waste. The medical center has a leadership role in the community and is expected to administer programs that improve the overall environment of the community. As a generator of large quantities of waste material, a medical center is expected to reduce, recycle, or reuse material. Paper and plastics are prime for recycling, but often the cost of sending material for recycling far exceeds the costs of disposal.

The medical center must be diligent to assure that its activities do not pose a hazard to patients, visitors, staff, or passersby. Exhausts from treatment and diagnostic procedures must be located so as not to adversely affect the health of patients and staff. Consideration must be given to the possibility that routine activities within medical center can create a life-threatening situation for a patient. This is most likely to occur among patients with hypersensitivity to chemicals or allergic responses to latex.

To assure clean air for the future the EPA has issued regulations under the Clean Air Act and other regulations that control the amount and type of emission that can be released into the atmosphere. The ban on chlorofluorocarbons or difluoroethane (Freon) has had the greatest effect on medical centers. This ban has caused a substantial changes in the delivery systems for ethylene oxide sterilizers, a decrease in the use of bromodifluoromethane (Halon) fire-fighting systems, and an increase in the cost of therapeutic inhalers. These regulations also have caused changes in how refrigeration units are repaired and discarded. Title V of the Clean Air Act requires recording of and obtaining permits for all emissions from a site. Sources of emissions under Title V at medical centers are boilers, emergency generators, and incinerators. Other sources that may be regulated depending on the amount of emission include ethylene oxide sterilizers and laboratory procedures, or they may be exempted with four pages of exempted emissions that include rest rooms, flora, fauna, and secretarial areas. A medical center has to decide whether it can handle the permit internally or needs consultants. This responsibility is determined on the basis of cost and expertise. Diligence is needed to determine the effect of these and other regulations of the Clean Air Act.

Newly proposed regulations on medical waste incinerators may affect facilities that incinerate their own medical waste and have a monetary impact on those that use contracted incinerators. Under proposed regulations, three categories of incinerators are based on the amount of material burned in an hour, as follows:

Less than 240 pounds/hour (108 kg/hour)—no emission controls required
More than 240 pounds/hour but less than 600 pounds/hour (270 kg/hour)—low-pressure wet scrubber
More than 600 pounds/hour—high efficiency wet scrubber

WORKER SAFETY

OSHA regulations that protect workers from environmental hazards at work place considerable responsibility on the EHO. OSHA was formed by the Occupational Safety and Health Act and was signed into law by President Nixon in 1970. The act states that every employer must provide its employees with a workplace free from recognized hazards. This requirement is better known as the general duty clause. As part of its mandate, OSHA is required to publish standards for worker protection from workplace hazards. A complete compilation of the OSHA standard can be found in 29 CFR 1910 for general industry, which includes medical centers. Contractors doing renovations or construction within the medical center are covered under the construction standard 29 CFR 1926. The EHO must keep abreast of changes in the regulations. However, many of the criteria OSHA uses to evaluate medical centers are not spelled out specifically in the general industry standards. Criteria can be found by reviewing the OSHA technical and compliance manuals or at the OSHA Web site (www.osha.gov/). The availability of the OSHA, CDC, and National Institute of Occupational Safety and Health (NIOSH) Web sites allows the EHO to keep abreast of changes in regulations, recommendations, and interpretations.

The general duty clause of the Occupational Safety and Health Act states that every employer must provide a workplace free of recognized hazards. What is a recognized hazard? Any situation that any national organization has deemed to be hazardous to an employee's health fits the definition of a recognized hazard. Violations of the general duty clause have resulted in citations for failure to protect health care workers from tuberculosis. Although, it has not issued a final tuberculosis standard, OSHA has adopted the 1990 CDC tuberculosis control guidelines. Hospitals have been cited for not providing adequate respiratory protection, even though the hospital provided the minimum respiratory protection recommended in the CDC guidelines. Citations have been issued for inadequate testing of dust mist respirators against the particle size that equates to a tuberculosis droplet nuclei and not providing dust mist respirators small enough for female hospital workers. These citations put medical centers on notice that they cannot rely on literature from a respirator company stating that a respirator meets required protection standards. Information from other hospitals and from federal, state, and local safety regulatory agencies can be useful. When obtaining compliance guidance from a regulatory agency, the EHO needs to follow any telephone conversation with a letter of understanding that restates the information or decision agreed upon.

OSHA part 1910 Occupational Safety and Health Standards subpart Z—Toxic and Hazardous Substances lists permissible exposure limits for employees exposures. These are listed in a series of tables known as the Z tables, which include substances for which specific standards are in place, and those for which a standard has not been generated. In 1990 OSHA attempted to update many of the chemicals exposure limits on the Z table for which specific standards have not been developed and place exposure limits on substances that previously have not been regulated. The American Conference of Governmental Industrial Hygienist (ACGIH) threshold limit values (TLVs) were the basis for the new OSHA permissible exposure limits (PELs) for many of the substances that had not been updated or regulated. The OSHA attempt to adopt the TLVs as PELs was met with an outcry and court actions by both the industry and unions. The court stated that the Occupational Safety and Health Act required assessment of each chemical for its hazard potential to workers and the economic effect of the proposed regulation. OSHA was forced to vacate the new PELs. Several states, however, have adopted the revised PELs as part of their programs for occupational health and safety. These are in effect because they were not subject to federal court action.

OSHA is reviewing the changes it had proposed and is selecting certain chemicals for evaluation before rule making. Evaluation is based on worker exposure, the effectiveness of engineering controls, the number of persons and facilities affected, and the cost of the new exposure limit on the industry. Evaluation of the chemical in a facility involves several days of on-site monitoring that details work practices, engineering controls, and worker exposures. Information on the costs of engineering controls and alternative procedures is included in a formal report that becomes the basis for promulgating a proposed standard. The proposed standard is published for review and public comment. OSHA must respond to comments and objections raised. On the basis of these comments, revisions are made to the proposed rule, and a final rule is issued. Even after a final rule is issued, changes can be made to the standard. OSHA is conducting an evaluation of glutaraldehyde. In 1990, the PEL was set at a 0.2 ppm ceiling, which was the ACGIH TLV. Since 1990, the ACGIH has changed the TLV to 0.04 ppm. OSHA has yet to propose a new PEL or standard for the use of glutaraldehyde.

The need to comply with environmental and worker safety regulations must not result in patient discomfort from exposure to a hazardous material, such as a disinfectant. EHOs often are asked to approve a particular substance as a safe disinfectant in the medical center. The role of the EHO is to determine the proper procedures to protect staff and patients from exposure, including personal protective equipment and engineering controls. Before a new product is brought into use, procedures to be used in the event of a spill or accident in a patient room should be determined. Whenever possible, hazardous material should not be brought into a patient room. If hazardous material must be brought close to a patient, the smallest amount possible should be used.

Chemical sensitivity is another situation that requires coordinated effort on the part of the EHO, patient care staff, facilities, and housekeeping. Once it is ascertained that a patient is sensitive to a chemical, every one in the medical center should be advised of procedures for providing a nonirritating environment. It is also advisable to develop procedures for handling the needs of hypersensitive staff, latex being the latest concern. Staff members identified as allergic to latex should be evaluated to determine the restricting factors for their particular latex exposure. On the basis of these restrictions, the workplace should be evaluated to determine measures needed to meet the restrictions and allow the person to return safely to work.

Maintaining compliance with the numerous regulations and issues that affect a medical center is a responsibility that cannot be delegated to any one person. A successful program of compliance with myriad regulations takes commitment and effort on the part of all within a medical center.

SUGGESTED READING

Code of Federal Regulations. Title 10.

Code of Federal Regulations. Title 29, parts 1900 to 1910.

Code of Federal Regulations. Title 40.

Code of Federal Regulations. Title 49.

Code of Federal Regulations. Title 42, part 84.

Code of Federal Regulations. Title V, part 70.

Erickson P. *Practical guide to occupational health and safety*. New York: Academic Press, 1996.

Guideline for protecting the safety and health of healthcare workers. US Department of Health and Human Services, Public Health Service, Center for Disease Control and Prevention, National Institute for Occupational Safety and Health. Washington, DC: US Government Printing Office, 1988.

Joint Commission on Accreditation of Healthcare Organizations. *Comprehensive accreditation manual for hospitals.* Oakbrook Terrace, IL: JCAHO, 1995.

McDairmid MA, Kessler ER. *The health care worker. Occup Med* 1997;12(4).

Plog B, ed. *Fundamentals of industrial hygiene*, 4th ed. Itasca, IL: National Safety Council, 1996.

Probst K, Portney P. *Assigning liability for superfund cleanups.* Washington, DC: Resources for the Future, 1992.

Medical Center Occupational Health and Safety, edited by Robert J. McCunney.
Lippincott Williams & Wilkins, Philadelphia © 1999.

18

Environmental Audits

Perry D. Cooper

The Johns Hopkins University, Homewood Safety Campus, Baltimore, Maryland 21218

Is your health care facility prepared to be audited? Between October 1995 and September 1996, general medical and surgical hospitals (Standard Industrial Classification 8062) received 458 citations from the Occupational Safety and Health Administration (OSHA) with total penalties in excess of $253,000. The three most commonly cited violations pertaining to OSHA standards (Table 18-1) were related to blood-borne pathogens, formaldehyde, and hazard communication (1–3). Most citations were for no written programs, no site-specific training, no use of personal protective equipment, and no postexposure management programs. OSHA cited the blood-borne pathogen standard 38 times during 16 inspections with total penalties in excess of $167,000. This chapter presents a view of what an environmental, health, and safety audit may include, documentation to be reviewed, and exercises to complete the audit. It also explains how certain environmental factors may affect patients, staff, and visitors.

ENVIRONMENTAL HEALTH AND SAFETY

The process begins with defining the environmental, health, and safety audit and determining the areas of the facility to review. An audit addresses records and procedures to assure a safe environment for patients, staff, and visitors. Environmental, health, and safety factors include air and water quality, the physical structure (i.e., asbestos, lead, radon), nosocomial infections, exposure latex allergen, chemicals used in housekeeping, such as disinfectants, disposal of chemicals, staff training, and exposure monitoring for biologic, chemical, and radiation hazards. These audits are one of the principal methods of identifying areas in

TABLE 18-1. *Top ten leading OSHA citations for general medical and surgical hospitals*[a]

Standard cited	Description of standard	No. of citations
1910.1030	Blood-borne pathogen	38
1910.1048	Formaldehyde	27
1910.1200	Hazard communication	23
1910.147	Lockout, tagout, control of hazardous energy	17
1910.303	Electrical system design, general requirements	19
1910.37	Means of egress, general	17
1910.134	Respiratory protection equipment	18
1910.132	Personal protective equipment, general requirements	11
1910.146	Permit-required confined spaces	16
1910.120	Hazardous waste operations and emergency response	15

[a]October 1995 through September 1996. From ref. 2.

need of attention and determining where improvement is necessary.

The health care environment is subject to various audits. Surveys performed by the Environmental Protection Agency (EPA) and OSHA address similar factors with different levels of emphasis. For example, when the EPA audits a facility, it addresses air, water, radiation, hazardous waste, and solid waste issues. The EPA also focuses on maintenance of the environment within the facility and how the operations affect the surrounding environment. An OSHA audit evaluates the management of facilities and staff in regard to work practices and controls, management leadership and employee participation, workplace assessment, accident records analysis, hazard prevention and control measures, emergency response, and training. An environmental audit traditionally falls under regulations set by the EPA (Table 18-2).

Who should perform the environmental audit? The auditor can be an employee or an outside consultant. Internal auditors are more apt to understand the facility and concentrate on specific areas. An outside consultant should provide unbiased evaluation of the entire process. In either case, the auditor must have a working knowledge of federal, state, and local regulations that affect the facility. The information obtained in the audit may be needed in legal cases. Audit information obtained as a result of day-to-day operations is considered discoverable information in a legal action. If, however, the information is requested by legal counsel for a specific case, the environmental audit is considered privileged, although such claims may be challenged.

An audit begins with a management assessment to determine whether management is an active participant in environmental quality. Are policies written and enforced so staff easily complies? Operational processes should be reviewed. What are the specific steps of each operation within the facility? What is the outcome of these operations? What waste products are generated, and what is done with them? Certain items of interest may include potable water supplies, waste water discharge, ambient air quality, emissions from incinerators or boiler operations, chemical, biologic, and radioactive wastes produced and disposed, and recycling operations (4). A simple checklist is outlined in Table 18-3.

After surveying facility processes, the persons preparing for the audit need to determine which environmental regulations apply by evaluating the facility's records. How many times has the facility been out of compliance with regulations? What efforts were done to comply? Accidents that have happened have to be investigated, and actions that could have been taken to reduce their severity have to be determined. Are employees trained in pollution prevention practices? An untrained employee can pour a hazardous material down a drain

TABLE 18-2. *Environmental Protection Agency regulations addressed in an environmental audit*

Federal regulation	U.S. code reference
Clean Air Act	42 USC s/s 7401 et seq 1970
Clean Water Act	33 USC s/s 1251 et seq 1977
Comprehensive Environmental Response Compensation & Liability Act (CERCLA)	42 USC s/s 9601 et seq 1980
Superfund Amendments and Reauthorization Act (SARA)	42 USC s/s 9601 et seq 1986
Resource Conservation and Recovery Act (RCRA)	42 USC s/s 321 et seq 1976
Toxic Substances Control Act (TSCA)	42 USC s/s 2601 et seq 1976
Federal Insecticide Fungicide and Rodenticide Act (FIFRA)	7 USC s/s 135 et seq 1972
Emergency Planning and Right to Know Act	42 USC s/s 11011 et seq 1986
Pollution Prevention Act	42 USC 13101, 13102 s/s et seq 1990

From ref. 3.

TABLE 18-3. *Simple checklist for an environmental audit*

Evaluation of management participation
Evaluation of written policy and procedures
Blood borne and pathogens
Hazard communication
Confined space program
Fire safety plans
Hazardous waste management
Lockout, tagout programs
Respiratory protection programs
Personal protective equipment
Evaluation of operational procedures
Documentation of requirements
Training records and programs
Follow-up programs to ensure compliance

and pollute the local sewer system and possibly nearby surface and ground water supplies.

Training of staff in emergency preparedness is required by the EPA Superfund Act Reauthorization Amendment. Can the staff handle a large hazardous material spill? First responders must be trained in proper procedures to protect themselves and the facility. The facility should keep training records, reports of incident investigations and outcomes, and records of compliance and corrective actions on safety- and health-related issues. Without documentation, evidence of compliance or corrective actions cannot be demonstrated. Failure to comply with the EPA regulations may lead to felony convictions and large fines and imprisonment. Recent examples of citations and penalties issued by OSHA include the North County Regional Hospital in Bemidji, Montana, which received citations and penalties in excess of $15,000. St. Charles Medical Center in Bend, Oregon, received 15 citations and penalties for noncompliance with the blood-borne pathogens, formaldehyde, and eye and face protection standards. Valley Hospital in Palmer, Arkansas, received a citation and penalty of $1,300 for noncompliance with the formaldehyde standard.

OSHA AUDITS

Health and safety audits fall under the realm of OSHA. When OSHA performs an audit, it addresses six core elements. The Program Evaluation Profile form OSHA-195 is divided into the following six categories: management leadership and employee participation, workplace analysis, accident and record analysis, hazard prevention and control, emergency response, and training (Table 18-4) (5). The Program Evaluation Profile can

TABLE 18-4. *OSHA audit categories*

Management leadership and employee participation
Management leadership: Does management actively support and participate?
Employee participation: Do employees have active roles in decision making and performing specified procedures?
Implementation: Are policies and procedures implemented effectively?
Contractor safety: Are outside service providers informed of current policy and procedures that must be followed?
Work analysis
Survey and hazard analysis: Are potential hazards recognized effectively?
Inspection: Are inspections regularly performed to identify hazards?
Reporting: Are reports of work activities made and analyzed?
Accident and record analysis
Accident investigation: Is each accident investigated to determine cause?
Data analysis: Are data analyzed statistically and accurately?
Hazard prevention and control
Hazard control: Are preventive measures taken to reduce the chance of future occurrences?
Maintenance: Is regular preventive maintenance performed to ensure proper operation of equipment?
Medical program: Are required medical evaluations of employees performed and maintained?
Emergency response
Emergency preparedness: Are employees prepared to handle an emergency?
First aid: Are employees trained in first aid techniques?
Safety and health training
Training: What kind of safety and health training is given? Is it appropriate and effective? Are training records maintained?

From ref. 5.

be obtained from the OSHA Internet site at http://www.osha.gov/.

When it conducts an audit, a regulatory organization begins with record keeping, an essential component of compliance with environmental, health, and safety standards. Documentation can support the adequacy and effectiveness of a program. Detailed management plans and record keeping can indicate accident trends, high-hazard areas, and the frequency and severity of incidents involving patients, staff, visitors, and equipment. Computer software record management programs simplify record keeping. The American College of Occupational and Environmental Medicine publishes a software directory that can be obtained from ACOEM, 55 West Seegers Rd., Arlington Heights, IL 60005, (847) 228-6850.

Policy, procedure, and management plans must be obtained. These plans specify the environmental issues important to the institution; how the plans function; the purpose of the plans and how normal operations should be performed according to written procedure. These documents should be reviewed at least annually to correct mistakes or revise protocols and to comply with regulations. Table 18-5 is a list of protocols and management plans that may be scrutinized.

Separate but coordinated records on accidents involving employees, patients, and visitors must be maintained. An effective and thorough system of record keeping can indicate areas in need of improvement and provide supportive evidence in litigation. Photographic evidence of particular incidents and activities may be helpful as part of the documentation process. Continuous review and updating of these documents can help identify problems overlooked in earlier environmental auditing processes.

TABLE 18-5. *Protocols and management plans assessed in OSHA and EPA audits*

Indoor/outdoor air quality management protocol
Water quality and sanitation management
Asbestos management
Lead paint management
Nosocomial infection prevention plans
Infection control plans
Chemical exposure plans
Hazardous waste management plans
Training documents
Postexposure management plans
Fire protection protocols

TABLE 18-6. *Recommended documentation and record keeping in preparation for audits*

OSHA form 200 accident reporting log
OSHA form 141 Summary Occupational Injuries and Illness
List of occupational hazards and their locations
Current list of hazardous materials and material safety data sheets
Hazardous materials management plan
Hazard communication plan
Universal precaution plan
Infection control plan
Radiation safety plan
Ergonomic evaluation plan
Results of mandatory exposure monitoring (noise levels, ultraviolet light, respiratory protection program)
OSHA issued citations and notices
Employee training program summary class outlines, attendance sheets, and test results
Equipment and facility inspections and subsequent repairs

Effective documentation cannot be overemphasized. Table 18-6 identifies various types of documents and record-keeping responsibilities. It is required by law that most of these records be maintained on a regular basis with updated information. Prudent practice for documentation is to have a written protocol for each operation within the facility whether or not it is required by law. Environmental health and safety issues should be evaluated uniformly to ensure the effectiveness of compliance programs. In preparation for an audit, it can be helpful to review an environmental issue with potential for affecting patient care and proceed through the auditing steps. For example, immunocompromised patients must have adequate room ventilation free of contaminants to reduce risk for transmission of airborne illnesses. Because air quality within patient care areas is a central component of an environmental audit, it is used as an example.

THE AIR QUALITY AUDIT

Preparation for a possible audit begins with a thorough review of previous air quality investigation documents that may be available in various organizational units, including occupational safety, legal, infection control, workers' compensation, facility, and maintenance. Each unit may have reports pertaining to varied issues related to the air quality. The safety department may have detailed analytic reports on specific air contaminants. The legal department may have governmental reports or citations. Infection control may have reports of past outbreaks of airborne disease. Workers' compensation records may include specific employee incidents or disease claims. Facility design and maintenance can provide construction and operational data.

A site survey should be performed on the part of the facility in which the indoor air quality problem surfaced. Current conditions, occupancy rates, and use of the area should be documented. Is the area designed to function as currently used? Modifications of the original design should be documented. Architectural drawings or blueprints should be made available. It has to be determined whether modifications of the building design or operation are contributing to the air quality. Adjacent areas should be investigated to determine whether they have potential effect on the air quality in the area being audited.

The audit may include environmental sampling to determine air quality. The first step is to engage a person with specific knowledge of potential air contaminants, ventilation operation, and possible infection transmission to evaluate the air requirements and components to be investigated. If not on staff, this person, usually an industrial hygienist, can be found through the American Conference of Governmental Industrial Hygienists. Sampling results must be evaluated by qualified individuals so the data are truly represented. Complete reports of analysis must be made, reported, and retained for future reference.

When the results of an air quality study are reported to management, steps must be taken to reduce or eliminate the hazard. Combined activities between the offices of environmental health and safety, infection control, facility maintenance, and departments located in the problem area are essential for remediation to be successful. Corrective actions should be documented and maintained on file to demonstrate the efforts of the organization to reduce, prevent, and eliminate hazards. Follow-up investigations are recommended to ensure closure and resolution of the problem. Regular reevaluation is performed to maintain a healthy air quality environment.

After understanding the basic environmental, health, and safety audit components of a facility, one can identify areas of health care concern and begin the evaluation process. Components of the entire organization should work together to maintain a balanced, healthy, functioning environment. Management, staff, patients, and visitors must take an active role in maintaining the physical and workplace environment.

REFERENCES

1. US Department of Labor, Occupational Safety and Health Administration. Standards cited for SIC 8062. Available at http://www.osha.gov.
2. US Department of Labor, Occupational Safety and Health Administration. http://www.osha.gov.
3. US Department of the Environment, Environmental Protection Agency. http://www.epa.gov.
4. *Safety guide for health care institutions.* Itasca, IL: American Hospital Association & National Safety Council, 1983.
5. The white papers. *Industrial Safety & Hygiene News* October 1996, November 1996, December 1996, January 1997.

SUGGESTED READING

American Conference of Governmental Industrial Hygienists. http://www.acgih.org.

Audit policy: incentives for self-policing. *Federal Register* 1995 Dec 22 60:66706.

Chemical health and safety: appropriate limits on OSHA review—employer-conducted self audits. Washington, DC: American Chemical Society, January/February 1998.

McCunney RJ. The environmental audit. In: McCunney RJ, ed. *A practical approach to occupational and environmental medicine.* Boston: Little, Brown, 1994:693–696.

National Research Council. *Prudent practices in the laboratory, handling and disposal of chemicals.* Washington, DC: National Academy Press, 1995.

Salvato JA. *Environmental engineering and sanitation.* New York: Wiley, 1992.

US Department of Labor. OSHA Form-195. Washington, DC: OSHA/OSHA Publications.

Medical Center Occupational Health and Safety,
edited by Robert J. McCunney.
Lippincott Williams & Wilkins, Philadelphia © 1999.

19

Safety Considerations for the Clinical Laboratory

Daniel F. Liberman and *Michael H. Ziskin

Boehringer Ingelheim Pharmaceuticals, Inc., Ridgefield, Connecticut 06877;
**Field Safety Corporation, Guilford, Connecticut 06437*

Many published studies and surveys have documented the hazards and risk of occupational illness among clinical laboratory workers (1–6). These studies invariably focus on laboratory-associated infections and the laboratory and facility practices shown to be effective in controlling or preventing exposure to infectious agents. However, the death of a laboratory research chemist (7,8) who was working with and apparently exposed to dimethyl mercury has served as a sobering warning about the importance of health and safety procedures, practices, and use of personnel protective equipment and clothing when working with toxic chemicals in laboratories.

The exposure occurred when one to several drops of dimethyl mercury were spilled on the back of the researcher's gloved left hand during transfer of the chemical between two containers. The transfer was conducted inside a chemical fume hood, and the researcher was wearing disposable latex gloves (7,8). The researcher removed the gloves promptly on completion of the activity and gave no further thought to the incident at the time. No medical monitoring or other follow-up evaluation was conducted until 5 months later when the researcher experienced progressive difficulty characterized by numbness and tingling in both lower extremities and difficulty in vision, walking, speaking, and hearing.

When informed that the symptoms were consistent with mercury poisoning, the researcher recalled the spill. When biologic monitoring was performed, the mercury level in the researcher's urine was 234 μg/L. The blood mercury level was 4,000 μg/L 5 months after the exposure. Background levels in unexposed populations are on the order of 4 to 5 μg/L and 1 to 8 μg/L, respectively. Results of hair analysis for mercury were consistent with a single or short exposure, such as the reported spill, and peaked 54 days after exposure followed by a subsequent slow decline in mercury levels (8). Full diagnostic evaluation identified organometallic toxicity as a result of exposure to dimethyl mercury. Because mercury levels in hair are believed to reflect blood mercury level at the time the hair was formed, analysis of level versus time (hair length where sample was taken) provided a history of mercury exposure before recognition of the problem. Despite aggressive chelation treatment, the researcher went into a coma and died 10 months after exposure. Diagnosis at the time of death was encephalopathy as a result of mercury intoxication (7).

The gloves used in this incident were disposable latex examination gloves. Subsequent permeation testing of the gloves by a certified, independent testing laboratory indicated that the chemical permeates latex, polyvinyl chloride, and neoprene almost instantaneously. While we may never really know whether this incident could have been prevented, this case serves as a sentinel event in laboratory safety and underscores the importance of a safety management program in laboratory-associated illness prevention.

SAFETY MANAGEMENT PROGRAM

To provide laboratory environments that protect employee health, organizations must develop and maintain a comprehensive program. An environmental health and safety program that prevents occupational injuries and illnesses, monitors the workplace environment (e.g., dust, vapor, chemical hazard, radiation, noise), and uses these data as the basis for engineering and work practice controls is essential. To be effective, this effort must have the commitment and support of management. The following elements are important components of an effective environmental health and safety plan (9,10):

- Management leadership
- Assignment of responsibility and accountability
- Design and maintenance of safe working conditions
- Accident investigation and analysis
- Safe-operating rules and procedures
- Safety training and education
- Recognition, evaluation, and control of occupational hazards
- Safety administration

Management Leadership

The institution must realize that the commitment of upper management is invariably reflected in the attitude of the supervisory force toward health and safety. Management therefore must demonstrate a sincere interest in the safety program if employee cooperation and participation are to be achieved. Management must issue clear statements of policy for the guidance of supervisors and employees. If safety is a shared responsibility, management must do its share.

Assignment of Responsibility

Although the prime responsibility for the safety and health of all employees by law is vested in the chief executive, the day-to-day responsibility rests with supervisors. This means that each supervisor has the responsibility to monitor the safety performance of all employees that report to him or her. Each employee is responsible for following the safety rules and requirements applicable to his or her responsibilities. Management should encourage employee participation in the development of safety promotion programs, goals, and objectives. Employees have the responsibility to make others aware of safety problems.

Design and Maintenance of Safe Working Conditions

The supervisor is responsible for checking out all new equipment and processes and initiating the standard operating procedures, including relevant safety precautions, before authorizing use of such equipment. Workplace inspections are essential for the maintenance of safe working conditions and operating practices and for the detection of causes of accidents and harmful exposures. Safety inspections of the entire facility should be conducted periodically, at least annually. Written reports should be prepared after inspections, and appropriate corrective action should be initiated to correct identified deficiencies. The person responsible for employee safety should conduct follow-up inspections to evaluate the corrective action taken.

Accident Investigation and Analysis

Employees must be encouraged to report all accidents, injuries, and occupational illness. These events should be investigated to determine the cause and to establish corrective measures to prevent reoccurrence. It is required by the Occupational Safety and Health Administration (OSHA) that an accident investigation and injury report be completed for all work-related injuries or illnesses. Supervisors are responsible for investigating incidents, accidents, and injuries that occur within their areas of supervision (11–14).

Safe-Operating Rules and Procedures

Safe-operating rules and procedures must be established as a guide to employees for the prevention of accidents, injuries, illness, or exposure to harmful substances (see Appendix A). These rules and procedures have to be reviewed periodically by employees with their supervisors. It may be necessary to establish new safety rules to cover new equipment or operations or to revise existing rules to improve conditions or procedures. When any safe-operating rule or procedure is violated, appropriate disciplinary action must be taken. Personnel must be advised of and required to comply with these rules and procedures.

Safety Training and Education

OSHA recognizes that adequate protection of employees goes beyond the provision of safe equipment and safe working conditions. Human factors must be considered, and action must be taken to encourage proper work practices. Education, training, and safety promotion programs are the means of developing a spirit of safety consciousness and good attitudes in the work place. OSHA and the Environmental Protection Agency include a worker training section as part of every standard they promulgate (11).

All new and transferred employees must be oriented and trained in their jobs. This basic orientation usually is followed by frequent on-the-job safety instructions by supervisors during the first few days on the job. Potential hazards, if any, in the area are identified, and precautions to avoid injury are defined. Information on fire and emergency procedures, reporting of injuries and accidents, and available health care should be covered. Attention to the integration of safe and healthy work practices into daily tasks is an important factor in this follow-up training. Safety reviews should be conducted periodically to assess the environment of safety. The reviewers are safety teams composed of representatives of senior management and employees.

Recognition, Evaluation, and Control of Occupational Health Hazards

The association of potential hazards with modern technology and the increasing use of new biologic and chemical reagents necessitate vigilance in the recognition, evaluation, and control of hazardous biologic and chemical reagents and of physical stresses in the workplace. Each supervisor must be diligent in recognizing biologic, chemical, and physical hazards. Supervisors must evaluate the hazards associated with each procedure and process to determine where exposures exist or may occur; evaluate actual exposure through air sampling, analysis, or other techniques as necessary; conduct medical surveillance programs for employees exposed to hazardous materials as necessary; and control hazards through substitution or elimination of materials, modification of equipment, addition of ventilation, use of personal protective equipment, or administrative changes.

Administration

Each organization should establish a safety committee responsible for the administration and monitoring of the health and safety program. This committee should include representatives from each laboratory area, nontechnical support staff, facility management, senior management, and the safety office in accordance with all applicable federal, state and local requirements. Specific duties and responsibilities include investigation of serious and lost-time injuries; formulation of safety policies and procedures; inspections and audits of safety conditions; development of training, education, and safety promotion programs; reports to management and employees on the status of the program; and development of emergency response teams.

BASIC PRACTICES

The rules presented herein are minimum requirements for typical laboratory conditions. Employees should use good judgment in dealing with conditions not covered by these basic rules and rely on their supervisors for guidance whenever questions about safety arise.

Employee Conduct and Performance

Employees who are called on to perform work they consider hazardous or for which they feel inadequately trained or protected should make their concerns known to their supervisor before starting the work (15). Employees should make certain that they can do the task without injuring themselves or others and without causing an accident or incident. Before starting a job, employees should inspect all materials and equipment and ensure their safety. Employees are not to take short cuts when working. They are to use only approved procedures. They are to use, adjust, and repair equipment only if they are qualified and authorized to do so.

Laboratory doors are to be kept closed when work is in progress. All work areas are to be maintained in a neat and clean manner. All liquid and solid wastes containing microorganisms are to be decontaminated before disposal. Reusable materials that have come in contact with research organisms are to be decontaminated before reuse or recycling. Eating, drinking, smoking, applying cosmetics, and storage of food in the work area is prohibited. Needles and syringes are to be disposed of promptly and properly.

Training Requirements

All technical staff members must be adequately trained before beginning any work with tissue or potentially hazardous materials (11). Each staff member should demonstrate a good working knowledge of laboratory protocols before initiating work involving hazardous materials. This review should be performed annually.

This training must include the biologic and chemical characteristics of the systems used; good laboratory technique; proper techniques for decontamination and disinfection; emergency procedures; and appropriate procedures and practices for handling hazardous and toxic chemicals. Employees should demonstrate a working knowledge of all relevant safety practices and an understanding of the work assignment and its potential hazards. Before they begin work, employees should be familiar with the institution's health and safety program (2,3).

All nontechnical employees should be familiar with the potential hazards associated with the laboratory. Such workers are typically shown the universal biohazard and chemical safety signs and instructed to avoid, if possible, areas posted with such signs. In general, nontechnical staff should not enter the laboratory unless properly supervised by a technical staff member. Participation in the medical surveillance program usually is not required for nontechnical workers (16).

Security, custodians, and glassware washers must be familiar with the laboratory area where they perform their duties. They must be instructed not to handle containers designated for radioactive, biohazardous, or chemical waste and to avoid refrigerators, freezers, and other containers designated for storage of biologic, chemical, or radioactive materials. All nontechnical staff should be prohibited from any areas designated for hazardous activity while such work is in progress (3). Glassware washers must be fully informed of all waste disposal procedures, particularly autoclaving methods, and emergency procedures for handling spills of chemicals and biologic materials.

MEDICAL REQUIREMENTS

It may be necessary to arrange for occupational medical surveillance services for some employees (16). This program is usually designed to monitor potential health hazards associated with the work activity (16). Such programs may include a preplacement physical examination and medical history for each employee in the laboratory environment. The examination includes several laboratory tests to determine baseline organ functions. Although it is frequently considered an option, a chest radiograph is highly recommended for persons with positive results of a tuberculin skin test.

The preplacement examination usually is designed to ascertain whether workers have medical conditions that may render them susceptible to the potential hazards of working with microorganisms, biologically active proteins, and hazardous chemicals. Certain medical conditions may place a worker at increased risk from workplace exposures. These conditions must be evaluated to provide the worker with a clear understanding of the associated risks.

Changes in the health status of personnel or unexplained illnesses should be reported to the supervisor. If there is any suspicion of work involvement, a physician must be consulted to determine whether the illness is work related and whether it must be reported to management. At some institutions an annual questionnaire is completed by each employee and reviewed by management. These questionnaires can be monitored for unusual illnesses. If the rate of illness is unusually high or if clusters of unusual illnesses are identified, an effort should be made to determine the cause.

ACCIDENTS

Accidents that might occur in laboratories include spills in containment cabinets (chemical fume hoods or biosafety cabinets) or on laboratory work surfaces and accidental exposure to hazardous agents. Spills and exposures should be reported for monitoring of frequency of accidents and for help in developing procedures or methods for prevention. It also helps to determine which types of accidents result in exposure of laboratory workers and whether such exposures are accompanied by overt illness. Important criteria in determining the need for reporting are the nature of the agent involved, the amount involved (concentration, volume), and the likelihood that an exposure might result in illness. In the event of any question regarding reporting, a member of the safety committee should be consulted and determination made regarding the incident and initiation of further investigation.

Reporting Incidents, Accidents, Injuries, Illnesses, or Emergency Actions

It is the responsibility of each employee to report all accidents and incidents, injuries, or illnesses. For serious accidents, injuries, or illnesses, the supervisor is responsible for notifying management. No matter how slight it may seem, all accidents, illnesses, or injuries must be reported as soon as possible. In this way, a record of the incident will be on file in the event that medical treatment is required at a later date.

Reporting Laboratory Hazards, Exposure, and Accidents

The procedures, activities, attitudes, and equipment that create conditions that favor occupational laboratory illness are similar to those that lead to the occurrence of industrial accidents. Laboratory events that might create hazards, exposures, or accidents can be classified into two categories. The first includes events during work with hazardous materials or in a hazardous area that can cause injury. The second includes events during the handling of hazardous agents or infected specimens that could allow release of the agent to the environment or to employees. In the first category, the injury site can be contaminated with a hazardous agent. In the second category, illness or cross contamination can occur without physical injury. Mechanisms of infection typical of the second category are ingestion of contaminated fluids, exposure to aerosols, and penetration of agents through unbroken skin.

An employee who is accidentally exposed to a hazardous agent must initiate decontamination procedures and then report to the immediate supervisor. If an injury accompanies an exposure or a substance enters the eye, mouth, or lungs or penetrates or comes in contact with the skin, the supervisor, if present, must direct disinfecting or decontaminating procedures and assist the employee in obtaining attention, if appropriate. If the exposure is not substantial, the employee should still report the exposure, if requested. If substantial exposure involves three or more persons, the person most familiar with all details should prepare a list of all exposed persons.

The laboratory supervisor should develop an emergency plan that covers contingencies that may arise in the event of an accidental exposure. This plan includes the name of a physician aware of the agents used, the use of the agents, and the procedures for treatment if accidental exposure occurs. The supervisor is required to inform all laboratory personnel of the name of and the procedure for contacting the physician. This information is kept on file.

MEDICAL EVALUATIONS

In the event of an exposure to a hazardous agent, the supervisor or employee is to contact the physician. The physician determines whether the exposure is of sufficient risk to require medical treatment. If the physician cannot be reached, the supervisor or employee needs to contact the emergency department at the nearest hospital and provide information on the agent and the nature of the exposure. Depending on whether a safety officer is present, the supervisor should investigate a laboratory accident. The goal is to prevent similar accidents and to obtain information about the circumstances and number of employees exposed to the agent or substance in question.

MATERIALS HANDLING IN THE LABORATORY

The dimethyl mercury tragedy highlights the need for laboratories to develop protective health and safety rules that include adequate guidance on the appropriate selection of personal protective equipment and engineering controls. If laboratory workers have sufficient knowledge to identify the potential hazards associated with the work and to institute procedures and practices necessary to conduct the activity in as safe a manner as possible, they will be prepared to take the necessary precautions to protect themselves, their coworkers, and the environment. Highly placed or very well-qualified researchers should not be assumed to have adequate health and safety information. All laboratory workers must recognize that the nature of their work may lead to diverse and often severe health hazards, and occupational health and safety must be regarded as important as the work activity itself. The following information is intended to serve as a practical guideline for the protection of laboratory workers from chemical and physical agents with which they may come in contact during the course of their laboratory activity.

Chemical Safety Training

The foundation of the chemical safety training program is the material safety data sheet (MSDS). An MSDS is a document prepared by the manufacturer in accordance with the OSHA hazard communication standard and contains chemical hazard and safe handling information (13). Chemical manufacturers and distributors must provide an appropriate MSDS for each hazardous chemical that they sell or distribute. If an MSDS is not provided with the shipment of a hazardous chemical, one can be requested in writing from the manufacturer or distributor. Each organization must maintain MSDSs on file for each current chemical in the organization's inventory. By law, workers have the right to know which chemicals in their workplace are classified as hazardous. Employers are required to make MSDSs available to employees on request. Employees must be provided chemical safety training. This training typically includes the following:

- The physical and health hazards of the chemicals in the laboratory

- The methods and observations that may be used to detect the presence or release of a hazardous chemical, including the visual appearance and odor of the substance and possible monitoring devices
- The selection and correct use of personal protective equipment, including instructions in the safe handling of the substance
- The procedures to be followed in the event of a spill or any other emergency
- The details of the hazard communication program, an explanation of the labeling system, and the location of the MSDS. The program consists of the following:
- A list of all chemicals present in each laboratory to be maintained by a member of the laboratory who periodically reviews the accuracy of the list
- MSDSs on file for each chemical substance in the various laboratories
- Information on label requirements and a prohibition on removing or defacing labels on bottles containing original chemical materials. If an empty bottle is to be reused with a new substance, labels must be replaced accordingly.
- Specific training literature that describes employer and employee rights and responsibilities, educational programs, a section by section description of MSDSs, and labels
- Specific toxicologic information that enables workers to understand the hazard warning statements, effects of chemicals, and the various hygienic standards
- Health and safety considerations in handling chemicals in the workplace, such as physical and physiologic classifications, basic personnel protective practices, and chemical storage and spill considerations

Basic Chemical Handling Procedures

Laboratory workers must be instructed to read the label on the chemical container and the MSDS before using a chemical. The MSDS frequently contains special handling information or instructions (13,14). Employees should adopt the following basic safe handling procedures (15).

Chemical Waste Disposal

Chemical disposal is an issue for those who generate chemical waste and those who are responsible for disposing of waste. Selection of a disposal method depends on the nature of the compound and the quantity to be disposed of. Prompt disposal of waste materials helps to reduce fire hazards and unnecessary exposure of personnel to toxic vapors and disagreeable odors. Disposal methods are intended to serve as a guide to laboratory workers in the disposal of small quantities of waste chemicals. The physical and chemical properties of any substance must be carefully considered before disposal. All workers should contact their supervisors for disposal of large quantities of waste chemicals.

Waste Disposal Guidelines

Flammable and combustible hazardous waste must be placed in a safety can. Nonflammable and noncorrosive waste may be placed in a temporary plastic container. Corrosive waste may be placed in a temporary glass container. This waste must later be transferred to an approved department of transportation container. Plastic or glass waste containers must be placed in boxes before being transported. Temporary waste containers must be labeled properly (organic solvent waste, chromic acid waste). A manifest of the identity and quantity of all hazardous waste must be kept.

Hazardous Waste Precautions

It is essential to keep the following precautions in mind as part of the laboratory effort:

- Do not dispose of any hazardous waste in the sink.
- Do not dispose of glass or plastic gallon chemical containers containing hazardous waste residue. Dispose of residue in the waste safety can. Rinse containers with water or appropriate solvent and empty diluted contents into a waste safety can.
- Make sure containers are thoroughly cleaned and the original labels removed before disposing of containers in a Dumpster.

- Contact the supervisor regarding questions or uncertainties about disposal of hazardous waste.
- Label waste containers with the category of waste. For example, label a container with organic waste solvents *Organic Solvents*. Avoid adding incompatible waste, which may result in fire, explosion, or release of flammable gases.

Chemical Hazards

A chemical compound is generally regarded as toxic if it can cause any disturbance of normal physiologic processes. Absorption of toxic materials can occur by means of inhalation, ingestion, or skin contact. Concentrations of some chemicals as low as 1 ppm in the atmosphere can cause considerable harm (e.g., arsine, phosgene, xylene). Materials inhaled through the nose and mouth can be partially dissolved in saliva and enter the stomach. Inhalation exposures can be controlled with proper ventilation and the use of respirators. Employees must receive training on the hazards of chemicals and on the measures they can take to protect themselves. They should be provided with the available information on toxicity studies. Employees should be instructed to ask their supervisors about the chemicals being used.

The dimethyl mercury tragedy highlights the need for laboratories to develop a protective chemical safety plan that includes adequate chemical safety training with an on-the-job component and guidance on the selection of personal protective equipment and engineering controls. All chemicals, unless proved otherwise, must be regarded as potentially hazardous and be handled accordingly. Workers must proceed with caution when handling chemicals. Their lives might depend on it.

PERSONAL PROTECTIVE EQUIPMENT

Clinical laboratory workers are exposed to an assortment of known (chemical) and unknown (specimen) risks. Some of these risks can be reduced or controlled through the proper use of personal protective equipment (14). Personal protective equipment is designed to prevent personal injury. Specific items include safety glasses, goggles, face shields, glass-blowing goggles, safety shields, rubber and asbestos gloves, rubber aprons, laboratory coats, protective creams, and respirators. If in doubt about the potential danger of any experiment, workers should speak to their supervisors.

Eye Safety

Eye protection is required for all personnel and visitors in areas where there is risk for eye exposure to hazardous materials. All areas where such hazards exist must be identified and signs posted accordingly—CAUTION: EYE PROTECTION MUST BE WORN BEYOND THIS POINT.

Safety Shields

Whenever breakage or a violent reaction might occur, a safety shield must be used. Safety shields must be used whenever solvent or vacuum distillations are being run in glass equipment, large glass vessels are subjected to a vacuum, and reactions will occur the characteristics of which are unknown.

Protective Gloves

Because many chemicals are readily absorbed through the skin, skin contact with chemicals is a common route of exposure. Review of the dimethyl mercury incident indicated that absorption of as little as 0.1 mL dimethyl mercury represented a severely toxic dose (7). Laboratory workers can avoid exposures by developing proper methods for handling hazardous materials. This includes wearing appropriate gloves, keeping hands off the rest of the body during the handling period, and washing hands promptly after the handling period.

Laboratory workers must be provided with appropriate personal protective clothing to prevent exposure. This means that permeability test data be reviewed to ensure that appropriate gloves and other personal protective clothing are selected on the basis of performance and not cost. The researcher who was exposed to dimethyl mercury was wearing latex gloves while performing a transfer operation with this chemical in a chemical fume hood (7). Unfortunately, rubber and plastics are both permeable to dimethyl mercury; therefore latex, neoprene, and butyl gloves constitute inappropriate glove choices (7,8).

Contaminated gloves should be removed and discarded as soon as possible. No glove protects against all chemicals. Where laboratory workers may come into contact with solvents and hazardous chemicals, depending on permeation nitrile, butyl rubber, or polyvinyl alcohol gloves should be considered and worn over latex gloves. These types of gloves offer more protection from a wide variety of solvents than do others. However, once gloves are contaminated, traces of the contaminant eventually permeate the glove material and contaminate the inner lining. Employees must remove gloves before leaving the laboratory area to prevent contamination of door knobs, light switches, telephones, and other surfaces.

Respirator Protection

Engineering controls offer more reliable and constant protection than do respirators. These controls can eliminate the need for respirators; therefore engineering controls should be used before a respirator program is put into effect. However, employees sensitive to certain chemicals must be supplied with a respirator if they are required to work in areas where they might be at risk.

Laboratory Clothing

Laboratory clothing must be confined to the laboratory. Laboratory clothing provides an extra layer of protection during work with hazardous materials. Wearing a laboratory coat helps prevent the spread of microorganisms and radioactive and carcinogenic materials from the work area.

GENERAL LABORATORY SAFETY PRACTICES

Certain safety practices apply to all employees regardless of where they are working (15). Among these are rules that apply to such items as housekeeping, exits, drains, disposal of waste materials, gas cylinders, use of flammable materials, use of gas, water, and electricity, labeling of bottles, opening and pouring from bottles, and disposal of chemicals.

Good Housekeeping

Good housekeeping is more than cleanliness; it is cleanliness and order. It is essential for both safety and efficiency that a laboratory be kept neat and orderly. Floors, shelves, and benches should be free from dirt and unnecessary apparatus and tools. Infrequently used equipment should be kept in cabinets. Apparatus should be set well back from the edge of the table to leave more room for work. Equipment should never be allowed to stand in the halls or otherwise obstruct exits or passages. Spills or leaks of radioactive, toxic, or flammable material should be reported to the safety officer. They should be cleaned up promptly using proper procedures. If the material is flammable, every precaution should be taken to avoid igniting the material by extinguishing all flames and turning off any source of electric heat during clean up. If the spilled material is toxic, personnel should leave the area promptly

Working after Hours or Working Alone

No one should work in a laboratory after working hours unless another person is working in the same or adjacent laboratory. Employees should receive permission from their supervisor to work after hours. No one should work alone with highly hazardous chemicals. There should be a spotter whenever there is an open transfer of these materials between containers to ensure that spills or contact with protected surfaces such as gloves and laboratory coats is reported.

Unattended and Unauthorized Experiments

Employees should request and receive permission from their supervisor to leave apparatus running unattended after hours. Unauthorized experiments are not to be conducted at any time. Only experiments approved by the supervisor are acceptable.

Regulated Areas

Certain laboratories and rooms may be designated regulated areas. The doors to these rooms usually are marked with a special sign that reads, AUTHORIZED PERSONNEL ONLY, RESTRICTED AREA, NO ADMITTANCE, or something similar. Employees should not enter these rooms without first consulting the supervisor responsible for the room.

Employee Rights and Responsibilities

Employees who may be exposed to hazardous chemicals must have access to (13) chemical exposure information, workplace chemical lists, and MSDSs. By law, employees have the right to know the hazards associated with the material with which they work. Employers must provide a compliance program that meets the requirements of the OSHA hazard communication standard, the OSHA chemical laboratory standard, or both. Workers have the right to file a complaint against their employers regarding alleged violations of the hazardous chemical information act. If a complaint is filed, the act protects the worker from discharge, cause for discharge, discipline, discrimination, loss of pay, position, seniority, or benefits. Although alleged violations of the standard should be referred to supervisors, employees always have the right to file a complaint with OSHA. Providing workers with information does not eliminate the liability of the employer with regard to the health and safety of employees. Each employer has the responsibility to take action to prevent the occurrence of occupational disease and unnecessary exposure.

Employer Rights and Responsibilities

Employers have the right to take disciplinary action against employees who do not follow established safety policies and procedures (13). Employers ought further to consider the employee safety record of management and supervisory personnel when making decisions about salary and promotions. Employers have both the right and responsibility to protect workers with unique susceptibilities by placing them in alternative positions of employment. The considerations for exercise of this kind of placement decision are as follows:

- Decisions are for protection and placement only, not for job hiring or firing,
- Alternative job placement for personal protection does not adversely alter personal income.
- Alternative job placement for uniquely susceptible workers is not seen as an alternative to prudent health and safety practice. Generally dangerous practices, such as exposures to toxic substances above recommended thresholds, should be met by engineering rather than personnel manipulations.
- Civil rights may not be abused.

Even within these considerations, employers might want to protect the health and well-being of some employees in certain types of jobs by finding alternative jobs for them.

EDUCATIONAL PROGRAMS

Employers are required to provide training, at least annually, to employees using or handling hazardous materials (11). New or newly assigned employees must receive training before working with or in a work area containing hazardous materials. The training program includes the following:

- Location of hazardous materials
- Acute and chronic effects of exposure

- Safe handling procedures
- Personal protective equipment
- First aid
- Clean up procedures
- Waste disposal

Employers are required to keep a record of training sessions provided to employees. Employees usually are requested to sign an attendance sheet to verify their presence at a training session. Employers are responsible for providing training and information that allow employees to work safely. It is the right and responsibility of the employer to require that both supervising and supervised personnel comply with the safety policies that have been developed to meet this responsibility.

CONCLUSION

The potential threat of illness in the laboratory has long been recognized by the medical community as an ever-present occupational hazard. Published reports of the occurrence of laboratory-acquired infections have served as reminders that the potential can easily become an actuality. The dimethyl mercury episode points out how tragic the outcome can be and the need for unremitting adherence to appropriate precautionary measures. Only in recent years have we come to appreciate the importance of the problem of laboratory-acquired illness and the many factors, both human and environmental, that may be involved (2,4–6). Laboratory safety is an exercise in recognizing the risks and introducing procedures, practices, equipment, and facilities to control the identified risks or hazards or reduce them to acceptable levels.

Safe laboratory practice requires an objective evaluation of the hazard potential associated with each aspect of work activity. Such an evaluation must include consideration of the materials involved; the procedures and practices associated with their use; the adequacy of equipment and facilities required to carry out the program in a safe and prudent manner; a review of available information on related laboratory-acquired illness; the training and experience of personnel; and the appropriateness of vaccination or other medical surveillance requirements before program initiation (1,2,16).

The purpose of this chapter is to emphasize the need for adequate safety precautions in the planning, initiation, and termination of laboratory activities that represent a real or potential hazard to workers and to provide basic chemical health and safety information. This approach was adopted because it is not possible for safety specialists to anticipate each use of potentially hazardous biologic or chemical systems and to monitor every operation that involves hazardous materials. Workers need to know what they can do to protect their health and well-being. It is intentional that parts of this chapter are written in the form of a generic health and safety manual. Clinical laboratory workers are required to work in an environment and with materials that place them at risk. Readers are encouraged to consider, modify, rewrite, or use this text as is to develop a health and safety program responsive to their specific needs and those of their institutions.

APPENDIX A

Safety Rules and Procedures

- Do not work alone in the laboratory.
- Use required personal protective equipment.
- Label all containers with appropriate hazard information.
- Keep your hands and face clean. Wash thoroughly with soap and water after handling any chemical.
- Avoid direct contact with any chemical.
- Keep chemicals off your hands, face and clothing, including shoes.
- Never smell, inhale, or taste a hazardous chemical.
- Never smoke, drink, eat, or apply cosmetics in an area where hazardous chemicals are in use.
- Do not dispense more of a chemical than is needed for immediate use.
- Always use chemicals with adequate ventilation or in a chemical fume hood, as appropriate. Refer to the MSDS.

- Use hazardous chemicals only as directed and for their intended purpose.
- Inspect equipment or apparatus for damage before adding any chemical. Do not use damaged equipment.
- Never use mouth suction to fill a pipette. Use a pipette bulb or other pipette aid.
- Electrically ground and bond containers using approved methods before transferring or dispensing a flammable liquid from a large container.
- Do not store chemicals in alphabetical order.
- Separate hazardous chemicals in storage as follows. Once separated into hazard classes, chemicals may be stored alphabetically.
- Solids
- Oxidizers
- Flammable solids
- Water-reactive substances
- Liquids
- Acids
- Caustic substances
- Oxidizers
- Perchloric acid
- Flammable or combustible substances
- Gases
- Toxic gases
- Flammable gases
- Oxidizers and inert gases
- Do not store incompatible chemicals close to each other
- Use only approved storage containers and safety cans for flammable liquids.
- Use spill trays under containers of strong acidic or basic reagents.
- Write the date received and the date opened on each chemical.
- Dispose of old chemicals promptly and properly.
- Do not store liquids above eye level.
- Label all containers properly.
- When in doubt, ask your supervisor

Chemical Incompatibilities

Certain hazardous chemicals cannot be safely mixed or stored with other chemicals because a severe reaction can take place or an extremely toxic reaction product can result. The label and MSDS contain information on incompatibilities. Solvents can be volatile, harmful when inhaled or absorbed through the skin, and flammable. Flammable liquids are more hazardous at elevated temperatures because of rapid vaporization.

- Read the label and MSDS for special hazards involving a given solvent.
- Electrically ground and bond containers using approved methods before transferring or dispensing a flammable liquid from a large container.
- Transfer only the amount necessary for immediate use.
- Use only approved flammable-liquid containers and storage cabinets.
- Keep flammable liquids away from heat sources.
- Do not store flammable liquids stored near oxidizing agents (e.g., chromic acid, permanganates, chlorates, or perchlorates).
- Avoid skin contact and inhalation of solvents.
- Do not dispose of solvents in sinks or drains.
- Use solvents only with adequate ventilation or in a fume hood.
- Use assigned personal protective equipment.

REFERENCES

1. Grist NR. Epidemiology and control of virus infections in the laboratory. *Yale J Biol Med* 1982;55:213–218.
2. Liberman DF. Identification and control of human health hazards associated with current and emergency biotechnology. In: Draggan S, et al, eds. *Environmental impacts on human health*. New York: Praeger, 1987:193–219.
3. Liberman DF, Harding AL. Biosafety: the research/diagnostic laboratory perspective. In: Liberman DF, ed. *Biohazards management handbook*, 2nd ed. New York: Marcel Dekker, 1995:151–172.
4. Martin JC. Behavioral factors in laboratory safety personnel characteristics and modification of unsafe acts. In: Fuscaldo AA, et al, eds. *Laboratory safety, theory, and practice*. New York: Academic Press, 1980:321–342.
5. Phillips GB. *Causal factors in microbiological laboratory accidents and infections*. Fort Detrick, Frederick, MD: US Army Biological Laboratories, 1965.
6. Phillips GB. Human factors in microbiological laboratory accidents. Research Triangle Park, NC: Becton Dickinson Research Center, 1973.
7. Blayney MB, Winn JS, Nierenberg DW. Letters: Chemical safety—handling dimethylmercury. *Chem Eng News* 1997; May 12.

8. Toriba TY, Clarkson TW, Nierenberg DW. Letters: More on working with dimethylmercury. *Chem Eng News* 1997; June 16.
9. Raouf A, Dhillon BS. *Safety assessment*. Boca Raton, FL: CRC Press/Lewis Publishers, 1994.
10. Roland HE, Moriarty RB. *System safety engineering and management*, 2nd ed. New York: Wiley, 1990.
11. Collert J. *Environmental health and safety CFR training requirements*. Rockville, MD: Government Institutes, 1995.
12. US Department of Labor, Occupational Health and Safety Administration. Occupational exposure to blood-borne pathogens: final rule. *Federal Register* 1991;56: 64004–64182.
13. US Department of Labor, Occupational Health and Safety Administration. Health and safety standards: chemical hazards communication; final rule; 29CFR part 1910.120. *Federal Register* 1991;228:53280–53348.
14. US Department of Labor, Occupational Health and Safety Administration. Health and safety standards: occupational exposure to hazardous substances in laboratories; 29CFR. *Federal Register* 1993;51: 22600–22684.
15. *Prudent practices in the laboratory.* Sections 5C; 5D. Washington, DC: National Academy Press, 1995.
16. Goldman RH. Medical surveillance program. In: Liberman DF, ed. *Biohazards management handbook*, 2nd ed. New York: Marcel Dekker, 1995:173–192.

Medical Center Occupational Health and Safety,
edited by Robert J. McCunney.
Lippincott Williams & Wilkins, Philadelphia © 1999.

20
Operating Rooms

Brian G. Forrester and *Victor S. Roth

Department of Occupational Medicine, Regional First Care, Athens, Georgia 30601;
**University of Michigan Occupational Health Services, Ann Arbor, Michigan 48103-5827*

The operating room environment deserves special consideration because of the myriad occupational hazards concentrated in a relatively confined area. Almost every hazard present in medical centers may be found in operating rooms, including chemical hazards (anesthetic gases), biologic hazards (bloodborne and other infectious agents), physical hazards (electrical, radiation, fire, compressed gas, laser, and noise), and psychologic hazards (time pressure, stress). These hazards are compounded by the fact that the primary focus of the operating team is on the welfare of the surgical patient, not on personal safety. However, if proper attention is paid to these hazards with engineering and administrative controls, personal protective equipment, and employee training, the result will be mitigation of the occupational risk associated with operating room work.

ANESTHETIC GASES

Anesthetic gases have been used in surgery for more than 150 years (1), but reports of adverse health effects caused by exposure to waste anesthetic gases were not published until 1967 (2). Over the next 20 years, interest in the nonnarcotic health effects of anesthetic gases spiraled, and numerous studies were published (3–12). Beginning in the mid 1970s, professional societies and government agencies recommended that scavenging systems be used to reduce exposure to waste anesthetic gases (13). Since that time research interest appears to have waned; however, occupational medicine physicians practicing in a medical center continue to be consulted about operating room anesthetic exposures stemming from concerns about safety. The inhalation anesthetics likely to be encountered today include desflurane, enflurane, halothane, isoflurane, sevoflurane, and nitrous oxide (14) (see Chapter 9).

Exposure to anesthetic gases has been suggested to have mutagenic, carcinogenic, and teratogenic effects (15). Increased frequencies of chromosomal abnormalities have been found among operating room personnel (16,17), as has increased mutagenic activity in the urine of anesthesiologists (18). Although increased rates of cancer have been reported among female operating room workers (19), there is insufficient evidence at this time to support a carcinogenic effect of waste anesthetic gases among humans (20).

Volatile anesthetics such as nitrous oxide and halothane have been shown to have a number of cellular effects, including decreased production of white blood cells (21), decreased cell division (22) possibly related to reduced mitochondrial oxygen uptake (23), and inhibition of DNA synthesis (24). Lassen et al. (25) described bone marrow suppression among patients with prolonged periods of nitrous oxide sedation as early as

1956. Megaloblastic changes have been seen in the bone marrow of patients who have undergone cardiac bypass operations exposed to 50% nitrous oxide for as little as 5 hours (8).

Animal studies have found adverse health effects from exposure to anesthetics. Rats exposed to halothane at 12 ppm for 40 hours per week showed irreversible learning deficits and neuronal damage (26). These effects were more pronounced among immature rats, suggesting increased susceptibility in developing central nervous systems.

Central nervous system effects, such as increased prevalence of headache, fatigue, irritability, and sleep disturbances, have been reported among operating room personnel (2,27). Subanesthetic doses have been associated with psychomotor impairment (3, 28–32). Habitual abusers of nitrous oxide and chronically exposed dental patients have developed a neuropathy syndrome characterized by paresthesias and ataxia (5–7).

Halothane has been reported to cause reversible hepatitis among anesthetists exposed to low doses in operating rooms (33,34), possibly through a hypersensitivity mechanism (35). Recrudescence after return to exposure and remittance after avoiding halothane are well documented (12).

Many studies have described an increased incidence of spontaneous abortion and congenital malformations among offspring of female operating room personnel (36–40). However, confounding these results are many other exposures present in the operating room environment (shift work, irregular working hours, stress, infections, prolonged standing, and others), which were not taken into account (1,12). Selection and reporting bias also may have been present (41). Many of the original fears concerning exposure to low-level anesthetics during pregnancy may have been unwarranted (42).

Operating room personnel may be exposed to anesthetic gases from a variety of sources (43–45) (Table 20-1). Exposure levels to these gases may be greatly reduced by following certain recommended protocols, such as proper equipment maintenance, preanesthesia equipment checks (46), proper anesthetic technique (47), use of a laryngeal mask (48), improved ventilation (46), and engineering controls consisting of various scavenging systems, including the double mask (46,49) or gas scavenging mask (44) (Table 20-2).

The efficacy of control measures may be verified by the use of personal sampling devices, which measure the levels of anesthetic gases present in the anesthetist's breathing

TABLE 20-1. *Sources of anesthetic gas exposure in operating rooms*

Carbon dioxide absorber gasket leaks
Leaks in anesthesia ventilator bellows
Leaks at pressure relief (pop-off) valve
Leaks in the reservoir bag
Leaks from high-pressure gas connections at central gas manifold
Leaks from beneath the edge of the anesthesia mask during inhalational anesthesia
Anesthetic gases exhaled by patient
Leaks around endotracheal tube cuffs insufficiently inflated
Uncuffed tubes in children
Poorly fitting face masks in edentulous or bearded patients
Turning gas flow to on position before mask placement on patient
Refilling vaporizers in the on position

Information from refs. 43–45.

TABLE 20-2. *Methods of control for waste anesthetic gases*

1. Do not use excessive gas flow.
2. Use closed circuit anesthetic systems.
3. Use standardized apparatus and safety equipment.
4. Use appropriate scavenging devices, including gas-scavenging masks.
5. Maintain proper ventilation and follow national standards for room air changes per hour.
6. Inspect equipment before each use.
7. Develop a preventive maintenance schedule for all equipment.
8. Train all anesthetists in good anesthesia administration technique to minimize excessive gas leakage into the environment.

Information from refs. 1, 46, 47.

zone. Personal monitoring appears to be superior to general area monitoring for detecting peak exposure levels (46). The anesthetist, typically the worker in the operating room who has the greatest exposure, should be the focus of the sampling strategy (47,50–52). Anesthetists are closest to the anesthetic machine and the patient's airway, both primary sources of waste anesthetic gases. Monitoring for nitrous oxide appears to be a useful surrogate for all other anesthetic gases present. The National Institute for Occupational Safety and Health recommends an 8-hour time-weighted average exposure limit of 25 ppm for nitrous oxide, primarily to prevent "decrements in performance, cognition, audiovisual ability, and dexterity" (53). Unfortunately, it appears that this recommended exposure limit often is exceeded during the routine practice of anesthesia administration (47,54). Table 20-2 lists methods suitable for reducing exposure to waste anesthetic gases in operating rooms.

BLOOD-BORNE PATHOGENS

Exposure to blood and body fluids is common in many health care settings but is magnified in operating rooms because of the invasive surgical procedures that take place there. Such exposure has become of increasing concern to all health care providers since the beginning of the human immunodeficiency virus (HIV) epidemic in the early 1980s. Tremendous potential for blood exposure exists in the operating room. Many times it is held in check only by the skill of a surgeon's technique. Nevertheless, important methods exist for preventing blood-borne disease among health care workers. Proper use of these methods in the operating room can diminish the risk of occupationally acquired blood-borne infection.

The infectious agents of greatest concern in the operating room are the blood-borne agents hepatitis B virus (HBV), HIV, and hepatitis C virus (HCV). Less frequent transmission of other viral, bacterial, parasitic, rickettsial, and fungal agents occurs after percutaneous exposure to blood in a health care setting. Accidental exposure to blood among health care workers has resulted in occupational infections by at least 20 different pathogens, including arbovirus, cytomegalovirus, hepatitis delta virus, and the pathogens that cause malaria, syphilis, brucellosis, babesiosis, leptospirosis, Creutzfeldt-Jakob disease, and toxoplasmosis (55,56). Risk factors for blood contamination of operating room personnel include the volume of blood loss during surgery, the use of fingers to hold tissue while suturing, the duration of an operation, the surgical specialty involved, the number of needles used, and the volume of irrigation fluid used (57–59).

Body contamination and percutaneous exposure to blood or body fluids occurs at a surprisingly high rate during surgical procedures. One hundred percent of orthopedists performing total joint arthroplasty were found by Smith et al. (60) to have body contamination with blood, body fluids, or bone particles. A large observational study found that 6.9% of all surgical procedures had at least one percutaneous exposure during the procedure (57). Resident physicians had higher rates of exposure than physician faculty, and obstetric and gynecologic surgeons had higher rates of exposure than other surgical specialties. The aggregate mean injury rate per surgeon was 2.5 percutaneous injuries per 100 procedures. Anesthetists also are at risk. A study by Kristensen et al. (61) found that contamination with body fluids occurs in 36% of common anesthetic procedures.

The Occupational Safety and Health Administration (OSHA) passed the Bloodborne Pathogens Standard in 1991 to address occupational exposure to human blood and body fluids (62; see Chapter 3). As part of this standard, employers are required to develop an exposure control plan and to adhere to universal precautions as specified by the Centers for Disease Control and Prevention (CDC). Engineering and work practices controls for preventing exposure must be developed and used, and personal protective equipment (eye and face protection, gowns, gloves) must be provided. Employers must provide the hepatitis B vaccination series free of charge and offer postexposure counseling and medical follow-up care.

Hepatitis B Virus

Occupationally acquired hepatitis has been recognized as a health hazard for health care workers for more than 40 years (63,64). The risk for acquiring HBV from a single percutaneous exposure is approximately 30% for hepatitis e antigen–positive sources (65); this greatly exceeds the risk for contracting HIV from a single exposure. The consequences of HBV infection may be serious. Approximately 5% of persons with the infection enter a chronic carrier state, which may lead to the development of cirrhosis, hepatocellular carcinoma, or both (66).

In seroprevalence studies, markers of previous infection with HBV are much more prevalent among health care workers than the general population of the United States. Studies performed in the 1970s and 1980s, before HBV vaccine became available, found the prevalence of HBV infection ranged from 10% to 28% among surgeons and 13% to 49% among anesthesiologists compared with 3% to 14% among the U.S. general population (67). Risk factors identified for the development of HBV infection include not receiving the hepatitis B vaccine, working in an area with a high prevalence of infection in the general population, reporting nine or more percutaneous injuries in the past year, being a general surgeon, and practicing surgery for at least 10 years (67,68). Unfortunately, even in an era when a safe, effective vaccine is available, substantial numbers of surgeons (14% to 50%) and other health care workers remain unvaccinated (68,69).

Hepatitis C Virus

The HCV is responsible for approximately 82% of all cases of non-A non-B hepatitis in the United States (70). The risk for transmission of HCV after a single percutaneous exposure, between 2.7% and 10%, appears to be less than that of HBV (71,72). Serious health consequences may occur after infection with HCV. As many as 50% of patients have evidence of chronic liver disease, and 20% of these patients go on to have cirrhosis (73). The epidemiologic characteristics of HCV infection among health care workers are under investigation. Only recently has a serologic test become available. It appears that the prevalence of HCV infection among orthopedic and other surgeons is less than 1% (68).

Human Immunodeficiency Virus

Although the risk for contracting HIV infection after a percutaneous exposure to infected blood is much less than the risk for contracting HBV or HCV infection after a similar exposure, much of the recent concern about occupationally acquired blood-borne infections coincided with the HIV epidemic in the early 1980s. The risk for contracting HIV after a single percutaneous exposure to infected blood is approximately 0.3%. It was calculated from prospective follow-up data on thousands of exposed health care workers (74–77). Most of this risk derives from exposure to hollow-bore needles, which cause deeper injuries and the transfer of considerably more blood than the solid suture needles used in surgery (78,79). Mucous membrane exposures are thought to carry considerably less risk for transmission of infection, approximating 0.09%, than are percutaneous injuries (76). Raahave and Bremmelgaard (80), using an actuarial probability technique, estimated the lifetime risk that a surgeon would occupationally acquire HIV infection. The estimate assumed a 0.46% chance of acquiring HIV after a single exposure, a patient population prevalence of HIV infection of 1%, and a 10% probability of injury for each operation. This resulted in an estimated 30-year lifetime probability of occupationally acquiring HIV of 2.72%. This risk is obviously unacceptable for a disease that is still assumed to be uniformly fatal and emphasizes the need for prevention of transmission.

Postexposure prophylaxis with zidovudine has been reported to result in 79% reduction in the odds of HIV transmission after a percutaneous exposure (81). The emergence of antiretroviral resistance makes the addition of newer antiretroviral agents (lamivudine) to the regimen a rational option (81). Knowledge of a patient's HIV status does not appear to reduce exposure rates during surgical procedures, therefore preoperative serologic testing is not indicated (82).

Prevention

Prevention of blood exposure is the most effective means of limiting occupational bloodborne infection. Prevention may be accomplished by considering all blood a toxic substance (universal precautions), instituting administrative, engineering, and work practice controls, and using appropriate personal protective equipment. The Surgical Infection Society (83) has published recommendations concerning conduct in the operating room that should limit exposure to blood and body fluids during operations (Table 20-3). Table 20-4 lists exposure control methods that have been

TABLE 20-3. *Conduct in the operating room recommended for limiting exposure to blood or body fluids during surgical procedures*

1. The number of personnel participating in an operation should be kept to an appropriate minimum.
2. Inexperienced (including residents), nonessential, or pregnant personnel should not participate in operations on patients known to harbor blood borne infection (HIV, HBV, or HCV).
3. Personnel with open wounds in areas that could be easily contaminated should not participate.
4. Disposable plastic aprons should be worn under operating gowns to avoid gross contamination if excessive exposure to blood or body fluids is anticipated.
5. Disposable scrub clothes and gowns should be worn so that they can be discarded at the end of the procedure.
6. Eye shields or eyeglasses always should be worn.
7. Masks that become contaminated should be changed immediately.
8. Contaminated underclothing or shoes should be soaked in a 1:10 diluted chlorine bleach solution and then washed. The use of rubber-soled canvas shoes is recommended.
9. Needles should not be recapped.
10. Suture needles should not be grasped with the fingers, only with needle holders, pickups, or other instruments.
11. The use of scalpels should be kept to a minimum.
12. Sharp instruments should be isolated from all other instruments and handled only by the surgeon and scrub nurse.
13. No member of the surgical team should remove instruments from or return instruments to the scrub nurse's tray.
14. No sharp or pointed instruments should be left lying on the surgical sheets, where they can injure someone.
15. The department of pathology should be informed ahead of time if a biopsy specimen is to be obtained so that the specimen can be handled appropriately.
16. All personnel should thoroughly wash their hands and arms at the end of the operation.
17. If skin contamination was possible, a warm shower should be taken immediately after the operation with an antimicrobial skin cleanser.
18. Consider scheduling procedures for the end of the operating room schedule to facilitate terminal cleaning procedures.

Information from ref. 83.

TABLE 20-4. *Exposure control methods for blood-borne pathogens in operating rooms*

1. Routinely use double gloving.
2. Use wraparound face shields or space helmets in procedures known to generate airborne blood or body fluids, such as the use of surgical power tools.
3. Replace sharp instruments with blunt instruments when feasible.
4. Keep sharp instruments in a neutral zone so that the nurse and surgeon touch the same sharp instrument at the same time.
5. Handle tissue with instruments only and minimize the use of fingers.
6. Use improved operating room gowns that limit blood strike-through.
7. Use protective garments, such as knee-high boots, for procedures known to require copious irrigation or expected to have considerable blood loss.
8. Develop a protocol for the handling of knives.
9. Do not recap contaminated needles unless absolutely necessary. If recapping must be done, use a mechanical device or a one-handed technique.
10. Place puncture-resistant needle disposal containers where they are easily accessible and properly seal and discard when three-fourths full.
11. Use needleless or protected needle products when suitable.
12. Wear gowns with impervious sleeves during operations requiring placement of hands and arms deep into body cavities.
13. Wear protective eyewear for all operations.
14. Use of an electrocautery rather than a surgical knife when possible to reduce accidental injuries.
15. Replace wire sutures used to close abdominal fascia with safer monofilament alternatives.

Information from refs. 55, 58–60, 62, 80, 113, 114.

recommended or proved to decrease exposure to blood or body fluids in operating rooms.

OTHER INFECTIOUS AGENTS

Tuberculosis

Occupational exposure to infectious agents is not confined to blood-borne pathogens for operating room personnel. Tuberculosis, especially strains resistant to multiple drugs, is an emerging problem for all health care workers (see Chapter 4). Operating room personnel involved in airway management (anesthetists) may be presumed to be at greatest risk. The CDC publishes guidelines concerning frequency of tuberculosis skin testing among health care workers (see Chapter 4). Other methods of control include using personal protective equipment (respirators) (84), maintaining adequate room air changes, and venting exhaust ventilation directly outside (see Chapter 4).

Papillomavirus

The use of carbon dioxide lasers in the management of warts has raised concerns about the transmittal of viral particles to operating room personnel in the laser plume (85,86). A report has been published of a case in which a surgeon acquired laryngeal papillomatosis after using a laser to treat a patient with anogenital condyloma (87). Although the incidence of warts among surgeons does not appear to exceed the incidence of warts in the general population, surgeons appear to be at site-specific increased risk for the development of nasopharyngeal lesions (88). Dispersion of virus in the laser plume appears to be limited to the immediate surroundings of the treatment fields (89). Control methods for the prevention of exposure to the laser-generated plume include use of a laser smoke evacuator and filter system positioned within 1 cm over the treatment field and use of a fit-tested laser mask by the surgeon (88,89).

Anesthetists run the risk for exposure to herpes simplex virus in tracheobronchial secretions. This may result in the formation of a herpetic whitlow through a cut in the finger (12,90).

PHYSICAL HAZARDS

Ionizing Radiation

A potential hazard exists when diagnostic or therapeutic ionizing radiation is used in the operating room. Ionizing radiation is defined as radiation that is powerful enough to produce ionization in matter. Radiation used in operating rooms is either x-rays (conventional radiography or fluoroscopy) or megavoltage electron radiation (radiation therapy). Although the use of x-ray fluoroscopy confers minimal risk to operating room staff if used properly, the risk is substantial with poor technique and improper shielding. Arnstein et al. (91) reported a case of multiple squamous cell carcinoma on the hands of a radiographer who used poor radiologic technique while performing fluoroscopy during the removal of foreign bodies from the hands.

The two components of radiation to which operating room staff may be exposed are the primary beam (radiation in the path between the x-ray tube and the image intensifier) and scattered radiation, mainly produced by the interaction of the primary beam with the patient or other objects in its path (91). Scattered radiation is the main radiation exposure among operating room staff. The eyes and hands of the surgeon are the tissues most likely to receive scattered radiation. The lens of the eye is especially sensitive to ionizing radiation, and exposure can lead to cataracts (92). Important measures of control while using diagnostic x-ray radiation in the operating room are listed in Table 20-5.

The use of intraoperative radiation therapy to deliver a single treatment of electron radiation to a surgically exposed target within a patient is becoming common (93). This method may be safely used in the operating room if more lead shielding is used in the portable accelerator treatment head than is used in conventional accelerators, polyethylene shielding is used to limit neutron radiation, and the operating room has additional lead shielding installed in the walls as necessary to limit penetration of the beam to areas outside the operating room (93).

TABLE 20-5. *Control measures for the intraoperative use of radiation*

1. Wear appropriate protective equipment (leaded aprons, thyroid shields, and eyewear).
2. Minimize radiation exposure time.
3. Leave the area if feasible if your presence is not essential.
4. Cone down the image to include only the area of immediate interest.
5. Remove the antiscatter grid whenever possible (reduces scattered radiation).
6. Avoid the primary beam at all times.
7. Use a remote positioning device when possible to minimize radiation dosage to operator, staff, and patient.

Information from ref. 91.

Nonionizing Radiation

Nonionizing radiation is defined as radiation not powerful enough to produce ionization in matter. Microwave radiation, a type of nonionizing radiation, is produced by the use of electrosurgical units in operating rooms. The primary hazard of microwave radiation is its nonspecific tissue-heating effects. The target organ of concern in the operating room is the lens of the eye, which is especially sensitive to the effects of microwave radiation (94). Microwave radiation is capable of producing marked lens opacification (cataracts) if the intensity and duration of exposure are sufficient. Paz et al. (95) found that measurements of the electrical field at the eyes, forehead, neck, chest, and arms of surgeons using an electrosurgical unit greatly exceed exposure levels recommended by the American National Standards Institute. Exposure of urologists performing transurethral prostate resection may be particularly intense, because the radiating active lead enters the cystoscope near the eye (96).

Fire

Fire requires an ignition source, an oxygen source, and a fuel source (97). In the operating room, the ignition source is controlled by the surgeon (electrosurgical units, lasers, and high-intensity light cords) and the oxygen source by the anesthetist (oxygen, nitrous oxide). The fuel may be a variety of materials, including surgical drapes, gowns, hair, skin, endotracheal tubes, and surgical preparation materials (97). Fires involving endotracheal tubes were reported soon after the introduction of lasers into the operating room environment (97). The medical products industry responded by developing several laser-safe endotracheal tubes that are resistant to fire (98).

Electrosurgical units are a potential ignition source. The cautery tip reaches a temperature of several hundred degrees during electrosurgery. If sufficient fuel and oxygen are presented to the tip of the cautery unit, a fire occurs. Fires in operating rooms have been caused by electrosurgical units. In one instance, an ignition of a surgical drape produced thick, black smoke and caused the nine-member surgical team to evacuate the operating room (97). High-intensity fiberoptic light sources also exceed the ignition temperature of most surgical drapes at the tip of the light cord (97). Table 20-6 lists practices that are essential for fire prevention in the operating room.

Gas Cylinders

Compressed gases in cylinders contain tremendous amounts of energy, and the cylinders may become lethal flying objects if the pressure is released rapidly in an uncontrolled manner. The jet-like force produced by instantaneous release of compressed oxygen can propel a cylinder through a concrete wall (99). To limit the potential for compressed gas accidents, all manufacturer and Food and Drug Administration (FDA) recommendations must be followed when handling compressed gas cylinders (100).

TABLE 20-6. *Fire prevention in the operating room*

1. Keep the electric cautery tip in a holster when not in use.
2. Turn on and turn off all high-intensity light sources after all connections have been made and just before their use.
3. Use appropriately protected endotracheal tubes when lasers are being used.
4. Use air or an air-oxygen mixture in the anesthetic gases when ignition is possible.
5. Tent surgical drapers so that pockets of oxygen cannot accumulate.
6. Use a water-soluble substance rather than petroleum-based ointments.
7. Use surgical drapes that resist ignition.
8. Know the location of the fire extinguisher and how to use it.
9. Practice using the extinguisher with real fires.
10. Know the location of all fire alarm pull stations and fire exits.

From ref. 97, with permission.

Lasers

The use of lasers in surgery was first reported in 1971 (101). Most surgical lasers in use today are class IV lasers (the most powerful) and are capable of causing damage to the eye even after a partial reflective exposure (102). Brodman et al. (103), reporting on 141 consecutive cases involving laser use, found that 13 cases (9%) were complicated by inadvertent morbidity associated with use of lasers. All of the accidents were associated with human error (dragging an activated laser tip off the field or accidentally activating the laser when it was not directed at the surgical site). None of the accidents was caused by laser equipment failure. Table 20-7 lists practices essential for safe use of laser during operations.

Noise

Occupational exposure to excessive noise is well known to have physiologic and psycho-

TABLE 20-7. *Safety procedures for laser use in surgery*

1. All physicians operating a laser should satisfactorily complete a certified laser course, including sections on laser physics and safety.
2. Safety goggles specific for the wavelength of laser in use should be worn by all operating room personnel.
3. Drapes used in the operating field should be wet or laser resistant.
4. A laser technician should run the laser control panel continuously and have a carbon dioxide fire extinguisher at hand.
5. Instruments should be anodized.
6. Reflective surfaces in operating rooms should be covered during laser surgery or replaced with brushed surfaces to reduce the risk of reflection.

Information from refs. 102, 103, 115.

logic effects, including hearing loss (104), cardiovascular effects (vasoconstriction, elevated heart rate and blood pressure) (105), and increased levels of psychologic stress (106). Noise may impair complex intellectual functions and the performance of complex tasks, reduce accuracy, and decrease capability to respond to the unexpected (107). These are serious considerations in the operating room.

Noise levels are measured on the logarithmic decibel scale. An increase of 3 dB is associated with a doubling of the sound pressure (intensity) of the noise. OSHA has set 90 dB as the time-weighted average allowable for a worker over an 8-hour period; 115 dB is the absolute exposure intensity allowable for any period of time (108).

The average noise levels in operating rooms are usually well below the OSHA standard (107). However, the use of power tools during surgical procedures is becoming increasingly common. In orthopedic surgery, powered bone-cutting tools are often used. Occupational hearing loss among orthopedic surgeons and their assistants has been associated with the use of power tools (109,110). Ray and Levinson (110) found noise levels as high as 118 dB in the operating room during use of high-speed, gas turbine bone-cutting drills, which is double the OSHA maximum allowable limit. Suction tips with internally trapped tissue reached noise levels of 96 dB (quadruple the OSHA 8-hour limit). Table 20-8 shows noise levels of common exposures and operating room exposures for comparison purposes. Table 20-9 lists measures recommended for limiting exposure of operating room personnel to high-intensity noise.

TABLE 20-8. *Environmental and operating room noise levels*

Exposure	Noise level (dB)
Threshold of hearing	0
Soft whisper at 5 feet	30
Large, busy office	50 dB
Operating room average noise (no power tools)	60–65
Automobile running	75
Noisy restaurant	80
Suction tip with trapped tissue	96
Chain saw	110
Rock-and-roll band	110
High-speed gas turbine bone-cutting drill	118
Jet taking off nearby	140

Information from refs. 107, 110.

Psychologic Stress

Stress is present in many health care environments, including the operating room. Surgeons score higher than the general population on standardized measures of anxiety, but much of this anxiety appears to be related to interference of the practice of surgery with the surgeon's personal and family life (111). Anesthetists appear to suffer more work-related stress in the operating room than do surgeons. Anesthetists' stress may be related to alternating periods of acute anxiety associated with managing a life-threatening crisis with periods of frustrating boredom (12). Anesthetists also are more likely to suffer drug addiction (12) and commit suicide (112) than are other physicians. Factors that may limit stress in the operating room include maintaining adequate staffing to limit the number of hours worked per week, presurgical medical screening of patients to decrease acute intraoperative crises, appropriate preoperative planning for long or difficult operations, and the availability of confidential employee assistance programs for workers with signs of increased stress, anxiety, depression, or substance abuse.

TABLE 20-9. *Noise reduction measures for the operating room*

1. Architectural design of operating rooms should include noise-reducing measures (use of sound-insulating materials for floors, ceilings, and walls).
2. All noise-producing machines should undergo routine maintenance for noise reduction.
3. All operating room personnel should wear OSHA-certified hearing protection when power tools capable of generating excessive noise levels are to be used.

Information from refs. 107, 110.

SUMMARY

The operating room environment is a microcosm of the occupational hazards present in medical centers—the hazards are concentrated in one area by time and place. Careful planning, use of engineering and administrative controls, worker training, counseling, and vigilance are required to limit the adverse health effects that can result from operating room exposures. Each operating room hazard presented in this chapter can be prevented or ameliorated by the use of the described measures. Operating room workers and surgical patients will benefit from the use of such preventive practices.

REFERENCES

1. Bihari V, Srivastava AK, Gupta BN. Occupational health hazards among operation room personnel exposed to anesthetic gases: a review. *J Environ Pathol Toxicol Oncol* 1994;13:213–219.
2. Vaisman AI. Working conditions in surgery and their effects on the health of anesthesiologists. *Eksp Khir Anesteziol* 1967;3:44–49.
3. Bruce DL, Bach MJ, Arbit J. Trace anesthetic effects on perceptual, cognitive, and motor skills. *Anesthesiology* 1974;40:453–458.
4. Davenport HT, Halsey MJ, Wardley-Smith B, Wright BM. Measurement and reduction of occupational exposure to inhaled anesthetics. *Br Med J* 1976;2:1219–1221.
5. Sahenk Z, Mendell JR, Couri D, Nachtman J. Polyneuropathy from inhalation of N_2O cartridges through a whipped cream dispenser. *Neurology* 1978;28:485–487.
6. Layzer RB, Fishman RA, Schafer JA. Neuropathy following abuse of nitrous oxide. *Neurology* 1978;28:504–506.
7. Layzer RB. Myeloneuropathy after prolonged exposure to nitrous oxide. *Lancet* 1978;2:1227–1228.
8. Amess JAL, Burman JF, Rees GM, Nancekievill DG, Mollon DL. Megaloblastic haemopoiesis in patients receiving nitrous oxide. *Lancet* 1978;2:339–342.
9. Cohen EN. *Anesthetic exposure in the workplace.* Littleton, MA: P.S.G. Publishing, 1980.
10. Brodsky JB. Adverse effects of nitrous oxide. *Med Toxicol* 1986;1:362–374.
11. Sweeney B, Bingham RM, Amos RJ, Petty AC, Cole JPV. Toxicity of bone marrow in dentists exposed to nitrous oxide. *Br Med J* 1985;291:567–569.
12. Redfern N. Morbidity among anaesthetists. *Br J Hosp Med* 1990;43:377–381.
13. Gray WM. Scavenging equipment. *Br J Anaesth* 1985;57:685–695.
14. Stevens WC, Kingston HGG. Inhalation anesthesia. In: Barash PG, Cullen BF, Stoelting RK, eds. *Clinical anesthesia*, 3rd ed. Philadelphia: Lippincott–Raven, 1997.
15. IARC monographs on the evaluation of carcinogenic risk of chemicals to man. General considerations on volatile anesthetics. Lyon: IARA, 1976;11:285–293.
16. Bigatti P, Lamberti L, Ardito G, Armelino F, Malanetto C. Chromosome aberrations and sister chromatid exchanges in occupationally exposed workers. *Med Lav* 1985;76:334–339.
17. Karelova J, Jablonicka A, Garova J, Hano L. Chromosome and sister-chromatid exchange analysis in peripheral lymphocytes, and mutagenicity of urine in anesthesiology personnel. *Int Arch Occup Environ Health* 1992;64:303–306.
18. McCoy EC, Hankel R, Rosenkranz HS, Gluffrida JG, Bizzari DV. Detection of mutagenic activity in the urine of anesthesiologists: a preliminary report. *Environ Health Perspect* 1977;21:221–223.
19. Cohen EN, Brown BW Jr, Bruce DL, et al. American Society of Anesthesiologists Ad Hoc Committee on the Effects of Trace Anesthetics on the Health of Operating Room Personnel. Occupational diseases among operating room personnel: a national study. *Anesthesiology* 1974;41:321–340.
20. IARC monographs on the evaluation of carcinogenic risk to humans. Overall evaluations of carcinogenicity: an updating of IARC monographs volumes 1 to 42, suppl 7. Lyon: IARA, 1987:93–95.
21. Perić M, Vraneš Z, Marušić M. Immunological disturbances in anesthetic personnel chronically exposed to high occupational concentrations of nitrous oxide and halothane. *Anaesthesia* 1991;46:531–537.
22. Anderson NB. The effects of CNS depressants on mitosis. *Acta Anaesthesiol Scand* 1966;10:2–36.
23. Jackson SH. Anesthetics and cell multiplication. *Clin Anesth* 1975;11:75–92.
24. Skacel PO, Hewlett AM, Lewis JD, et al. Studies on the hematopoietic toxicity of nitrous oxide in man. *Br J Haematol* 1983;53:189–200.
25. Lassen HCA, Henriksen E, Neukirch F, Kristensen HS. Treatment of tetanus: severe bone marrow depression following prolonged nitrous oxide inhalation. Lancet 1956;1:527–530.
26. Quimby KL, Aschkenase LJ, Bowman RE, Katz J, Chang LW. Enduring learning deficits and cerebral synaptic malformation from exposure to 10 parts of halothane per million. *Science* 1975;185:625–627.
27. Uhlirova A, Pokorny J. Results of questionnaire survey of the health hazards of anesthesiologists [Czech]. *Rozhl Chir* 1974;53:761–770.
28. Bentin S, Collins GI, Adam N. Effect of low concentrations of enflurane on probability learning. *Br J Anaesth* 1978;50:1179–1183.
29. Bruce DL, Bach MJ. Psychological studies of human performance as affected by traces of enflurane and nitrous oxide. *Anesthesiology* 1975;42:194–196.
30. Cook TL, Smith M, Winter PM, Starkweather JA, Eger EI. Effect of subanesthetic concentrations of enflurane and halothane on human behavior. *Anesth Analg* 1978;57:434–440.
31. Smith G, Shirley A. A review of trace concentrations of anaesthetics on performance. *Br J Anaesth* 1978;50:701–711.
32. Bruce DL, Bach MJ. Effects of trace anaesthetic gases on behavioral performance of volunteers. *Br J Anaesth* 1976;48:871–876.
33. Klatskin G, Kimberg DV. Recurrent hepatitis attributable to halothane sensitization in an anaesthetist. *N Engl J Med* 1969;280:515–522.
34. Stock JG, Strunin L. Unexplained hepatitis following halothane. *Anesthesiology* 1985;63:424–439.

35. Lings S. Halothane related liver affection in an anaesthetist. *Br J Ind Med* 1988;45:716–717.
36. Cohen EN, Bellville JW, Brown BW Jr. Anesthesia, pregnancy, and miscarriage: a study of operating room nurses and anesthetists. *Anesthesiology* 1971;35:343–347.
37. Knill-Jones RP, Rodrigues LV, Moir DD, Spence AA. Anesthetic practice and pregnancy: controlled survey of women anesthetists in the United Kingdom. *Lancet* 1972;1:1326–1328.
38. Rosenberg P, Kirves A. Miscarriages among operating theatre staff. *Acta Anaesthesiol Scand [Suppl]* 1973;53:37–42.
39. Corbett TH, Cornell RG, Enders JL. Birth defects among children of nurse-anesthetists. *Anesthesiology* 1974;41:341–344.
40. Pharoah PO, Alberman E, Doyle P, Chamberlain G. Outcome of pregnancy among women in anaesthetic practice. *Lancet* 1977;1:34–36.
41. Perry GF. Occupational medicine forum. *J Occup Med* 1994;36:498–500.
42. Halsy MJ. Occupational health and pollution from anaesthetics: a report of a seminar. *Anaesthesia* 1991;46:486–488.
43. Allander C, Carlsson P, Hallen B, Ljungqvist B, Norlander O. Thermocamera, a macroscopic method for the study of pollution with nitrous oxide in operating theatres. *Acta Anaesthesiol Scand* 1981;25:21–24.
44. Schapera A. An anesthesia mask gas-scavenging system. *J Occup Environ Med* 1993;35:1138–1141.
45. Brown DG, Wetterstrom N, Finch J. Anesthetic gas exposure. *AORN J* 1985;41:590–608.
46. Schuyt HC, Verberk MM. Measurement and reduction of nitrous oxide in operating rooms. *J Occup Environ Med* 1996;38:1036–1040.
47. Wood C, Ewen A, Goresky G. Exposure of operating room personnel to nitrous oxide during paediatric anaesthesia. *Can J Anaesth* 1992;39:682–686.
48. Lambert-Jensen P, Christensen NE, Brynnum J. Laryngeal mask and anaesthetic waste gas exposure. *Anaesthesia* 1992;47:697–700.
49. Reiz S, Gustavsson AS, Haggmark S, et al. The double mask: a new local scavenging system for anaesthetic gases and volatile agents. *Acta Anaesthesiol Scand* 1986;30:260–265.
50. Rajhans G, Brown DA, Whaley D, Wong L, Guirguis SS. Hygienic aspects of occupational exposure to waste anaesthetic gases in Ontario Hospitals. *Ann Occup Hyg* 1989;33:27–45.
51. Sass-Korstak AM, Purdham JT, Bozek PR, Murphy JP. Exposure of hospital operating room personnel to potentially harmful environmental agents. *Am Ind Hyg Assoc J* 1992;53:203–209.
52. Tran N, Elias J, Rosenberg T, Wylie D, Gaborieau D, Yassi A. Evaluation of waste anesthetic gases, monitoring strategies, and correlations between nitrous oxide levels and health symptoms. *Am Ind Hyg Assoc J* 1994;55:36–41.
53. NIOSH. Criteria for a recommended standard-occupational exposure to waste anesthetic gases and vapors. DHWE(NIOSH) publication no. 77-140. Cincinnati, OH: National Institute for Occupational Safety and Health, 1977.
54. US Department of Health and Human Services. National Institute for Occupational Safety and Health alert: request for assistance in controlling exposures to nitrous oxide during anesthetic administration; DHHS (NIOSH) publication no. 94–100. Washington, DC: US Government Printing Office, 1994.
55. Berry AJ, Greene ES. The risk of needlestick injuries and needlestick-transmitted diseases in the practice of anesthesiology. *Anesthesiology* 1992;77:1007–1021.
56. Udasin IG, Gochfeld M. Implications of the Occupational Safety and Health Administration's bloodborne pathogen standard for the occupational health profession. *J Occup Med* 1994;36:548–555.
57. Tokars JI, Bell DM, Culver DH, et al. Percutaneous injuries during surgical procedures. *JAMA* 1992;267:2899–2904.
58. Quebbeman EJ, Telford GL, Hubbard S, et al. Risk of blood contamination and injury to operating room personnel. *Ann Surg* 1991;214:614–620.
59. Quebbeman EJ, Telford GL, Wadsworth K, et al. In-use evaluation of surgical gowns. *Surg Gynecol Obstet* 1992;174:369–375.
60. Smith RC, Mooar PA, Cooke T, Sherk HH. Contamination of operating room personnel during total arthroplasty. *Clin Orthop* 1991;271:9–11.
61. Kristensen MS, Sloth E, Jensen TK. Relationship between anesthetic procedure and contact of anesthesia personnel with patient body fluids. *Anesthesiology* 1990;73:619–624.
62. Occupational Safety and Health Administration. Bloodborne pathogens. 29CFR 1910.1030.
63. Kuh C, Ward WE. Occupational viral hepatitis: an apparent hazard for medical personnel. *JAMA* 1950;143:631–635.
64. Trumbell ML, Greiner DJ. Homologous serum jaundice: an occupational hazard to medical personnel. *JAMA* 1951;145:965–967.
65. Werner BG, Grady GF. Accidental hepatitis B surface antigen positive inoculations: use of e antigen to estimate infectivity. *Ann Intern Med* 1982;97:367–369.
66. Seef LB, Koff RS. Evolving concepts of the clinical and serologic consequences of hepatitis B virus infection. *Semin Liver Dis* 1986;6:11–22.
67. Short LJ, Bell DM. Risk of occupational infection with bloodborne pathogens in operating and delivery room settings. *Am J Infect Control* 1993;21:343–350.
68. Panlilio AL, Shapiro CN, Schable CA, et al. Serosurvey of human immunodeficiency virus, hepatitis B virus, and hepatitis C virus infection among hospital-based surgeons. *J Am Coll Surg* 1995;180:16–24.
69. Williams WW, Hickson MA, Kane MA, et al. Immunization policies and vaccine coverage among adults: the risk for missed opportunities. *Ann Intern Med* 1988;108:616–618.
70. Alter MJ, Margolis HS, Krawczynski K, et al. The natural history of community-acquired hepatitis C in the United States. *N Engl J Med* 1992;327:1899–1905.
71. Kiyosawa E, Sodeyama T, Tanaka E, et al. Hepatitis C in hospital employees with needlestick injuries. *Ann Intern Med* 1991;115:367–369.
72. Mitsui T, Iwano K, Masuko K, et al. Hepatitis C virus infection in medical personnel after needlestick accident. *Hepatology* 1992;16:1109–1114.
73. Rubin RH, Tolkoff-Rubin NE. Post-transfusion viral infections. *Transplant Proc* 1988;20:1112–1117.
74. Henderson DK, Fahey BJ, Willy M, et al. Risk for occupational transmission of human immunodeficiency

virus type I (HIV-I) associated with clinical exposures. *Ann Intern Med* 1990;113:740–746.

75. Tokars JI, Marcus R, Culver C, et al. Surveillance of HIV infection and zidovudine use among health care workers after occupational exposure to HIV-infected blood. *Ann Intern Med* 1993;118:913–919.
76. Ippolito G, Puro V, De Carli G. The risk of occupational human immunodeficiency virus infection in health care workers: Italian multicenter study. *Arch Intern Med* 1993;153:1451–1458.
77. Geberding JL. Management of occupational exposures to bloodborne viruses. *N Engl J Med* 1996;332: 444–451.
78. Mast ST, Woolwine JD, Geberding JL. Efficacy of gloves in reducing blood volumes transferred during simulated needlestick injury. *J Infect Dis* 1993;168: 1589–1592.
79. Shirazian D, Herzlich BC, Mokhtarian F, et al. Needlestick injury: blood, mononuclear cells, and acquired immunodeficiency syndrome. *Am J Infect Control* 1992;20:133–137.
80. Raahave D, Bremmelgaard A. New operative technique to reduce surgeon's risk of HIV infection. *J Hosp Infect* 1991;18[Suppl A]:177–183.
81. Geberding JL. Prophylaxis for occupational exposure to HIV. *Ann Intern Med* 1996;125:497–501.
82. Geberding JL, Littell C, Tarkington A, Brown A, Schecter WP: Risk of exposure of surgical personnel to patient's blood during surgery at San Francisco General Hospital. *N Engl J Med* 1990;322:1788–1793.
83. Davis JM, Demling RH, Lewis FR, Hoover E, Waymack P. The Surgical Infection Society's policy on human immunodeficiency virus and hepatitis B and C infection: the ad hoc committee on acquired immunodeficiency syndrome and hepatitis. *Arch Surg* 1992;127:218–221.
84. Jarvis WR, Bolyard EA, Bozzi CJ, et al. Respirators, recommendations, and regulations: the controversy surrounding protection of health care workers from tuberculosis. *Ann Intern Med* 1995;122:142–146.
85. Andre P, Orth G, Evenou P, et al. Risk of papillomavirus infection in carbon dioxide laser treatment of genital lesions. *J Am Acad Dermatol* 1990;22:131–132.
86. Garden JM, O'Banion MK, Shelnitz LS, et al. Papillomavirus in the vapor of carbon dioxide laser-treated verrucae. *JAMA* 1988;259:1199–1202.
87. Hallmo P, Naess O. Laryngeal papillomatosis with human papillomavirus DNA contracted by a laser surgeon. *Eur Arch Otorhinolaryngol* 1991;248:425–427.
88. Gloster HM, Roenigk RK. Risk of acquiring human papillomavirus from the plume produced by the carbon dioxide laser in the treatment of warts. *J Am Acad Dermatol* 1995;32:436–441.
89. Ferenczy A, Bergeron C, Richart RM. Human papillomavirus DNA in CO_2 laser-generated plume of smoke and its consequences to the surgeon. *Obstet Gynecol* 1990;75:114–118.
90. Tuxen DV, Cade JF, McDonald MI, Buchman MRC, Pain MCF. Herpes simplex virus from the lower respiratory tract in adult respiratory distress syndrome. *Am Rev Resp Dis* 1982;125:98.
91. Arnstein PM, Richards AM, Putney R. The risk from radiation exposure during operative x-ray screening in hand surgery. *J Hand Surg* 1994;19B:393–396.
92. Nonstochastic effects of ionizing radiation. International Commission on Radiological Protection (ICRP) publication no. 41. *Annals of the ICRP.* Vol. 14, no. 3. Oxford, UK: Pergamon Press, 1984.
93. Mills MD, Almond PR, Boyer AL, Ochran TG, Madigan W, Rich TA, Dally EB. Shielding considerations for an operating room based intraoperative electron therapy unit. *Int J Radiat Oncol Biol Phys* 1990;18: 1215–1221.
94. Lipman RM, Tripathi B, Tripathi R. Cataracts induced by microwave and ionizing radiation. *Surv Opthalmol* 1988;33:200–210.
95. Paz JD, Milliken R, Ingram WT, Frank A, Atkin A. Potential ocular damage from microwave exposure during electrosurgery: dosimetric survey. *J Occup Med* 1987;29:580–583.
96. Fox JWC, Knadle RT, Brook RH. Radiofrequency in the operating theatre [Letter]. *Lancet* 1976;1:962.
97. Norris JL. Fire safety in the operating room. *J Am Assoc Nurse Anesthetists* 1994;62:342–345.
98. Bond PM, ed. *Health Devices* 1992;21:1.
99. Petty WC. AANA journal course: update for nurse anesthetists—medical gases, hospital pipelines, and medical gas cylinders; how safe are they? *J Am Assoc Nurse Anesthetists* 1995;63:307–324.
100. Center for Drug Evaluation and Research Division of Manufacturing and Product Quality. Compressed Medical Gases Guideline; HFD-320. Rockville, MD: Office of Compliance, Food and Drug Administration, 1989.
101. Hall RR, Hill DW, Beech AD. A carbon dioxide surgical laser. *Ann R Coll Surg Engl* 1971;48:181–218.
102. Toon S. Doctors using lasers risk problems without proper training, protection. *Occup Health Saf* 1988;57: 30–31.
103. Brodman M, Port M, Friedman F, Sperling R, Dottino P, Thomas AG. Operating room personnel morbidity from carbon dioxide laser use during preceptored surgery. *Obstet Gynecol* 1993;81:607–609.
104. Ward WD. General auditory effects of noise. *Otolaryngol Clin North Am* 1979;12:473–491.
105. Falk SA, Woods NF. Hospital noise-levels and potential health hazards. *N Engl J Med* 1973;289:774–781.
106. Gloag D. Noise: hearing loss and psychological effects. *Br Med J* 1980;281:1325–1327.
107. Kam PCA, Kam AC, Thompson JF. Noise pollution in the anesthetic and intensive care environment. *Anaesthesia* 194;49:982–986.
108. Occupational Safety and Health Administration. Occupational noise exposure. 29CFR 1910.95
109. Willett KM. Noise-induced hearing loss in orthopaedic staff. *J Bone Joint Surg* 1991;73B:113–115.
110. Ray CD, Levinson R. Noise pollution in the operating room: a hazard to surgeons, personnel, and patients. *J Spinal Disord* 1992;5:485–488.
111. Green A, Duthie HL, Young HL, Peters TJ. Stress in surgeons. *Br J Surg* 1990;77:1154–1158.
112. Neil HAW, Fairer JG, Coleman MP, Thurston A, Vessey MP. Mortality among male anaesthetists in the United Kingdom 1957–83. *Br Med J* 1987;295:360–362.
113. Telford GL, Quebbeman EJ. Assessing the risk of blood exposure in the operating room. *Am J Infect Control* 1993;21:351–356.
114. Berridge DC, Lees TA, Chamberlain J, Jones NAG. Eye protection for the vascular surgeon. *Br J Surg* 1993;80:1379–1380.

115. Laser Institute of America. *American national standards for the safe use of lasers in health care facilities* (ANSI Z 136.3-1988). Toledo, OH: Laser Institute of America, 1988.

SUGGESTED READING

Berry AJ, Katz JD. Hazards of working in the operating room. In: Barash PG, Cullen BF, Stoelting RK, eds. *Clinical anesthesia*, 3rd ed. Philadelphia: Lippincott–Raven, 1997:69–91.

An excellent in-depth review of operating room hazards. The focus is on the anesthetist with special emphasis on human factors, psychologic stress, and drug addiction.

Berry AJ, Greene ES. The risk of needlestick injuries and needlestick-transmitted diseases in the practice of anesthesiology. *Anesthesiology* 1992;77:1007–1021.

An in-depth overview of blood-borne pathogens, needlestick injuries in the operating room, preventive recommendations, and regulatory standards.

Bihari V, Srivastava AK, Gupta BN. Occupational health hazards among operation room personnel exposed to anesthetic gases: a review. *J Environ Pathol Toxicol Oncol* 1994;13:213–219.

A review of the toxicology of inhalation anesthetics.

Redfern N. Morbidity among anaesthetists. *Br J Hosp Med* 1990;43:377–381.

A general overview of the occupational hazards of anaesthetists.

Telford GL, Quebbeman EJ. Assessing the risk of blood exposure in the operating room. *Am J Infect Control* 1993;21:351–356.

A review article describing the risks of blood contamination in the operating room and important preventive strategies to limit such exposure.

Medical Center Occupational Health and Safety,
edited by Robert J. McCunney.
Lippincott Williams & Wilkins, Philadelphia © 1999

21

Bronchoscopy: Health and Safety Issues in the Medical Center Environment

Daniel E. Banks, Samuel Skarote, and *Philip Harber

*Department of Medicine, Section of Pulmonary and Critical Care Medicine, West Virginia University School of Medicine, Morgantown, West Virginia 26506; *Department of Medicine, Division of Occupational and Environmental Medicine, University of California at Los Angeles, Los Angeles, California 90024-7027*

Bronchoscopy with a flexible fiberoptic bronchoscope allows direct visualization of the tracheobronchial tree to the level of subsegmental bronchi. Fiberoptic technology has been a great advance over the previously used rigid bronchoscopes. It is much easier for patients to tolerate the procedure, and in many instances, the optics are better and one can visualize more of the tracheobronchial tree. Table 21-1 lists common indications for fiberoptic bronchoscopy. Performed by an expert bronchoscopist, this procedure has proved to be an essential diagnostic and therapeutic intervention in the appropriate clinical setting. Inherent in the procedure, however, are risks to the patient (the complications of the procedure, most commonly bleeding and pneumothorax) and inhalational risks to the bronchoscopist and bronchoscopy suite personnel (exposure risks associated with the procedure and cleaning of the instruments). The latter are the focus of this chapter.

TABLE 21-1. *Common indications for fiberoptic bronchoscopy*

Evaluation of chronic cough
Evaluation of hemoptysis
Assistance in intubation
Evaluation of an abnormal chest radiograph, especially to assess for lung cancer or infection
Collection of specimens for laboratory investigation in the setting of respiratory infections, especially for an immunocompromised host
Evaluation and biopsy of interstitial lung disease
Evaluation of the anatomy of the upper and lower respiratory tract
Therapeutic intervention: foreign body removal, mucous plug clearance, laser intervention for malignant airway obstruction
Research

EXPOSURE RISKS

Risk to bronchoscopists and associated personnel include respiratory infection due to inhalation of infectious aerosols and sensitization or irritant responses due to exposure to chemical or organic allergens (1). Adverse effects attributable to laser injury may be encountered if this specialized procedure is performed. Ergonomic hazards may be present but have been poorly studied. The physical posture of the bronchoscopist and the need to maintain a static position may constitute ergonomic hazards.

Infectious Exposure Risks

Inherent to a surgical procedure is risk for spread of infectious agents to medical personnel. In the bronchoscopy suite, exposure can occur through venipuncture for blood draws, initiation of venous access, or administering medication; splashing of body fluids; handling of a contaminated endoscope; handling and processing of specimens; cleaning of the endoscope; inhalation of infectious agents; and contact with contaminated surfaces. Although information is available to describe cross contamination of endoscopes and patient-to-patient transmission of infectious agents, relatively small amounts of data exist regarding risk to the operator for the transmission of infectious agents. Although the bronchoscopist may not be in direct contact with a patient undergoing bronchoscopy, coughing with aerosolizing secretions potentiates disease transmission. Placement of the suction channel near the eyepiece of nonvideo bronchoscopes makes possible splattering of human material onto an unprotected bronchoscopist's face.

Tuberculosis is principally a pulmonary infection caused by the bacterium *Mycobacterium tuberculosis*. After introduction of antituberculous therapy in the mid-twentieth century, the number of tuberculosis cases declined until 1985, when principally because of the human immunodeficiency virus HIV epidemic, the number of cases of tuberculosis again began to increase in the United States. *M. tuberculosis* is an aerobic, nonmotile, non–spore-forming, slow-growing bacillus 2 to 4 μm long by 0.2 to 5 μm wide. Humans serve as its only reservoir. This organism is most often spread through the air, a mechanism enhanced by closely crowded living conditions. Almost all primary infection is caused by transmission and inhalation of infectious bacteria aerosolized from the respiratory tract of the infected person by means of coughing, sneezing, or talking. In an enclosed space such as a room or airline compartment (2), air surrounding a person with active pulmonary tuberculosis is infectious, and the risk for infection increases with repeated or prolonged exposure and an increased number of organisms in the aerosol. The risk for infection is enhanced among persons with compromised immune function. Persons with HIV infection may suffer very rapid progression from inoculum to active pulmonary and multisystem disease.

Mycobacterial infection, especially tuberculosis, is clearly a risk to health care workers. Outbreaks of tuberculosis in health care institutions have been reported and have been attributed to the increased incidence of HIV disease; inadequate negative-pressure ventilation in the hospital rooms of patients with active disease; increased use of procedures that cause aerosolization of sputum; failure to diagnose or delay in the diagnosis of active tuberculosis in a patient admitted with pulmonary symptoms; rapid progression to active tuberculosis after exposure, especially among patients with HIV; and persistent or prolonged infectivity in the setting of multidrug-resistant tuberculosis despite therapy (usually 2 weeks of therapy for tuberculosis not resistant to multiple drugs is accepted as the period of treatment after which a patient is not considered infective).

To control the spread of organisms in the health care environment, a high index of suspicion for active tuberculosis among patients admitted with symptoms of pulmonary infection is needed, especially when these patients are in high-risk groups. This level of clinical suspicion necessitates respiratory isolation in negative-pressure rooms. Such rooms are required in the care of patients who might have active tuberculosis if procedures that aerosolize airway secretions are anticipated. These include aerosol bronchodilator therapy, sputum induction maneuvers, chest physiotherapy, and bronchoscopy.

The transmission of mycobacterial organisms and infection by flexible bronchoscopes is well documented. A number of investigators (3,4) showed transmission of *M. tuberculosis* through a bronchoscope that had apparently not been sufficiently cleaned after bronchoscopy of a patient with active tuberculosis. In two instances, transmission was attributed to cleaning a bronchoscope with a solution that had insufficient antitubercular properties (a povidone-iodine solution inadequate to disinfect the bronchoscope of mycobacterial organisms). In the third instance, transmission was attributed to poor cleaning of the removable valves of the bronchoscope, even though a 2% glutaraldehyde solution was used and manufacturer guidelines followed. Steam cleaning of these valves has been encouraged. Like *M. tuberculosis,* atypical mycobacterial organisms have been recognized to contaminate flexible bronchoscopes (5–7).

Centers for Disease Control and Prevention (CDC) recommendations for respiratory protection in attempts to diagnose active mycobacterial infection in a patient believed to have this illness require that health workers wear particulate respirator masks and ultraviolet air filtration until the diagnosis of tuberculosis is ruled out with three normal results sputum smears. Obtaining negative results of acid-fast bacillus (AFB) staining of sputum smears collected by means of spontaneous coughing before bronchoscopy minimizes the likelihood of performing an aerosolizing procedure on an infected patient.

Bacterial and fungal species such as *Salmonella, Pseudomonas, Serratia,* and *Staphylococcus* have been implicated in patient-to-patient pseudoepidemics through contaminated endoscopes but have not been reported to play a role in infective transmission from patient to bronchoscopist (8,9).

Viruses such as HIV, cytomegalovirus, herpesvirus, and hepatitis B virus have not been recognized to have been transmitted from patient to bronchoscope in association with bronchoscopy but can pose such a risk. HIV can be isolated from most body fluids, including alveolar fluids, but is readily inactivated with endoscope-cleaning agents. The annual incidence of hepatitis B among health care workers is estimated at 12,000. Hepatitis may have been transmitted from patient to patient through a contaminated endoscope but not from patient to endoscopist.

Chemical Exposure Risks

Flexible fiberoptic bronchoscopes may be damaged by heat or gas sterilization with ethylene oxide at temperatures exceeding 55°C. Therefore effective cold sterilization is most important. However, inhalational exposures to cleaning agents have the potential to induce lung injury when the agent is used in excess or without sufficient ventilation in the bronchoscopy suite.

Alkaline glutaraldehyde is a low-molecular-weight substance used as an antimicrobial agent in the cold sterilization of bronchoscopes. Like formaldehyde, it has a low odor threshold and can serve as a potent irritant and sensitizer. After exposure, irritation of the eyes, nose, throat, and skin, wheezing, and chest tightness can occur with the potential for sensitization and the development of occupational asthma among previously nonsensitized health care workers (10). Appropriate ventilation of the disinfecting station and a special cabinet for storage of the chemical are recommended. Advised additional measures include use of gloves, gowns, and eye protection for those using the solutions.

Axon et al. (11) were the first to write about the skin and respiratory difficulties associated with use of glutaraldehyde. They described the cases of 36 workers (37% of all employed) in 16 endoscopy units. In a second report, 8 of 9 employees employed in the endoscopy unit had skin irritation, eye watering, and nasal congestion in work areas where a 2% glutaraldehyde solution was in use (12). Corrado et al. (13) examined four nurses working in endoscopy units who had respiratory symptoms on exposure to alkaline glutaraldehyde used as a disinfectant for fiberoptic endoscopes. Although an irritant effect could not be completely discounted, provocation test results were positive for two nurses. This finding implied a relation between exposure to glutaraldehyde and respiratory disease. All four nurses were atopic by history and three of the four had positive skin prick test reactions to common allergens.

Chan-Yeung et al. (14) documented asthma in an atopic respiratory technologist who had worsening of childhood asthma after employment in a bronchoscopy unit. In addition to helping with the procedures, it was her job to clean bronchoscopes with Sporicidin (Sporocidin International Ltd., Rockville, MD), a commercial cleaning agent containing 3.6%

glutaraldehyde, 7% phenol, and 1.2% sodium phenolate. Workplace challenge testing showed a clinically significant decrement in forced expiratory volume in 1 second (FEV_1) after exposure to the commercial agent. The authors found that the specific component causing asthma was likely glutaraldehyde, although tests with individual components of the commercial product were not undertaken. Because levels of glutaraldehyde were not measured, it was not possible to determine whether the worker had been sensitized *de novo* to Sporocidin or the asthma was associated with irritant exposure of a person with underlying asthma. A worker employed in a similar role contracted asthma in association with recurrent exposures to a 2% solution of glutaraldehyde (15).

Provocation challenge testing with glutaraldehyde, a very potent irritant, can lead to difficulties in proving sensitivity. Stenton et al. (16) addressed this complex question in the evaluation of a 46-year-old endoscopy nurse who contracted what was thought to be glutaraldehyde-induced asthma. An initial inhalation challenge test in the endoscopy suite caused a dramatic, immediate decrease in FEV_1. More detailed evaluation with double-blind exposures to a placebo and nonirritant doses of glutaraldehyde vapor in the laboratory suggested marked dual asthmatic reactions after challenges with 0.032 ppm glutaraldehyde but with similar declines on placebo days and increased airway responsiveness to methacholine. These data were potentially confounded by an intercurrent respiratory tract infection and by technically poor FEV_1 recordings, so the challenge was repeated several weeks later. A second series of double-blind inhalation challenges with carefully controlled exposures to glutaraldehyde showed no obvious asthmatic reactions and only a slight increase in airway responsiveness. The authors concluded that the results illustrate the potential for misdiagnosis of occupational asthma when unblinded challenge tests are used and show that sophisticated investigatory techniques may not define the diagnosis. A sophisticated chamber has been developed for challenge testing with aldehydes (17).

To show that glutaraldehyde has acted as a sensitizer and induced asthma it may not be enough to provoke asthma with exposure to aldehyde fumes. To prove sensitivity one must be certain that the exposures are nonirritating and that atmospheres provided in challenge tests are less than the permissible exposure limit. Gannon et al. (18) provided important convincing evidence for glutaraldehyde as a sensitizer. They showed that 7 of 8 hospital workers with respiratory problems exposed to glutaraldehyde contracted asthma after challenge tests in which the mean level of glutaraldehyde in air was 0.068 mg/m^3, about one-tenth the short-term occupational exposure standard of 0.7 mg/m^3.

Curran et al. (19) compared the immunologic responses of subjects with occupational asthma or work-related respiratory symptoms and exposed to glutaraldehyde with the responses of unexposed workers. They found evidence of immunologic sensitization among some workers exposed to glutaraldehyde. A series of glutaraldehyde-modified proteins were characterized, and a significant difference was recognized between level of glutaraldehyde-specific immunoglobulin E (IgE) antibodies in exposed subjects and the level in unexposed subjects who had normal levels of serum IgE. Approximately one third of exposed workers with occupational asthma had antibody levels exceeding those in the unexposed population. False-positive results were obtained with serum from unexposed workers who had high total IgE levels. It appears that the behavior of glutaraldehyde is like that of a number of other low-molecular-weight chemicals in that specific antibodies are detected in only a small percentage of exposed workers with work-related respiratory symptoms. Therefore antibody detection cannot be used in a reliable diagnostic test.

Like formaldehyde (20,21), glutaraldehyde can sensitize workers. Those at greatest risk appear to be those employed in health care. Workers in the bronchoscopy suite are particularly at risk. In the workplace, the use of steam sterilization whenever possible and minimizing glutaraldehyde exposure by providing appropriate ventilation in areas where this agent must be used as a disinfectant appear to be the best ways to prevent sensitization. There appears to be poor correlation between the presence of specific antibodies and respiratory symptoms, making the importance of the presence of these antibodies and their role in the mechanism of asthma unclear.

Workers in the bronchoscopy suite, like other health care workers, are at risk for natural rubber latex allergy. With recognition of the need to contain the spread of infectious agents in the health care environment over the past 10 years, natural rubber latex has become increasingly recognized as a high-molecular-weight sensitizing agent (22). Repeated exposure to natural rubber latex gloves or inhalation of natural latex particles in the workplace can lead to sensitization. Additional exposure causes anaphylaxis, urticaria, asthma, or rhinoconjunctivitis. Frequent exposure appears to be an important risk factor for sensitization.

In one report, the prevalence of latex allergy among health care workers approximated 10% (23). Overall, one population of atopic health care workers had a 24% prevalence of positive skin test reactions to natural latex rubber allergens; approximately half the workers had no symptoms (24). The risk for progression to latex allergy among workers with positive skin test results and no symptoms is not known.

Reaction to natural rubber latex usually is type IV delayed hypersensitivity presenting contact dermatitis, usually on the dorsum of the hands. However, severe type I, IgE-mediated reactions have been reported. Avoidance is the cornerstone of therapy. The first step is a change to vinyl or latex-free gloves. In many hospital suites there remains potential for exposure to other latex devices (e.g., catheters, adhesives, tourniquets, and possibly anesthetic devices). Once sensitized, a worker must recognize that the potential for exposure to latex-containing products in any given area of the hospital is unpredictable. An unexpected exposure can provoke a serious allergic event. Even though direct exposure might be controlled, inhalational exposure may be sufficient to provoke an allergic reaction (25). For example, in our bronchoscopy suite, we primarily use Olympus instruments. Although some balloon catheters made by Olympus contain natural latex rubber, the bronchoscope and material used in association with bronchoscopy do not (Hiroshi Ichikawa, Olympus America, Inc., personal communication).

CONTROL OF RISKS ASSOCIATED WITH LASER BRONCHOSCOPY

Our bronchoscopy suite is designated as a laser controlled area within the hospital. There are no windows to modify. Extensive warning signs are permanently posted in the room and area. A team of nurses and personnel credentialed in laser procedures and precautions assist in the procedure. A system of checks and oral commands is in force when laser bronchoscopy is performed in the bronchoscopy suite.

In laser bronchoscopy the thermal effect of laser radiation is used to achieve controlled tissue destruction with minimal surrounding edema. The laser beam vaporizes obstructing masses of the central airway. The main risks to the medical staff from laser use are optical and respiratory problems.

Optical radiation damage to the eye can occur faster than the blink reflex can respond to either the intense light or the corneal thermal injury that might be induced by laser energy. The operator and the staff are at risk. Because the laser is a collimated beam of light and depending on the wavelength of the laser light, energy may be transmitted onto the cornea or lens. It also may be transmitted through the cornea to focus intensely on the retina in a spot 10 to 20 μm in diameter with resultant damage. This small spot can be surrounded by areas of thermal damage. Retinal foci such as the fovea may be quite sensitive to even small areas of damage before vision is affected. Retinal light damage (loss of color vision) from retinal exposure to intense halogen-xenon light has been recognized. Neodymium:yttrium-aluminum-garnet (Nd:YAG) lasers (wavelength 1.064

nm) tend to be most hazardous to the retina, xenon chloride excimer lasers (wavelength 308 nm) to the lens, and carbon dioxide lasers (wavelength 10.6 μm) to the cornea.

Because the different lasers project and reflect laser light at different wavelengths, different eye protection may be indicated on the basis of the laser in use (26,27). Accidental ocular exposure can be caused by reflected laser light beams and the direct beam. Although in general laser light is attenuated through the optics of an operating endoscope, it is recommended that the bronchoscopist and medical staff in the vicinity of a laser procedure use appropriate eye protection for the wavelength of the laser being used. Eye protection is mandatory in the suite during the procedure. For Nd:YAG lasers, eye protection consists of attenuation level in the 1060-nm wavelength. A shield with the same attenuation is fitted to the eyepiece of the scope to minimize backscatter risk to the endoscopist's eye. Protective eyewear can be spectacles, wraparound lenses, or goggles.

Pyrolysis of tissues releases toxic products, including nitrosamines and carcinogens, and intact viral particles into the laser plume. In vitro work has shown that using laser energy on tissue may generate the intact viral DNA of papillomavirus (but no viable cells) and proviral HIV DNA. This raises concern about exposure of the bronchoscopy suite staff to products of disease (28,29). Thus the laser plume is more than just malodorous smoke that affects the field of view. Both vaporized viral particles and particles generated from carbon dioxide lasers are reported to approximate 0.3 μm in diameter. Short-term exposure (a total of 32 minutes over 4 days) to such particles in a rat model produced bronchiolitis, emphysema, and interstitial pneumonia (30). Long-term effects have not been characterized. High-volume suction is available to minimize collection of laser smoke or plume (31). Because the average standard surgical mask can filter at 99% efficiency for 5.0-μm particles but at only 25% efficiency for 0.3-μm particles, even double masking is unlikely to appreciably block inhalation of such small particles. More aggressive airway protection is necessary (32).

General guidelines for risk control center on the after concepts, which are as follows: (a) orientation and continuing medical education for medical personnel regarding risks and safety issues in the bronchoscopy suite; (b) provision of appropriate equipment and supplies to implement protective measures; and (c) monitoring and enforcement of compliance with safety guidelines. The principal aspects of prevention are shown in Table 21-2.

Bronchoscope Disinfection

Cleaning of a scope is defined as removing organic material or soil from a device. Cleaning is begun with water and detergent. Disinfection of a scope is defined as killing most microorganisms on or in a device using a liq-

TABLE 21-2. *Major preventive measures for bronchoscopy*

Training
Bronchoscopists
Support staff
Engineering controls
Bronchoscopy suite design
Ventilation
Air disinfection
Control of chemical exposures during equipment disinfection
Laser system enclosure
Personal protection
Respirators
Gloves, gowns, and goggles to limit expsoure to blood and respiratory secretions and to scope-cleaning materials
Goggles during laser procedures
Work practices
Bronchoscope cleaning
Identification of patients at high risk
Selection of patients and timing of procedures
Care of patients after bronchoscopy (while cough is increased)
Screening of employees
Tuberculosis
Administrative controls
Limiting number of persons present
Limiting exposure of employees at high risk for infection
Exposure control during patient transport

uid germicide. High-level disinfection, as defined by the CDC, involves using a liquid germicide to kill all vegetative microorganisms, tubercle bacilli, and small nonlipid viruses but not necessarily bacterial spores. This is the minimal accepted standard for endoscope sterilization. Steam autoclaving is not possible for a flexible fiberoptic scope, but ethylene oxide can be used with aeration of the scope after sterilization. Instruments such as biopsy forceps should be autoclaved after each use (33).

Stonehill et al. (34) in 1963 described the infecting and sterilizing properties of an aqueous solution of 2% alkaline glutaraldehyde (34). Since then this agent has been confirmed by many investigators to be an effective sterilizing agent (35).

We are unaware of transmission of HIV with a bronchoscope. Sattar and Springthorpe (36) reviewed the relation between HIV survival and disinfectants. Although solutions of the glutaraldehyde-phenate product Sporicidin were not as bactericidal as 70% alcohol, the authors recognized data showing that endoscope disinfection with 2% glutaraldehyde is much more efficient at viral inactivation than disinfection with either 1% glutaraldehyde or 70% alcohol (37). Weller et al. (38) came to a similar conclusion. Infectivity testing showed that exposed to liquid glutaraldehyde, HIV is quickly deactivated; hepatitis B virus is deactivated after 10 minutes.

Bacterial decontamination of flexible fiberoptic endoscopes is accomplished with detergent cleaning followed by a 5, 10, or 20 minute glutaraldehyde soak; there was no statistically significant difference between results with the different soaking periods. However, forced-air drying of channels does significantly reduce bacterial contamination. *M. tuberculosis v. bovis* activity occurs within 10 minutes of submersion. Stabilized 2% glutaraldehyde solution remains effective as a germicidal agent for 14 days before it becomes necessary to change the solution. When a series of disinfectants were tested against *M. tuberculosis* in a bench laboratory, the most effective agents were 2% glutaraldehyde solution and a glutaraldehyde-phenol solution (39–41).

Guidelines for cleaning and disinfecting bronchoscopes were published in 1989 by The Working Party of the British Thoracic Society and are described in Table 21-3.

Spach et al. (42) commented on four potentially important flaws associated with the guidelines in Table 21-3. They include glutaraldehyde-induced side effects; flaws in automatic endoscope washers; inherent difficulties in cleaning and disinfecting endoscopes; and lack of compliance with current guidelines. There remains a concern about leaving glutaraldehyde in bronchoscope channels. In the gastrointestinal literature, postcolonoscopic chemical proctitis was attributed to spraying residual glutaraldehyde from the colonoscope into the rectum (43). Bloody cramps after sigmoidoscopy were attributed to exposure to glutaraldehyde from a sigmoidoscope (44). To our knowledge, al-

TABLE 21-3. *Guidelines for cleaning and disinfecting the bronchoscope*

1. Cleaning and disinfecting the bronchoscope should occur at the beginning of the first procedure each day and immediately after each procedure.
2. The valve should be dismantled, and all parts of the bronchoscope should be washed and brushed in detergent to prevent drying of secretions, development of a biofilm, or fixation of blood and secretions by glutaraldehyde.
3. The bronchoscope should be immersed in 2% glutaraldehyde solution for at least 20 minutes.
4. After the glutaraldehyde soak, the channel should be rinsed with sterile water or 70% alcohol, not tap water.
5. If the scope is to be used to examine an immunocompromised host, the scope should be prepared as above but with a 60-minute glutaraldehyde soak.
6. Nonimmersible scopes should be phased out; dedicated scopes for immunocompromised patients are not necessary with the above cleaning procedures.

(Published in 1989 by The Working Party of the British Thoracic Society).

though exposure to glutaraldehyde can occur in association with bronchoscope use, such inflammatory changes have not been described, perhaps because of the potentially smaller reservoir of a bronchoscope.

Automated disinfecting machines were initially received with considerable enthusiasm because they relieved endoscopic laboratory personnel from the time-consuming manual disinfection process and from irritating and potentially sensitizing glutaraldehyde exposure (45). In addition to being expensive, noisy, and heavy (46), these machines have fallen out of favor because contamination (especially with *Pseudomonas* species) of gastrointestinal endoscopes cleaned in these machines has been implicated in transmission of infectious disease (47). Despite cleaning with glutaraldehyde solution, only by means of manual rinsing of machine-cleaned endoscopes with 70% alcohol followed by forced-air drying has reliable disinfection been achieved (48). Overall, automatic cleansing machines have not satisfactorily replaced manual cleaning. They are not used in our laboratory.

Because of the small diameter of the channels in a bronchoscope, considerable time and attention must be spent on cleaning this instrument. Residual tissue and blood clots must be removed. Brushes obtained from bronchoscope manufacturers are optimal for cleaning. The bronchoscope, biopsy forceps, and reusable catheters must be cleaned with care.

Personal Protection

Bronchoscopists and support staff should protect themselves against inhalation of infectious agents by using appropriate respirators. The level of protection required determines the type of respirator to be used. A typical surgical mask provides a minimal level of protection; it is not effective for small particles, such as those of many bioaerosols. A single use respirator of the N-95 class provides a greater degree of protection and is the minimum recommended when substantial infectious risk is present. High-efficiency particulate air (HEPA) filter respirator masks are effective but expensive. In particularly high-risk situations, such as bronchoscopy of a patient with possible untreated cavitary tuberculosis or laryngeal tuberculosis, a powered air-purifying respirator (PAPR) may be needed. PAPRs have a fan to force air through the filtration medium rather than relying on negative pressure generated by the user. The fan decreases inward leakage at the seal between face and mask. Unfortunately, PAPRs are bulky and may interfere with the vision and agility necessary for bronchoscopy. Video-assisted bronchoscopy, in which the operator need not maintain close contact with the scope eyepiece may overcome this limitation.

Use of respirators requires a complete infection control program. Program elements are described in Chapter 5. Risk for infectious aerosol exposure does not end when the procedure ends. Airborne droplets may remain suspended for prolonged periods; as the aerosol ages, the water evaporates, particle size decreases, and the likelihood of inhalation increases. Suite personnel should not remove their masks as soon as the patient leaves the room. Use of respiratory protection should continue until air changes and air disinfection are likely to be effective.

Gloves, protective clothing, and goggles are needed to protect against blood-borne pathogens, such as HIV and hepatitis viruses. This is discussed in detail in Chapter 25. A single-use respirator that becomes soiled by blood or respiratory secretions should be discarded and replaced.

Engineering Controls: Design and Maintenance of Bronchoscopic Facilities

Proper design of the suite used for bronchoscopy can decrease risk for infectious and other exposures. Adequate ventilation of the room and maintenance of pressure gradients between the room and the exterior are key elements (see Chapter 24). In general, 6 to 12 air changes per hour are recommended to dilute any bioaerosols produced. The higher number of air changes per hour is needed when the infectious risk is greater. Airflow should be distributed to assure adequate dilution in the highest-risk areas (e.g., near the bronchoscopist's breathing zone). Most systems include recirculation of air; single-pass systems, in which there is no recirculation, are expensive because of the high volume of air that must be conditioned (heated or cooled) and moved. In selected circumstances, recirculated air can be treated with ultraviolet germicidal irradiation, or passed through HEPA filters, or both.

In addition to proper design and construction, ventilation systems require periodic maintenance. The adequacy of airflow and balance of pressures must be checked periodically. Physical separation of the scope-cleaning operations can decrease exposure to glutaraldehyde and other agents. Flow of patients should be planned. Patients often cough after the procedure, and therefore an area with adequate ventilation is needed for postprocedure recovery.

Bronchoscopy is occasionally performed as a bedside procedure rather than in a designated suite. In such settings, ventilation and other controls may be less than optimal. Personal respiratory protection (respirators) becomes particularly important. It should be used by the bronchoscopy team and by other staff working in the area.

The design and operation of the bronchoscopy suite at the West Virginia University Medical Center illustrate the application of the principles described herein. The bronchoscopy suite includes a preprocedure holding area where patients are admitted and receive both preprocedure and postprocedure care; a procedure room where bronchoscopy is performed; and a cleanup room where the bronchoscope is cleaned and prepared for the next procedure.

Universal precautions are in force hospital-wide for care of all patients. In the preprocedure area, intravenous access, phlebotomy, and initial administration of medication are undertaken by surgical nurses. Further sedation of the patient in the procedure room is administered by a physician only. In the bronchoscopy suite, development of and adherence to risk control guidelines is supervised by the physician-director and nurse-director of the pulmonary suite supplemented by hospital infection control personnel.

Bronchoscopes are cleaned and stored hanging in a room physically separate from the procedure room. This decontamination room, which has separate ventilation and washing facilities, contains glutaraldehyde-based cleaning solutions and appropriate garb to protect technicians. The procedure room contains (a) cabinets that store protective garb, including wraparound eye protection, HEPA and other respirators, and fluid-resistant gowns and shoe covers, (b) secured medication storage, (c) appropriate monitoring and resuscitation equipment, (d) a wash area for accidental exposures and postprocedure cleanup, (e) a radiographic viewing box, (f) bronchoscopic equipment and sterilized instruments to be used in the immediate procedure, (g) a fluoroscopy table, (h) containers for the disposal of sharp instruments and contaminated waste, (i) a fire extinguisher (laser bronchoscopy can start fires), and (j) an operating theater light. At the end of each procedure, collected specimens are sealed and delivered to the appropriate laboratory. Contaminated scopes and instruments are removed to the cleaning area adjacent to the suite, and the room and surfaces are cleaned before the next procedure. Personnel remove all protective garb before leaving the room.

At our institution bronchoscopy not performed in the operating room or intensive care unit takes place in a single-purpose suite

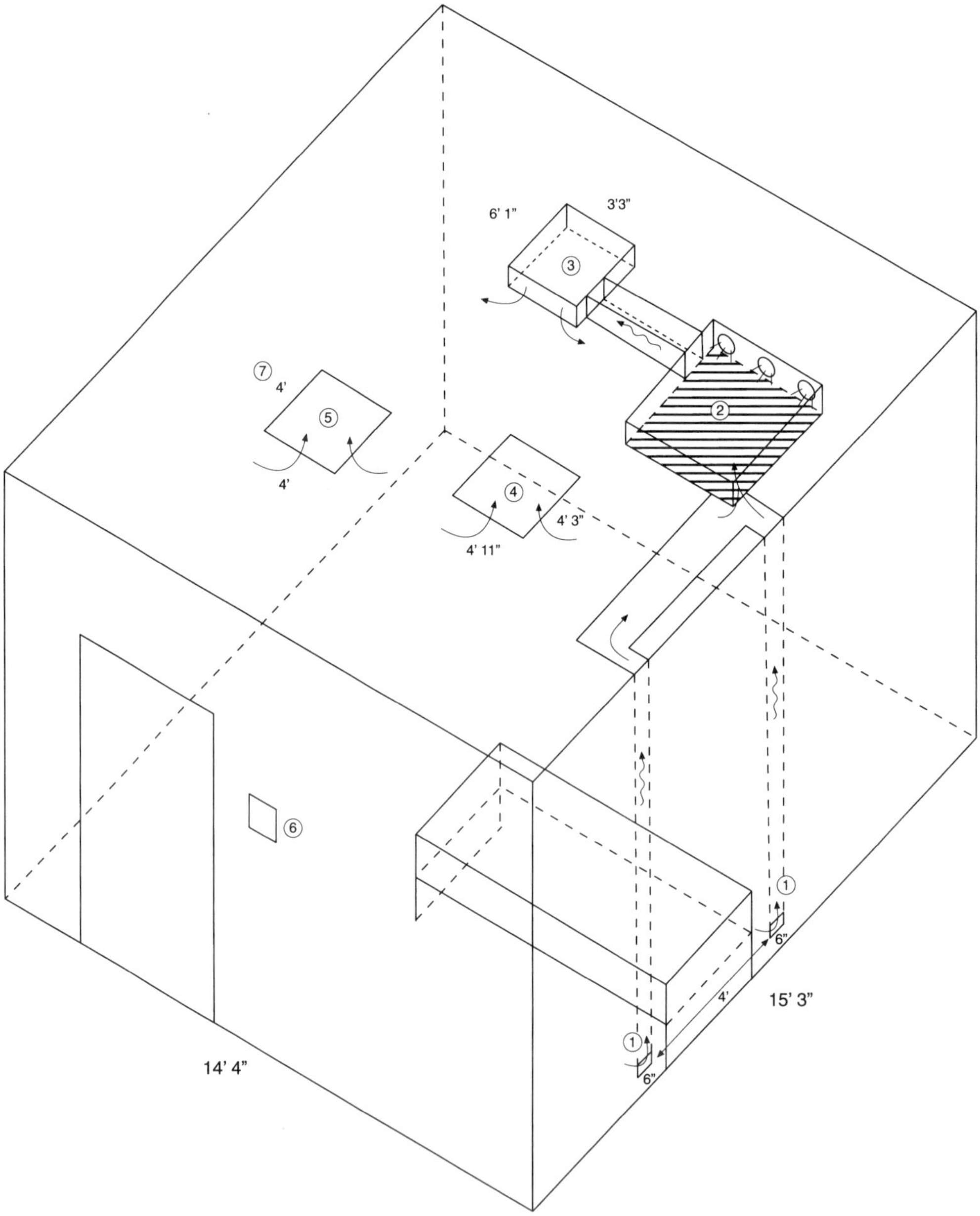

6' 1"
3'3"
③
②
⑦
4'
⑤
4'
④
4' 3"
4' 11"
⑥
①
6"
4'
15' 3"
①
6"
14' 4"

in the pulmonary function laboratory. Figure 21-1 shows the room configuration in detail. Several principles are important in understanding the design of this room. The suite is constructed for use as a positive or negative airflow room. Bronchoscopy under positive-flow conditions usually is reserved for patients for whom active mycobacterial infection has been absolutely ruled out. Clean airflow is directional (see Fig. 21-1). If negative air flow is necessary, the door must be closed or an audible alarm is triggered.

Although more than 6 air exchanges per hour in a room is likely to reduce the concentration of aerosolized respirable pathogens, current CDC recommendations for new construction or renovation recommend 12 air exchanges per hour. The acceptable equivalent of these air exchanges can be accomplished with an existing ventilation system or with auxiliary means such as flow through a HEPA filter. Exhausted air cannot be recirculated into the general circulation unless first ventilated through a HEPA filter. Figure 21-2 demonstrates the result of implementing new technology in designing isolation systems for ventilation when external ventilation is not available because of building constraints. Figure 21-3 is an enlargement of the functional unit in the cabinet.

Work Practices and Administrative Controls

The risk that an employee will contract a disease is related to the duration of exposure. Therefore the number of employees exposed should be minimized. In one outbreak of tuberculosis in a hospital, 13 persons were present at a bronchoscopy; 10 (77%) had conversion of purified protein derivative (PPD; tuberculin) test results (49). Employees at particularly high risk for infectious airborne disease (e.g., those with suppressed immune

FIG. 21-1. Schematic of a bronchoscopy suite. Overall, we are pleased with the design and ventilation characteristics; however, if we had it to do over again, we would make the room larger. With the current dimensions of this room, a flow rate of 500 cubic feet per minute (cfm) approximates 16 air exchanges per hour. Although this may not work out mathematically, considerable dead space in the room (e.g., cabinets and desk space) makes it relatively smaller. Neither cleaning of the bronchoscope nor storage of volatile chemicals (such as glutaraldehyde or other agents) takes place in this room. *1,* Air intakes 6 inches from the floor at the head of the bronchoscopy bed. *2,* Above-ceiling collection device includes a fan with an intake rate of 1,150 cfm, a prefilter, a primary HEPA filter, and germicidal ultraviolet irradiation. This system effectively filters infectious particles and disinfects the air of mycobacteria. This device is sold as a unit by Medical Air Technology Corp. (Canton, MA) and is labeled SSI series 20. *3,* Once the air is cleaned it passes through ductwork to reenter the bronchoscopy suite at a rate of 1,150 cfm. *4,* An additional 400 cfm fresh air flow is brought into the room directly from the hospital's ventilation system through a high-velocity diffuser. The flow pattern progresses from the ceiling downward over the bronchoscopist's head, over the patient, and toward the floor. *5,* 500 cfm air flow is returned to the hospital's auxiliary general exhaust. This air bypasses all other conduits and is vented directly to the outside. This system is considered a closed system, meaning there is no chance of contamination of the main in-hospital ventilation system. The difference between the 400 cfm entering the room and 500 cfm exhaust produces the negative pressure system. *6,* Negative pressure isolation room management system (Medical Air Technology, Canton, MA) is monitored in the bronchoscopy suite with local and remote alarms. The alarms alert the bronchoscopist to loss of negative pressure within the bronchoscopy suite. *7,* Around the ceiling vents and fans several measurements reflect the distance from the outside of the vent or fan to the nearest wall.

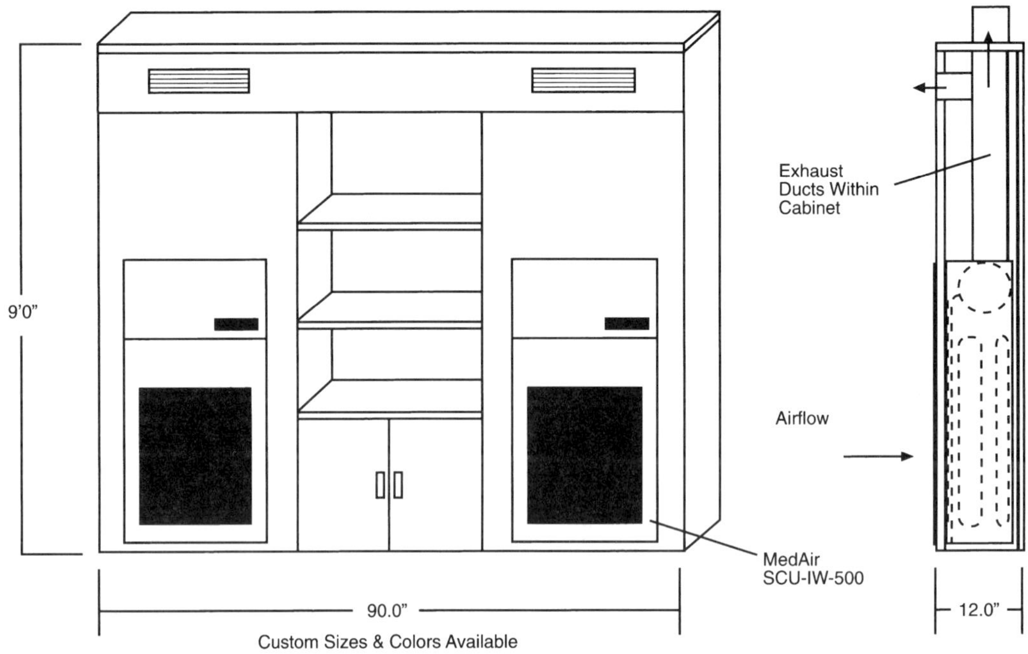

FIG 21-2. Results of implementation of new technology in designing isolation systems for ventilation when external ventilation is not available because of building constraints. For rooms in a hospital or health care center where external ventilation options are limited, this unit can provide acceptable air cleaning of airborne pathogens and germicidal irradiation. The central part of this unit can also serve as a storage area. The attraction of this design is based on the ability to retrofit existing spaces without extensive cost or building modifications. The two side panels function in ventilation, filtration, and sterilization. Air enters from the room at the base of the unit and is cleaned and exhausts at the upper vent. Part of the exhaust must be exhausted externally to produce negative pressure in the bronchoscopy suite. (Courtesy of Joanne O'Keefe, Medical Air Technology Corp., Canton, MA.)

function) should be counseled about the risk and the need for increased personal protection. The decision about placement of health care workers in at-risk situations requires sensitivity and understanding of the actual risks (see Chapter 1).

Patients with tuberculosis that has not been diagnosed constitute the main source of risk to bronchoscopy employees. A clear policy is needed to ascertaining which patients are likely to have tuberculosis. Such a policy would allow adequate protection to be instituted. In some instances, delay of bronchoscopy until antituberculosis drug therapy has been initiated may be advisable.

Screening of Employees

The frequency of screening of bronchoscopy employees should depend on the overall risk at the institution. Particularly because of the high possibility of aerosolization of organisms during bronchoscopy, bronchoscopists and support staff in settings with a high prevalence of tuberculosis may warrant PPD testing more often than annually. For example, pulmonary trainees have been found to be at greater risk for PPD conversion than infectious disease trainees, possibly because of performance of procedures such as bronchoscopy.

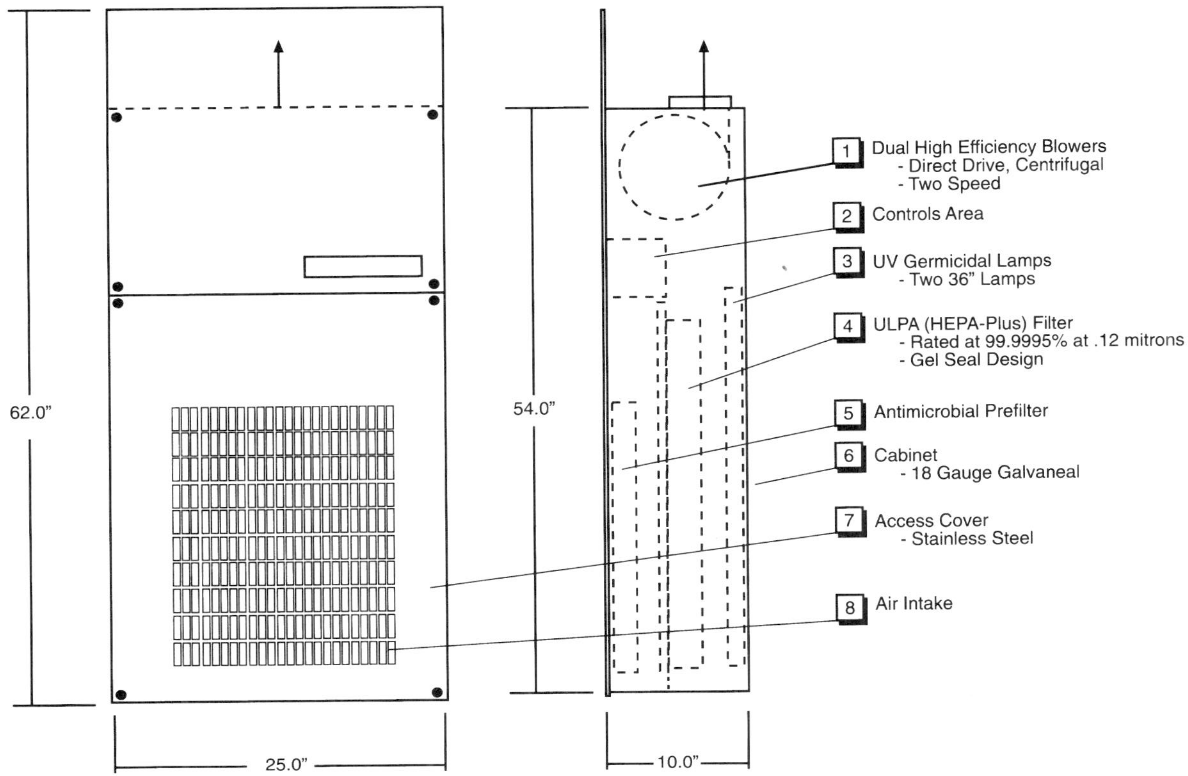

FIG. 21-3. Enlargement of functional unit within the cabinet. The components of this system are identified individually. (Courtesy Joanne O'Keefe, Medical Air Technology Corp., Canton, MA.

SUMMARY

The performance of bronchoscopy possesses inherent risks, not only to the patient but also to a lesser degree to the bronchoscopist. There is direct risk for infection from the patient to the bronchoscopist and bronchoscopy suite team and for aerosolization of both infectious and allergenic materials into the work environment. Risk for exposure during cleaning and disinfection of the bronchoscope must be recognized and meticulously addressed. The new generation of bronchoscopes in which the face of the operator is no longer as close to the patient as in the past may lessen infectious risk to bronchoscopists. However, no information is available, and any lessening of potential exposures may be balanced by potential exposures to increasingly virulent organisms. Use of universal precautions and education regarding recognition of risks remain the best way to protect the bronchoscopy team.

REFERENCES

1. Hirschowitz BI. The cost of doing business: occupational hazards for endoscopists. *Endoscopy* 1994;26: 559–561.
2. Kenyon TA, Valway SE, Ihle WW, Onorato IM, Castro KG. Transmission of multidrug-resistant *Mycobacterium tuberculosis* during a long airplane flight. *N Engl J Med* 1996;334:933–938.
3. Nelson KE, Larson PA, Schraufnagel DE, Jackson J. Transmission of tuberculosis by flexible bronchoscopes. *Am Rev Respir Dis* 1983;127:97–100.
4. Wheeler PW, Lancaster D, Kaiser AB. Bronchopulmonary cross-colonization and infection related to mycobacterial contamination of suction valves of bronchoscopes. *J Infect Dis* 1989;159:954–958.
5. Pappas SA, Schaaf DM, DiConstanzo MB, King FW Jr, Sharp JT. Contamination of flexible fiberoptic bronchoscopes. *Am Rev Respir Dis* 1983;127:391–392.
6. Steere AC, Corrales J, von Graevenitz A. A cluster of *Mycobacterium gordonae* isolates from bronchoscopy specimens. *Am Rev Respir Dis* 1979;120:214–216.
7. Dawson DJ, Armstrong JG, Blacklock ZM. Mycobacterial cross-contamination of bronchoscopy specimens. *Am Rev Respir Dis* 1982;126:1095–1097.
8. Hussain SA. Fiberoptic-bronchoscope related outbreak of infection with *Pseudomonas* [Letter]. *Chest* 1978; 74:483.
9. Webb SF, Vall-Spinoza A. Outbreak of *Serratia marcescens* associated with the flexible bronchoscope. *Chest* 1975;68:703–705.
10. Abbott L. The use and effects of glutaraldehyde: a review. *Occup Health (Lond)* 1995;47:238–289.
11. Axon ATR, Banks J, Cockel R, et al. Disinfection in upper-digestive-tract endoscopy in Britain. *Lancet* 1981;1:1093–1094.
12. Jachuck SJ, Bound CL, Steel J, et al. Occupational hazard in hospital staff exposed to 2 per cent glutaraldehyde in an endoscopy unit. *J Soc Occup Med* 1989;39:69–71.
13. Corrado OJ, Osman J, Davies RJ. Asthma and rhinitis after exposure to glutaraldehyde in endoscopy units. *Hum Toxicol* 1986;5:325–327.
14. Chan-Yeung M, McMurren T, Catonio-Begley F, et al. Occupational asthma in a technologist exposed to glutaraldehyde. *J Allergy Clin Immunol* 1993;91:974–978.
15. Benson WG. Case report: exposure to glutaraldehyde. *J Soc Occup Med* 1984;34:63–64.
16. Stenton SC, Beach JR, Dennis JH, et al. Glutaraldehyde, asthma, and work: a cautionary tale. *Occup Med (Oxf)* 1994;44:95–98.
17. Lemiere C, Cloutier Y, Perrault G, et al. Closed-circuit apparatus for specific inhalation challenges with an occupational agent, formaldehyde, in vapor form. *Chest* 1996;109:1631–1635.
18. Gannon PF, Bright P, Campbell M, et al. Occupational asthma due to glutaraldehyde and formaldehyde in endoscopy and x-ray departments. *Thorax* 1995;50: 156–159.
19. Curran AD, Burge PS, Wiley K. Clinical and immunologic evaluation of workers exposed to glutaraldehyde. *Allergy* 1996;51:826–832.
20. Hendrick DJ, Lane DJ. Occupational formalin asthma. *Br J Ind Med* 1977;34:11–18.
21. Hendrick DJ, Rando RJ, Lane DJ, et al. Formaldehyde asthma: challenge exposure levels and fate after five years. *J Occup Med* 1982;24:893–897.
22. Sussman GL, Beezhold DH. Allergy to latex rubber. *Ann Intern Med* 1995;122:43–46.
23. Turjamaa K. Incidence of immediate allergy to latex gloves in hospital personnel. *Contact Dermatitis* 1987; 17:270–275.
24. Arellano R, Bradley, Sussman G. Prevalence of latex-sensitization among hospital physicians occupationally exposed to latex gloves. *Anesthesiology* 1992;77: 905–908.
25. Landwehr LP, Boguniewicz M. Current perspectives on latex allergy. *J Pediatr* 1996;128:305–312.
26. Sliney DH, LeBodo H. Laser eye protectors. *J Laser Appl* 1990;2:9–13.
27. Holst GC. Proper selection and testing of laser protective materials. *Am J Optom Physiol Opt* 1973;50:477–483.
28. Baggish MS, Elbakry M. The effects of laser smoke on rat lungs. *Am J Obstet Gynecol* 1987;156:1260–1265.
29. Garden JM, O'Banion K, Shelnitz LS, et al. Papillomavirus in the vapor of carbon dioxide laser-treated verrucae. *JAMA* 1988;259:1199–1202.
30. Baggish MS, Polesz BJ, Joret D, Williamson P, Refai A. Presence of human immunodeficiency virus DNA in laser smoke. *Lasers Surg Med* 1991;11:197–203.
31. Sliney DH. Laser safety. *Lasers Surg Med* 1995;16: 215–225.
32. American National Standards Institute. Safety code for head, eye, and respiratory protection; ANSI, Z-2.1. New York: American National Standards Institute, 1978.
33. Elford B. Care and cleansing of the bronchoscope. *Chest* 1978;73[Suppl]:761–763
34. Stonehill AA, Krop S, Borick PM. Buffered glutaraldehyde: a new chemical sterilizing solution. *Am J Hosp Pharm* 1963;20:458–465.

35. Miner NA, McDowell JW, Willcockson GW, et al. Antimicrobial and other properties of a new stabilized alkaline glutaraldehyde disinfectant/sterilizer. *Am J Hosp Pharm* 1977;34:376–382.
36. Sattar SA, Springthorpe VS. Survival and disinfectant inactivation of the human immunodeficiency virus: a case review. *Rev Infect Dis* 1991;13:430–437.
37. Hanson PJ, Gor D, Jeffries DJ, Collins JV. Chemical inactivation of HIV on surfaces. *Br Med J* 1989;298: 862–864.
38. Weller IVD, Williams CB, Jeffries DJ, et al. Cleaning and disinfection of equipment for flexible gastrointestinal flexible endoscopy: interim recommendations of a Working Party of the British Society of Gastroenterology. *Gut* 1988;29:1134–1151.
39. Best M, Sattar SA, Springthorpe VS, Kennedy ME. Efficacies of selected disinfectants against Mycobacterium tuberculosis. *J Clin Microbiol* 1990;28:2234–2239.
40. Rutala WA, Cole EC, Wannamaker NS, Weber DJ. Inactivation of *Mycobacterium tuberculosis* and *Mycobacterium bovis* by 14 hospital disinfectants. *Am J Med* 1991;91[Suppl 3B];267S–271S.
41. Collins FM, Montalbine V. Mycobacterial activity of glutaraldehyde solutions. *J Clin Microbiol* 1976;4: 408–412.
42. Spach DH, Silverstein FE, Stamm WE. Transmission of infection by gastrointestinal endoscopy and bronchoscopy. *Ann Intern Med* 1993;118:117–118.
43. Qizilibash A, Castelli M, Seaton T. Post-colonoscopy chemical proctitis. *Lab Invest* 1986;54:51A.
44. Durante L, Zulty JC, Israel E, et al. Investigation of an outbreak of bloody diarrhea: association with endoscopic cleaning solution and demonstration of lesions in an animal model. *Am J Med* 1992;92:476–480.
45. Reichert M. Automatic washers/disinfectors for flexible endoscopes. *Infect Control Hosp Epidemiol* 1991;12: 497–499.
46. Bottrill PM, Axon AT. Cleaning and disinfection of flexible endoscopes and ancillary equipment: use of automatic disinfectors. *J Gastroenterol Hepatol* 1991;61:45–47.
47. Allen JI, Allen MO, Olson MM, et al. Pseudomonas infection of the biliary system resulting from use of a contaminated endoscope. *Gastroenterology* 1987;92: 759–763.
48. Alvarado CJ, Stolz MK, Maki DG. Nosocomial infections from contaminated endoscopes: a flawed automatic endoscope washer—an investigation using molecular epidemiology. *Am J Med* 1991;91:[Suppl 3B]:277S–280S.
49. Catanzaro A. Nosocomial tuberculosis. *Am Rev Resp Dis* 1982;125:559–562.

Medical Center Occupational Health and Safety,
edited by Robert J. McCunney.
Lippincott Williams & Wilkins, Philadelphia © 1999.

22

Hazards of Anatomic Pathology

Jonathan Silver Rutchik

Division of Occupational and Environmental Neurology, Occupational Health and Rehabilitation, Inc., Boston, Massachusetts 02210

A medical center aims to evaluate and diagnose medical illness and to educate and conduct research. The anatomic pathology laboratory is a vital component of a medical center. Its services include postmortem storage and autopsy and diagnostic evaluation of blood, body fluids, and tissue and organ specimens. A university medical center also teaches students human anatomy, which requires preparation and storage of human remains for dissection. Occupational hazards exist for those who work in this department. This chapter outlines the potential occupational exposures and known associated adverse health effects for pathologists, embalmers, histologists, cytologists, laboratory technicians, medical center staff, and medical students during dissection. Professional organizations and government agencies that regulate and accredit these areas of the medical center for quality, health, and safety standards are discussed. Important considerations and suggestions to reduce adverse health effects are described.

PROCESSES INVOLVED IN ANATOMIC PATHOLOGY AND THE CORRESPONDING HAZARDS

After death, a human body is bagged and transported to the morgue before it is determined that an autopsy is to be performed. If the medical center has been asked to perform these services, the body is transported to the autopsy room, where it is dissected as a fresh specimen. Workers must adhere to universal precautions by wearing respirators, full body suits, gowns, gloves, glasses, masks, and boots to protect themselves from exposure to blood and body fluids. Organs are collected from the body and placed in a preservative solution of formaldehyde. Small specimens may be frozen and analyzed with a microtome. Surgical specimens may be prepared and analyzed in these laboratories. Many blood and cytologic specimens are prepared in xylene and alcohol solutions to make slides. Workers involved in all stages of this process have potential inhalation exposure to these chemicals.

Formaldehyde exposure has been found to be excessive for personnel engaged in the examination of preserved tissue compared with those working with fresh specimens (1). Estimated weekly time-weighted average (TWA) exposures for pathologists, residents, and technicians were between 0.61 and 1.32 ppm for the three groups, but technicians were exposed to a baseline level for a prolonged period of time. Formaldehyde vapor was found to be the main occupational chemical exposure of embalmers in another study (2). Air monitoring revealed TWA concentrations of 0.1 to 0.4 ppm and 0.5 to 1.2 ppm during embalming of intact and autopsied bodies, respectively. The Occupational Safety and Health Administration (OSHA) permissible exposure limit (PEL) for formaldehyde at a TWA of 8 hours is 0.75 ppm; a short-term limit is 2 ppm (3). The National Institute for Occupational Safety and Health (NIOSH) threshold limit value (TLV) is 0.016, the ceiling 0.1 ppm, and the immediately dangerous to life and health value 20 ppm (4).

Some medical schools have embalmers in the anatomy laboratory who perform body preparation for anatomic dissection. Others receive bodies from local funeral directors. Embalming requires mixing a water-based solution of embalming fluid that contains preservatives, germicides, anticoagulants, perfuming agents, surfactants, dyes, modifying agents, and other solvents. Although the complete quantity of toxic substances is small, skin contact and inhalation exposure potential exist for all these chemicals. Table 22-1 lists the common components of embalming fluid. Many of these items are produced by chemical companies and material safety data sheets are available for all of them.

A quantity of 2 to 3.5 gallons (8.44 to 14.77 L) of embalming mixture is poured into a machine connected to an intravenous pumping device that enters one of the cadaver's large arteries, often the cervical carotid artery. Embalmers may have individual preferences for the primary injection site. Secondary injection sites are selected to ensure complete perfusion of the embalming agent. In some instances a six-point injection procedure is done through both carotid arteries, both axillary or brachial arteries, and both femoral or external iliac arteries. One or more cut-down procedures to access the large artery for infusion and a lower extremity vein for drainage is necessary. Exsanguination and perfusion of the body must be complete. Visceral air evacuation and introduction of other prepared solutions into the abdominal cavity follow. Injection with a needle or trocar to other areas of the body may be necessary. The embalmer risks blood-borne exposure when using sharp objects to perform the cut-down procedure and intravenous and abdominal insertion and again when exsanguinating the body's blood into a sink drain (usually at the foot end of the metal table on which the specimen lies). Inhalation and dermal exposure may occur while the embalmer pours the embalming mixture of hazardous chemicals into the pumping device (5). Because medical schools rarely knowingly purchase infected, deformed, or cut bodies, embalmers and body handlers in the anatomy laboratory in theory are at minimal risk for infectious contamination.

After a week, the body is ready for dissection. Because the body is stored in a refrigerated area, mold can become a problem. Chemicals can be used to spray or bathe bodies to alleviate this complication. The formulas are not known, but the products are available as proprietary items sold by chemical companies. Moldex and Antisept are two that

TABLE 22-1. *Common components of embalming fluid*

Quality	Chemical
Preservatives and germicides	Aldehydes: formaldehyde, paraformaldehyde (a polymer), trioxane (polymer), glutaraldehyde, and acetaldehyde Alcohols: methanol and phenol Quaternary ammonia compounds: zepharin chloride
Anticoagulants	Citrates, oxalates, borates, EDTA, magnesium sulfate, sodium chloride, sodium sulfate and sodium phosphate
Perfuming additives	Natural flower-based compounds
Coloring agents	Natural and synthetic ingredients
Osmotic agents	Moisturizers or dehydraters: glycerine, sorbital or lanolin Buffers and conditioners: carbonates, borates, and inorganic salts
Embalming fluid vehicles	Alcohols
Other important additives	Alkyl or arylsulfonates, sulfated alcohols, oils, and condensation products of ethylene oxide, amides, and fatty acids

Information from Hanzlick R. Embalming, body preparation, burial, and disinternment: an overview for forensic pathologists. *Am J Forensic Med Pathol* 1994;15:122–131 and Bradbury SA, Hoshina K. An improved embalming procedure for long-lasting preservation of the cadaver for anatomical study. *Acta Anat (Basel)* 1978; 101:97–103.

contain a high content of alcohol. Mold accumulation can erode an entire body in a short time. Humidity, temperature, ventilation, hydration, and laboratory cleanliness directly contribute to the optimum growth of mold.

EXPOSURE RISKS OF INFECTIOUS AND CHEMICAL HAZARDS

Occupational hazards for workers in an anatomic pathology laboratory, a morgue, or a medical school anatomy laboratory include infectious and chemical agents. Infectious agents borne by blood and body fluids include human immunodeficiency virus (HIV), hepatitis viruses, and pathogens that cause transmissible spongiform encephalopathy, such as Creutzfeldt-Jakob disease. Respiratory infections include tuberculosis. Chemical hazards present risks from inhalation or dermal contact. Formaldehyde and xylene are used in varying quantities and in many different processes. Phenols, alcohols, aldehydes, including glutaraldehyde, glycerol, and estrogen and acrylic creams are used in smaller quantities and fewer processes but also represent potential exposure risks.

Blood-borne Pathogens

All hospital personnel are at risk from blood-borne pathogens. HIV, hepatitis B and C viruses (HBV, HCV), and other infectious agents (see Chapter 3) are of concern. Anatomy and pathology laboratory staff who handle corpses before embalming are at risk for exposure to all transmissible infectious agents. In a study involving 539 morticians, 39% reported needle-stick injuries in the past 12 months, and 3% reported percutaneous exposure to the blood of a decedent with acquired immunodeficiency syndrome (6). Among 36 pathologists, 56% sustained a cut or needle-stick injury in 1989. It was calculated that a needle-stick injury occurred once for every 2,639 surgical specimens handled and for every 37 autopsies performed. Resident physicians reported a fivefold increase in injuries compared with staff pathologists. Of these injuries, 67% were to the distal thumb, index finger, and middle finger of the nondominant hand. These injuries have been called *dissector's digital injury* because they occur mainly during dissection when the nondominant hand is used to retract. Splash injuries to the face and eyes and glove punctures were frequently reported (7).

Johnson et al. (83) in 1997 reported autopsy-acquired HIV infection of a pathologist who sustained a scalpel wound to the hand. Controversy, however, exists about how long HIV survives after death. One study found no culturable HIV-1, 21.25 hours after death (8). Other investigators have isolated HIV-1 from brain 24 hours post mortem and from bone, spleen, brain, and blood up to 6 days post mortem (9–11). These studies emphasize the point that risk for HIV infection might be present when postmortem evaluation is delayed. Delaying autopsy reduces risk for exposure to infectious agents. Universal precautions must be observed by all hospital staff (3).

A study involving 11 funeral directors concluded that the highest risk for exposure to infectious agents and formaldehyde occurred during the following three tasks required in this process: the mixing of arterial embalming concentrates in the embalming pump reservoir, trocar introduction of cavity fluid in routine embalming procedures, and introduction of cavity fluid to the viscera in posted (after autopsy) embalming procedures (5).

Airborne Pathogens

Respiratory precautions are important preventive measures because oral and respiratory matter may be expelled from a body after death as air escapes the gastrointestinal tract. Tuberculosis testing and prophylactic medication, when appropriate, are useful as preventive and control measures. In 1979, 8 of 35 medical students with negative Mantoux test results who attended an autopsy of an immunosuppressed patient with unsuspected active tuberculosis became infected, and one contracted active disease. These students had viewed the procedure for approximately 1 hour (12). Masking a body while it is being handled and transported can prevent contamination of the immediate areas and personnel.

Creutzfeldt-Jakob Disease

Creutzfeldt-Jakob disease is a poorly understood progressive, dementing illness that has been characterized as transmissible spongiform encephalopathy. Iatrogenic transmission is well documented (13,14). This neuropathologic diagnosis has been made among 24 health care workers, including six physicians (14,15). One physician was a pathologist and two were neurosurgeons. A case of an internist with 1 year of training in pathology 30 years before becoming ill has been reported (16). Transmission has been documented through contact with central nervous system organs (brain, spinal cord, meninges, cerebrospinal fluid) and through corneal transplantation, dural grafting, intracerebral placement of electrodes for stereotactic operations, and administration of pooled human pituitary growth hormone (17). Noncerebral tissues such as lung, liver, lymph node, kidney, and leukocytes have low titers of infectivity and have been transmissible to nonhuman primates and small laboratory animals by many methods of inoculation. Although blood and urine have been found to be infectious in humans, other excretory products such as saliva and stool have not been found to contain the Creutzfeldt-Jakob pathogen (18).

Until recently, the common clinical presentation of Creutzfeldt-Jakob disease was a rapidly progressive dementing illness in an adult older than 50 years. Latency of more than 20 years from an initial exposure is suspected in these cases. Since 1996, however, Creutzfeldt-Jakob disease has been diagnosed among more than a dozen Europeans 30 years and younger who became ill with a syndrome that began with depression and abnormal movements. The diagnosis of spongiform encephalopathy was made by means of brain biopsy in each case. Ingestion of beef from animals infected with bovine spongiform encephalopathy has been suspected and suggests an animal-to-human vector for this disease.

The pathogen responsible withstands many customary sterilization methods, including heat, formaldehyde, and ultraviolet radiation, that typically eradicate viral and bacterial pathogens (19). Because many neurologic and psychologic symptoms may herald clinical presentation of Creutzfeldt-Jakob disease, pathologists and laboratory staff must exercise extreme caution when approaching cadavers with unclear neurologic or psychiatric diagnoses.

Many methods of disinfection have been tested (19). Formaldehyde diluted to 10% has been shown to be ineffective (20). A 1.0 Eq/L solution of sodium hydroxide bathed for 60 minutes then steamed at 121°C for 30 minutes has proved to be effective in at least two studies (21). Thus hospitals often incorporate additional measures to ensure complete disinfection. Recommendations are as follows (22): recipients of pituitary hormone of Creutzfeldt-Jakob disease should not be organ donors; tissues should be labeled clearly; gloves should be worn by all personnel, and skin should be rinsed immediately with 1 Eq/L sodium hydroxide for several minutes if skin contact occurs. Families should be counseled to use cremation. Operating and autopsy rooms should restrict traffic, and unnecessary supplies should be removed. Workers should use no supplies that require ethylene oxide sterilization. All personnel should double glove. Manual saws not power tools should be used to minimize splash and jetting of materials. The corpse should be cleaned and all surfaces disinfected with 1 Eq/L sodium hydroxide. After exposure, rinsing with sodium hydroxide for several minutes then rinsing with water is advised. Decontamination includes wiping off instruments before sterilization. Steam sterilization should be used with a prevacuum for 18 minutes at 134°C. Steam sterilization should be at standard gravity for 60 minutes at 134°C. Trash, sharp instruments, and tissue remnants should be incinerated. If the foregoing measures are not possible, instruments should be soaked for 1 hour in 1 Eq/L sodium hydroxide followed by 1 hour of steam sterilization at 121°C standard gravity. When equipment has come into direct contact with contamination and the foregoing procedures are not possible, the equipment should be soaked for 1 hour in 1 Eq/L sodium hydroxide. Liquid waste, including wash water, should be contained and incinerated.

Reporting exposure to Creutzfeldt-Jakob disease is important. Disinfection processes that are adequate to inactivate the pathogen include autoclaving at 121°C or higher, bathing in 0.5% sodium hypochlorite (a 10-fold dilution of household bleach) both for 1 hour and require decontamination with soap and water. Surfaces contaminated by the Creutzfeldt-Jakob pathogen should be disinfected, cleaned, and disinfected a second time (20).

Formaldehyde

Formaldehyde, a widely used agent for embalming, organ preservation, and disinfection, is used mainly in diluted form, known as formalin, an aqueous solution that is 37% formaldehyde by weight. Formaldehyde, a single carbon molecule with a double-bonded oxygen and two hydrogen molecules attached, is also known as methanal, methyl aldehyde, and methylene oxide. A natural gas with a pungent suffocating odor, formaldehyde is a common component of foods and cosmetics and a product of combustion from car exhaust, wood- and coal-burning fires, and cigarette smoke.

Formaldehyde exposure commonly occurs by means of inhalation or dermal absorption. In the liver and blood, the enzyme formaldehyde dehydrogenase rapidly metabolizes to formic acid (half life, 1.5 minutes), carbon dioxide, and a one-carbon metabolite (23). In aqueous solution, formaldehyde combines with free unprotonated amino groups to form a methylol amino acid and a liberated proton (24), which is thought to be responsible for the bacteriocidal properties. In higher concentrations (5% to 10%) formaldehyde precipitates protein. This property allows use of formaldehyde as a fixative of histologic specimens. The mechanism of the effects of formaldehyde as an irritant is unknown but is thought to relate to formaldehyde's acting as a low-molecular-weight compound, a hapten, that combines with a carrier protein to form a complex that induces an immune reaction (24–26).

Acute inhalation exposure leads to upper respiratory and eye irritation at levels between 1 and 5 ppm. Although the odor threshold for formaldehyde is between 0.05 and 1 ppm (27), rapid adaptation by olfaction occurs among persons exposed to low and high levels (24). At 6 ppm, eye irritation is intolerable to all (27). Pulmonary edema occurs at levels greater than 50 ppm. Short-term inhalation and dermal-contact exposure have been associated with allergic dermatitis and sensitization. Dermatitis has been found to occur at greater than 2% liquid solution (28). Dryness, reddening of the skin, maculopapular lesions, hyperesthesia, and angioneurotic edema have been reported. Liquid splashes into the eyes have caused permanent corneal damage, even after immediate washing.

OSHA Formaldehyde Standard

The formaldehyde standard, CFR 1910.1048 (3), is a comprehensive document that establishes a PEL and short-term excursion limit (STEL) and regulations for exposure monitoring for workers exposed at or above the STEL. It also specifies respiratory protection depending on the condition and concentration of exposure to formaldehyde, as follows: for exposure to up to 10 times the PEL, a full facepiece with approved canisters; for up to 100 times PEL, type C supplied-air respirator, pressure demand or continuous flow type with full facepiece, hood, or helmet; and for greater than 100 times PEL and firefighting, a self-contained breathing apparatus. The standard lists other relevant regulations, as follows: protective clothing and equipment are to be stored separately and cleaned before reuse; quick-drench showers and eyewash stations are to be available for immediate use; and regular visual inspections are mandatory to detect leaks and spills. A medical surveillance plan must be in place for workers who may be exposed to levels at or above the STEL. This includes examinations if the physician believes the employee may be at increased risk from exposure. Otherwise a questionnaire must be available before exposure, annually, and if an employee experiences signs or symptoms indicative of exposure. The standard also outlines provisions for removal of an employee from the workplace, restrictions in the workplace, and the requirement that the employer comply.

Appendix A of the OSHA formalin standard describes technical guidelines for use of formalin. This includes all chemical properties, health hazard data, emergency and first aid procedures, monitoring methods, protective equipment and clothing, and engineering controls. Appendix B describes sampling strategies and analytic methods for use of formaldehyde. Appendix C concentrates on medical surveillance. Appendix D contains a nonmandatory medical disease questionnaire. Appendix E describes qualitative and quantitative fit-testing procedures.

Formaldehyde Mortality Studies

Epidemiologic studies have assessed mortality due to cancer. A review of the UK registrar general's mortality tables for 131 pathologists found more deaths from lymphoid tumor (8 found, 3.3 expected) and less-than-expected rates of mortality from respiratory cancers. The authors could not exclude the possibility that occupational exposure to formaldehyde was responsible (28). A review of the Danish Cancer Registry for physicians in pathology, anatomy, or forensic medicine since 1943 found no increased incidence of nasal or lung cancer (29). Other mortality studies involving pathologists and medical laboratory technicians found a lack of evidence of an increased incidence of nasal cancer. One author remarked that because all the studies were retrospective, they do not exclude potential carcinogenicity (27). Embalmers licensed in California were found to have a mortality elevated for total cancer [proportionate mortality ratio (PMR) 111], arteriosclerotic heart disease, and suicide (PMR 112) but deficits for mortality from diseases of the respiratory and genitourinary systems. Deaths from cancer of the colon (PMR 143), brain (PMR 156), and prostate (PMR 91), and leukemia (PMR 140) were higher than expected. A parallel study of embalmers in New York State showed similar findings (30,31).

In 1984, Harrington and Oakes (32) conducted a study with nearly 2,800 members of the Royal College of Pathologists and found an excess of brain tumors (6 observed, fewer than 2 expected, $p > .02$) but not of deaths from lymphatic or hematopoietic neoplasms. Etiologic hypotheses included previous exposure to organic solvents or tuberculosis. No nasal or nasal sinus tumors were reported. A cohort study of 1,477 male Canadian undertakers licensed between 1928 and 1957 revealed that cirrhosis of the liver [standardized mortality ratio (SMR) 238] and chronic rheumatic heart disease (SMR 199) were the only causes of death significantly in excess. The authors suggested that alcohol intake could be the rationale for these findings. They also presented the opinion that formaldehyde is not likely to be correctly implicated in the causation of cancer at distant sites because it is highly reactive and rapidly detoxified. The importance of formaldehyde as a human carcinogen was questioned because of present-day exposure levels (33). In 1990, Hayes et al. (34) reported a statistically significant excess of cancer of the colon (PMR 127), lymphatic and hematopoietic systems (white subjects PMR 131, nonwhite subjects PMR 241) in a population of more than 4,000 U.S. embalmers.

In 1991, Hall et al. (35) found the number of deaths from cancer of the lymphatic and hematopoietic systems among a population of more than 4,500 members of the Royal College of Pathology to be in excess but not significantly so compared with the number of deaths among the general population. An excess of brain cancer was marginally significant for men [observed 6, expected 2.5, SMR 240, 95% confidence interval (CI), 88–522].

The authors thoroughly reviewed other mortality studies and warned that although consistent results have been demonstrated for leukemia and other malignant diseases in various studies involving professionals, selection bias could not be ruled out nor could disease risk be attributed to specific work practices or exposures. Scant information on duration of employment, actual material used, and duties performed were limiting.

Formaldehyde Morbidity Studies: Acute and Short-term Effects

Acute and short-term inhalation of formaldehyde in health care settings may cause respiratory symptoms. Productive cough, breathlessness, and chest tightness were more frequent in a group of 74 workers from anatomy and pathology departments in India compared with age- and sex-matched controls who were exposed to an average of 1 ppm ($p < .01$) (36). Lung function values such as forced vital capacity and forced expiratory velocity were also significantly decreased in this population, suggesting a bronchoconstriction effect of formaldehyde exposure.

Chronic bronchitis ($p = .03$), dyspnea ($p = .04$), and nasal, eye, and skin irritation ($p = .003$, .02, and .09) was more frequent among 84 embalmers compared with 38 controls evaluated with symptom questionnaires, pulmonary function, and patch testing. Airborne formaldehyde levels averaged 0.36 ppm during 22 embalming procedures. No change in forced vital capacity or forced expiratory volume was found. Patch testing, however, found 4% of embalmers sensitive to formaldehyde and 10% to glutaraldehyde compared with zero for controls (37). In another study, however, although 46% of pathologists indicated they had problems with formaldehyde, no subject had detectable circulating immunoglobulin E (IgE) specific to formaldehyde (38). A third study found that 50% of 66 workers ($p < .001$) experienced nasal discomfort from formaldehyde. Two had a positive radioallergosorbent test for formaldehyde. Concentrations averaged 0.26 ppm. Atopic workers were not found to be overrepresented in the group with nasal symptoms. The authors concluded that some pathologists may experience symptoms of a type 1 allergic reaction, but in most cases this is caused by hyperreactivity (39).

Students enrolled in an anatomy dissection course were found to have itchiness and paresthesias of the hands, headache, burning eyes, and dizziness at the end of one month. The mean indoor air concentration of formaldehyde was 0.124 ppm. Specific IgE against formaldehyde or phenol was found in none of the students at the beginning or end of the course. Sensitization to these chemicals was deemed not responsible for their symptoms (40). In another cross-sectional study 34 workers in a gross anatomy laboratory were evaluated by means of pulmonary function testing for exposure, symptoms, and acute pulmonary response. Ninety-four percent were exposed to levels above the American Conference of Governmental Industrial Hygienists (ACGIH) ceiling value of 0.3 ppm, and 31% experienced exposures above the OSHA action level of 0.5 ppm. Irritation of the eye was reported by 88% of workers, of the nose by 74%, of the throat by 29%, and of the airways by 21% (41). A thorough review by Smedley in 1996 (26) concluded that inhaled formaldehyde rarely induces a specific immune response and the relation between the response and respiratory symptoms is poor. Exposure has not been proved as a clear cause of immunologically mediated respiratory disease among adults. In a 1984 study in which questionnaires and pulmonary function tests were used to evaluate licensed white male morticians, relatively high exposure was not associated with chronic bronchitis or pulmonary function deficits. It was concluded that long-term intermittent exposure to formaldehyde gas exerted no meaningful chronic effect on respiratory health (42).

Exposure to formaldehyde is associated with neurobehavioral changes. In one study, women working in histology laboratories who were exposed to formaldehyde, xylene, and toluene, mood equilibrium and sleep disturbances were found to to be associated more with formaldehyde than with the other two chemicals (43,44).

Formaldehyde Morbidity Studies: Carcinogenicity, Mutagenicity, and Reproductive Effects

Formaldehyde has been deemed a potential carcinogen because of studies that found it to be a cancer promoter and initiator in animals. These studies helped to establish a weak association with cancers of the lung, nasopharynx, oropharynx, and nasal passages among humans. NIOSH was the first government agency to label formaldehyde as a potential carcinogen on the basis of its ability to produce cancer in experimental animals (45). A case-control study in France could not separate wood dust exposure as a confounding variable but found that exposure to formaldehyde along with wood dust may increase risk for nasal adenocarcinoma over risk from exposure to wood dust alone (46).

Mutagenicity has been explored among humans exposed to formaldehyde in occupational settings. Sister-chromatid exchanges measured in the peripheral lymphocytes of 8 nonsmoking students after exposure to formaldehyde embalming solution during a 10-week anatomy class revealed a small but statistically significant increase in exchanges with exchanges among controls. In this study, mean breathing zone concentrations were found to be 1.2 ppm (47). No increase in sister-chromatid exchanges or chromosomal aberrations was found in another study of a small group of pathology workers (48). Chromosomal aberrations were not elevated among workers engaged in formaldehyde manufacturing and processing compared with controls (49). A higher frequency of micronucleated cells and squamous metaplasia was found in the respiratory nasal mucosa of a group of plywood factory workers exposed to formaldehyde compared with controls. Mean exposure levels were 0.23 mg/m^3 in the warehouse area and 0.73 mg/m^3 during sawing operations. Wood dust exposure, however, was not controlled (50). A measure of DNA repair found to be inhibited by formaldehyde in vitro, *O*-6 alkylguanine DNA alkyltransferase activity, was assessed in the peripheral blood lymphocytes of 23 mortuary science students before and after 9 weeks of a laboratory course on embalming techniques. No clear link was found (51). Chromosomal damage in human exfoliated cells from the oral cavity was shown to be increased after exposure to embalming solution. The authors concluded that these data helped confirm the genotoxic properties of formaldehyde (52). Long-term effects were assessed among 164 workers exposed daily to the chemical during the production of urea formaldehyde resins. No evidence was found of excess respiratory symptoms or decline in lung function (53).

Hospital staff workers and laboratory workers have been evaluated for reproductive and development effects in a number of studies. Many focused on those exposed to formalin, glutaraldehyde, and ethylene oxide while sterilizing instruments. A study by Taskinen et al. (54) in 1994 focused on women working in laboratories in Finland. Information on various habits of work and leisure were collected during the first trimester of pregnancy. The odds ratio for spontaneous abortion was increased among women who had been exposed to formalin for 3 days a week or more. A greater proportion of these had been working in pathology and histology laboratories. Most of these women who were exposed to formalin also were exposed to xylene. The authors cautioned that exposure in these settings is to a host of chemicals simultaneously. No association was found between formalin exposure and congenital malformations.

Other Chemical Hazards

Workers in anatomic pathology laboratories may come into contact with xylene, glutaraldehyde, phenol, methanol, ethanol, ethylene glycol, glycerin, and various other chemicals. These substances are often used in conjunction with formaldehyde (Table 22-2).

TABLE 22-2. *Chemical hazards of anatomic pathology*

Hazard (CAS #)	Properties	OSHA PEL	NIOSH REL	ACGIH
Formaldehyde 50-00-0	Single-carbon molecule with one ketone group attached (double-bonded oxygen). Known also as methanal, methylaldehyde, methylcne oxide. Nearly colorless gas with a pungent, suffocating odor.	0.75 ppm. STEL 2 ppm. Action level 0.5 ppm	Cancer 0.016 ppm Ceiling 0.1 (15 minute) IDLH 20 ppm	Ceiling 0.3 ppm or 0.37 mg/m^3
Xylene 1330-20-7; 95-47-6; 108-38-3; 106-42-3	Benzene ring with two methyl substitutions at various positions specific for the ortho, meta, and para forms. Also known as 1,2; 1,3; or 1,4 dimethylbenzene and ortho, meta, or para xylol. Colorless liquid with aromatic odor.	100 ppm (435 mg/m^3)	REL 100 ppm STEL 150 ppm (655 mg/m^3) IDLH 900 ppm	TLV 100 ppm (434 mg/m^3) STEL 150 ppm (651 mg/m^3) BEI end of shift urine methyl-hippuric acids ≥1.5 g/g creatinine
Glutaraldehyde 111-30-8	Five-carbon molecule with two double-bonded oxygens and one single-bonded hydrogen at each end of the chain. Also referred to as glutaric dialdehyde or 1,5 pentanedial. Colorless liquid with a pungent odor.	None	Ceiling (15 minutes) 0.2 ppm (0.8 mg/m^3)	Ceiling 0.05 ppm (0.2 mg/m^3)
Methanol 67-56-1	One-carbon molecule with a hydroxyl group attached. It is referred to as carbinol, columbian spirits, methyl alcohol, pyroligneous spirit, wood alcohol, wood naphtha, and wood spirit. Colorless liquid with a characteristic pungent odor.	200 ppm (260 mg/m^3)	REL 200 ppm (260 mg/m^3) STEL 250 ppm (325 mg/m^3)	Skin TLV 200 ppm (262 mg/m^3) STEL/ceiling 250 ppm (328 mg/m^3) BEI End of shift urine methanol ≥15 mg/L
Phenol 108-95-2	Benzene-ring molecule with one substituted hydroxy group. Also known as carbolic acid, hydroxybenzene, mono- hydroxy-benzene, phenyl alcohol, and phenyl hydroxide. Colorless to pink crystalline solid with a sweet, acrid odor. Naturally liquifies by mixing with 8% water.	5 ppm (19 mg/m^3)	REL 5 ppm (19 mg/m^3) Ceiling 15.6 ppm (60 mg/m^3) IDLH 5 ppm (19 mg/m^3)	TWA with a skin designation 5 ppm (19 mg/m^3)
Glycerine (mist) 56-81-5	Three-carbon molecule with three substituted hydro groups, one on each carbon. Also called glycerol, glycyl alcohol, 1,2,3 propanetriol, and trihydroxypropane. Clear, colorless, odorless, syrupy liquid or solid.	15 mg/m^3 (total) 5 mg/m^3 (resp)	None	TLV 10 mg/m^3 (inhalable particles)
Ethylene glycol 107-21-1	Two-carbon molecule with hydroxy groups attached on each end. Referred to as 1,2 dihydroxyethane, 1,2 ethanediol, glycol, glycolalcohol, and monoethylene glycol. Clear, colorless, syrupy, odorless liquid.	None	None	Ceiling 100 mg/m^3
Ethanol 64-17-5	Two-carbon molecule with a hydroxyl group attached to one end. Also called alcohol, cologne spirit, ethyl alcohol, and grain alcohol. Clear, colorless with a weak, ethereal vinous odor.	1000 ppm (1,900 mg/m^3)	None	TWA 1000 ppm (1,880 mg/m^3)

CAS, chemical abstract service; PEL, permissible exposure limit; NIOSH, National Institute for Occupational Safety and Health; REL, recommended exposure limit; ACGIH, American Conference of Governmental Industrial Hygienists; STEL, short-term excursion limit; ILDH, immediately dangerous to life and health; TLV, threshold limit value; BEI, biologic exposure limit; TWA, time-weighted average.

Phenol

Phenol has been implicated as a possible skin irritant and asthma inducer (55). Although none of 45 medical students in one anatomy class were found to have IgE-specific antibodies to phenol, many had symptoms including itching and paresthesias of the hands (33 students), headache (15 students), burning eyes (13 students), and dizziness (8 students). Phenol has been studied for its carcinogenicity in animals and humans. Studies with animals have found that phenol may have an inhibitory effect on other carcinogens. At low levels, there is no clear evidence of carcinogenicity (5,6). An excess of cancer of the esophagus (SMR 1.4), kidney (SMR 1.1), and Hodgkin's disease (SMR 1.2) was found among 14,861 employees of factories using phenol. Lower mortality ratios were found for cancer of the buccal cavity and pharynx, stomach, and brain, arteriosclerotic heart disease, emphysema, and cirrhosis of the liver. Duration and cumulative phenol exposure were found to be inversely related to arteriosclerotic heart disease, emphysema, and cirrhosis of the liver. Phenol has been shown to interfere with the generation of oxidants in experimental systems, and there is biologic plausibility to account for this phenomenon (56,57).

Xylene

Xylene is used widely in the medical technology industry. Its principal metabolite in the urine, methyl hippuric acid, has been recommended as a strong indicator of exposure. A biologic exposure index has been standardized by the ACGIH (see Table 22-1). Xylene is absorbed rapidly from the lungs and as a liquid slowly through the skin. About 95% is metabolized in the liver to methyl hippuric acid, and 70% to 80% of this is excreted within 24 hours. Alcohol, exercise, coexposure, sex, size, lifestyle, and environmental factors may affect the physiologic effects (58).

Xylene may act as a narcotic and induce acute and chronic neuropsychologic and neurophysiologic dysfunction. Short-term exposure to 90 to 100 ppm may lead to coordination problems, although tolerance may develop (59,60). Visual evoked responses have been affected by increasing exposures. Xylene was found to counteract the deleterious effect of alcohol in some studies (61–63). Respiratory tract symptoms are common. Central nervous system toxicity from xylene exposure has not been well established (64). No deleterious effects were found on the electroencephalograms of volunteers exposed to 200 ppm for 4 hours (65). In a 1990 study Dudek et al. (66) found neurobehavioral disturbances among volunteers exposed to 100 ppm for 4 hours. Hematologic and liver disturbances have been evaluated in workers exposed to xylene. No clear association has been established for these health effects (60,67–70). Increased risk for spontaneous abortion has been reported with exposure to solvents in some studies. Xylene had been a part of these exposure profiles; however, the presence of confounding variables has made it difficult to implicate a particular solvent. International Agency for Research on Cancer documents show association between xylene exposure and cancer of the prostate, lymphosarcoma, lymphatic leukemia, adenocarcinoma of the lung, and primary central nervous system tumors, but the numbers of cases is small, there were inadequate controls, and multiple-solvent exposures occurred (71).

Glutaraldehyde

The highly reactive properties of glutaraldehyde give it strong disinfecting and sterilizing abilities. Many cleaning solutions containing irritants of the eyes and mucous membranes, contact dermatitis, and skin discoloration from occupational exposures have been reported. Respiratory distress and secondary infections from irritation and ulceration of exposed sites can occur. Glutaraldehyde has been deemed a sensitizing agent (72). Patch testing was positive for 8 of 84 funeral workers exposed to glutaraldehyde; none of the controls had positive results.

Chest wheezing was found among 9% of 150 hospital staff workers who responded to questionnaires about glutaraldehyde in Great Britain. None had abnormal lung function tests. The authors suggested that there was no evidence of chronic airway disease among these workers (73). The case has been described of a respiratory technician who had a decline in forced expiratory volume in 1 second when exposed to glutaraldehyde used as a sterilizing agent in her workplace and an improvement away from work (74). Although glutaraldehyde has been suspected of being teratogenic, human epidemiologic studies have found that exposure has not been associated with spontaneous abortions (75–77).

REGULATIONS APPROPRIATE TO ANATOMIC PATHOLOGY

The Occupational Safety and Health Act of 1970 established a government agency with regulatory authority to protect workers from occupational hazards. OSHA requires places of employment with more than 12 employees to abide by regulations that appear in the *Federal Register* and the Code of Federal Regulations (CFR). The blood-borne pathogens standard, CFR 1910.1030 (78), is applicable to all occupational exposure to blood or potentially infectious materials, including all types of body fluids and any unfixed tissues or organ from a human (living or dead). The hazard communication standard, CFR 1910. 1200 (79), is aimed at ensuring that hazards of all chemicals produced or imported are evaluated and that information about them is transmitted comprehensively to employers and employees by means of labeling, training, and material safety data sheets. The laboratory standard, CFR 1910.1450 (80), Occupational Exposure to Hazardous Chemicals in Laboratories, outlines procedures to minimize all chemical exposures, avoid underestimation of risk, provide adequate ventilation, institute a chemical hygiene program, and observe PELs and TLVs. This includes general rules for all laboratory work with chemicals, such as not eating, drinking, or smoking in the area and the use of a hood for operations that might result in the release of toxic chemical vapors or dust. Waste disposal is mentioned. The laboratory standard also outlines methods for working with allergens.

NIOSH and ACGIH have published recommended exposure limits and TLVs. These and the OSHA limits are listed in Table 22-2 for some selected chemical hazards of anatomic pathology laboratories. Those that are not listed may not have any recommended or published standards.

The Clinical Laboratory Improvement Act (CLIA) is a federal act that established that all laboratories need to be certified and inspected regularly to ensure quality test results. CLIA 1988 was passed in response to public concerns over laboratory quality. The College of American Pathology (CAP) was given the right to certify pathology laboratories. Before CLIA 1988 laboratories volunteered for CAP certification. The Joint Commission on Accreditation of Health Care Organizations (JCAHO) may inspect and certify laboratories for quality and safety and considers an entire facility its jurisdiction. Often the laboratory is evaluated yearly by CAP in place of JCAHO. CAP requires laboratories to fill out a detailed checklist for each area of the laboratory. It assures that its policies and procedures are visible and up to date and assesses for fire protection and control, reporting of occupational injuries, chemical hygiene, designation of officers for safety and health, personal protective equipment, exposure monitoring for specific chemicals, such as formaldehyde, necessary medical consultation, training, adherence to requirements of the OSHA hazard communication standard and laboratory standard, and handling of carcinogenic chemicals.

Medical schools and their anatomy laboratories are not under the influence of the foregoing associations. Many university policies, however, state that regulations applicable to their employees are also applicable to students and volunteers. The American Association of Medical Colleges (AAMC) establishes standards for medical schools. Its Liaison Committee on Medical Education is an

AAMC and American Medical Association cosponsored group that deals with issues such as policy guidelines for personal counseling and student health services, student exposure to infectious and environmental hazards, education about prevention, procedures for care and treatment exposure, definition for financial responsibility, and the effects of infectious and environmental disease or disability on student education activities. These policies are not necessary for accreditation.

Embalmers in medical schools are not required to be licensed in all states. They may or may not be members of the National Funeral Directors Association (www.nfda). This professional agency aims to educate and inform and support its members. The association has published recommendations related to health and safety issues and assists members with specific problems.

The American Association of Anatomists (www.faseb.anat) and professional societies such as the American Society of Clinical Pathologists, the American Clinical Laboratory Association, the American Society of Clinical Laboratory Science, the Clinical Laboratory Management Association, and the International Society of Clinical Laboratory Technology may be helpful resources regarding regulations, standards, and guidelines.

PREVENTION

Prevention requires personal protective equipment, engineering controls, and training. Those who frequently come in contact with blood or body fluids, organs, or specimens are required to use universal handling precautions (81,82) and adhere to the OSHA blood-borne pathogen standard. This approach usually includes sharp-instrument and needle capping policies and use of gowns, gloves, masks, and boot covers. The OSHA blood-borne pathogens standard outlines regulations that hospital staff must follow with the assistance of the employee health service to ensure protection from infectious agents.

Pathologists who perform autopsies should use caution to prevent cuts, needle punctures, and mucocutaneous exposure from splashes (83). Because scalpel wounds tend to be inflicted on oppositional areas during autopsy, protection of the retracting hand is critical. The use of Kevlar gloves with two pairs of latex gloves is a practical alternative to conventional double gloving (84). The use of gauntlet-type gloves to cover the forearms also helps. Reducing blood accumulation with proper drainage systems may decrease risk for an unexpected splash. Because the improperly placed aspirator discharge nozzles may generate blood aerosols, nozzles should be aimed below the water surface in the embalming sink. Excess embalming pump pressures or release of lodged venous clots used for drainage may lead to sprays of blood. These risks necessitate the use of personal protective equipment. Direct handling of organs should be avoided. Viscera bags should be of quality construction to prevent the possibility of breakage. Rounded scalpel blades and placement of towels over sharp, bony projections are other ideas to reduce risk. Preventing or reducing bone dust or aerosolization exposure with the use of hand saws instead of power tools within the confines of a biohazard bag is strongly recommended (85).

The potential for blood contact can be reduced with the use of a modified carotid tap or heart tap variations in routine embalming. This method minimizes accumulation of blood and embalming solution on the surface of the embalming table. Proper positioning of the aspirator discharge nozzle and proper selection and use of quality personal protective equipment are important. Routine inspections should address disinfection processes, waste disposal, sharp-instrument containers, product effluents, and functionality of eyewash stations and emergency preparedness.

A walk-through evaluation of 11 funeral facilities in Minnesota for potential exposure to infectious agents and formaldehyde revealed that 6 directors did not wear a protective mask or adequate eye protection or observe the universal precautions recommended by the Centers for Disease Control and Prevention

(CDC). Receptacles were not properly labeled in 10 of 11 sites, and training was inadequate in all 11. An eyewash facility was not available in 10 of 11, and proper spill, cleanup, and decontamination procedures had not been developed as required by CDC. Embalming room ventilation at 10 of the 11 sites ranged from 3.7 to 24.6 room air changes per hour. The highest 15-minute mortician formaldehyde exposures measured at the three posted (embalming after autopsy) sites ranged from 1.0 to 2.9 ppm with a mean of 1.7 ppm. One site exceeded the OSHA STEL of 2 ppm. Mean exposure during the 68 to 145 minute procedures was 0.55 ppm. For routine embalming, the mean exposure for these 36 to 110 minute procedures was 0.35 ppm. Because of the high level at one posted embalming site, an increase in dilution ventilation or local exhaust to remove formaldehyde vapor near the point of generation was required. Respiratory protection was necessary during the transition. Initiation of a medical surveillance program, including a medical examination to approve use of a respirator for the embalmer, and a training program also were required (5).

Technique may determine the level of exposure to formaldehyde during embalming of autopsied bodies (86). Exposure may be related to frequency and thoroughness of suctioning of pooled fluids from body cavities and washing away of spillage. The condition of bodies is variable; severed arteries and veins may have increased spillage of preservatives. The dilution of formaldehyde is important because it determines the concentration of vapor inhaled. A decomposing body may require more potent or higher quantities of embalming fluid, and these increases lead to additional routes of exposure. Paraformaldehyde, used as a powder, is less water soluble than formaldehyde and may be inhaled deeper into the lungs and alveoli. Formaldehyde may adsorb to these particles and cause additional injury to these structures (87). Exposure is different for workers who performed specific tasks. Technicians, for example, have baseline levels of exposure for a prolonged period of time. Physicians are exposed to shorter but higher levels during tissue sectioning and examination. Evaluation of work procedures is encouraged for autopsy services to reduce exposure to vapors.

Increasing ventilation of dissection rooms is one method of reducing exposure to inhalable hazards. Recommendations in one study included a fan on an outside wall opposite the embalming area to reduce fumes. The fan should produce a minimum of 12 to 15 air exchanges per hour (87). A toxicity survey in the study demonstrated that respiratory irritation occurred at levels slightly greater than 2 ppm formaldehyde. Fumes frequently were found not to bother workers because the workers had become accustomed to them. The authors emphasized that this olfactory numbing effect was potentially detrimental, because the workers would not be able to detect the fumes when concentrations were above the safe level. Respiratory protection may be necessary if systems are antiquated or the industrial hygiene department has demonstrated levels higher than the action level for formaldehyde or other regulated hazardous chemicals (88).

The TWA ranged from 0.07 to 2.94 ppm during dissection operations in one gross anatomy laboratory. Irritation of the eyes was a prominent symptom for 30 of 34 workers. A novel solution was use of a dissection bed with an internal motor that causes downflow of the formaldehyde vapor, which is then absorbed into a replaceable carbon filtration system. Vapor levels were found to be greatly reduced in one study and allowed the laboratory to comply with safety and health regulations and provide an excellent working environment (89). Local exhaust ventilation combined with good work practices is the control method of choice.

To improve the air quality in the dissection room environment, a method has been introduced to reduce use of phenol and formaldehyde by substituting phenoxyethanol as a postfixation long-term preservative for cadavers. Phenoxyethanol, a nontoxic, lightly scented common chemical often used in cosmetic and first aid products, has no environmental agency restrictions. It acts as an effective solvent to remove formaldehyde from fixed tissues. It is inexpensive, nonflammable, slow to evaporate, and effective as an antimicrobial and tissue preservative and softener. The technique initially developed required large volumes of formaldehyde and long and cumbersome preparation. A study of 138 cadavers preserved with phenoxyethanol in a more rapid modified method showed good tissue integrity that resulted in good prosection specimens. No mold or fungal growth occurred in 3 years of soaking. Formaldehyde and phenol vapors were low, 0.07 ppm of formaldehyde and 0.65 mg/m^3 for phenol. This procedure has a shorter embalming process and lower volumes and concentrations of formaldehyde, shortens or eliminates phenoxyethanol immersion, greatly reduces the time, facility, and cost associated with embalming fluids, and provides for a toxic free environment. It appears to be an excellent alternative to use of conventional formaldehyde- and phenol-based embalming or wetting fluids for long-term postfixation preservation of anatomic materials (90).

CONCLUSION

The hazards of anatomic pathology—blood-borne and airborne pathogens, transmissible encephalopathies, and health effects from chemical exposures—may be reduced with adherence to universal precautions, altering technique to minimize spillage of body fluids and embalming fixatives, diluting fixative concentrations, and using personal protective equipment. Laboratory ventilation is necessary to reduce exposures below OSHA PELs and ceiling levels. Workers should be aware that odors may not be noticeable because of olfactory desensitization. Respiratory symptoms of the health effects of formaldehyde exposures are well documented for acute and short-term problems; for chronic exposure and reproductive effects, they are less certain. Animal research has led to concerns about cancer and government regulation. More than one human mortality study of professionals in these work settings revealed increased prevalence of cancer of the brain and hematopoietic, lymphatic, and gastrointestinal systems. The authors warned, however, that study design problems should limit enthusiasm for their results. National professional organizations can provide information. More research is needed to answer the serious questions about occupational exposure for those in the field of anatomic pathology.

REFERENCES

1. Coldiron VR, Ward JB, Trieff NM, et al. Occupational exposure to formaldehyde in a medical center autopsy service. *J Occup Med* 1983;25:544–548.
2. Williams TM, Levine RJ, Blunden PB. Exposure of embalmers to formaldehyde and other chemicals. *Am Ind Hyg Assoc J* 1984;45:172–176.
3. Occupational Safety and Health Administration. Formaldehyde standard. 29 CFR 1910.1048;1995, 1996, 1998.
4. National Institute of Occupational Health and Safety (NIOSH). *Handbook of chemical hazards*. Cincinnati, OH: NIOSH, 1994.
5. Wasvick JL, Anderson DE. Evaluation of mortician exposure to formaldehyde and infectious agents with recommended controls relative to new OSHA standards. Report to the Minnesota Department of Health, http://www.osha-slc.gov/, 1988.
6. Beck-Sague CM, Jarvis WR, Fruehling JA, et al. Universal precautions and mortuary practitioners: influence on practice and risk of occupational acquired infection. *J Occup Med* 1991;33:874–878.
7. O'Brian DS. Patterns of occupational hand injury in pathology: the interaction of blades, needles, and the dissector's digits. *Arch Pathol Lab Med* 1991;115:610–613.
8. Bankowski MJ, Landay AL, Staes B, et al. Postmortem recovery of HIV-Type 1 from plasma and mononuclear cells. *Arch Pathol Lab Med* 1992;116:1124–1127.
9. Ho DD, Rota TR, Schooley RT, et al. Isolation of HTLV-III from cerebrospinal fluid and neural tissues of patients with neurologic syndromes related to the acquired immunodeficiency syndrome. *N Engl J Med* 1985;313:1493–1501.
10. Nyberg M, Suni J, Haltia M. Isolation of HIV at autopsy one to six days postmortem. Am J Clin Pathol 1990;94: 422–425.
11. Henry K, Dexter D, Sanneru K. Recovery of HIV at autopsy. *N Engl J Med* 1989;321:1833–1834.
12. Wilkins D, Woolcock AJ, Cossart YE. Tuberculosis: medical students at risk. *Med J Aust* 1994;160:395–397.
13. Gadjusek DC, Gibbs CJ, Asner DM, et al. Precautions in medical care of and in handling materials from patients with transmissible virus dementia (Creutzfeldt-Jakob disease). *N Engl J Med* 1977;297:1253–1258.
14. Miller DC. Creutzfeldt-Jakob disease in histopathology technicians. *N Engl J Med* 1988;318:853–854.
15. Sitwell L, Lach B, Atack E, Atack D, Izukawa D.

Creutzfeldt-Jakob disease in histopathology technicians. *N Engl J Med* 1988;318:853–854.
16. Berger JR, Noble NJ. Creutzfeldt-Jakob disease in a physician: a review of the disorder in health care workers. *Neurology* 1993;43:205–206.
17. Brown P. Iatrogenic Creutzfeldt-Jakob disease. *Aust N Z J Med* 1990;20:633–634.
18. Rosenberg RN, White CL III, Brown P. Precautions in handling tissues, fluids, and other contaminated materials from patients with documented or suspected CJD. *Ann Neurol* 1986;19:75–77.
19. Steelman VM. Creutzfeldt-Jakob disease: recommendation for infection control. *Am J Infect Control* 1994:22:312–318.
20. Brown P, Gibbs CJ, Amyx HL, et al. Chemical disinfection of Creutzfeldt-Jakob disease virus. *N Engl J Med* 1982;306:1279–1282.
21. Taguchi F, Tamai T, Uchida K. Proposal for a procedure for complete inactivation of the CJD agent. *Arch Virol* 1991;119:297–301.
22. Committee on Health Care Issues, American Neurological Association. Precautions in handling tissues, fluids, and other contaminated materials from patients with documented or suspected Creutzfeldt-Jakob disease. *Ann Neurol* 1986;1:75–77.
23. Bernstein RS, Stayner LT, Elliot J, et al. Inhalation exposure to formaldehyde: an overview of its toxicity, epidemiology, monitoring, and control. *Am Ind Hyg Assoc J* 1984;45:778–785.
24. Loomis TA. Formaldehyde toxicity. *Arch Pathol Lab Med* 1979;103:321–324.
25. Frigas E. Testing for bronchial sensitivity to formaldehyde gas. (Clinical brief). *Mayo Clin Proc* 1981;56:277.
26. Smedley J. Is formaldehyde an important cause of allergic respiratory disease? *Clin Exp Allergy* 1996;26:247–259.
27. Pabst R. Exposure to formaldehyde in anatomy: an occupational health hazard. *Anat Rec* 1987;219:109–112.
28. Clark RP. Formaldehyde in pathology departments. *J Clin Pathol* 1983;36:839–846.
29. Jensen OM, Andersen SK. Lung cancer risk from formaldehyde. *Lancet* 1982;1:913.
30. Walrath J, Fraumeni JF. Mortality patterns among embalmers. *Int J Cancer* 1983;31:407–411.
31. Walrath J, Fraumeni JF. Cancer and other causes of death among embalmers. *Cancer Res* 1984;44:4638–4641.
32. Harrington JM, Oakes D. Mortality study of British pathologists 1974–1980. *Br J Ind Med* 1984;41:188–191.
33. Levine RJ, Andjelkovich DA, Shaw LK. The mortality of Ontario undertakers and a review of formaldehyde-related mortality studies. *J Occup Med* 1984;26:740–746.
34. Hayes RB, Blair A, Stewart PA, Herrick RF, Mahar H. Mortality of U.S. embalmers and funeral directors. *Am J Ind Med* 1990;18:641–652.
35. Hall A, Harrington JM, Aw TC. Mortality study of British pathologists. *Am J Ind Med* 1991;20:83–89.
36. Khamgaonkar MB, Fulare MB. Pulmonary effects of formaldehyde exposure. *Indian J Chest Dis Allied Sci* 1991;33:9–13.
37. Holness DL, Nethercott JR. Health status of funeral service workers exposed to formaldehyde. *Arch Environ Health* 1989;44:222–227.
38. Salkie ML. Allergens in the workplace. *Clin Biochem* 1994;26:81–85.
39. Wilhelmsson B, Holmstrom M. Possible mechanisms of formaldehyde-induced discomfort in the upper airways. *Scand J Work Environ Health* 1992;18:403–407.
40. Wantke F, Focke M, Hemmer W, et al. Formaldehyde and phenol exposure during an anatomy dissection course: possible source of IgE-mediated sensitization. *Allergy* 1996;51:837–841.
41. Akbar-Khanzadeh F, Vasquerano U, Akbar-Khanzadeh M, Bisesi MS. Formaldehyde exposure, acute pulmonary response, and exposure control options in a gross anatomy laboratory. *Am J Ind Med* 1994;26:61–75.
42. Levine RJ, DalCorso RD, Blunden PB, Battigelli MC. The effects of occupational exposure on the respiratory health of West Virginia morticians. *J Occup Med* 1984;26:91–98.
43. Kilburn KH, Seidman BC, Warshaw R. Neurobehavioral and respiratory symptoms of formaldehyde and xylene exposure in histology technicians. *Arch Environ Health* 1985;40:229–233.
44. Kilburn KH, Warshaw R, Boylen CT, et al. Pulmonary and neurobehavioral effects of formaldehyde exposure. *Arch Environ Health* 1985;40:254–260.
45. Clark RP. Formaldehyde in pathology departments. *J Clin Pathol* 1983;36:839–846.
46. Luce D, Gerin M, Leclerc A, et al. Sinonasal cancer and occupational exposure to formaldehyde and other substances. *Int J Cancer* 1993;53:224–231.
47. Yager JW, Cohn KL, Spear C, Fisher JM, Morse L. Sister chromatid exchanges in lymphocytes of anatomy students exposed to formaldehyde solutions. *Mutat Res* 1986;174:135–139.
48. Thomson EJ, Shackelton S, Harrington JM. Chromosomal aberrations and sister chromatid exchange frequencies in pathology staff occupationally exposed to formaldehyde. *Mutat Res* 1984;141:89–93.
49. Fleig I, Petri N, Stocker WG, Theiss AM. Cytogenic analysis of blood lymphocytes of workers exposed to formaldehyde in formaldehyde manufacturing and processing. *J Occup Med* 1982;24:1009–1012.
50. Ballarin C, Sarto F, Giacomelli L, Bartolucci GB, Clonfero E. Micronucleated cells in nasal musosa of formaldehyde-exposed workers. *Mutat Res* 1992;280:1–7.
51. Hayes RB, Klein S, Suruda A, et al. O6-Alkylguanine DNA alkyltransferase activity in student embalmers. Am J Ind Med 1997;31:361–365.
52. Titenko-Holland N, Levine AJ, Smith MT, et al. Quantification of epithelial cell micronuclei by fluorescence in situ hybridization (FSH) in mortuary science students exposed to formaldehyde. *Mutat Res* 1996;371:237–248.
53. Nunn AJ, Craigen AA, Darbyshire JH, Venables KM, Taylor AJN. Six-year follow-up of lung function in men occupationally exposed to formaldehyde. *Br J Ind Med* 1990;47:747–752.
54. Taskinen H, Kyyronen P, Hemmenki K, et al. Laboratory work and pregnancy outcome. *J Occup Med* 1994;3:331–319.
55. Mitchell F. Hazardous waste. In: Rom WN, ed. *Environmental and occupational medicine*, 2nd ed. Boston: Little, Brown, 1992:1275–1284.
56. Bruce MR, Santonodato J, Neal MW. Summary review

of the health effects associated with phenol. *Toxicol Ind Health* 1987;3:535–568.
57. Dosemeci M, Blair A, Stewart PA, Chandler J, Trush MA. Mortality among industrial workers exposed to phenol. *Epidemiology* 1991;2:188–193.
58. Langman JM. Xylene: its toxicity, measurement of exposure levels, absorption, metabolism, and clearance. *Pathology* 1994;26:301–309.
59. Riihimaki V, Savolainen K. Human exposure to m-xylene, kinetics and acute effects on the central nervous system. *Ann Occup Hyg* 1980;23:411–422.
60. Riihimaki V, Hanninen O. Xylenes. In: Snyder R, ed. *Ethyl Browning's toxicity and metabolism of industrial solvents*. Amsterdam: Elsevier, 1982:64–84.
61. Sepalainen AM, Laine A, Salmi T, Riihimaki V, Verkkala E. Changes induced by short-term xylene exposure in human evoked potentials. *Int Arch Occup Environ Health* 1989;61:443–449.
62. Savolainen K. Riihimaki V, Linnoila M. Effects of short-term xylene exposure on psychophysiological functions in man. *Int Arch Occup Environ Health* 1979; 44:201–211.
63. Savolainen K, Riihimaki V, Vaheri E, Linnoila M. Effects of xylene and alcohol on vestibular and visual functions in man. *Scand J Work Environ Health* 1980;6: 94–103.
64. Uchida Y, Nakatsuka H, Ukai H, et al. Symptoms and signs in workers exposed predominantly to xylenes. *Int Arch Occup Environ Health* 1993;64:597–605.
65. Seppalainen AM, Laine A, Salmi T, et al. Electroencephalographic findings during experimental human exposure to xylene. *Arch Environ Health* 1991;46: 16–24.
66. Dudek B, Gralewicz K. Jakubowski M, Kostrzewski P, Sokal J. Neurobehavioral effects of experimental exposure to organic solvents in house painters. *Pol J Occup Med* 1990;3:109–116.
67. Low LK, Meeks JR, Mackerer CR. Health effects of alkylbenzene, II: xylenes. *Toxicol Ind Health* 1989;5: 85–101.
68. Angerer J, Wolf H. Occupational chronic exposure to organic solvents. XI: alkylbenzene exposure of varnish workers—effects on hematopoietic system. *Int Arch Occup Environ Health* 1985;56:307–321.
69. Guzelian P, Mills S, Fallon HJ. Liver structure and function in print workers exposed to toluene. *J Occup Med* 1988;30:791–796.
70. Kurppa K, Husman K. Car painter's exposure to a mixture of organic solvents: serum activity of liver enzymes. *Scand J Work Environ Health* 1982;21:137–140.
71. IARC monograph on the evaluation of carcinogenic risk to humans. *Some industrial chemicals*. Vol 60. Lyon: IARA, 1994.
72. Beauchamp RO, St. Clair MBG, Fennel TR, et al. A critical review of the toxicology of glutaraldehyde. *Crit Rev Toxicol* 1992;22:143–174.
73. Waldron HA. Glutaraldehyde allergy in hospital workers. *Lancet* 1992;339:880.
74. Chan-Yeung M, McMurren T, Catonio-Begley F, Lam S. Occupational asthma in a technologist exposed to glutaraldehyde. *J Allergy Clin Immunol* 1993;91:974–978.
75. Hemminki K, Kyroenen P, Lindbohm M. Spontaneous abortions and malformations in the offspring of nurses exposed to anesthetic gases, cytostatic drugs, and other potential hazards in hospitals, based on registered information of outcome. *J Epidemiol Community Health* 1985;39:141–147.
76. Hemminki K, Mutanen P, Saloniemi I, Miemi ML, Vainio H. Spontaneous abortions in hospital staff engaged in sterilizing instruments with chemical agents. *Br Med J* 1982;285:1461–1463.
77. Le Leu L. Glutaraldehyde. *Med J Aust* 1992;157:356.
78. OSHA. CFR 1910.1030.
79. OSHA. CFR 1910.1200.
80. OSHA. CFR 1910.1450.
81. Centers for Disease Control and Prevention. Update: universal precautions for prevention of transmission of human immunodeficiency virus, hepatitis B virus, and other bloodborne pathogens in health care setting. *MMWR Morb Mortal Wkly Rep* 1988;36:377–382,387.
82. Centers for Disease Control and Prevention. Recommendations for prevention of HIV transmission in health care settings. *MMWR Morb Mortal Wkly Rep* 1987;36:(S2S).
83. Johnson MD, Schaffner W, Atkinson J, Pierce MA. Autopsy risk and acquisition of human immunodeficiency virus infection. *Arch Pathol Lab Med* 1997;121:64–66.
84. Lucas S. Glove punctures in the postmortem room. *J Clin Pathol* 1992;45:548.
85. Geller AS, Gerber MA. Guidelines for high-risk autopsy cases. In: Hutchins CM, ed. *Autopsy performance and reporting*. Skokie, IL: College of American Pathologists, 1990:67–75.
86. Williams TM, Levine RJ, Blunden PB. Exposure of embalmers to formaldehyde and other chemicals. *Am Ind Hyg Assoc J* 1984;45:172–176.
87. Keerfoot EJ, Mooney TF. Formaldehyde and paraformaldehyde study in funeral homes. *Am Ind Hyg J* 1975;36:533–537.
88. Moore LL, Ogrodnik EC. Occupational exposure to formaldehyde in mortuaries. *J Environ Health* 1985;49: 32–35.
89. Coleman R. Reducing the levels of formaldehyde exposure in gross anatomy laboratories. *Anat Rec* 1995;243: 531–533.
90. Wineski LE, English AW. Phenoxyethanol as a nontoxic preservative in the dissection laboratory. *Acta Anat* 1989;136:155–158.

Medical Center Occupational Health and Safety,
edited by Robert J. McCunney.
Lippincott Williams & Wilkins, Philadelphia © 1999.

23
Control of Health Hazards

Louis Joseph DiBerardinis

Environmental Medical Service, Massachusetts Institute of Technology, Cambridge, Massachusetts 02139-4307

Occupational health professionals have generally relied on the following hierarchy of control techniques to eliminate or minimize worker exposures: substitution, isolation, ventilation, work practices, personal protective clothing. The first three are sometimes called engineering controls. Usually a combination of two or more of these techniques are applied. The occupational health professional should always think of the concept of source-path-receiver. The source is the location of the generation of the contaminant. The path is the route, usually the air, that the contaminant travels after generation. The receiver is the person exposed as a result of migration of the contaminant. The primary focus should be control at the source; control of the path is second. Control at the receiver should be considered the last choice. It is likely that all or most of these control strategies will be needed. Implementation of these control techniques cannot be successful without an understanding of the particular hazards being generated and the work activities that hospital personnel need to perform. The affected hospital workers should be involved in selection of the appropriate control techniques.

CONTROL TECHNIQUES

Substitution

The principle of substitution is to eliminate or reduce a hazard by using nontoxic or less toxic materials or redesigning the task or process to eliminate escape of contaminants into the workplace. Because this is not always possible, the other controls in the hierarchy are attempted. Examples of substitution technique used in hospitals are listed in Table 23-1. Extreme care should be taken to assure that substitution does not result in a more hazardous condition. Although the focus is on the toxicity hazard, the flammable and chemical reactivity of substitutes must be considered in assessment of risk. One should not replace a toxic material with a less toxic but highly flammable one when the conditions of use will result in higher risk for fire or explosion.

Isolation

The principle of isolation is to eliminate or reduce a hazard by separating the process emitting the contaminant from the worker. This is accomplished by completely enclosing the process or locating it a safe distance away from the people. The process may have to be operated or controlled remotely. Isolation is particularly useful for jobs requiring few workers and when control by other methods is difficult. Another approach is to perform hazardous operations on off shifts when less workers may be exposed. Sometimes isolation does not eliminate exposure but reduces the number of people exposed. Examples are provided in Table 23-2.

TABLE 23-1. *Examples of substitution technique*

Substitution	Examples	Comments
Eliminate toxic chemical	Substitute aqueous based cleaner for organic based cleaner Replace chromic acid with No-Chromix or Alconox cleaner Replace mercury thermometers with digital or alcohol thermometers	May not be possible for specific activities but should be investigated first
Substitute less toxic chemical	Toluene for benzene Chlorinated anesthetics halothane, enflurane, or fluorothane for anesthetic gases such as nitrous oxide Local anesthetic for general anesthetic Replace glutaraldehyde as a sterilant with peracetic acid Nitric acid for perchloric acid for sample digestion Nonignitable solvents for xylene in scintillation fluids Ethanol or Notox for formalin as a fixative or preservative	Care must be taken to determine that the toxicity is indeed lower
Change process	Use automated staining process to replace open bench operations Use closed systems in place of open systems Use microscale techniques	Also a laboratory isolation technique
Change physical condition of raw materials	Purchase preweighed dyes	Use pellet or briquette forms of material that produce less dust
Eliminate process	Have another facility conduct the process	This does not eliminate the hazard but gives it to some one else who may be more capable of doing the process safely

Ventilation

Two types of exhaust ventilation are commonly used to minimize airborne exposure levels of contaminants. The first is called *general* or *dilution ventilation.* The second is *source control* or *local exhaust ventilation* and is discussed in detail later. These two types of exhaust ventilation should not be confused with comfort ventilation, the main purpose of which is to provide measured amounts of outdoor air for breathing and to maintain design temperature and humidity (see Chapter 24).

TABLE 23-2. *Examples of isolation techniques*

Use of glovebox or other enclosures
Placement of ethylene oxide sterilizers in separate room
Use of isolation rooms for highly infectious agents, such as *Mycobacterium tuberculosis,* or susceptible patients

Work Practices

Work practices encompass the methods workers use to perform operations and the extent to which they follow correct procedures. Examples of this control procedure are given throughout this book whenever general or specific processes are discussed. Important components of health and safety programs that facilitate the effectiveness of this technique are training and management support. It is critical that hospital workers be aware of the potential hazards of the materials and equipment they use and the proper procedures for reducing or eliminating these hazards. These procedures include proper use of laboratory ventilation and protective clothing. Management must demonstrate its commitment by providing the appropriate control equipment and enforcing the rules.

Personal Protective Equipment

Personal protective equipment is considered the last line of defense for control of worker exposure. It encompasses the use of respiratory protection and protective clothing. It is frequently used in conjunction with other control practices, particularly to minimize the effects of unexpected releases or accidents (see Chapter 25).

VENTILATION

Purpose of Ventilation

Laboratory ventilation is needed to provide an environment that is safe and comfortable. This is accomplished by providing controlled amounts of supply and exhaust air and provisions for temperature, humidity, and velocity control. *Comfort ventilation* is a means of supplying measured amounts of outdoor air for breathing and maintaining design temperature and humidity. This is sometimes referred to as general exhaust. It can be used for control of nonhazardous odors by diluting them to unobjectionable levels. *Local exhaust ventilation* is designed specifically for health and safety protection. The laboratory chemical hood (sometimes erroneously called a fume hood; it contains gases, vapors, and some aerosols in addition to fumes) is an example of local exhaust ventilation. Good laboratory local exhaust ventilation captures toxic contaminants at the source before they escape into the laboratory. It transports the contaminants out of the building through ductwork and a fan that do not contaminate other areas of the building through recirculation from discharge points to clean air inlets or creation of negative pressure in the building that subjects inactive hoods to downdrafts. A laboratory ventilation system frequently is a combination of comfort and local exhaust ventilation.

Types of Local Exhaust Ventilation

The most efficient and cost-effective form of contaminant control is local exhaust ventilation. This involves capture of the chemical contaminant at its source of generation. There are three types of local exhaust ventilation systems—enclosures, exterior hoods, and receiving hoods. The type of system selected depends on the activity to be performed, the toxicity of the materials, and the design of the facility (1).

Enclosing Hoods

An enclosing hood is a specialized form of local exhaust that totally encloses the emission source. The more complete the enclosure the more likely it is that a contaminant will be contained. Laboratory chemical hoods and biologic safety cabinets are examples of enclosing hoods because they primarily contain materials generated within the enclosures. These are the most common type of hoods in hospital laboratories. They are considered partial enclosures because one side usually is open during use. Examples of total enclosures include glove boxes, toxic gas cylinder storage cabinets, and equipment enclosures. Enclosing hoods control only the toxic materials generated within the enclosure.

Enclosures are the preferable type of hood. The design of enclosures is more art than science. The basic principle is to design a hood with the smallest opening possible. This requires input from workers regarding the access needed for the activity performed. The volume of air required usually is based on the area of all openings and maintenance of airflow velocity into the opening of 50 to 200 feet per minute (fpm) (15 to 60 meters/min). The control velocity chosen depends on the characteristics of the operation, including the temperature and the degree to which the contaminant is propelled or generated. For complex enclosures extreme care must be taken to assure the exhaust flow is evenly distributed throughout the enclosure, particularly if the openings are distributed. Many enclosure designs are evaluated experimentally and if demonstrated to be effective are included as design plates in the American Conference of Governmental Industrial Hygienists (ACGIH) industrial ventilation manual (2). Use of a totally enclosed and ventilated glove box is recommended for handling extremely hazardous materials (Fig. 23-1). Use of glove boxes min-

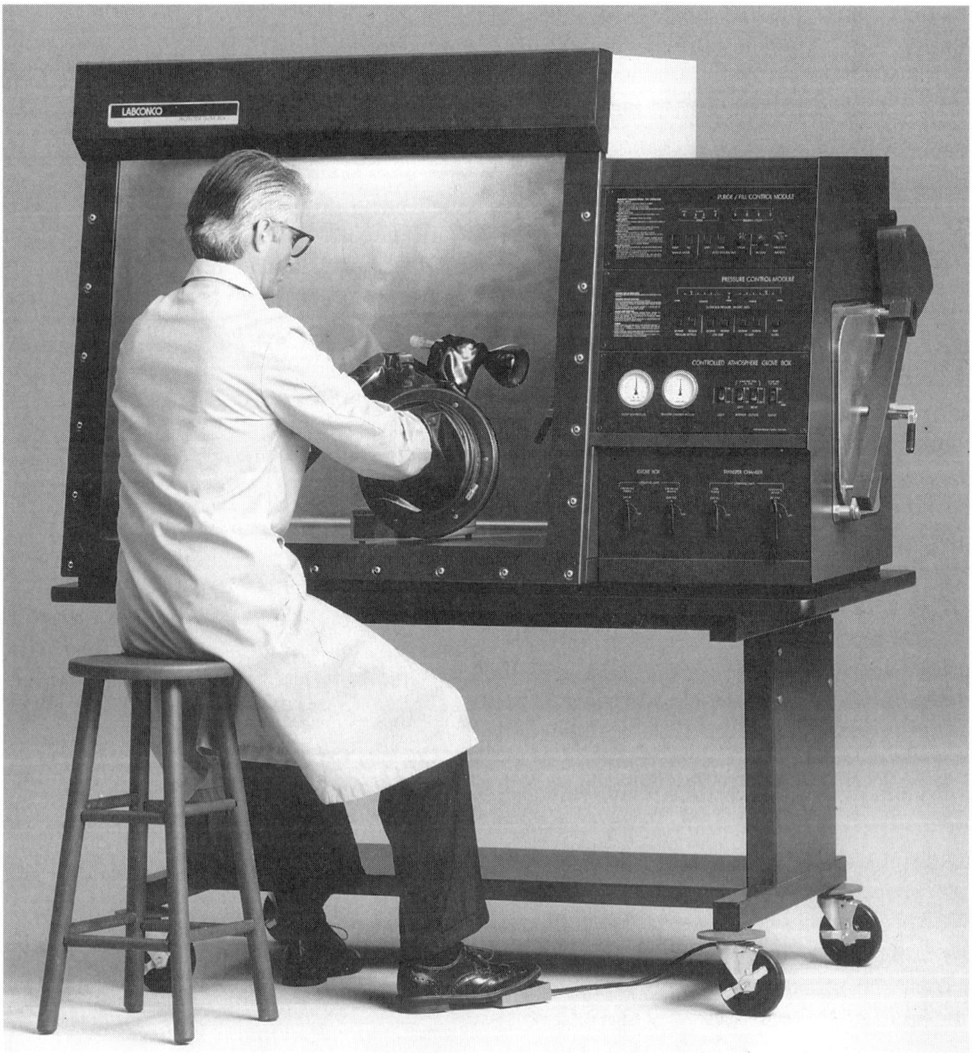

FIG. 23-1. Ventilated glove box. (Courtesy Labconco Corporation, Kansas City, MO.)

imizes air volume and simplifies air treatment for environmental protection.

Chemical Fume Hoods

Laboratory hoods, sometimes called chemical fume hoods or fume cupboards, are a form of local exhaust ventilation commonly found in laboratories that use toxic, corrosive, flammable, or malodorous substances. The purpose of a laboratory fume hood is to prevent or minimize escape of contaminants from the hood to the laboratory air and to provide containment. Successful performance depends on an adequate and uniform velocity of air moving through the hood face, commonly called *face velocity.* Hood performance is adversely affected by high-velocity drafts across the face, large thermal loads inside, bulky equipment in the hood that obstructs the exhaust slots at the rear or creates eddy currents at the opening, and poor operating procedures on the part of personnel by their failing to work 6 inches (15 cm) or more inside the hood face. With the sash closed, the hood can minimize the effects of small explosions, fires, and similar events that may occur, but it should not be depended upon to contain fires or explosions other than trivial ones. To function correctly, a chemical fume hood must be designed, installed, and operated according to well-established criteria.

A laboratory chemical hood is a laboratory worker's all-purpose safety device. It is probably the single item that most definitively characterizes a laboratory, and its importance for the safety and health protection of laboratory workers cannot be overstated. It is essential for users of laboratory hoods to understand thoroughly the functions that characterize a satisfactory laboratory hood and the several designs on the market. Not all are equally effective or efficient in utilization of airflow or in function.

Well-designed chemical hoods have the following important characteristics: (a) Uniform air velocity, i.e., the velocity at any point is less than 20% above or below the average velocity over the entire work access opening. (b) All hood surfaces surrounding the work access opening are smooth, rounded, and tapered in the direction of airflow to minimize air turbulence at the hood face. (c) Average face velocity is a minimum of 100 fpm (30 m/min) for work with any of the chemical, biologic, or radioactive materials usually encountered in university, government, and industrial research and commercial consulting laboratories. When handling substances associated with a somewhat higher hazard level, 120 fpm (36 m/min) average face velocity is recommended. Under the laboratory standard promulgated in 1990 (3), OSHA did not specify a hood face velocity, recognizing that face velocity alone may not be a good indicator of protection. Hood face velocities in excess of 120 fpm are not recommended because they cause disruptive air turbulence at the perimeter of the hood opening and in the wake of objects placed inside the work area of the hood (4–6). (d) The face velocity of hoods with an adjustable front sash is kept constant (within reasonable limits) by means of an inflow air bypass that proportions the air volume rate entering the open face to the open area or by some other method that produces a similar result. (e) An indicator is provided that continuously monitors airflow and triggers an alarm if airflow decreases more than 20% from the original design.

Standard Laboratory Chemical Hoods

Bypass Type

The basic laboratory chemical hood (Fig. 23-2) incorporates the principles that characterize a well-designed fume hood. Most laboratory furniture suppliers have one or more models that meet the criteria. Important characteristics of a bypass hood are as follows:

- Bottom and side airfoils around the open face to produce turbulence-free airflow into the hood.
- A mechanism to minimize excessive velocities (300 fpm; 90 m/min) when the total opening is 6 inches (15 cm) or less. This may be accomplished with an air bypass or by means of switching the fan to a lower speed.
- Sash constructed of shatterproof material.
- Hood constructed of material that is resistant to damage by the materials used in the hood.
- Adequate containment. This can be evaluated qualitatively by means of setting off a 30-s smoke candle or other heavy smoke generator inside the hood with the sashes fully open and then with the sashes fully closed. The smoke is totally and quickly removed, and there is no reverse flow out of the hood.
- Inward airflow across the entire opening. Reverse flow can be detected by means of passing a smoke stick or equivalent smoke generator across the entire perimeter of the face opening and looking for flow out of the hood.
- No velocity measurement across the hood face less than 80 fpm (24 m/min) or greater

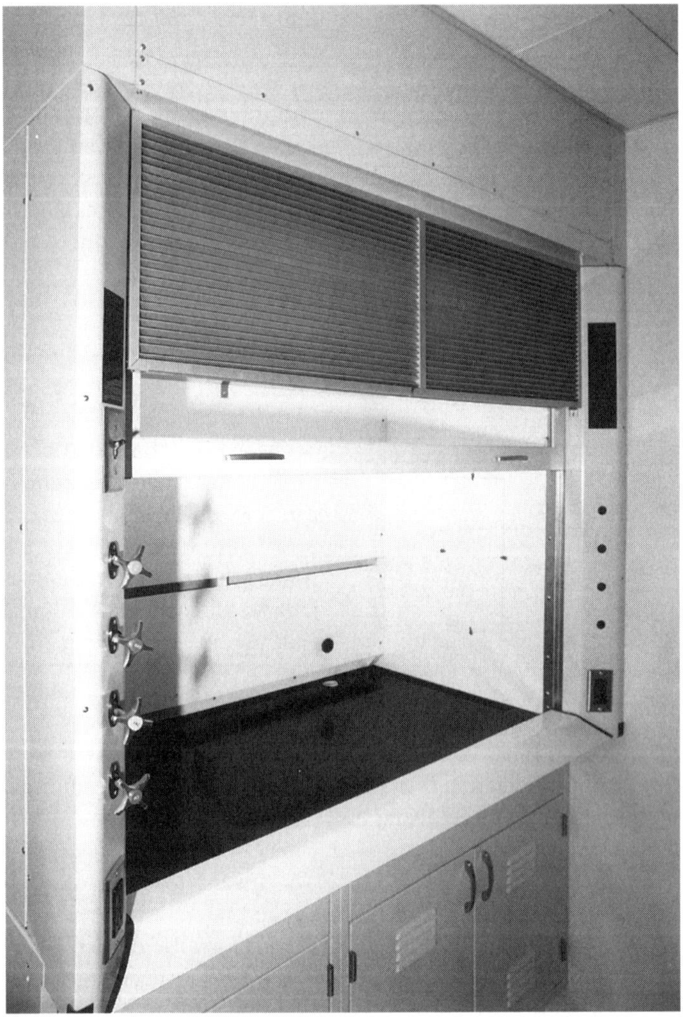

FIG. 23-2. Bypass chemical hood. (Courtesy Fisher Hamilton Industries, Inc., Two Rivers, WI.)

than 120 fpm (36 m/min) when the sashes are positioned to ensure the maximum opening.

- Airflow through the hood that provides an average face velocity of 100 fpm (30 m/min) at the maximum face opening allowed.
- Monitoring of airflow through the system with an in-line measurement device (Pitot tube, orifice meter) or by means of static pressure measurements in the duct just downstream of the hood and calibrated to the specific hood system or other equivalent means. The dial of the measurement instrument should be visible to the hood user.
- Modification of existing fume hoods during renovations, when they are to remain. This includes providing a bottom airfoil and a means of controlling face velocity at all sash positions by means of a bypass or air volume control and providing an airflow monitoring system.

Auxiliary Air Type

Auxiliary air hoods (Fig. 23-3) are a basic type of fume hood that is acceptable for laboratory use. The main difference between a standard chemical fume hood and an auxil-

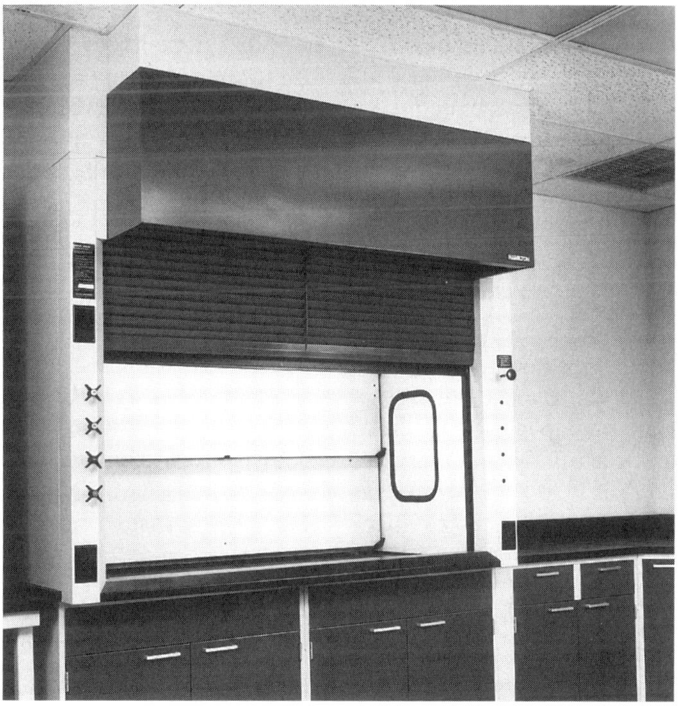

FIG. 23-3. Auxiliary air chemical hood. (Courtesy Fisher-Hamilton Industries Inc., Two Rivers, WI.)

iary air hood is the method used to provide makeup air to the hood. For standard hoods, all of the makeup air is provided by the room heating, ventilation, and air-conditioning (HVAC) system. For auxiliary air hoods, sometimes called supply air hoods, part of the air is introduced from a supply air grille just above and outside the hood face. Some manufacturers recommend up to 70% of the total hood exhaust volume be supplied in this manner with the remainder coming from the laboratory HVAC system. It is recommended that the percentage of air delivered in this manner be kept less than 60%. When auxiliary supply air is introduced behind the sash (an incorrect hood design), the hood chamber is likely to become pressurized and blow toxic contaminants out the open front into the laboratory. The only kinds of auxiliary air hoods recommended are those that introduce the auxiliary air exterior to and above the hood face.

Auxiliary air hoods have two advantages. First, the air supplied to the hood does not have to be cooled in warm climates, a substantial energy saving. Second, auxiliary air hoods can be used in laboratories that contain so many hoods that the volume of supply air, were they all standard chemical fume hoods, would result in many more room air changes per hour than are desirable. Providing auxiliary supply air, even to only some of the hoods, reduces room air velocities and supply air quantities to more acceptable levels.

There are disadvantages to the use of the auxiliary supply air hoods. First, they are more complex in design than the usual chemical fume hood, and their correct installation is more critical to safe and efficient operation. Often only a small imbalance between room air and auxiliary air supplies can result in unsafe operating conditions. Second, unsafe conditions occur when the velocity of external auxiliary air supplied to the face of the hood is excessive. High-velocity air sweeping down across an open hood face can produce a vacuum effect and draw toxic contaminants out of the hood. Third, this type of hood must have two mechanical systems (separate exhaust and supply systems) for each hood. Inasmuch as some supply air has to be added to the laboratory anyway, the auxiliary air hoods require two supply air systems instead of the one supply system required by standard chemical fume hoods.

The use of auxiliary air hoods is generally discouraged by safety and health professionals (4). When the advantages outweigh the disadvantages, auxiliary air fume hoods should be used because energy savings through reductions in summer cooling and winter heating can be realized even in moderate climates. Energy savings during the heating season occur because the auxiliary air need not be heated to as high a temperature as the comfort ventilation air. Use of auxiliary air hoods is particularly attractive for renovations when one or more fume hoods must be added to a laboratory with limited capacities of supply air. Because of the complexity of this type of hood, the performance specifications are more stringent than for standard chemical fume hoods. It is extremely important to choose an auxiliary air hood before the supply air system is designed because not all auxiliary air hoods have the same requirements for room and auxiliary air volumes; some must use less than 60% auxiliary air to meet performance requirements.

Horizontal Sliding Sash Hoods

Economy in the use of conditioned air for laboratory hoods can be achieved most satisfactorily by maintaining the required face velocity but restricting the open area of the hood face. A transparent horizontal sliding sash (Fig. 23-4) arrangement can cut overall air requirements by 50% if two half-width panels are used. Similarly, if three panels are used, the maximum open area reduction is 67% for a two-track setup and 33% for a three-track arrangement. This design has an advantage

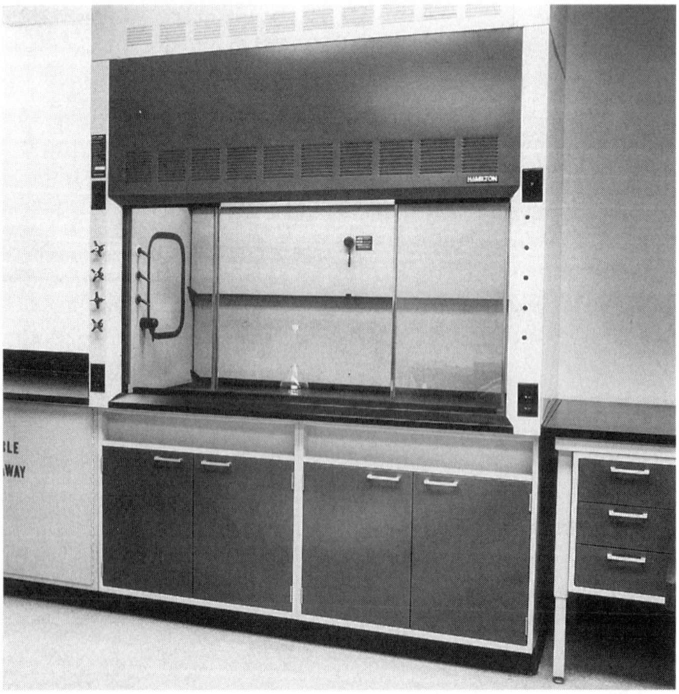

FIG. 23-4. Bypass hood with horizontal sliding sash. (Courtesy Fisher Hamilton Industries, Inc., Two Rivers, WI.)

over the conventional vertical sash because the full height of the hood opening is available. If panels 14 to 16 inches (36 to 41 cm) wide are used, they can serve as safety shields.

Under most conditions, a conventional fume hood with horizontal sliding sashes gives personnel protection equal to that of a hood with a vertical sash, provided it is designed and operated to have a minimum average face velocity of 100 fpm (30 m/min) at the maximum face opening. All velocities in the plane of the hood face should be greater than 80 fpm (24 m/min) but less than 120 fpm (36 m/min) under operating conditions. Turbulence sometimes occurs at sharp panel edges when inflow velocities exceed design values. Visual smoke trails may be used to test for inward airflow across the entire face opening and an absence of turbulence at sash edges. Removing the panels decreases face velocity and seriously compromises the safety of hood performance.

Perchloric Acid Hoods

Perchloric acid hoods require special construction, construction materials, and internal waterwash capability. Problems reported with hoods heavily used for perchloric acid digestions are associated with the consolidation of explosive organic perchlorate vapors that condense while passing through the hood exhaust system. They can detonate on contact during cleaning, modification, or repair. Therefore specially designed fume hoods are required for use with perchloric acid at elevated temperatures or in a manner that produces an aerosol. Perchloric acid hoods should meet the same contaminant fume retention capabilities as chemical fume hoods. They should be constructed of stainless steel and have welded seams throughout. No taped seams or joints and no putties or sealers can be used in the fabrication of the entire hood and duct system. Perchloric acid hoods also require an internal waterwash system to eliminate buildup of perchlorates. The waterwash system should consist of a water spray head in the rear discharge plenum of the hood and as many more as are needed to ensure complete washdown of all surfaces of the ductwork from the hood work surface to the discharge stack on the roof. To drain all of the water to the sewer in a satisfactory way during normal washdown operations, it is important that the exhaust duct go straight up through the building with no horizontal runs. A straight vertical duct run also facilitates periodic examination for maintenance purposes.

When small amounts of perchloric acid are used, it is possible to construct an air scrubber in the hood. This can be done if the point of generation of perchloric acid fumes can be identified and a small capture hood designed. The National Safety Council recommends such a system (7).

Biological Safety Cabinets

A biological safety cabinet is a special form of containment equipment used for work with cell and tissue cultures and parenteral drugs when the materials being handled must be maintained in a sterile environment and the operator must be protected from toxic chemicals and infective biologic agents. The dual functions of protecting the worker and maintaining sterility are achieved with two separate cabinet flows: turbulence-free downward flow of sterile air through a high-efficiency particulate air (HEPA) filter inside the cabinet for work protection and an inward flow of laboratory air through the work opening for worker protection. All air exhausted from biological safety cabinets is filtered through HEPA filters to provide environmental protection. The inward airflow and the downward airflow are delicately balanced in the biological safety cabinet, and great care must be exercised to maintain the design flow rate of each and the ratio between the two. Biological safety cabinets have achieved widespread use in the last two decades for recombinant DNA research and work with highly infectious agents. A more detailed discussion of biological safety cabinets is found in Chapter 6 and in Centers for Disease Control and Prevention guidelines (8).

Variable Air-volume Hoods

Variable air-volume hoods can be any one of the standard hoods discussed earlier. The main difference is that the exhaust quantity is not constant. Exhaust quantity decreases as the hood face opening decreases. This can be accomplished by means of a variety of techniques. The main advantage of this type of system is a reduced operating cost in the form of energy savings. The disadvantages relate to the relative sophistication of the control equipment, maintenance, and long-term repeatability of some control systems. Variable air-volume systems can be installed on a single hood or as part of a manifold system that exhausts multiple hoods. Some of the advantages of the variable-volume fume hood exhaust systems are as follows:

1. It reduces the number of exhaust fans in a building. With a conventional system, one or two fume hoods are connected to an exhaust fan, requiring a large number of fans depending on the facility. Combining hoods to a central system reduces the need to one or two large fans.
2. One or more central fans can be installed as a backup to provide continuous ventilation if the other fans fail. In this manner, some ventilation is guaranteed to all fume hoods at all times. With a conventional system in which one fan is installed to one fume hood, there is no ventilation in that one fume hood if the fan fails.
3. When the fume hood stacks are decreased in number they can be inexpensively increased in height. This reduces the possibility of reentrance of exhaust contaminants into the building or surrounding buildings. This is attractive in a hospital complex.
4. If a bypass damper is provided at the inlet side of exhaust fans on the roof, the air exhausted is further diluted thereby minimizing the chemical concentration of air exhausted.
5. As the number of fume hoods increases, the concentration of a particular chemical is diluted.
6. A variable-volume exhaust and makeup air system can be installed, which reduces energy utilization by varying air volume with respect to demand.

The main disadvantages of a variable air-volume system are as follows:

1. To balance the system, there are manual or automatic dampers in the exhaust system. These dampers can fail. If this happens, one or more fume hoods can be without proper exhaust for some time.
2. Although unlikely, it is possible that mixing various or different types of chemicals and products in the exhaust stream may cause an unsafe situation.
3. The control equipment used may consist of a hotwire element in a direct exhaust stream, which may be hazardous when certain chemicals are exhausted. The element also may become corroded and nonfunctional.
4. The complex nature of the control system may be beyond the capabilities of the maintenance staff.

Airflow Monitors

For safety, especially when working with hazardous materials that give no sensory warning by odor, visibility, or prompt mucous membrane irritation of their escape into the workroom from the laboratory hood, it is advisable to provide each hood with an airflow monitor capable of giving an easily observed visual display of functional status. Use of a monitor is required by the American National Standards Institute (4) and is inferred by OSHA (3). Installation of a hood airflow gage at the site of use has the special advantage of placing responsibility for day-by day monitoring of hood function with the primary users. Devices that may be used to monitor hood function include liquid-filled draft gauges or magnehelic gauges, which measure hood static pressure. Other devices measure airflow velocity in the exhaust duct where velocity is high or at some point at the side of the hood opening as a surrogate measurement of total exhaust. In all cases, the type and location of monitors should be evaluated carefully because incorrect positioning of static pressure taps can give false readings, and inline airflow devices may become clogged or corroded.

Exterior Hoods

Total enclosure of a source often is not possible or is not necessary. In these cases, another form of local exhaust, an exterior or capture hood, can be used. An exterior hood prevents release of toxic materials into the laboratory by capturing or entraining them at or close to the source of generation, usually a workstation or laboratory operation. Considerably less air volume is required than for the standard chemical hood. However, because the contaminant is generated outside the hood, it must be designed and used properly to be as effective as an enclosure.

To work effectively, the air inlet of a capture hood must be of proper geometric design and placed near the point of chemical release. The maximum distance between the hood and the source depends on the size and shape of the hood and the velocity of air needed at the generation source to capture the contaminant and bring it into the hood—the closer to the generation source the better. Design face velocities typically are 50 to 200 fpm (15 to 60 m/min) and slot velocities are 1,000 to 2,000 fpm (90 to 180 m/min). Many design guidelines exist for this class of exhaust hoods (2,9). Two types of capture hoods that find frequent application in the hospital laboratory are canopy hoods and slot hoods.

Canopy hoods are used primarily for capture of gases, vapors, and aerosols released in one direction with a velocity that can be used to aid capture. These are sometimes called receiving hoods. This type of hood is used when the process to be controlled is at elevated temperatures to make use of the thermal updraft or when emissions are directed upward by the process. Examples of operations that may be controlled include ovens, gas chromatographs, autoclaves, and atomic absorption spectrophotometers. Many equipment manufacturers recommend specific capture hood configurations that are suitable for their units. They should be consulted for advice. Design guidelines are provided in the ACGIH industrial ventilation manual (2). For example, for use of an autoclave or oven (Fig. 23-5) when the distance between the hood and the hot source does not exceed approximately the diameter of the source or 3 feet (90 cm), whichever is smaller, the hood may be considered a low canopy hood. Under such conditions, the diameter or cross section of the hot air column is approximately the same as the source. The diameter or side dimensions of the hood therefore needs to be only 1 foot (30 cm) larger than the source. The total flow rate for a circular low canopy hood is as follows:

$$Q_t = 4.7\,(D_f)^{2.33}\,(\Delta t)^{0.42}$$

where Q_t is total hood air flow in cubic feet per minute (cfm), D_f is the diameter of hood in feet, and Δt is the difference between temperature of the hood source and the ambient temperature in degrees Fahrenheit. Similar relations exist for rectangular hoods and high canopy hoods.

Slot hoods are used for control of laboratory bench operations that cannot be per-

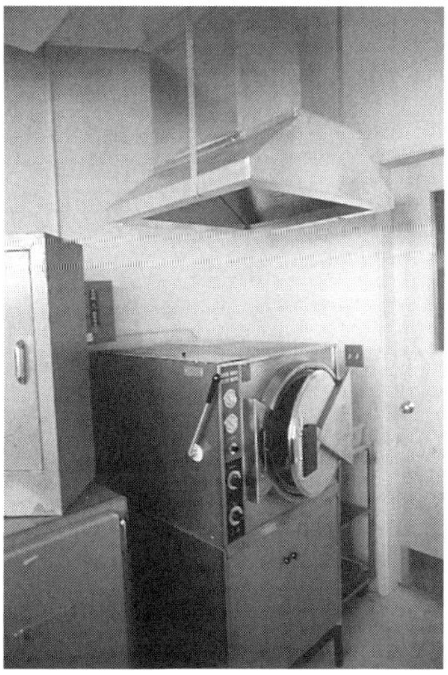

FIG. 23-5. Canopy hood.

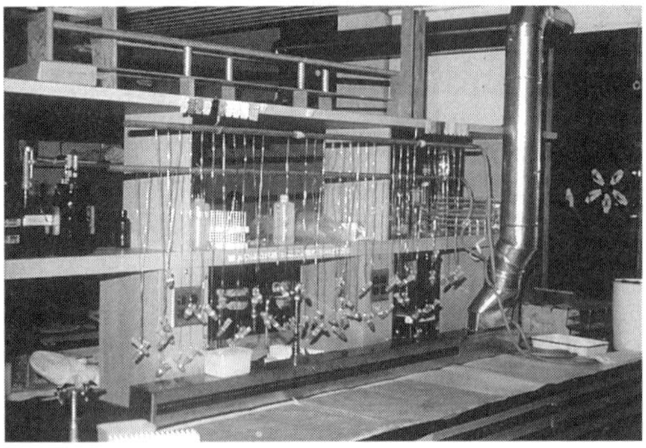

FIG. 23-6. Slot hood.

formed inside a containment hood (chemical fume hood) or under a canopy hood. Typical operations include slide preparation, microscopic examinations, preparation of biologic specimens, and chemical mixing. An example is shown in Fig. 23-6.

The required flow can be calculated from a series of equations determined empirically depending on the size and shape of the hood and the distance of the hood from the source. For example for a flanged slot hood, the flow is determined as follows:

$$Q = 3.7\ LVX$$

where Q is total hood air flow in cfm, L is the length of the slot in feet, V is the velocity needed at the source to capture it measured in fpm, and X is the distance from the source to the slot in feet. The velocity needed at the source is sometimes called capture velocity and is usually 50 to 500 fpm (15 to 150 m/min). Guidelines for selecting an appropriate capture velocity are provided in the ACGIH industrial ventilation manual (2). Some examples are given in Table 23-3. For areas with excessive cross drafts or for high-toxicity materials, the upper end of the range should be selected. For particulates, higher capture velocities are necessary.

Another laboratory operation that needs special consideration is the weighing of highly toxic materials. Because of the nature of the materials used, it is advantageous to do this in a ventilated enclosure. A chemical laboratory hood is not the best location because its relatively high airflow may disrupt the weighing process, and it is not an efficient use of ventilated space. A ventilated weighing station has been developed as part of the National Toxicology Program (Fig. 23-7). Because this is almost a full enclosure, relatively little airflow (100 to 400 cfm; 3 to 12 m^3) is needed compared with that needed for a laboratory chemical fume hood (1,000 to 1,500 cfm; 30 to 45 m^3).

Some hoods may be a combination of enclosure, exterior, and receiving hoods. For example, a grinding hood is a partial enclosure that is also a receiving hood. It is designed to provide efficient capture of particles generated by making use of the particle momentum created by the rotating grinding wheel in the direction of the hood.

Care must be used in selecting and designing local exhaust systems. Considerations should include ability to enclose the operation, source characteristics, such as point source versus widespread source and how the contaminant is generated, capacity of existing ventilation systems, space requirements, and toxicity and flammability of contaminants.

TABLE 23-3. *Range of capture velocities*

Condition of generation	Example	Capture velocity (m/s)	Capture velocity (ft/min)
Released with practically no velocity into quiet air	Evaporation from containers	0.25–0.50	50–100
Released at low velocity into moderately still air	Pouring of chemicals	0.50–1.0	100–200
Active generation into zone of rapid air motion	Spraying, vigorous mixing	1.0–2.5	200–500
Released at high initial velocity into zone at very rapid air motion	Grinding	2.5–10.0	500–2,000

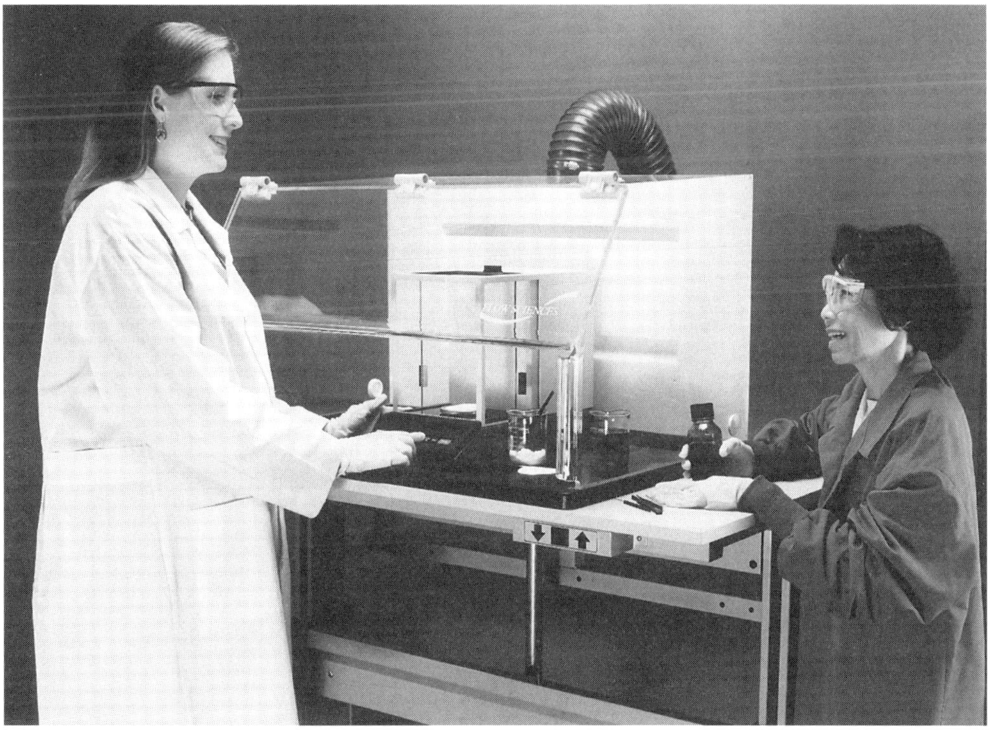

FIG. 23-7. Ventilated weighing station. (Courtesy Flow Sciences, Inc., Wilmington, NC.)

Ventilation Program

Once a hood is installed, a routine monitoring and maintenance program for the systems is implemented to assure its effectiveness in preventing exposure to workers (3). Monitoring of laboratory chemical hoods has been standardized during the last two decades (4). However, there is no standard for other forms of local exhaust; therefore users must devise their own procedures. The most effective is continuous flow monitoring. This can be done with a device as simple as a magnehelic or water pressure gage that measures static pressure at the hood. The required hood static pressure (inches of water) is known from the design calculations, and flow measurements can be made at the time of installation to verify them. Whether or not a continuous flow monitor is present, there should be periodic evaluation of the hood performance. This can be done with smoke at the hood to visualize capture and by measuring total flow in the system and comparing it with design flow. For enclosures it is usually advantageous to measure face velocity through the openings (10). Biological safety cabinets have specific testing requirements as defined by the National Sanitation Foundation (11).

Personnel must be instructed in the proper use of hoods, particularly when the distance from the source and the hood can be easily changed by the user. If local exhaust systems are designed, installed, and used properly, they can be an effective and economical means of controlling toxic exposures.

REFERENCES

1. *Guidelines for laboratory design: health and safety considerations.* New York: Wiley, 1993.
2. Committee on Industrial Ventilation, American Conference of Governmental Industrial Hygienists. *Industrial ventilation: a manual of recommended practices*, 23nd ed. Cincinnati, OH: American Conference of Governmental Industrial Hygienists, 1998.
3. US Department of Labor, Occupational Safety and Health Administration. Health and safety standard: occupational

exposure to hazardous substances in laboratories; 29 CFR 1910.1450. *Federal Register* 51:22660–22284.
4. ANSI/AIHA. Standard Z9.5: laboratory ventilation. Fairfax, VA: American Industrial Hygiene Association, 1993.
5. Chamberlin R, Leahy J. Development of quantitative containment performance tests for laboratory fume hoods. EPA contract no. 68-01-6197, June 1982.
6. Ivany R, First MW, DiBerardinis LJ. A new method for quantitative, in-use testing of laboratory fume hoods. *Am Ind Hyg J* 1989;50:275–280.
7. Controlling perchloric acid fumes, research and development section fact sheet. Chicago: National Safety Council, 1986.
8. US Department of Health and Human Services, Centers for Disease Control and Prevention, and National Institutes of Health, Biosafety in microbiological and biomedical laboratories, 3rd ed. Washington, DC: US Government Printing Office, 1993.
9. Burgess WA, Ellenbecker MJ, Treitman RD. *Ventilation for control of the work environment*. New York: Wiley, 1989.
10. Hallock MF, Martin KP, Mendes BL, et al. Development of a program for performance evaluation of university specialty local exhaust systems for compliance with OSHA laboratory standard. *Appl Occup Hyg* 1995;11:170–177.
11. National Sanitation Foundation. Standard no. 49 for class II (laminar flow) biohazard cabinetry. Ann Arbor, MI: National Sanitation Foundation, 1992.

Medical Center Occupational Health and Safety,
edited by Robert J. McCunney.
Lippincott Williams & Wilkins, Philadelphia © 1999.

24
Ventilation

Robert K. McLellan

Center for Occupational and Environmental Health at Exeter Hospital, Exeter, New Hampshire 03833

Hippocrates counseled early physicians to study the winds of a city to understand its occupants' health. In today's cultural parlance, fresh air evokes an image of health; *sick room* connotes stale air or worse. Behind the semiotics lies sound science. The germ theory of disease helped launch a variety of improvements in medical center hygiene that promoted the function of ventilation in controlling nosocomial infection. In the general community, an epidemic of building-associated health problems beginning in the 1970s prompted the phrase *tight building syndrome* and the hypothesis that poor ventilation was its cause. In the same decade, an outbreak of legionnaires' disease underscored the role of mechanical ventilation in spreading disease in mundane indoor environments. Over the last decade, the maturation of building science has elucidated the complex role of ventilation in indoor air quality. Beginning with fundamental principles and mechanics, this chapter explores the effect of general ventilation on comfort and health in medical centers.

PURPOSE AND PRINCIPLES OF GENERAL VENTILATION

Ventilation removes indoor stale air and replaces it with cleaner air. This process occurs naturally in buildings, but may be enhanced and controlled mechanically. General mechanical ventilation allows heat and humidity control, removal or dilution of a contaminant, and replacement (makeup) of air. Facility managers may use these features of mechanical ventilation to optimize the comfort and health of occupants, reduce risk for fire and explosion, and preserve building contents and structural integrity.

Natural General Ventilation

Variation in pressure across a building envelope results in air migration. When air pressure outside exceeds that inside a building, air infiltrates through incidental (cracks) and purposeful (doors, windows, ventilation louvers) breaches in the integrity of the walls. In the reverse case, positively pressurized interiors push air out through the building shell—a process known as *exfiltration* (Fig. 24-1). Similar pressure dynamics naturally operate within a building, resulting in air movement. Natural ventilation fails to control the migration of contaminants and water vapor across the building envelope.

A wide variety of factors influence building pressure dynamics. Naturally ventilated buildings usually operate under negative pressure because of the combined effects of three factors: weather effects, stack effect, and combustion air effects. Wind creates negative pressures in the lee of a building and positive pressures on the windward side. Temperature differentials between soil and building air drive infiltration through the stack effect (Fig. 24-2). The building acts like a large chimney—warm air escaping upward through vertical penetrations of the structure draws cooler

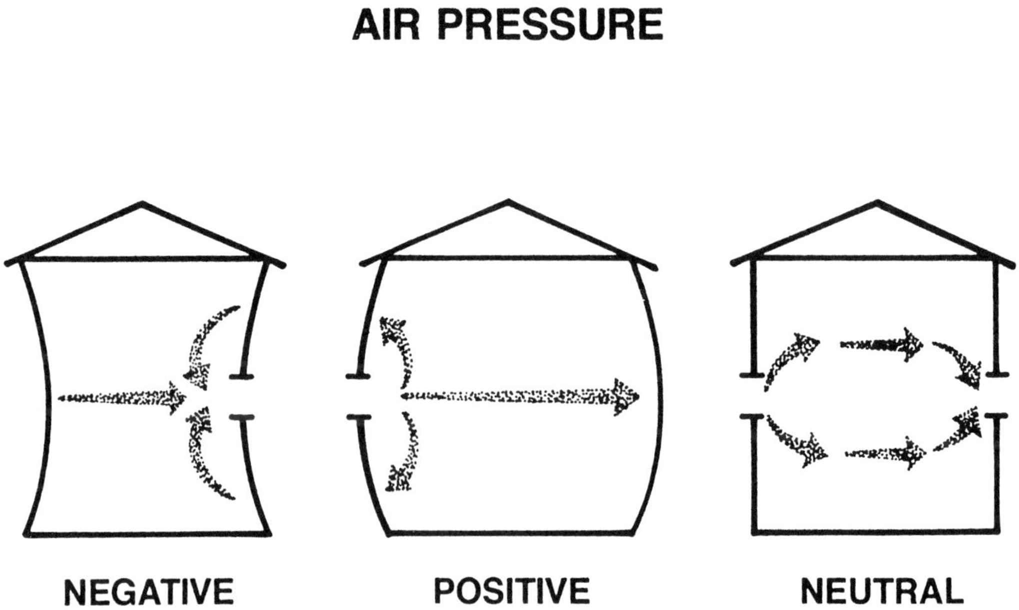

FIG. 24-1. Air pressure. (Reproduced from: Reducing Radon in Structures, Visual Aids. US Government Printing Office 1986; 716-002/60557.)

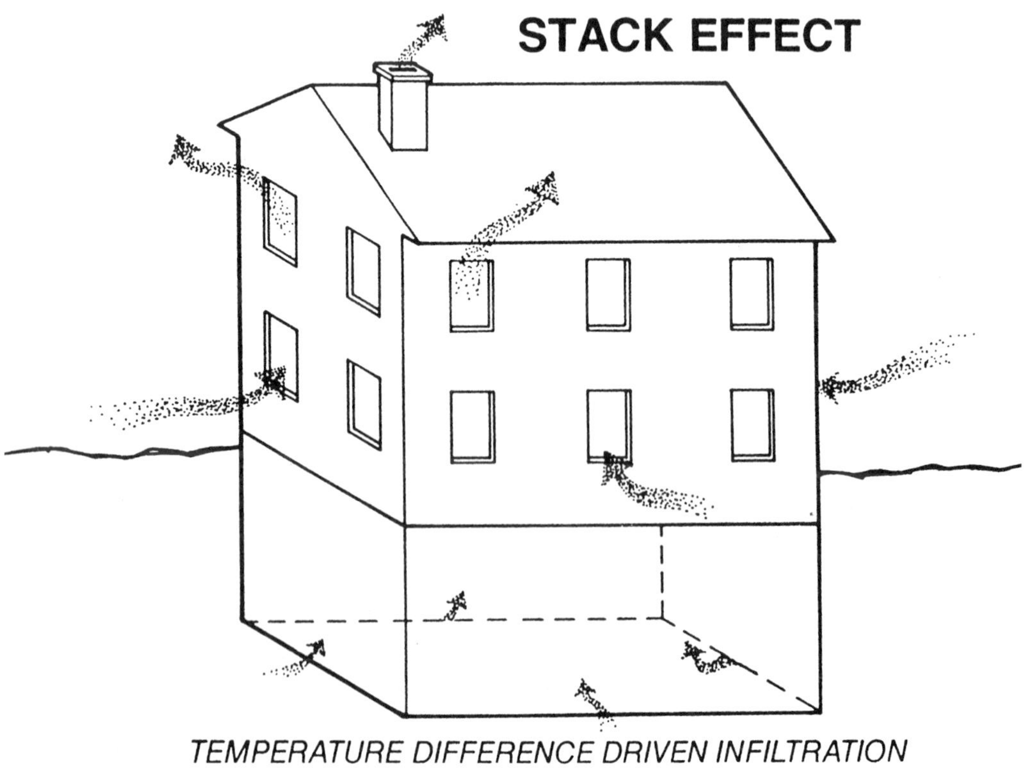

FIG. 24-2. Stack effect. (Reproduced from: Reducing Radon in Structures, Visual Aids. US Government Printing Office 1986; 716-002/60557.)

air into the bottom. As combustion devices consume air and fuel, they create negative pressures, which generate uncontrolled infiltration unless makeup air is provided (Fig. 24-3). The addition of exhaust fans produces similar effects unless engineers design for equal replacement air. Infiltration and exfiltration (uncontrolled ventilation) also occur in mechanically ventilated buildings because building envelopes are never absolutely sealed.

Mechanical Ventilation

Mechanical ventilation greatly augments opportunities for accomplishing the fundamental goals of ventilation. Engineers may control pollution at its source with local exhaust and through the dilution effects of general ventilation. Filters and other air treatment devices may be added to the system to remove contaminants. Fans pressurize or depressurize rooms or buildings depending on exhaust to makeup air ratios. For example, in a positively pressurized building, fans bring in outdoor air (makeup air) at rates that exceed exhaust rates. Building designers commonly use positive pressurization to minimize infiltration. In an isolation room designed to minimize exfiltration of bioaerosols such as the tubercle bacillus, exhaust exceeds makeup air to create a negatively pressurized room. Older systems may rely only on exhaust fans with replacement air entering the building passively. This approach increases risk for downdrafting of combustion devices and infiltration of soil gasses and water vapor. Some systems may restrict mechanical ventilation to the supply side, and risk uncontrolled exfiltration of moisture into exterior walls in cold climates. To optimally control infiltration and exfiltration of pollutants and moisture, mechanical ventilation uses fans to supply and exhaust air through designated intakes and exhausts. Architects and building engineers must use several strategies to prevent moisture accumula-

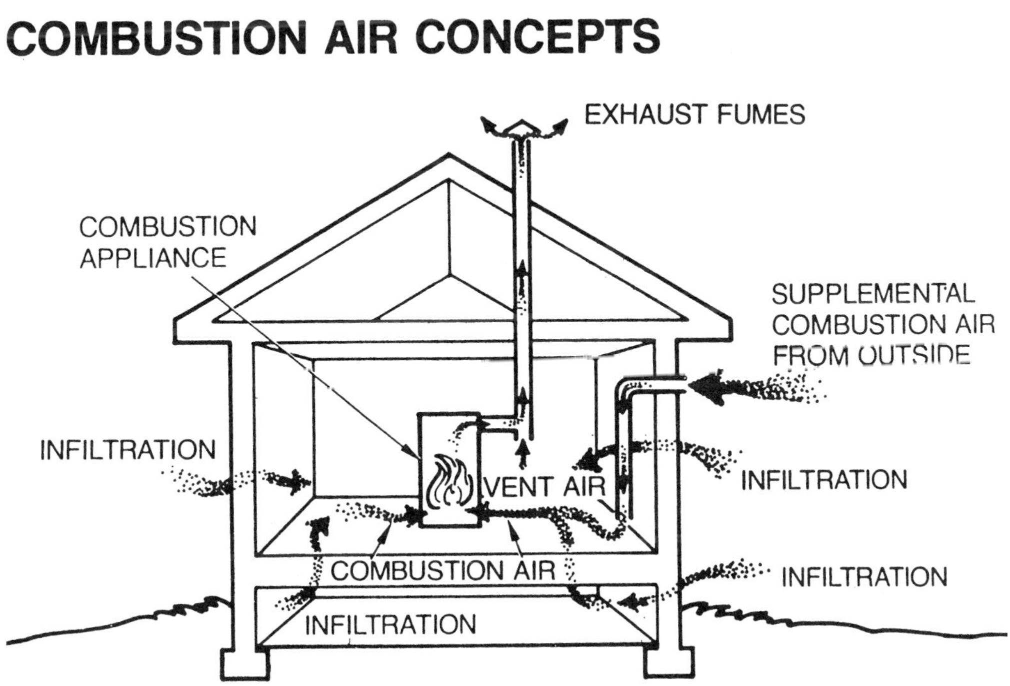

FIG. 24-3. Combustion air concepts. (Reproduced from: Reducing Radon in Structures, Visual Aids. US Government Printing Office 1986; 716-002/60557.)

tion in the building envelope as the result of uncontrolled air movement (1).

Description of Heating, Ventilation, and Air-conditioning Systems

Although a medical center may separate thermal conditioning functions from ventilation, engineers commonly design systems that combine ventilation with equipment capable of heating, cooling, humidifying, and dehumidifying air. These assemblages are known as HVAC (heating, ventilation and air-conditioning) systems. Because HVAC systems present special conditions that affect general ventilation and air quality, the configuration of a typical HVAC system is described.

Constant-volume HVAC systems deliver a constant amount of air to each space. Thermal needs are met by means of varying the temperature of the ventilation air or cycling the system on and off. Engineers usually design constant-volume systems to operate with a fixed amount of outside air or to rely on an economizer as described later. Variable air-volume systems control thermal comfort through variation in the amount of heated or cooled air provided to a space. Demand-controlled ventilation is a new approach designed to overcome the difficulties of variable air-volume and constant-volume systems in assuring adequate ventilation. In demand-controlled ventilation key parameters of indoor air quality are monitored. Exceeding contaminant concentrations, such as that of carbon dioxide, a measure of occupant-generated pollution, triggers ventilation.

The HVAC systems of large buildings such as medical centers typically consist of multiple air-handling units assigned to distinct building zones. Separating the HVAC system into zones allows better handling of varying thermal and pollution demands in different areas. Kitchens, bathrooms, operating rooms, airway procedure rooms, and isolation rooms exemplify areas with pollution sources that require special exhaust and higher ventilation rates than those of waiting rooms or offices. Thermal burdens on rooms on the building perimeter differ from those in the core. Consequently, perimeter hot water piping or independent, auxiliary devices known as fan coil or induction units commonly service perimeter rooms. These units provide additional thermal conditioning and may be designed to introduce additional outside air. Without periodic cleaning of the units, accumulated debris is redistributed into indoor air.

Outdoor intakes serve as the source of outdoor air (Fig. 24-4). Location of intakes and the quality of the outdoor air critically determine whether ventilation dilutes or increases indoor pollution. To avoid reentrainment of building contaminants, intakes should be placed where outdoor air is likely to be cleanest—away from parking garages, loading docks, and building exhausts. Typical weather patterns should help determine intake placement because winds can carry exhaust contaminants substantial distances to intakes. If outdoor air is predictably and unavoidably contaminated, it should be filtered before mixture with building air. Insect or animal screens usually cover outdoor intakes. Unless these screens are regularly cleaned, they become fouled and restrict intake of outdoor air. Because birds and other animals may frequent rooftops near outdoor air intakes, the regularity of roof cleaning may determine indoor air quality.

Outdoor air mixes with return air from occupied spaces in a confined area called a *mixing plenum.* The ratio of outdoor to recirculated air helps determine the ability of an air-handling unit to dilute indoor pollution. Mechanics can control this ratio by changing damper settings manually. In modern HVAC systems, economizers automatically control dampers in outdoor intakes and exhausts to minimize energy costs. If thermostats call for cooling and outdoor air is cooler than indoor air, the economizer opens dampers widely to benefit from the free cooling. In many climactic circumstances, however, economizers close dampers to reduce energy use to condition air. Inadequate outdoor air ventilation may occur if minimum outdoor air intake is not maintained under all conditions.

As air exits the mixing plenum it travels through filters. When chosen, installed, and

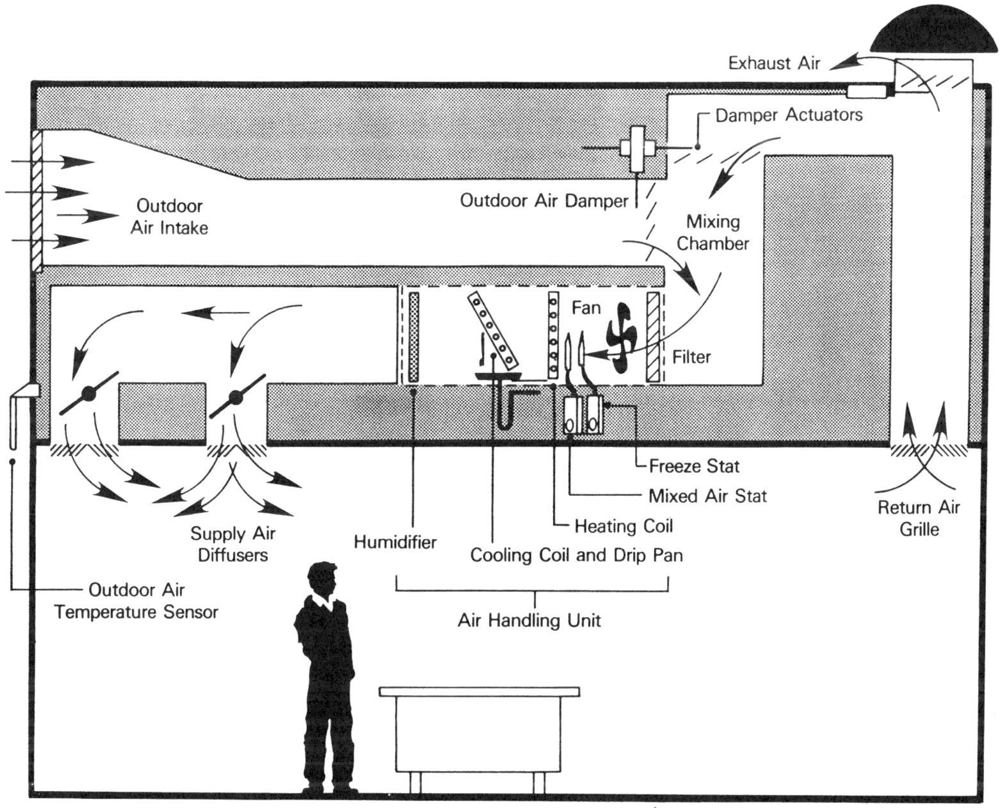

FIG. 24-4. Typical components of an HVAC system. (Reproduced from: Building Air-quality. A Guide for Building Owners and Facility Managers. EPA 400/1-91/033, DHHS (NIOSH) Publication no. 91-114, December 1991.)

maintained correctly, filters clean air before delivery to the occupied space. HVAC engineers select filters for removal of gross debris to protect the HVAC system, for removal of finer particulates that may affect health, and rarely to adsorb gaseous contaminants from the airstream. Air cleaners remove particulates mechanically or by means of electrostatic precipitation, whereas gas removal occurs through adsorption to a chemical medium, such as activated charcoal, selected specifically for particular contaminants. Because all filters become loaded over time, only regular maintenance can prevent discharge of contaminants downstream. Because even large filters designed to adsorb gasses saturate quickly, indoor air quality professionals rarely recommend filters to control gaseous indoor air contaminants.

The efficiency of a filter is its capacity to remove contaminants from air passing through it. The American Society of Heating, Refrigerating, and Air-conditioning Engineers (ASHRAE) has established two methods for testing the efficiency of air-cleaning devices (2). The ASHRAE arrestance test is generally used to rate low-efficiency filters. The dust-spot efficiency test is used to evaluate high-efficiency filters. Arrestance and dust-spot efficiency ratings are not equivalent. A 25% dust-spot efficiency filter may be adequate to protect mechanical equipment, but 90% and higher efficiencies are needed to impede the transport of the fine particles injurious to health. As filter efficiency increases, the rate of contaminant loading increases. Pressure drop across the filter increases and necessitates use of larger fans to maintain ventilation rates.

Filters may be combined and variously located in the airstream for different purposes. Coarse screens cover outdoor intakes to block insects and animals. A low-efficiency filter placed in an air-mixing plenum helps protect mechanical equipment and high-efficiency filters from gross debris. High-efficiency filters should be set downstream of humidifiers, heat exchangers, and other equipment. From the mixing plenum, air moved by fans travels through a heat exchanger, where thermal conditioning occurs by means of contact with heating and cooling coils. During warm weather, coils containing chilled liquid cool and dehumidify moisture-laden warm air. Water condenses moisture and drips to a drain pan. The condensate then drains or is pumped out of the air-handling unit. Inadequate drainage of the condensate promotes microbial growth. During heating season, hot liquid or steam flows through the coils and heats air passing by. HVAC engineers often use air-to-air heat exchangers to recover heat from exhaust air. Because the heat exchange occurs by means of passing supply air by exhaust air, use of these devices carries some risk for cross-contamination.

Located at some distance from the air-handling units, cooling towers or water chillers remove heat from fluids circulated through cooling coils. Proper operation and maintenance of this equipment reduces the risk that bioaerosols or heat exchange fluids will contaminate indoor air. Boilers reheat water used in the heating coils. Careful attention to providing adequate outdoor air for combustion, design and location of boiler stacks, and maintenance of gaskets help decrease the likelihood that combustion gasses will pollute indoor air.

After the heat exchanger, HVAC systems in medical centers in cold climates may have humidifiers. Engineers choose from two basic types of central humidification systems for commercial buildings. One type involves passing air through a screen or aerosol of cool water. Excess water recirculates back into the airstream. The water reservoir serves as a potential reservoir for amplification of microbial organisms. The other type, recommended for medical centers, involves introduction of steam into the airstream. Though free of microbial contamination itself, steam can condense in ductwork and microbial growth can occur.

Using supply fans, the air-handling unit delivers conditioned air to occupied spaces through ducts. In theory, ducts can convey all outdoor air processed by the air-handling unit to building occupants. However, ducts are not airtight, and resistance to air flow may be caused by long and tortuous runs. As a result, air may not be fully or equally distributed. HVAC designers may insulate ducts to dampen vibration noise and reduce energy costs. Manufactured mineral fiber duct lining may degrade, and fibers are released into the airstream. Duct insulation may become wet and serve as a reservoir for microbes. Duct lining may emit chemicals used for its manufacture or for suppression of microbial growth or physical degradation. Air distribution may occur through elements of the building structure such as pressurized supply air plenums above false ceilings.

Terminal devices control the distribution and collection of air within an occupied space. Incorrect placement of supply diffusers and return grilles leads to incomplete room air mixing, which may substantially degrade ventilation effectiveness. Without careful attention to the location of terminal devices, installation of partitions and other furniture after HVAC commissioning may seriously impair air mixing. Tampering with diffuser controls by occupants dissatisfied with air flow commonly produces an imbalance in airflow distribution to adjacent areas.

When air exits occupied spaces through return grilles, it is either exhausted or reconditioned in the air-handling unit for recirculation. Air may first pass through a common return plenum above suspended ceilings or directly through return ducts. Some HVAC systems have fans to assist air return. When agitated by the vibration of HVAC machinery or human activities, particulates in the return plenum may shower the occupied space.

Building codes require dedicated passive or mechanically assisted exhaust of rooms with intense contaminant sources, such as bathrooms. Chapter 23 describes the critical role of localized exhaust in controlling the many hazards associated with the specialized activities of a medical center.

A variety of manual and automatic controls regulate the performance of an HVAC system. Proper placement, calibration, and maintenance of all controls are needed to assure optimal performance of equipment. In practice, facility managers balance ventilation requirements with energy costs. Costs can be reduced through devices that recapture energy, variable speed fans, variable air-volume controls, and scheduling of ventilation on the basis of building occupancy and circadian and weekly activity fluctuations. Facility managers scheduling HVAC operation with reference only to occupancy may not ventilate appropriately for nonoccupant sources of indoor pollution. Because a variable air-volume system links its operation with thermal demands, ventilation may be inadequate to control indoor air pollution unless the system guarantees a minimum outside air ventilation.

SPECIAL CHARACTERISTICS OF MEDICAL FACILITIES

The characteristics of medical facilities place special demands on ventilation to control indoor air quality. The activities and occupants of medical centers differ substantially from those of residential and most public buildings. With ages ranging from neonate to elderly and a diversity of disease, patients and staff represent the entire spectrum of susceptibility to indoor contaminants. Staff, though generally healthy, come from a broad socioeconomic spectrum and perform widely varying tasks. In addition to health status, demographic features, personal lifestyle, and job control factors influence building-related complaint rates (3–6).

The multiplicity of hazardous processes and materials housed in medical centers complicates ventilation requirements. Diagnostic and treatment procedures vary widely in generating indoor pollution. Urgent care outpatient settings stand in stark contrast to the airborne hazards generated in operating rooms, animal facilities, laboratories, and procedure rooms where bronchoscopy or administration of pentamidine may generate intense showers of bioaerosols. Patients with compromised immune function need special protection from airborne infectious agents. The pungent odors of disease and uncontrolled excretion require attention. Facilities must provide appropriate ventilation for chemical storage, public access spaces, areas for storage, preparation and eating of food, and office suites. To avoid cross contamination between different areas, engineers must in many cases provide distinct ventilation systems.

As health care institutions struggle to keep up with changing social and economic realities, their managers remodel and transform buildings for new uses. These times of transition in a building usually generate intense pollution loads that demand specific ventilation approaches (7). Changing use and configuration of rooms demands reassessment of ventilation needs. Unfortunately, contemporary health care budgetary restrictions place more pressure on facility managers to cut expenses. Historically, ventilation has suffered despite well-supported arguments that question this economic wisdom (8). As health care organizations, modern medical centers arguably have a special role in the community as model healthy environments. Front page attention to epidemics of building-associated illnesses in health care centers adds a public relations nightmare to the inherent disruptions caused by these epidemics.

VENTILATION GUIDELINES: HISTORICAL PERSPECTIVE

Well before the germ theory of disease, the sixteenth century French surgeon Paré attributed military wound infections to noxious battlefield air. Medieval Europeans used incense and garlic to prevent the spread of the plague. In later years, the popular opinion arose that drafts of fresh air caused illness. With Koch's discovery of the tubercle bacillus, however, emerged the association of contagion with overcrowded housing (9). On the basis of this discovery, nineteenth century ventilation experts made recommendations that large amounts of outdoor air could help dilute infectious agents. In 1895, the newly formed American Society of Heating and Ventilation Engineers promulgated a guideline of 30 cubic feet per minute (cfm) of outside air per occupant to dilute contagion and thereby lower risk for diseases such as tuberculosis. At the same time, some health professionals recommended ventilation rates as high as 60 cubic feet per minute per person (cfm/p) (10).

As the twentieth century unfolded, ventilation recommendations were tied to varying degrees of concern about comfort, building-associated illness, tobacco smoke, and energy costs. In the 1930s, the research of Yaglou concluded that 10 to 30 cfm of outdoor air per occupant was necessary to control odor annoyance related to human bioeffluents (11). With the discovery that thermal conditions greatly affect occupant comfort and the advent of air-conditioning, outdoor air requirements of 10 to 15 cfm/p were typically recommended. In the context of the energy concerns precipitated by the 1975 Arab oil embargo, ASHRAE lowered recommended minimum rates to as little as 5 cfm/p of outdoor air. Designed to protect occupants from exposure to carbon dioxide concentrations exceeding the Occupational Safety and Health Administration (OSHA) standard, this recommendation downplayed concerns about other bioeffluents and tobacco smoke (12). Partially correcting this error, ASHRAE standard 62-1981 raised minimum outdoor air ventilation rates to 20 cfm per occupant in spaces where smoking was permitted (13). This standard also allowed engineers to conserve energy by providing less outdoor air as long as levels of indoor pollutants were maintained below specified thresholds (the air quality procedure). Practical difficulties in differentiating nonsmoking from smoking-permitted areas along with controversy over the formaldehyde guideline led to a revised standard (14).

CURRENT GUIDELINES AND LAWS

ASHRAE standard 62-1989 sets the current foundation for the design, operation, and performance of mechanical general ventilation (15). It specifies "minimum ventilation rates and indoor air quality that will be acceptable to human occupants and are intended to avoid adverse health effects." By convention and empirical practicality, ASHRAE has defined acceptable air quality as that which satisfies at least 80% of exposed people and which contains no contaminants at harmful concentrations. The standard retains the two procedures for ventilation design previously promulgated—the ventilation rate procedure that prescribes minimum ventilation rates or the alternative air-quality procedure described earlier. As before, recommended ventilation rates depend on occupant density, a minimum of 20 cfm per occupant of office space. As the population of a room increases, ventilation rates per square foot increase. The standard specifies different ventilation rates for areas with uses differing from the usual office. Rates per person recommended for areas unique to medical centers include 25 cfm/p for patient rooms; 15 cfm/p for medical procedure areas, physical therapy departments, intensive care units, and recovery rooms; and 30 cfm/p for operating rooms. With the ASHRAE recommended minimum ventilation rates it is assumed that there are no unusual sources of contaminants and that all outdoor air supplied reaches and mixes well with the air of the occupied zone. It also is assumed that intense point sources, such as bathrooms, are directly exhausted outdoors.

ASHRAE and other organizations address special ventilation requirements of other hazardous areas, such as research laboratories (16,17). Animal laboratories, for example, require a variety of stringent ventilation controls and procedures to protect the health of both humans and animals. ASHRAE recommends minimum general ventilation rates between 10 to 15 air changes per hour and that an animal facility not recirculate its air. Ventilation of animal laboratories must prohibit migration of air to other parts of a medical center. Laboratory designers must provide temperature and humidity conditions appropriate for the specific animal species.

ASHRAE standard 62-1989 responds to the threat of outdoor air pollution. If outdoor air does not conform to local outdoor air standards and thresholds set by ASHRAE for indoor air contaminants, it must be treated before being mixed with recirculated air. The 1989 standard recognizes that operating conditions may vary from design specifications. To avoid this risk, it requires documentation for system operation and design. In 1989, ASHRAE published a separate guideline for the commissioning of HVAC systems (18).

To reduce the risk that excessive moisture will amplify biologic contamination, the ventilation standard calls for maintenance of humidity in habitable spaces between 30% and 60%. These recommendations dovetail with ASHRAE standard 55-1981, which provides an envelope for indoor thermal comfort under varying climactic conditions (19). Standard 55, revised in 1992, identifies values for temperature, humidity and air movement that will satisfy 80% or more of building inhabitants (20).

In 1996, ASHRAE released a long-awaited revised ventilation standard for public comment (21). Ongoing controversy regarding some of its provisions continues to delay promulgation of a new standard. To overcome some of these concerns, ASHRAE decided to divide the proposed revision into two separate standards. One committee is preparing a standard that will address all buildings except low-rise residential buildings. The standards committee authorized a second project committee to revise portions of standard 62-1989 that relate to low-rise residential buildings.

Besides ASHRAE, a number of other organizations have established nonregulatory guidelines and standards relevant and in some cases specific to the HVAC systems of medical centers (22–24). Many of these standards have been adopted by local jurisdictions as building codes and thereby acquire the force of law. Some states have promulagated indoor air quality laws that address ventilation. The National Fire Protection Association 99 standard for health care facilities sets ventilation criteria to minimize the hazards of fire, explosion, and electricity in health care facilities (17). OSHA standards and National Institute of Occupational Safety and Health (NIOSH) recommendations prescribe ventilation as a method for the control of specific hazards in health care centers, such as tuberculosis, ethylene oxide or anesthetic agents. Although OSHA has as yet to issue a standard on indoor air, it can issue citations under the general duty clause with reference to ventilation recommendations of recognized authoritative organizations. OSHA has published a proposed standard that goes well beyond ventilation design by addressing HVAC operation, maintenance, and effectiveness (25).

With ASHRAE standard 62-1989 as a reference point, the American Institute of Architects (AIA) has published ventilation requirements for areas that affect patient care in hospitals and outpatient facilities. The published ventilation rates are meant to offer asepsis, odor control, and comfort. The guides allow lowering rates to zero when a room is unoccupied and ventilation is not otherwise needed. The AIA also addresses other aspects of HVAC systems, such as filtration, humidification, and location of outdoor air intakes, room air supply diffusers, and returns. Two filter beds are required for any ventilation air supplied to patient care areas with a minimum prefilter of 25% and second filter of 90% dust-spot efficiency. The guidelines recommend a minimum of one filter bed of 25% efficiency for HVAC systems servicing administrative areas. The AIA prohibits reservoir spray–type central humidifiers and sets placement of humidifiers in the HVAC system as to prevent water droplets from reaching filters and supply duct takeoffs. The guides mention the need for education of operators and proper commissioning of the HVAC system before occupying the area served. The guidelines apply to construction and equipment, not to operation and maintenance.

ASSESSING VENTILATION

With respect to indoor air quality, evaluation of a ventilation system should answer two questions: Is sufficient outdoor air supplied to the building occupants? What is the quality of the air delivered? The assessment relies on three tools—review of design, maintenance, and operation documentation; visual examination; and analytic measurements. Cost effectiveness and accuracy necessitate a phased approach. Ventilation measurements should follow a thorough history and physical inspection of the HVAC system and be taken only when they will add useful information. A number of checklists have been published for HVAC evaluation that aid a comprehensive investigation of the following issues (1,26, 27):

1. Has the ventilation system been adequately designed for the current building configuration, occupant density, and use?
2. Is HVAC operation scheduled appropriately?
3. Has the HVAC system been constructed as designed?
4. Has the HVAC system been commissioned, operated, and maintained correctly?
5. Does the HVAC system function as designed with respect to thermal comfort, air supply, and ventilation effectiveness (air mixing)?
6. Are potent pollution sources present that were not anticipated by the engineers who designed the ventilation?
7. Does the outdoor air intentionally drawn into the building conform with air quality acceptability?
8. Does the air infiltrating into the building conform with air quality acceptability?
9. Is the HVAC system hygienic?
10. Does the ventilation satisfy at least 80% of the building occupants?

Assessment begins with a review of building blueprints and ventilation design specifications for comparison with ASHRAE standards, the AIA guide, and other relevant codes. Natural and mechanical ventilation are considered. Remodeling and other building interventions may lead to new ventilation designs that should be studied. More commonly, the investigator finds that ventilation has not been redesigned as building modifications have been made, frequently creating problems. If the system does not run continuously, does the design adequately anticipate changing pollution loads related to the people and the building? Reference to local ambient outdoor air pollution monitoring data helps ascertain the quality of outdoor air supplied by the ventilation system.

Physical inspection of the HVAC system consists of visualization of the complete pathway of building air beginning with the condition of outdoor air intakes and their proximity to point sources of pollution, through air-handling units, filters, heat exchange units, ductwork, and supply diffusers. The examiner looks for incorrectly sized, wrongly installed, poorly maintained, missing, or malfunctioning equipment. Because degradation or biologic contamination of ductwork lining is common, its presence and condition are documented. Investigators particularly attend to possible biologic reservoirs—areas where moisture collects by design or accident, such as condensate trays, spray cooling units, humidifiers, and ductwork. HVAC configuration often impedes this inspection. At times the investigator uses fiberoptic scopes to see areas such as duct interiors that cannot otherwise be examined. Location of supply diffusers with respect to air returns provides insight into the effectiveness of ventilation. Improper placement leads to short circuiting and inadequate mixing of recirculated air. Examiners look for sources of contaminants in the occupied space and record whether the contaminants are exhausted or recirculated. Because unintentional passive infiltration often occurs, the investigation includes a survey of penetrations of the building envelope (windows, doors, loading docks) and their proximity to pollution sources. Smoke from a smoke stick held at an opening provides a rough test for passive infiltration by traveling in the direction of the air stream.

Because of ventilation inefficiencies, simple tests of the amount of air drawn into outdoor intakes do not indicate the volume of air supplied to occupants. A wide variety of analytical measurements can help in assessment of the adequacy of ventilation (28–30). Three basic methods are used to ascertain whether adequate outdoor air is being supplied to the occupied space: measurement of carbon dioxide, monitoring the decay of a tracer gas such as sulfur hexafluoride or carbon dioxide, and calculations based on measurements of supply air quantity and a determination of percentage of outdoor air in the supply air.

As an inexpensive and robust method for assessing the adequacy of outdoor air supply for human occupancy, the principles of carbon dioxide monitoring are described. The technique depends on the relation between the generation of carbon dioxide through respiration, occupant density, and the ability of ventilation to dilute this contaminant with outdoor air. Carbon dioxide levels in a building vary with outdoor air supply and changes in occupancy and time required to achieve equilibrium. At equilibrium carbon dioxide levels can be used directly to calculate outdoor air supply as explained in ASHRAE standard 62-1989.

The interpretation of carbon dioxide levels obtained at a single point in time must reflect circadian occupancy trends. Multiple measurement locations and continuous recording of carbon dioxide offers the opportunity to assess effects of variation in population density by time and location, HVAC operation, and combustion sources. Comparison of carbon dioxide in return air with occupied space air can help assess adequacy of ventilation mixing. With good mixing the carbon dioxide concentrations in the two locations closely match. With poor mixing, the amount of carbon dioxide in the return air is lower than the average found in the occupied zones. Additional testing to rule out infiltration of outdoor air directly into the return air plenum is needed to confirm the hypothesis of poor ventilation effectiveness.

Outdoor air carbon dioxide levels are normally about 370 ppm. The current ASHRAE standard is 1,000 ppm. As indoor carbon dioxide levels rise above 800 ppm, the likelihood of building-associated health complaints increases. Carbon dioxide itself is not toxic in this range (the OSHA Standard is 5,000 ppm), but the level of carbon dioxide serves as an index of the adequacy of ventilation. Interpretation of carbon dioxide levels is complex because of the need to account for possible changing occupancy, time to reach equilibrium, and effects of variable air-volume systems, which provide ventilation air on thermal demands. Carbon dioxide generation rates tend to parallel rates of generation of other human bioeffluents, but not of contaminants generated by the building and its inanimate contents. Therefore a normal carbon dioxide level should not be used as a sole indicator of adequate ventilation.

COMMON VENTILATION PROBLEMS

Ventilation can improve or degrade indoor air depending on its configuration, operation, and maintenance. Investigators of problem buildings frequently find ventilation deficiencies (Table 24-1). NIOSH investigators collated the results of hundreds of building investigations conducted since 1971. The earliest reports identified ventilation problems in about 50% of the structures (31,32). More recently NIOSH has reported the results of more systematic evaluations of 104 problem office buildings (33). About 90% had at least one recommendation concerning deficiencies in HVAC design, operation, or maintenance. The most common difficulties included inadequacies in HVAC design, maintenance, and operation.

Comparison of HVAC design plans with applicable standards may quickly clarify ventilation inadequacies. Unless provision for a constant minimum ventilation has been made,

TABLE 24-1. *Common ventilation problems*

- Design
  - Documentation not available
  - Ventilation design inadequate for occupant density
  - General ventilation design inadequate to control occupant activities or point sources of pollution
  - Local exhaust not used to control intense pollution sources
  - Ventilation not redesigned to accommodate remodeling, changes in occupant density, or use of occupied space
  - Improper placement of outdoor intakes allowing entrainment of contaminants from point pollution sources or reentrainment of building exhaust air
  - Inadequate filters
  - Improperly placed supply and return air ducts leading to decreased ventilation effectiveness
- Construction
  - Ventilation not built as designed
  - Incorrectly pitched condensate pans, improperly placed humidifiers, building structural or plumbing problems that allow moisture build-up
- Commissioning
  - Space occupied before commissioning completed
  - ASHRAE guidelines (57) for commissioning not followed
- Maintenance
  - Malfunctioning or blocked outdoor intakes
  - Loaded, poorly maintained filters
  - Moisture accumulation due to building or plumbing leaks, humidification system problems, inadequate drainage of condensate
  - Microbial contamination of AHU or ductwork due to moisture accumulation
  - Debris in AHU, ductwork, fan coil, and induction units
  - Improperly balanced air supply system
  - Malfunctioning equipment and controls
  - Degrading duct lining
  - Inadequate or improper treatment of cooling tower water with biocides and scale and corrosion inhibitors
  - Inadequate training of maintenance personnel
- Operation
  - Incorrectly scheduled ventilation operation
  - Variable air-volume systems inadequately ventilating when thermal demands are low
  - Inadequate training of operators
  - Occupant tampering with controls, supply diffusers
- Building Activities
  - Failure to protect air returns during remodeling, extermination, hazardous materials incidents, or other polluting activities
  - Failure to schedule building maintenance and construction at times of least occupant density
  - Failure to choose least polluting consumer products
  - Failure to choose least polluting consumer products
  - Change in building activities without reassessment of ventilation needs

ASHRAE, American Society of Heating, Refrigerating and Air-conditioning Engineers; AHU, air-handling unit.

variable air-volume systems risk inadequate ventilation. Placement of outdoor air intakes near pollution sources means that outside air contaminates rather than improves indoor air quality. Ventilation effectiveness may decline substantially when return and supply air diffusers too closely approximate each other. A glance at HVAC design specifications may reveal that the system was not reconfigured with changes in occupant density, remodeling, or division of common office space with partial partitions.

An HVAC engineer's vision for a building may not have been realized. Contractors may loosely interpret ventilation blueprints or frankly botch construction and installation. Construction funds may run low, and ventilation may be shortchanged. Architects or on-site supervisors may make structural changes from original drawings without consulting the HVAC engineer.

The commissioning of an HVAC system tests its mechanics and allows an opportunity to correct problems before people begin using a space. Seemingly inevitable construction delays may put pressure on facility managers to occupy a space before adequate commissioning. As a result ventilation may not function as designed as a new area is occupied. With new construction or extensive remodeling, special ventilation provisions may not have been made to protect ductwork from contamination with construction debris. Facility managers may not have made provisions to use temporary exhaust fans or provide 100% outside air to wash out volatile organic chemicals emitted from new products.

Insufficient preventive maintenance ruins the potential of the best ventilation system. Worse, a contaminated mechanical ventilation system excels at delivering pathogenic substances to the breathing zone. When occupant complaints multiply as ventilation rates increase, HVAC contamination is the suspect. Manipulation of dirty ductwork, filters, and air-handling units can generate showers of bioaerosols and other particulates. Ventilation debris also may serve as sinks and sources for volatile organic chemicals.

Poorly trained operators or building occupants fiddling with controls or blocking supply air diffusers and outdoor intakes may defeat the effectiveness of a ventilation system. Misguided attempts to save energy by minimizing HVAC operation lead to inadequate ventilation. If ventilation is shut down while a space is unoccupied, indoor pollutants from building sources may accumulate and cause uncomfortable or even hazardous exposures for people who reoccupy the space.

Building activities may contaminate HVAC systems, which can then redistribute these pollutants to other occupied spaces. Hazardous materials incidents, renovations, and other processes that generate substantial air pollution may expose large numbers of people to hazards because of lack of attention to special ventilation requirements during these operations. These requirements may include negative pressurization and 100% exhaust of air from the work area, attention to air movement through common return air plenums, and at a minimum sealing air returns.

Specific activities, such as photocopying, and variations in occupant density in combination with incomplete air mixing lead to multiple microenvironments in a building (34). The same ventilation system may provide different levels of satisfaction within a common space because of these variations.

INTERACTION OF GENERAL VENTILATION AND HEALTH

Ventilation problems commonly lead the list of specific findings during building environmental audits, but to what extent can poor ventilation be correlated with occupant health concerns? Research to answer this question has taken three approaches. First, cross-sectional surveys have identified characteristics of building ventilation that correlate with complaints. Second, experimenters have tracked changes in occupant complaints with manipulation of ventilation rates. Third, investigators have linked epidemics to specific indoor air contaminants.

Authorities have conventionally divided building-associated health complaints into two broad categories, sick-building syndrome and building-related illnesses. Sick-building syndrome describes a panoply of transient, nonspecific symptoms precipitated by entering a particular building and relieved by leaving it. Causes of sick-building syndrome remain speculative but are probably multifactorial. Popular theories have linked thermal variables, the presence of bioaerosols and particulates, total volatile organic chemical levels, noise, lighting, ergonomics, personal factors, work organization, and ventilation rates to sick-building syndrome (35,36). Building-related illnesses have defined pathophysiologic characteristics frequently attributable to a specific building contaminant. Though they may occur in isolation, building-related illnesses frequently occur in the context of an epidemic of sick-building syndrome; this suggests an etiologic relation (32).

By design, ventilation systems aim to provide a comfortable and clean indoor air environment. Bowing to practical experience, however, ASHRAE air quality standards anticipate that as many as 20% of a building's occupants are not satisfied by a system built and operated to standard. Occupant complaints are pandemic. Epidemiologic research on both sides of the Atlantic has consistently documented that symptom reports in buildings vary considerably but invariably exceed 20% (34). At the extreme, a British study of 4,373 office workers in 42 office buildings found that 80% of the occupants had at least one building-related symptom (37).

Field and experimental research provides a rationale for prescriptive minimum ventilation rates. Laboratory manipulation of ventilation rates in experimental chambers occupied by volunteers has consistently supported the relation between ventilation and human comfort (38). Several field studies have associated ventilation rates and other characteristics of HVAC systems with nonspecific health problems. A metaanalysis of this literature indicated that sealed, mechanically ventilated, humidified, and air-conditioned buildings are more likely to generate complaints than naturally ventilated buildings (39). Both cross-sectional and experimental studies have specifically assessed the relation between outdoor air ventilation rates and occupant symptoms (40–43). In reported research, the ability of increasing mean ventilation rates to control occupant symptoms reaches an asymptote at 21 cfm/p. Higher rates had little added benefit. At lower rates, studies found increased symptom prevalence. By contrast, in a well-controlled, double-blind, multiple cross-over study, Jaakkola et al. (42) found no significant differences in symptom prevalence between ventilation rates of 13 and 42 cfm/p of outside air. Differences in study methods confound attempts to draw simple conclusions from the reported investigations. Inexact measurement of outdoor air ventilation leads to possible misclassification. Classifying buildings on the basis of mean ventilation rates neglects the effect of local variations in ventilation. Differences in indoor pollution sources within and between buildings further complicate simple assessment of mean ventilation rates and symptoms.

The premise that ventilation can decrease the number of complaints about indoor air quality rests on the theory that ventilation with clean outdoor air dilutes indoor air pollution. ASHRAE standard 62-1989 offers the indoor air quality procedure as an alternative approach to its prescriptive ventilation rates (44). Using this option, HVAC engineers calculate ventilation requirements to achieve an acceptable level of exposure as defined by a variety of standard-setting organizations.

Although questions remain about the relation between outdoor air ventilation rates and building occupant complaints, HVAC problems have been linked to unacceptable concentrations of air contaminants. NIOSH investigators studied associations between environmental factors and work-related health conditions for 2,435 respondents in 80 office buildings evaluated as part of the Health Hazard Evaluation program. The incidence of asthma and the prevalence of nonspecific multiple lower respiratory and atopic symptoms were associated with many HVAC system design and maintenance variables, such as presence of debris within air intakes, poor drainage from condensate pans, inadequate maintenance of HVAC filters, absence of regularly scheduled inspections of air-handling units, and presence of an outdoor air intake within 25 feet (7.5 m) of a pollution sources (45). Negative building pressure has caused downdrafting of combustion gasses and infiltration of outdoor air pollutants and soil gases (46). Contaminants from renovation projects have been distributed to occupied spaces through ventilation ducts. Degrading duct lining has led to epidemics of dermatologic complaints. Biologic contamination of various aspects of an HVAC system has triggered building epidemics such as legionnaires' disease, humidifier fever, Pontiac fever, and hypersensitivity pneumonitis (47). Ventilation equipment and design may affect latex aeroallergen concentrations (48). Recommendations for protecting persons who are highly sensitive to latex include HVAC interventions such as air duct cleaning and installation of clean high-frequency particulate air (HEPA) filters (49).

Although far from robust, there are data to support the role of general ventilation in controlling the transmission of airborne infection and exposure to immunogenic bioaerosols (50,51). Studies of nosocomial infection and epidemic spread of tuberculosis are particularly relevant to medical centers. Everett and Kipp (52) observed variations of operating room infections resulting from changes in ventilation and temperature. Merisi et al. (53) investigated air microbial contamination in hospital wards. Though the authors were unable to demonstrate causation, several observations suggested a link between air contamination and nosocomial infection. Nardell et al. (50) reviewed an epidemic of tuberculosis in an office building and used mathematical models to conclude that increasing levels of ventilation as high as 35 cfm/p would have minimized the epidemic. Aside from impracticality, they calculated that higher rates would have resulted in progressively smaller increments of protection.

Much remains unclear about the role of building ventilation in occupant complaints. Research in experimental chambers, epidemiology, and problem building investigation support a minimum outside air ventilation rate in the range currently recommended by ASHRAE. Minimum ventilation standards, however, are not protective. Ventilation interacts with other components of an HVAC system. The thermal factors controlled by HVAC systems substantially determine human comfort and indoor air quality (54,55). The source of contamination frequently is the HVAC system itself. Proper operation and maintenance of HVAC systems critically determine the effect of the system on the pollution load of a building. Because general ventilation cannot overcome strong contaminant sources, source control must remain high on the list of necessary steps to assuring optimal indoor air quality. However, ventilation will never improve other factors related to occupant complaints, such as lighting, noise, work organization, and psychosocial considerations.

RISKS TO HVAC TECHNICIANS

The work of HVAC technicians involves potential exposure to a variety of hazards associated with the design, construction, maintenance, and operation of air handling and conditioning equipment. Hazardous particulates such as asbestos or manufactured mineral fibers may be disturbed as the technicians perform their work. Maintenance activities may cause exposures to chemicals such as biocides, disinfectants, duct cleaners, and sealants. Cleaning and maintenance of filters, humidifiers, condensate pans, and ductwork may lead to intense bioaerosol exposures. Air-handling unit equipment rooms may concentrate contaminants in ventilation exhaust. HVAC work may also require entry into confined spaces. HVAC work involves physical hazards associated with working at heights, with thermal extremes, with moving and noisy equipment, and with awkward postures.

With attention to hazards unique to their workplaces, employers should provide HVAC technicians with appropriate hazard communication, personal protective equipment, and safe work practice instruction. Steps may be taken during the design and construction of HVAC systems that facilitate easy and safe access to equipment for cleaning and maintenance.

CONCLUSION

Medical care cannot be divorced from the buildings in which it is delivered. The therapeutic role of medical centers in communities dictates special attention be provided to an indoor environment that supports, maintains, and promotes the health of its patients, staff, and visitors (56). General ventilation plays a critical part in meeting this goal. In this era of budgetary constraints, failure to provide adequate ventilation is a false economy. A successful HVAC system integrates good design, knowledgeable operation, and preventive maintenance. Changes in the use or configuration of an occupied space necessitate redesign of the HVAC system. Renovations, building maintenance activities, and hazardous releases demand special planning to avoid wide distribution of contaminants. Optimal general ventilation in medical centers cannot eclipse the necessity of controlling the sources of pollution or the need for administrative controls and personal protective equipment. Occupant satisfaction, however, does not depend solely on protection from indoor air pollution. A comprehensive approach to indoor environmental quality includes attention to aesthetics, noise, lighting, and organizational factors.

RESOURCES

Building air-quality: a guide for building owners and facility managers. EPA 400/1-91/033, DHHS (NIOSH) publication no. 91-114, December 1991.
An off-the-shelf, comprehensive guide for facility managers, maintenance personnel, and building investigators involved in preventing, evaluating, and correcting indoor air pollution problems.
Burton DJ. *Indoor air quality workbook.* Salt Lake City, UT: 1990.
A step by step guide for building investigators, this volume is packed with checklists and practical information.
Maroni M, ed. *Ventilation and indoor air quality in hospitals.* Boston: Kluwer Academic Publishers, 1996.
This book contains scientific presentations of a NATO Advanced Research Workshop held in Italy in 1995. Information about hospital indoor air quality is combined with general considerations about strategies and technical aspects of hospital air quality management.
Persily AK. Manual for ventilation assessment in mechanically ventilated commercial buildings. Portland, OR: NIST, 1994.
Written for technically competent indoor air quality investigators, this manual describes procedures for comparing ventilation performance with standards, guidelines, and design values and for investigating ventilation-related indoor air quality problems.
Principles of heating, ventilating and air conditioning. Atlanta: American Society for Heating, Refrigerating, and Air-conditioning, 1994.
Provides definitive, yet easy to understand coverage of all aspects of the indoor environmental control field.
Seltzer JM, ed. Effects of the indoor environment on health. Occup Med 1995;10:1–254.
A collection of articles concerning the source, control, and human impact of indoor air pollution.

GLOSSARY OF VENTILATION TERMINOLOGY

Air-handling unit The mechanical assembly that contains the fans that move conditioned air.

Constant volume A type of HVAC system that supplies a constant volume of air that meets thermal demands by varying the temperature of the supplied air.

Demand control volume A type of HVAC system that supplies air based on concentrations of specified parameters of indoor air quality.

Economizer A system that allows the use of outdoor air to decrease energy requirements to heat or cool air.

Exfiltration Uncontrolled exit of air from a room or building.

Fan coil unit An independent device designed to supplement heating of rooms on the perimeter of a building. A fan provides air movement across the heating coil and may also be used directly to draw in outside air (see Induction unit).

HVAC Heating, ventilation, and air-conditioning system that typically combines the thermal conditioning functions of heating, cooling, humidifying, dehumidifying, humidifying with mechanical ventilation that may or may not be designed to provide outdoor air and exhaust stale indoor air.

Induction unit An independent device designed to supplement heating of rooms on the perimeter of a building. Thermal convection induces air movement.

Infiltration Uncontrolled entrance of air into a room or building.

Intake An opening that allows controlled entrance of air into a building or room.

Lee The downwind, sheltered side of a building.

Makeup air Outside air that exactly replaces the amount of air exhausted from a room or building. Also called replacement air.

Plenum An area that allows mixing of air from several sources. A return air plenum mixes air from several return air grilles and delivers it to the air-handling unit. An air-handling unit may have a plenum that mixes outdoor with recirculated air.

Return air grille The opening through which air is returned to the HVAC system from a room.

Supply air diffusers The louvered opening at which air is supplied to a room with the goal of maximum air mixing or diffusion through the occupied space.

Variable air volume An HVAC system that varies the amount of air delivered on the basis of thermal demand.

REFERENCES

1. Building air quality: a guide for building owners and facility managers; EPA 400/1-91/033. DHHS (NIOSH) publication no. 91-114, December 1991.
2. American Society of Heating Refrigerating and Air-conditioning Engineers. Standard 52.1-1992: gravimetric and dust spot procedures for testing air-cleaning devices used in general ventilation for removing particulate matter (ANSI approved). Atlanta, GA: ASHRAE, 1992.
3. Baker DB. Social and organizational factors in office building-associated illness. *Occup Med* 1989;4:607–624.
4. Norbäck D, Michel I, Widström J. Indoor air quality and personal factors related to the sick building syndrome. *Scand J Work Environ Health* 1990;16:121–128.
5. Skove P, Valbjírn, Pedersen BV. Influence of personal characteristics, job-related factors, and psychosocial factors on the sick building syndrome. *Scand J Work Environ Health* 1989;15:286–295.
6. Norbäck D, Edling C. Environmental, occupational, and personal factors related to the prevalence of sick building syndrome in the general population. *Br J Ind Med* 1991;48:451–462.
7. Overberger PA, Wadowsky RM, Schaper MM. Evaluation of airborne particulates and fungi during hospital renovation. *Am Ind Hyg Assoc J* 1995;56:706–712.
8. Woods JE. Cost avoidance and productivity in owning and operating buildings. *Occup Med* 1989;4:753–770.
9. Magner LN. *A history of medicine.* New York: Marcel Dekker, 1992.
10. Turner WA, Bearg DW, Brennan T. Ventilation. *Occup Med* 1995;10:41–57.
11. Janssen JE. The V in ASHRAE: a historical perspective. *ASHRAE J* 1994;36:126–132.
12. Morey PR, Woods JE. Indoor air quality in health care facilities. *Occup Med* 1987;2:547–563.
13. American Society of Heating Refrigerating and Air-conditioning Engineers. Standard 62-1981: ventilation for acceptable indoor air quality. Atlanta: ASHRAE, 1981.
14. American Society of Heating Refrigerating and Air-conditioning Engineers. Standard 62-1981R: ventilation for acceptable indoor air quality. Atlanta: ASHRAE, 1986.
15. American Society of Heating Refrigerating and Air-conditioning Engineers. Standard 62-1989: ventilation for acceptable indoor air quality. Atlanta: ASHRAE, 1989.
16. American Society of Refrigerating and Air-conditioning Engineers. Laboratories. In: *HVAC applications.* Atlanta: ASHRAE, 1991.
17. American Industrial Hygiene Association. Laboratory ventilation standard. ANSI no Z9.5, 1992.
18. American Society of Heating Refrigerating and Air-conditioning Engineers. Guideline 1-1989: guideline for the commissioning of HVAC systems. Atlanta: ASHRAE, 1989.
19. American Society of Heating Refrigerating and Air-conditioning Engineers. Standard 55-1981: thermal environmental conditions for human occupancy. Atlanta: ASHRAE, 1981.
20. American Society of Heating Refrigerating and Air-conditioning Engineers. Standard 55-1992: Thermal environmental conditions for human occupancy. Atlanta: ASHRAE, 1981.
21. American Society of Heating Refrigerating and Air-conditioning Engineers. Standard 62-1989R draft for public review [unpublished). Available from ASHRAE, 1791 Tullie Circle, NE, Atlanta, GA 30329.
22. Klein BR, ed. *Health care facilities handbook,* 4th ed. Quincy, MA: National Fire Protection Association, 1993.
23. BOCA National Building Code/1993, 12th ed. Country Club Hills, IL: Building Officials & Code Administrators International, 1993.
24. American Institute of Architects Committee on Architecture for Health with the US Department of Health and Human Services. Guidelines for Construction and Equipment of Hospital and Medical Facilities, 1992-1993. Washington, DC: American Institute of Architects Press, 1993.
25. *Federal Register* 1994;59:15968–16039.
26. Burton DJ. *Indoor air quality workbook.* Salt Lake City, UT: IVE, 1990.
27. National Institute for Occupational Safety and Health. Indoor air quality and work environment symptoms survey. Available at http://www.cdc.gov/niosh/ieqpage.html.
28. Nagda NL, Rector HE, Koontz MD. Guidelines for monitoring indoor air quality. Washington, DC: Hemisphere Publishing, 1987.
29. Samimi BS. The environmental evaluation: commercial and home. *Occup Med* 1995;10:95–118.
30. Bisesi MS, Kohn JP. Industrial hygiene evaluation methods. Boca Raton, FL: CRC Lewis, 1995.
31. Melius J, Wallingford K, Keenlyside R, Carpenter J. Indoor air quality: the NIOSH experience. *Ann Am Conference Governmental Ind Hyg* 1984;10:3–7.
32. Seitz TA. NIOSH indoor air quality investigations: 1971 through 1988. In: Weekes DM, Gammage RB, eds. *Proceedings of the Indoor Air Quality International Symposium.* Akron, OH: American Industrial Hygiene Association, 1990:163–171.
33. Crandall MS, Sieber WK. The National Institute of Occupational Safety and Health indoor environmental evaluation experience, I: building environmental evaluations. *Appl Occup Environ Hyg* 1996;11:533–539.
34. Hodgson MJ, Frohliger J, Permar E, et al. Symptoms and microenvironmental measures in nonproblem buildings. *J Occup Med* 1991;33:527–533.
35. Kreiss K. The epidemiology of building-related complaints and illness. *Occup Med* 1989;4:575–592.
36. McLellan RK, McCunney RJ. Indoor air pollution. In: McCunney RJ, ed. *A practical approach to occupational and environmental medicine*, 2nd ed. Boston: Little, Brown, 1994:633–650.
37. Burge S, Hedge A, Wilson S, Bass JH, Robertson A. Sick building syndrome: a study of 4373 office workers. *Ann Occup Hyg* 1987;31:493–504.

38. Cain WS, Leaderer BP, Isseroff R, et al. Ventilation requirements in buildings, I: control of occupancy odor and tobacco smoke odor. *Atmos Environ* 1983;17: 1183–1197,
39. Mendell MJ, Smith AH. Consistent pattern of elevated symptoms in air conditioned office buildings: a reanalysis of epidemiologic studies. *Am J Public Health* 1990.80:1193–1199.
40. Menzies R, Tamblyn R, Farant JP, et al. The effect of varying levels of outdoor air supply in the symptoms of sick building syndrome. *N Engl J Med* 1993;328:821–827.
41. Mendell MJ. Nonspecific symptoms in office workers: a review and summary of the epidemiologic literature. *Indoor Air* 1993;3:227–236.
42. Jaakkola JK, Tuomaala P, Seppänen O. Air recirculation and sick building syndrome: a blinded crossover trial. *Am J Public Health* 1994;84:422–428.
43. Mendell MJ, Fine L. Building ventilation and symptoms: where do we go from here [Editorial)? *Am J Public Health* 1994;84:346–348.
44. Burton DJ. ASHRAE's indoor air quality procedure generates the dilution ventilation rate. *Occup Health Saf* 1993;62:35.
45. Sieber WK, Stayner LT, Malkin R, et al. The National Institute of Occupational Safety and Health indoor environmental evaluation experience, III: Associations between environmental factors and self-reported health conditions. *Appl Occup Environ Hyg* 1996;11:1387–1392.
46. Morey PR, Shattuck DE. Role of ventilation in the causation of building-associated illnesses. *Occup Med* 1989;4:625–641.
47. Seltzer JM. Biologic contaminants. *Occup Med* 1995; 10:1–25.
48. Swanson MC, Yunginger JW, Reed CE. Immunochemical quantification of airborne natural rubber allergens in medical and dental office buildings. In: Maroni M, ed. *Ventilation and indoor air quality in hospitals.* Boston: Kluwer Academic Publishers, 1996:257–262.
49. Culver JB. Latex sensitivity in healthcare workers. *J Assoc Occup Health Prof Healthcare* 1995;15:1–10.
50. Nardell EA, Keegan J, Cheney SA, Etkind SC. Airborne infection: theoretical limits of protection achievable by building ventilation. *Am Rev Resp Dis* 1991;144: 302–306.
51. Brundage JF, Scott RM, Lednar WM, et al. Building-associated risk of febrile acute respiratory diseases in army trainees. *JAMA* 1988;259:2108–2112.
52. Everett WD, Kipp H. Epidemiologic observations of operating room infections resulting from variations in ventilation and temperature. *Am J Infect Control* 1991;19: 277–282.
53. Merisi AM, Venezia R, Ciacco V, et al. Airborne microbial contamination and hospital infections. In: Maroni M, ed. *Ventilation and indoor air quality in hospitals.* Boston: Kluwer Academic Publishers, 1996:161–167.
54. McLellan RK. Optimal humidification in occupied buildings. *Occup Environ Med Rep* 1996;9:21–25.
55. Levin H Physical factors in the indoor environment. In: Seltzer JM. Effects of the indoor environment on health. *Occup Med* 1995;10:59–94.
56. Horsburgh CR. Healing by design. *N Engl J Med* 1995;333:735–739.
57. American Society of Heating, Refrigerating and air-conditioning Engineers. ASHRAE guideline 1-1996: the HVAC commissioning process. Atlanta: ASHRAE, 1989.

Medical Center Occupational Health and Safety, edited by Robert J. McCunney.
Lippincott Williams & Wilkins, Philadelphia © 1999.

25

Personal Protective Equipment

Victor S. Roth and *Timothy J. Key

*University of Michigan Occupational Health Services, Ann Arbor, Michigan 48103-5827; *Division of Occupational and Environmental Medicine, University of Alabama, Birmingham, Alabama 35294-2042*

Personal protective equipment, generally the least desirable way to control workplace hazards, places the burden of protection on the worker. Personal protective equipment is frequently uncomfortable, difficult to use, and needs to be adequately maintained and fit properly (1). The medical center environment can be considered a community in microcosm with employees working in areas as varied as food service, maintenance, custodial services, laundry, and security in addition to direct health care. Personal protective equipment for such a large variety of occupations is out of the scope of this chapter and is better described in resource pertinent to general industry. The focus of this chapter is personal protective equipment specifically for health care workers.

Health care workers are protected by the standards of the Occupational Safety and Health Administration (OSHA) and recommendations of the National Institute of Occupational Safety and Health (NIOSH) that apply to workers in other industries. These recommendations include the use of engineering, administrative, and work practice controls and employee education before resorting to personal protective equipment.

In the health care setting, unlike some other industries, personal protective equipment has become an integral part of conforming to well-established OSHA standards, including the laboratory standard (29 CFR 1910.1450) and the blood-borne pathogens standard (29 CFR 1910.1030). Unlike most other industries, medical centers have the ever-present risk for transmission of infectious disease to employees. This risk can be substantially reduced by the use of physical barriers, that is, personal protective equipment. If universal precautions and engineering and work practice controls are insufficient to prevent exposure to blood and body fluids, aerosol droplets, laboratory reagents, and potentially toxic medications in the daily course of duties, the employer is expected to provide and the employee is expected to wear personal protective equipment (2). In the medical center environment, and for the purpose of this discussion, recommended personal protective equipment for health care workers includes gloves, respirators, goggles, gowns, and arm sleeves. Lead aprons and back belts also are frequently used in the medical center environment and protect health care workers from illness and injury.

GLOVES

Virtually all hospital-related exposure to blood involves the hand (3). One study found that 88% of all high-level contacts were limited to the hands (4). High level and low level are based on likelihood of contact with blood or body fluids. The use of gloves as protective barriers by health care workers is effective in reducing risk for occupational exposure to blood and body fluids. An investigation into the effectiveness of an educational program on compliance with glove use cited a study in which it was found that that glove use significantly reduces risk for emergency department workers' exposure to blood during procedures such as intravenous catheter placement, venipuncture, and arterial blood sampling (3). Another study (5) cited in the article found that after implementation of universal precautions, physicians who complied with the recommended barrier precautions experienced significant reduction in risk for blood and body fluid exposures. The authors in the latter study concluded that "the use of gloves is the largest contributor to the efficacy of universal precautions."

The use of gloves to reduce transmission of microorganisms and blood-borne pathogens to and from the hands of health care workers has been mandated by OSHA and strongly recommended by the Centers for Disease Control and Prevention (CDC), American Hospital Association, and others. The principal rationale for gloving in most medical centers has been the implementation of universal precautions, designed to reduce risk for occupationally acquired blood-borne infections among health care workers. Another increasing use of gloving is body substance isolation, in which glove use is recommended when health care workers anticipate hand contact with blood or other body secretions, such as wound drainage or vomitus, to prevent hand contamination and cross infection of patients (6).

Types of Gloves

Both vinyl and latex examination gloves are used by health care personnel in a variety of clinical settings. An alternative glove material is a thermoplastic elastomer. This synthetic, nonlatex, nonvinyl, thermoplastic elastomer has a tensile strength equal to or superior to that of latex (7). In medical research settings, workers who handle a variety of potentially toxic chemicals and solvents need to use chemical protective gloves (Table 25-1) (8).

TABLE 25-1. *Common construction materials of chemical protective gloves*

Butyl, sobutylene-isoprene rubber
Natural rubber
Neoprene, chloroprene
Nitrile, acrylonitrile-butadiene rubber
Polyethylene
Polyvinyl alcohol
Polyvinyl chloride
Polyurethane
Vilton
Silver Shield

Glove permeability should be the main consideration for glove selection. This choice should be based on the chemicals handled by the worker. In tests of permeation, the glove material acts as a barrier that separates the chemical of interest from a medium that collects the chemical as it permeates. The collecting medium (liquid or gas) is analyzed quantitatively for its concentration of challenge chemical. The test procedure involves cutting a material specimen from the glove and clamping it onto a test cell, where it acts as a barrier membrane. The outside of the specimen is touched with the chosen chemical, and the collecting medium on the inside is tested at intervals for the presence of permeated chemical (8).

Several studies have compared leakage rates between vinyl and latex gloves (6,9). Most studies have demonstrated the superiority of latex over vinyl. Another factor shown to be important in leakage rates in these studies was brand of glove used, which suggests that quality control methods may vary from manufacturer to manufacturer (9).

In response to requests for more protection than gloves alone provide, several manufacturers have developed glove liners made from synthetic fibers or combinations of fibers (Kevlar, Spectra) (10). Some liners contain stainless steel fibers. All are designed to be used in combination with latex or vinyl gloves.

Latex allergy is an extremely important consideration in choosing a type of glove material (see Chapter 10). With most studies showing increased leakage rates for vinyl gloves, thermoplastic elastomer gloves may be a desirable choice in such cases.

Double Gloving

An important factor in glove permeability is thickness. A logical conclusion would be that double gloving can provide more protection than using one pair of gloves (10). Studies (11,12) have shown that double gloving can be beneficial in reducing the exposure of blood and body fluids to health care workers.

Double gloving, while increasing safety may compromise the comfort of the wearer and the sensitivity and dexterity needed for delicate procedures (13). However, a report of double gloving and surgical technique (14) claimed that surgeons performed operative tasks without significant impairment when double gloved compared with use of one pair of gloves. Most study participants preferred using a larger glove on the inside and their normal size glove on the outside. Another study of glove preferences of surgeons, however, indicated that most participants preferred a larger outside glove and a normal-size inside glove (15).

Recommendations regarding double gloving are based on the type of procedure performed and the type of glove used. Wearing double gloves gives no advantage during routine procedures in which glove use is not emphasized. Single gloving for latex and double gloving for vinyl should be used when the procedure involves blood-contaminated materials and when there is a great deal of manual manipulation (11).

Proper Use of Gloves

To be effective personal protective equipment has to be properly used. Despite extensive data supporting the efficacy of glove use and growing concern over risk for transmission of infectious diseases, some health care workers fail to wear gloves when in contact with patients until after a diagnosis of infectious disease is made. This constitutes a diagnosis-dependent isolation system (16). At the other extreme, some studies have shown a high percentage of glove use, mostly by nursing personnel, in the absence of exposure to blood or body fluids (9).

It is well acknowledged that gloves should be worn in exposure- prone procedures, that is, those that present recognized risk for percutaneous injury to the worker and involve potential exposure to infectious blood or other body fluids. Such exposure-prone procedures should be identified by the health care institution at which the procedure is performed (17).

Gloves should be changed between patients. Not changing gloves is analogous to not washing hands between patients, a direct violation of CDC guidelines. Gloves should not be washed, because washing tends to weaken their structural integrity (2).

Hand Washing after Glove Use

Despite proper use of gloves in recommended clinical settings, hand contamination after procedures has been detected among a high percentage of health care workers (6). Recommendations from the U.S. Food and Drug Administration allow for a 2.5% failure rate of unused gloves for surgical gloves and 4% for examination gloves. Some studies have demonstrated glove leakage rates as high as 8% for unused examination gloves (9). It is recommended that hand washing routinely follow removal of gloves at the completion of a potentially contaminating procedure.

Other Uses for Gloves in the Health Care Setting

In addition to protecting health care workers from contracting illnesses from patient blood and body fluids, gloves serve as a barrier against transmission of viral and bacterial infections from skin or mucous membrane lesions (e.g., herpes simplex type I, skin abscess) and reduce skin absorption of medications and chemicals (13). Gloves should be used when administering medications such as antineoplastic drugs. Studies have shown that use of personal protective equipment, including gloves, while handling antineoplastic drugs reduces the mutagens in urine specimens of these health care workers and results in a lower prevalence of side effects than among workers who do not use gloves (18). Skin contact with the drug was the best predictor of subsequent symptoms. OSHA suggests use of gloves, gowns, and a vertical laminar flow hood for drug preparation. The OSHA laboratory standard (29 CFR 1910.1450) mandates glove use by medical laboratory workers.

RESPIRATORS

Surgical masks historically have been worn to protect patients from being infected by pathogens emitted by health care personnel. Today emphasis has shifted from solely protecting the patient to protecting the health care worker as well. Of concern are aerosolized hazardous agents of submicrometer size that pose a threat to health care workers (19). Surgical masks provide insufficient protection to protect from these aerosols.

The infectious disease of most concern that can be controlled with respirator use is tuberculosis, especially multidrug-resistant tuberculosis. Exposure of health care workers to tuberculosis may come from patients with undiagnosed active disease but also can occur during procedures such as sputum induction, bronchoscopy, pentamidine administration, and cough induction (see Chapter 4). NIOSH favors portable powered air-purifying respirators (PAPRs) for protection against tuberculosis (20). The CDC refers to studies showing control of tuberculosis outbreaks without the use of PAPRs and suggests use of lighter mask respirators (21). OSHA recommends a compromise between the two positions and calls for use of a mask-like high-efficiency particulate air (HEPA) filter respirator by health care workers when their work puts them at risk for tuberculosis (22).

In 1995, NIOSH published a new regulation, 42 CFR 84, which replaced the Dust/Mist, Dust/Fume/Mist, and HEPA certifications with new classes of particulate respirators, N, P, and R. The N series is tested against a solid submicron sodium chloride particle. An N95 respirator has a filtration efficiency of 95% or more against the sodium chloride aerosol. The N95 respirators meet CDC performance specifications for respirators that can be used for tuberculosis exposure control, so N95 respirators can replace HEPA respirators for this purpose. The cost of N95 respirators will likely be considerably lower than that of HEPA respirators.

OSHA policy requires that health care employees wear appropriate respirators (N95, HEPA) for all high-exposure procedures, such as endotracheal intubation and suctioning, bronchoscopy, and aerosol treatments such as pentamidine therapy. The policy also requires that respirators be worn by persons who enter rooms occupied by patients with confirmed or suspected active tuberculosis. Also covered by this policy are emergency response personnel who transport in a closed vehicle patients with confirmed or suspected tuberculosis (23).

The OSHA respiratory protection standard requires that all respiratory protective devices used in the workplace be NIOSH certified. NIOSH-approved respirators (N95, HEPA) are air-purifying respirators that meet or exceed recommended performance criteria outlined in the CDC publication, Guidelines for Preventing the Transmission of *Mycobacterium tuberculosis* in Health Care Facilities, 1994 (see Chapter 4).

The OSHA requirement that health care workers in situations that place them at risk for exposure to patients with active tuberculosis must use N95 or HEPA respirators is not without controversy. Some experts believe that this approach is unnecessarily conservative and imposes an undue burden on patient care. Supporters of this view (24,25) do not consider tuberculosis to be a serious problem in some areas of the country and believe that less stringent and less expensive personal protective devices may provide adequate protection. On the other hand, reports of tuberculosis (many cases being multidrug-resistant tuberculosis) skin-test conversions among health care workers and the absence of what can be considered a safe level of exposure to bacilli have led many experts to conclude that OSHA-required respirators are an appropriate selection (23). Approval of the N95 respirator may serve to lessen this controversy.

A study has been conducted of health care workers' risk for acquiring tuberculosis while using different types of respiratory protection in low-exposure (present in the isolation room of a patient with tuberculosis under treatment for 1 hour a day, 60 days a year) and high-exposure (present during bronchoscopy of a patient with tuberculosis for 1 hour a month) situations (26). The 10-year cumulative risk with different types of respiratory protection in the low-exposure situation is shown in Table 25-2. On the basis of these results, the authors concluded the following:

- In high-exposure situations such as bronchoscopy, a health care worker may need to wear highly protective respirators, such as the N95 or HEPA filter PAPR.
- Elastomeric half-mask PAPRs with HEPA filters provide substantially better protection from airborne tuberculosis transmission than surgical masks and disposable dust-mist particulate respirators.
- One cannot rely solely on the use of air-purifying respirators (including PAPRs) to prevent transmission of occupational tuberculosis, as evidenced by the risk associated with different respirators.
- In addition to use of an appropriate respirator, primary exposure control measures (screening of patients at high risk, prompt initiation of chemotherapy, implementation of engineering controls) continue to be important in reducing aerosol transmission of tuberculosis bacilli to health care workers.

The OSHA recommendation for the use of respirators to protect against infectious agents in the medical center environment differs from respirator use in other industries in that a regular medical evaluation is not required. A questionnaire focused on the respiratory system is used as a screening device among health care workers who regularly use N95 or HEPA respirators in the clinical setting. The results of such a questionnaire should be used to indicate whether further evaluation, such as a medical examination or a pulmonary function test, is needed.

EYEWEAR

The occupational transmission of blood-borne disease through eye splatter is relatively unimportant in comparison with other modes of transmission, especially needle-stick injuries. On the other hand, the incidence of eye splatter among health care workers is relatively high, and prevention through the use of personal protective equipment such as eye shields and goggles is quite effective (27). The case of a nurse who contracted human immunodeficiency virus infection from a splash to the eye highlights the fact that though such incidents may be uncommon, potential risk for contracting infection through eye contact remains (28).

Blood splashes to the face commonly occur in emergency situations and during elective surgical procedures that last more than 2 hours (29). The frequency of such events may be much more common than first thought. A study of the effectiveness of different types of eyewear concluded that "many eye splatter events are not noticed by health care personnel" and "go unreported" (27). The OSHA blood-borne pathogens standard specifically states "eye protection devices, such as goggles . . . shall be worn whenever splashes, spray, spatter, or droplets of blood may be generated and eye . . . contamination can be reasonably anticipated" (30).

TABLE 25-2. *Ten-year cumulative risk for type of respiratory protection*

Respiratory protection	Low-exposure situation (%)	High-exposure situation (%)
No respirator	15	48
Surgical mask	6.7	24
Disposable dust-mist particulate	0.94	3.7
Elastomeric halfmask HEPA filter	0.33	1.3
Powered air purifying HEPA filter	0.064	0.26

Many different types of eyewear are effective in preventing eye splatter. Eye shields made of clear antifog plastic have a number of shapes and configurations. Important features in choosing eye protection products are complete covering of the frontal aspect of the eyes and lateral protection. A factor that contributes to increased eye exposure despite use of eyewear is splashing through the open top of protective shields during procedures that require the health care worker to bend over (27).

Goggles, compared with other eye protection devices such as eye shields, minimize risk for conjunctival exposure by forming a seal around the eyes. Most goggles, however, are not disposable and therefore have to be disinfected when contaminated. In a large medical center, goggle maintenance, presumably by means of soaking in glutaraldehyde then rinsing, has been described as a nuisance (28). Maintenance itself can lead to eye irritation and dermatitis if goggles are poorly rinsed. Eye and face protection, including spectacles, face shields, and goggles, are described in detail by the American National Standards Institute (31).

GOWNS AND ARM SLEEVES

Personnel in operating rooms have traditionally worn protective apparel to prevent contamination of the patient. In hospital emergency departments, staff physicians usually wear white coats over ordinary clothes or uniforms that can be easily changed when they become contaminated with blood or body fluid (32). Recommendations for protective gowns from professional organizations were discussed referred in a study of gown efficacy (33). The recommendations included such descriptive qualities as "should be resistant to blood and other liquids that may cause contamination" (Association of Operating Room Nurses) (34), "must resist the passage of aqueous liquids" (CDC) (35), and "appropriate only if they do not permit blood or other potentially infectious materials to pass through" (OSHA 29 CFR 1910.1030).

Emergency department personnel are at high risk for contamination of clothing and skin from patients' blood and body fluids. The variety of medical conditions encountered in emergency departments may result in unanticipated events, such as sudden vomiting, spurting blood, and oozing purulent drainage. This recognition has led to recommendations that consider it unhygienic for emergency department personnel to wear personal clothing or traditional uniforms during work duties (36). Use of a polyester, liquid-repellent suit was tested for a 14-month period in a study at an emergency department (36). In no instance did fluid splashed on the suit penetrate to the inner surface or cause skin contamination. Episodes that resulted in contamination among workers wearing the protective suits came from splashes on either exposed skin or between glove and sleeve. These results suggest that clothing of appropriate design and material repellent to blood and body fluids used properly in the high-risk environment of the emergency department affords skin protection from splashed blood and body fluids. One would therefore conclude that such apparel should be used either in place of or as a covering over personal clothing and traditional white coats and scrub suits.

Results of a study of surgical gowns (33) led to recommendations that such gowns be made completely resistant to liquid penetration by means of reinforcing the material with films, coatings, or membranes. These gowns would be worn when comprehensive liquid and microbial barrier protection is needed. The same study found that during procedures when risk for exposure to blood and body fluids is low, single-layer gowns and those reinforced with an additional layer of fabric can be used. Surgical gowns ideally should be single use and thermally comfortable to wear. Reusable gowns eventually lose their barrier protective properties because of normal wear and tear. However, if a decision is made to use this type of protective clothing, a quality assurance program in the medical center should establish a protocol to determine when the garment should be repaired or removed from service (33).

Arm sleeves used in conjunction with surgical gowns and worn over the gown sleeve should be made of waterproof material with a watertight connection between sleeve and glove to afford the health care worker additional protection from contamination by blood and body fluids. It is important that the sleeve cuff contain water-resistant adhesive tape to ensure a waterproof seal with the glove (37). This adhesive should prevent seepage of blood between glove and sleeve and prevent the sleeve from migrating up the forearm, as frequently occurs during exposure-prone procedures. The upper end (proximal portion) of the sleeve should be elastic to allow it to stay firmly in place on the upper arm. Additional protective apparel used to complement gowns and arm sleeves includes caps and shoe covers.

LEAD APRONS

A lead apron, by protecting radiologists and radiologic technicians from potentially harmful radiation, plays an important role in modern radiologic practice. Anecdotal experience among radiologists involved in long procedures has suggested that wearing this protective garment may carry risk for low back pain. Studies have not proved this assumption to be true (38).

BACK BELTS

Low-back pain is a common physical disorder that affects many occupational groups. Nurses and other patient care personnel, including nurse's aides and patient care technicians, have higher prevalence rates of back pain and a higher incidence of back injuries than most other occupational groups working in a medical center (39).

Back belts or spinal orthotics have gained popularity in the last few years under the assumption that their use will reduce low-back injuries (40). Lifting belts are not recommended for persons who do infrequent lifting, pushing, or pulling (41). A health care worker who performs regular heavy physical tasks has the potential to lose support in the lumbar region of the spine as a result of decreased muscle efficiency caused by an increased metabolism level, which leads to localized fatigue of the lower back muscles. In such cases, lifting belts can be used as additional support during heavy or extended physical exertion to prevent fatigue and give support to the stressed musculature (41).

Several studies have shown good results with back belt use (42,43) in the form of decreased numbers of back injuries among health care workers using this device. Other studies, however, have shown little or no difference in back injury rates whether or not back belts were used (40). The NIOSH Back Belt Work Group (44) analyzed biomechanical, physiologic, psychophysical, and epidemiologic studies and concluded that "there is insufficient scientific evidence that [back belts] actually deliver what is promised." The NIOSH group "does not recommend back belts to prevent injuries." In any case, back supports should not be used as a primary means of back injury prevention. Such prevention requires multidisciplinary collaboration and instruction in proper lifting techniques. A careful workplace evaluation of lifting, pulling, pushing, and twisting tasks should be made before the use of a back belt is advised (45).

SUMMARY

Regardless of the clinical setting in a medical center, better protection of all health care personnel from the risks of hazardous biologic, chemical, and physical exposures should be the goal (46). Such protection can be accomplished with appropriate use of personal protective equipment in conjunction with engineering and administrative controls. If exposure occurs despite proper preventive measures, a program to respond to such events should be in place. With conscientious use of methods to reduce exposure to patients' blood and body fluids, respiratory aerosol droplets, hazardous chemicals, potentially harmful medications, and ergonomically unsafe tasks and with the use of personal protective equipment playing an important role in this effort, the medical center should become a safer environment.

RESOURCES

1. US Department of Health and Human Services. Guidelines for protecting the safety and health of health care workers; DHHS (NIOSH) publication no. 88-119. September 1988.

   These general guidelines incorporate NIOSH, CDC, and OSHA documents. Includes an overview of hospital hazards, methods for developing hospital safety and health programs, a discussion of hazards, infectious diseases, and methods for disposing of hazardous wastes, and a list of occupational safety and health agencies and resource organizations.
2. Charney W, Schirmer J. *Essentials of modern hospital safety.* Vols. 1, 2. Boca Raton, FL: Lewis, 1993.

   Edited by industrial hygienists. Volume 2 includes tuberculosis, needle-stick injuries, exposure to blood, pentamidine, and ribavirin aerosols, shiftwork, and back injuries.
3. Johnson JS, Anderson KJ. *Chemical protective clothing.* Vols. 1, 2. Akron, OH: American Industrial Hygiene Association, 1990.

   A comprehensive treatment of the principal aspects of chemical protective clothing design, performance, and use.
4. American National Standards Institute. American national standard practice for occupational and educational eye and face protection; ANSI Z87.1-1989. Des Plaines, IL: American Society of Safety Engineers, 1989.

   A standard for eye and face protection with emphasis on performance. Contains descriptions, illustrations, and appropriate applications of this equipment.

REFERENCES

1. US Department of Health and Human Services, Centers for Disease Control. Guidelines for protecting the safety and health of health care workers; DHHS publication no. 88-119. September 1988.
2. Roup BJ. OSHA's new standard: exposure to bloodborne pathogens. *AAOHN J* 1993;41:136–142.
3. Friedland LR, Joffe M, Wiley II JF, Schapire A, Moore DF. Effect of educational program on compliance with glove use in a pediatric emergency department. *Am J Dis Child* 1992;146:1355–1358.
4. Lund S, Jackson J, Leggett J, Hales L, Dworkin R, Gilbert D. Reality of glove use and handwashing in a community hospital. *Am J Infect Control* 1994;22: 352–357.
5. Wong ES, Stotka JL, Chinchilli VM, Williams DS, Stuart CG, Markowitz SM. Are universal precautions effective in reducing the number of occupational exposures among health care workers? a prospective study of physicians on a medical service. *JAMA* 1991;265: 1123–1128.
6. Olsen RJ, Lynch P, Coyle MB, Cummings J, Bokete T, Stamm WE. Examination gloves as barriers to hand contamination in clinical practice. *JAMA* 1993;270:350–353.
7. Hamann CP, Nelson JR. Permeability of latex and thermoplastic elastomer gloves to the bacteriophage .X174. *Am J Infect Control* 1993;21:289–296.
8. Johnson JS, Anderson KJ. *Chemical protective clothing.* Vol. 1. Akron, OH: American Industrial Hygiene Association, 1990.
9. Korniewicz DM, Kirwin M, Cresci K, Larson E. Leakage of latex and vinyl exam gloves in high and low risk clinical settings. *Am Ind Hyg Assoc J* 1993;54:22–25.
10. Witmeyer RJ. Trends in glove product and process development. *Biomed Instrum Technol* 1992;26:235–238.
11. Korniewicz DM, Kirwin M, Cresci K. Barrier protection with examination gloves: double versus single. *Am J Infect Control* 1994;22:12–15.
12. Hansen ME, McIntire DD, Miller GL. Occult glove perforations: frequency during interventional radiologic procedures. *Am J Radiol* 1992;159:131–135.
13. Heller ET, Greer CR. Glove safety: summary of recent findings and recommendations from health care regulators. *South Med J* 1995;88:1093–1098.
14. Webb JM, Pentlow BD. Double gloving and surgical technique. *Ann R Coll Surg Engl* 1993;75:291–292.
15. Keeling NJ, Ataullah CM, Wastell C. A survey of glove preferences of general and orthopaedic surgeons in north west thames regional health authority. *J Hosp Infect* 1995;30:305–308.
16. Wilkinson WE. Medical center studies how consistently workers use gloves to prevent infection. *Occup Health Saf* 1992;61:35–43.
17. Bell DM, Shapiro CN, Ciesielski CA, Chamberland ME. Preventing bloodborne pathogen transmission from health-care workers to patients: the CDC perspective. *Surg Clin North Am* 1995;75:1189–1203.
18. Valanis B, Vollmer WM, Labuhn K, Glass A, Corelle C. Antineoplastic drug handling protection after OSHA guidelines. *J Occup Med* 1992;34:149–155.
19. Weber A, Willeke K, Marchioni R, et al. Aerosol penetration and leakage characteristics of masks used in the health care industry. *Am J Infect Control* 1993;21:167–173.
20. US Department of Health and Human Services, Centers for Disease Control and Prevention. NIOSH recommended guidelines for personal respiratory protection of workers in health care facilities potentially exposed to tuberculosis; 1992.
21. US Department of Health and Human Services, Centers for Disease Control and Prevention. Guidelines for preventing the transmission of tuberculosis in health-care facilities, with special focus on HIV-related issues. *MMWR Morb Mortal Wkly Rep* 1990;39:(RR-17).
22. Crow S. The lone ranger rides again, this time followed by a federal posse. *Infect Control Hosp Epidemiol* 1994; 15:673–676.
23. Vesley DL. Respiratory protection devices. *Am J Infect Control* 1995;23:165–168.
24. Nettleman MD, Fredrickson M, Good NL, Hunter SA. Tuberculosis control strategies: the cost of particulate respirators. *Ann Intern Med* 1994;121(1):37–40.
25. Decker MD. Respiratory protection standard: comments on OSHA's proposed revision. *Infect Control Hosp Epidemiol* 1995;16(6):365–371.
26. Nicas M. Respiratory protection and the risk of *Mycobacterium tuberculosis* infection. *Am J Ind Med* 1995;27:317–333.

27. Garrett SJ, Robinson JK. Disposable protective eyewear devices for health care providers. *J Occup Med* 1993; 35:1043–1047.
28. Berry K. Reducing the risk of eye contamination. *Nurs Stand* 1995;9:27–29.
29. Berridge DC, Lees TA, Chamberlain J, Jones NAG. Eye protection for the vascular surgeon. *Br J Surg* 1993;80: 1379–1380.
30. Occupational Safety and Health Administration. Occupational exposure to bloodborne pathogens. *Federal Register* 1991;56:64175–64182.
31. American National Standards Institute. American national standard practice for occupational and educational eye and face protection;ANSI Z87.1-1989. Des Plaines, IL: American Society of Safety Engineers, 1989.
32. Boon D, Wardrope J. What should doctors wear in the accident and emergency department? patients' perception. *J Accid Emerg Med* 1994;11:175–177.
33. McCullough EA. Methods for determining the barrier efficacy of surgical gowns. *Am J Infect Control* 1993; 21:368–374.
34. Association of Operating Room Nurses. Recommended practices: protective barrier materials for surgical gowns and drapes. *AORN J* 1992;55:832–835.
35. Garner JS. CDC Guidelines for prevention of surgical wound infections. *Am J Infect Control* 1986;14:71–80.
36. Steedman DJ. Protective clothing for accident and emergency personnel. *J Accid Emerg Med* 1994;11:17–19.
37. Kabukoba JJ, Pearce JM. The design, effectiveness and acceptability of the arm sleeve for the prevention of body fluid contamination during obstetric procedures. *Br J Obstet Gynaecol* 1993;100:714–716.
38. Moore B, vanSonnenberg E, Casola G, Novelline RA. The relationship between back pain and lead apron use in radiologists. *Am J Radiol* 1992;158:191–193.
39. Yassi A, Khokhar J, Tate R, Cooper J, Snow C, Vallentyne S. The epidemiology of back injuries in nurses at a large Canadian tertiary care hospital: implications for prevention. *Occup Med* 1995;45:215–220.
40. Mitchell LV, Lawler FH, Bowen D, Mote W, Asundi P, Purswell J. Effectiveness and cost-effectiveness of employer-issued back belts in areas of high risk for back injury. J Occup Med 1994;36:90–94.
41. Perry GF, ed. Occupational medicine forum: lumbar support belts. *J Occup Med* 1992;34:679–680.
42. Allen SK, Wilder K. Back belts pay off for nurses. *Occup Health Saf* 1996;59–62.
43. Votel T. Correct PPE helps alleviate persistent back injuries, compensation expenses. *Occup Health Saf* 1993; 65–70.
44. US Department of Health and Human Services, Centers for Disease Control and Prevention. Workplace use of back belts, review and recommendations 1994; DHHS publication no. 94-122.
45. Lusk SL, ed. Linking practice and research: use of back belts to prevent low back injury. AAOHN J 1995;43: 489–493.
46. Fry DE, Telford GL, Fecteau DL, Sperling RS, Meyer AA. Prevention of blood exposure:body and facial protection. *Surg Clin North Am* 1995;75:1141–1157.

Medical Center Occupational Health and Safety,
edited by Robert J. McCunney.
Lippincott Williams & Wilkins, Philadelphia © 1999.

26

Organization and Management of a Medical Center's Occupational Health, Safety, and Environmental Program

Edward Joseph Bernacki

Department of Medicine, Division of Occupational Medicine, Section of Health, Safety, and Environment, The Johns Hopkins University, Baltimore, Maryland 21287

Health care workers account for approximately 3% of the U.S. workforce, a labor force that grew from 4.2 million persons in 1970 to approximately 10.5 million persons in 1994 (1). Approximately half of these workers are employed in hospitals; the others are employed in long-term care facilities, physicians' offices, laboratories, and managed care organizations.

HEALTH, SAFETY, AND ENVIRONMENT PROBLEMS IN THE HEALTH CARE INDUSTRY

The hazards associated with employment in health care are numerous. They range from exposures to biologic, chemical, and physical agents to traumatic injuries. Biologic and physical stresses are the most important risks to health care providers, whereas physical and chemical hazards predominate among workers in nonclinical areas, such as laboratories, maintenance, and housekeeping.

A 1986 report prepared by the American College of Occupational and Environmental Medicine (ACOEM) Committee on Medical Center Employee Occupational Health described a number of infectious diseases that are of particular risk to health care workers (2). These include human immunodeficiency virus (HIV) infection, diphtheria, polio, tetanus, measles, mumps, infection by enteric pathogens, hepatitis B, hepatitis C, influenza, tuberculosis, and varicella (2–4).

In a 1976 survey, the National Institute for Occupational, Safety and Health (NIOSH) found that at least 135 chemicals frequently used in hospitals are mutagenic, carcinogenic, teratogenic, or a combination of these among animals and humans (5). Potentially hazardous chemicals include anesthetic gasses, asbestos, chemotherapeutic agents, ethylene oxide, formaldehyde, and mercury, among others (2–7).

According to the National Safety Council, the number of injuries per 100 health care workers, is about 4.25 and the number of lost-time days per 100 health care workers (an index of severity) averages between 70 and 90, depending on the year (8). The frequency and severity rate of injuries and illnesses among health care workers are considerably less than those in mining, construction, and farming but are considerably greater than those in other service industries (6,8–10). By far the most common occupational injuries in health care are sprains, strains, puncture wounds, abrasions, contusions, lacerations, burns, and fractures. However, musculoskeletal disorders of the low back and the neck are the leading causes of work-related lost time among health care workers (9). Workers' compensation per $100 of payroll for health care industry costs $1.00, close to the average workers' compensation cost of all industrial classifications in the United States (approximately $1.10 per $100 of payroll) (10). In addition to traumatic injuries, noise, heat, ionizing and nonionizing radiation, electrical hazards, unstable surfaces, poor lighting, and inadequate ventilation are important physical hazards in the health care environment (2,3,6,7).

Psychosocial factors contribute to a large amount of lost-time among health care workers. There are conflicting data regarding the incidence of psychosocial disease and substance abuse among health care workers as opposed to other occupational groups (11,12). However, subclassifications of health care workers such as physicians and nursing aides may be at comparatively higher risk than other occupational groups (11–14). Although the incidence or prevalence of mental disorders or substance abuse in health care may not exceed the incidence of such problems in other industries, programs to address absenteeism and poor job behaviors associated with them should and can be addressed in health care the way they are in nonservice settings (15).

REGULATION OF HAZARDS IN HEALTH CARE

The health care industry is regulated or credentialed by a variety of local, state, and federal agencies, including the Occupational Safety and Health Administration (OSHA), Joint Commission on Accreditation of Healthcare Organizations (JCAHO), Environmental Protection Agency (EPA), Nuclear Regulatory Commission (NRC), National Fire Protection Agency (NFPA), Department of Transportation (DOT), Equal Employment Opportunity Commission (EEOC), and state workers' compensation commissions, among others. The body of regulations is vast and intricate in both detail and interrelationships. The application of these regulations varies from state to state, and each health care institution must have a strong capability to respond to these regulations in an appropriate manner. The penalties for noncompliance can be onerous.

A number of new legislative mandates have increased the authority of OSHA and the EPA in overseeing the health, safety, and environmental problems in health care. OSHA has enacted standards that require training of employees, use of new types of personal equipment, hepatitis B vaccination, among a variety of other preventive measures to control blood-borne pathogens (16). The OSHA Occupational Exposures to Hazardous Chemicals in Laboratories Standard mandates that a chemical hygiene plan be devised to prescribe work practices, procedures, and policies that ensure that all employees are protected from hazardous chemicals in their work areas (17). OSHA adopted as regulation and began enforcing the 1990 Centers for Disease Control and Prevention (CDC) guidelines for preventing the transmission of tuberculosis in health-care facilities (18). It mandates surveillance of employees for tuberculosis, use of high-efficiency particulate air (HEPA) filters, use of respirators for contact with potentially infectious patients, and evaluation and management if infection does occur (19).

Under the Resource Conservation and Recovery Act (19), Comprehensive Environmental Response Compensation Liability Act (20), and Superfund Amendments and Reauthorization Act (21), environmental regulatory agencies were given great authority in promulgating regulations governing the generation, transport, treatment, storage, and disposal of hazardous waste. The Resource Conservation and Recovery Act defines hazardous waste as follows (19):

> solid waste because of its quantity, concentration or physical, chemical or infectious characteristics that may; (1) cause or slightly contribute to an increase in the mortality or an increase in the serious irreversible or incapacitating or reversible illness or, (2) poses substantial present or potential hazards to human health or the environment when improperly treated, stored or transported disposed of, or otherwise managed

Health care institutions, particularly academic health care institutions, generate large quantities of hazardous waste. Health care institutions, like other institutions that dispose their hazardous waste in permitted landfills, are liable for at least some portion of the cleanup of these hazardous waste sites if any wastes generated by the institution are within the site. This is true even if the site is fully licensed by the state and federal government to operate as a hazardous waste facility. The law imposes strict liability without regard to fault for costs of cleanup of an institution's hazardous waste stored at a site. The Land Disposal Rule of 1986 augments this authority by placing limitations on the wastes that can be placed into secured landfills (22). Because of the rule, many marginal landfills have closed, and institutions that store their waste in these facilities are bearing a large part of the expense of cleanup. These legislative efforts have forced medical centers and higher educational institutions to reevaluate the use and disposal of hazardous wastes (23,24). Programs aimed at waste minimization through destruction and recycling, rather than transport and storage in permitted landfills, are the most cost-efficient way of handling hazardous substances.

Radioactive waste management philosophy has changed remarkably in the past two decades. In the 1970s, there were six commercially operated disposal sites, and disposal fees were approximately $3.50 per cubic foot. By 1978, three of these sites had closed. Because the South Carolina site was the only site operating east of the Mississippi River, it became the primary repository for all low-level radioactive waste. The South Carolina government imposed volume limitations for that site and the governors of South Carolina, Nevada, and Washington initiated action that culminated in congressional passage of the Low-Level Radioactive Waste Policy Act of 1980 (25). This act gave states the right to form regional compacts and to deny access to waste generated outside the regional compact. The severe consequences of the act were realized in 1995, when most licensees were denied access to disposal sites. Now only two disposal sites in the United States accept radioactive waste from generators, ChemNuclear of South Carolina and Envirocare of Utah. The average 1998 cost for radioactive waste disposal is $400 per cubic foot. Closure of disposal sites and increased fees have forced health care and other waste generators to minimize radioactive waste and implement decay-in-storage programs. For radioactive waste to be disposed of as nonradioactive waste, it must be stored for ten half-lives (26). Long-lived radionuclides must be shipped for disposal or incinerated. Therefore, decay-in-storage programs, site-selection for storage sites, waste incineration programs, and waste monitoring have become important components of most academic medical center safety programs.

MINIMUM REQUIREMENTS OF AN ORGANIZED HEALTH, SAFETY, AND ENVIRONMENTAL EFFORT

Each health care enterprise should have in place the organization, personnel, and procedures to address prevention and management of a multitude of occupational injuries and illnesses, the avoidance of hazardous emissions to the environment, and compliance with federal and state regulations dealing with these issues. NIOSH developed nine criteria for what it calls effective occupational safety and health programs in hospitals, as follows (27):

1. Preplacement physical examination
2. Periodic health appraisal
3. Health and safety education
4. Immunization
5. Care for injury and illnesses
6. Health counseling
7. Environmental control and surveillance
8. A health and safety record system
9. Coordinated planning with hospital departments and services regarding safety

The ACOEM Committee on Medical Center Employee Occupational Health in a 1986 report recommended that the employee occupational health service should at a minimum provide preplacement examinations and periodic health assessments and render treatment of workers for occupational injuries and illnesses (2). The employee health service also should contribute to prevention of communicable diseases by instituting policies and procedures that include periodic evaluation, immunization programs, and care of personnel for work-related exposures to infectious diseases. The report also stated that "specific programs that address chemical hazards such as anesthetic gases, chemotherapeutic agents, ethylene glycol, formaldehyde and mercury should be developed." The committee also recommended that "the employee health department should be actively involved in coordinating the efforts of occupational physicians, occupational health nurses, safety professionals and industrial hygienists to develop an effective environmental control program." The report also indicated that employees who are "suspected to be under the influence of alcohol or drugs of abuse should be evaluated and treated for these disorders through an employee assistance program, clinically or chemically, whether or not the employee's function is impaired."

The OSHA Office of Occupational Health Nursing in its 1993 publication Framework for a Comprehensive Health and Safety Program in the Hospital Environment also outlines the essential components of a health and safety program in the health care setting (28). Like the ACOEM report, this document describes preplacement, occupational, and postexposure assessments and rehabilitation programs as core programs. The Office of Occupational Health Nursing goes farther, recommending programs to identify hazard categories, various surveillance procedures, health hazard analysis, exposure monitoring programs, and safety engineering programs. This report encourages the use of administrative controls and personal protective equipment to protect health care workers exposed to hazardous agents. Like ACOEM, the Office of Occupational Health Nursing encourages establishment of a variety of management and supervisory training programs to ensure that all health care workers are knowledgeable about safety practices.

Other than OSHA and NIOSH, there is little guidance from accrediting or regulatory agencies regarding health, safety, and environmental programs for health care institutions. The JCAHO only requires that a safe environment be provided health care workers, visitors, and patients, that a safety officer be appointed, and that the institution have a formal safety committee (29). However, the JCAHO environment of care standard is explicit regarding acceptable safety practices and training programs (Table 26-1).

TABLE 26-1. *1995 JCAHO Standards for management of the environment of care*

Safety
- Providing a physical environment free of hazards and managing staff activities to reduce the risk of human injuries. This is accomplished through
- Hospital and departmental safety policies and procedures
- Reporting of incidents that involve property damage, occupational illness, and patient, personnel, or visitor injury
- Orientation of new employees to safety policies and procedures
- Ongoing safety education of all employees
- Training of staff for specific job-related hazards

Security
- Security concerns regarding patients, visitors, personnel, and property. This is accomplished through
- Appropriate identification of patients, visitors, personnel, and property
- Access control to sensitive areas
- Reporting and investigation of all security incidents that involve patients, visitors, personnel, and property
- Orientation and ongoing training of personnel to reporting and emergency procedures to be followed during a security incident

Hazardous materials and waste
- Proper handling, storage, use, and disposal of hazardous materials
- Proper procedures to follow in cases of a hazardous material or waste spill
- Health hazards associated with mishandling of or exposure to hazardous materials
- Processes for reporting hazardous materials and waste incidents
- Orientation and training of staff regarding the above

Emergency preparedness
- Implementing specific procedures in response to a disaster. This is accomplished through employee orientation and training about
- Roles and responsibilities in disasters as defined in the departmental disaster plan
- Contingent methods of communicating during disasters and emergencies
- Method for obtaining supplies and equipment during a disaster

Life safety
- Protecting patients, personnel, visitors, and property from fire and products of combustion. This is accomplished through
- Fire safety training in orientation and annually
- Staff's knowledge of the locations of the fire alarms, extinguishers, nearest exits, and evacuation routes
- Staff's knowledge of their roles and responsibilities in fire and evacuation procedures
- Procedures to contain smoke and fire through building compartmentalization

TABLE 26-1. *Continued.*

Medical equipment
- A management program that promotes the safe, effective and efficient use of medical equipment in the environment of care. This is accomplished through clinical engineering participation in
- Selection and acquisition of medical equipment
- Inspection, testing, and maintenance of equipment
- Monitoring and reporting to the FDA incidents in which a medical device may have caused or contributed to a death, serious injury or illness as required by the Safe Medical Devices Act of 1990
- Investigation of equipment failures or user errors that have or may have an adverse effect on patient safety or quality of care
- Staff orientation and training regarding
- Basic operating and safety procedures for the equipment on the unit
- Procedures for reporting equipment malfunctions or failures or user errors
- Hospital procedures for inspection, preventive maintenance, and testing of medical equipment

Utility systems
- Management plans that ensure the reliability, minimize the risk, and reduce the failures of the electrical system, emergency power, heating, ventilating, and air conditioning, plumbing, boiler and steam, medical gas, medical or surgical vacuum, or communication systems. Orientation and training of staff should include:
- Proper emergency procedures staff should follow when utility systems fail
- For appropriate staff, the location and use of emergency shutoff controls or whom to contact in the event of an emergency
- Process for reporting utility system problems or failures

Guidance on health care occupational medicine programming is also contained in a number of monographs, books, and articles written by professionals practicing in the area. Two references (3,30) describe in detail virtually every component of a good program. Those unfamiliar with the general field of occupational medicine services and delivery can gain insight by reading books by Silver (31) and McCunney (32). The National Safety Council publishes a number of texts that may be used as a guide to setting up and managing safety and environmental programs (33,34). These texts focus primarily on safety and environmental programs and are recommended for persons who are not safety and environmental professionals who are charged with the responsibility of initiating these programs within a health care institution. Use of these resources should provide an understanding of the various components of health and safety program management that can be adopted in the health care setting.

DESIGN AND IMPLEMENTATION OF AN EFFICIENT HEALTH, SAFETY, AND ENVIRONMENT PROGRAM

The establishment of an occupational health and safety program can be and usually is a relatively straightforward task, a task for which a large body of data is available. How an organization manages these programs in the most cost-effective manner possible requires a great deal of planning, introspection, and a desire to monitor performance and change activities that do not meet their intended goals.

The recruitment of workers with the expertise necessary to address these issues is of foremost importance if truly efficient occupational medicine and environmental services are to be delivered. Occupational health nurses, occupational medicine physicians, industrial hygienists, biosafety officers, sanitarians, safety engineers, radiation safety officers, health physicists, claims adjusters, workers' compensation attorneys, psychologists, and social workers are professionals commonly employed in this area. A detailed description of the qualifications of each of these disciplines is outside the scope of this chapter, but certification in occupational medicine (American Board of Preventive Medicine), industrial hygiene (Certified Industrial Hygienist), occupational health nursing (Certified Occupational Health Nurse-Specialist), or safety (Certified Safety Professional) is evidence of competencies in some of these professions. Attorneys and insurance adjusters who specialize in the adjudication of workers' compensation cases and social workers or psychologists skilled at employee assistance programming round out the skill base of personnel in a comprehensive health and safety program. Although it may be alluring for a health care institution to hire a surgical nurse, internist, or plant engineer to run these programs, this strategy usually leads to the provision of adequate rather than exemplary services.

Small health care institutions with an employee population of fewer than 500 would not be justified in hiring more than a full-time occupational health nurse or safety professional. In such settings, consultant physicians, industrial hygienists, and ergonomists must supplement the expertise of those professionals. Smaller institutions have to depend on part-time workers with expertise in plant engineering and infection control to complement the limited number of occupational health and safety resources available. In larger institutions, a full complement of health and safety professionals can be hired to address the hazards inherent in the institution. Even in large institutions that are made up of many autonomous components, the organizational structure that would allow an integrated and therefore an efficient safety program may be lacking. By pooling resources multiple health care institutions can gain the critical population mass necessary to secure the professional expertise to handle most of the problems these institutions may encounter. A health care institution also may achieve a larger population base and thereby gain economies of scale by offering services to companies in the catchment area.

Occupational health programs rank among the main diversification strategies for hospitals (35). The number of physicians being recruited into a hospital or clinic-based program continues to increase, and this type of employment is displacing non-health-care corporate employment as the largest employer of occupational medicine physicians (36). Health care institutions have discovered the benefits of providing occupational health and nursing services to employees in their service areas.

In many communities the hospital or health care center is either the largest employer or among the largest employers in a community. It may be the only employer in a community that can assemble the personnel necessary to provide occupational, health, and safety programming on an ongoing basis. A health and safety program set up to provide occupational medicine, safety engineering, and industrial hygiene services to the institution itself can provide similar services to small and medium-sized businesses within the community. The provision of such services to companies in the health care organization's catchment area can leverage the fixed cost of the health care institution's own health, safety, and environmental organization and provide substantial revenues to offset the expense of the institution's internal program. The benefits of this strategy are as follows: (a) occupational health and safety services directed at outside clients' programs affords the health care institution direct contact with employers; (b) ongoing, close relationships with area businesses can create an opportunity to market the institution's nonoccupational medical services, such as pediatrics, gynecology, or urology, all of which can have a greater effect on hospital revenues than primary occupational health services; (c) it allows smaller employers in a community access to the skills of highly qualified occupational health and safety professionals.

PERFORMANCE MEASURES

An organization must measure its ability to minimize hazards to workers and the environment, meet its regulatory requirements, and minimize the cost of health care, litigation, and fines associated with hazards. Table 26-2 presents a number of variables that can be used to assess whether a program is meeting its objectives and whether it is doing so in a cost-effective manner. The measurement parameters focus on injury prevention, timely return to work, cost-effective service delivery, minimization of litigation and fines, and customer satisfaction. Depending on the breath or scope of the health and safety organization, some or all of these performance measures can be used. Many of these parameters can be compared over time or with those of other institutions to determine whether the organization is performing better or worse than it has in the past or than comparable institutions. Statistics for comparison can be obtained from the National Council on Accident Insurance, state workers' compensation boards,

TABLE 26-2. *Performance measures for health, safety, and environment*

Injury prevention	Timely return to work	Cost-effective services	Minimize litigation and fines	Maximize customer satisfaction
A. Labor force covered Parameters: 1. Population 2. NCCI classification code 3. Payroll 4. Age distribution 5. Sex distribution B. Claims incidence Parameters: 1. Total number of claims Medical only Lost-time Fatal claims 2. Nature of injury 3. Cause of injury 4. Part of body injured 5. ICDA classification Outcome variables: 1. Number of medical-only claims per 100 workers 2. Number of lost-time claims per 100 workers 3. Number of lost-time days per 100 workers C. Compliance with federal and state regulations Parameters and outcome variables: 1. Fines and citations by agencies (OSHA, EPA, NRC, etc.) 2. Workplace inspections 3. Surveillance examinations 4. Tuberculin tests D. Preventive practices Parameters and outcome variables: 1. Population immunity 2. Number of isolation rooms 3. Adequacy of ventilation systems 4. Personal protective equipment use	A. Information by benefit types Parameters: 1. Temporary/total disability days (TTD) 2. Total dollars expended on TTD 3. Work status at return to work (modified duty, full duty) 4. Permanent/partial disability (PPD) a. Total number of cases b. Total dollars expended 5. Total permanent disability a. Total number of cases b. Total dollars expended Outcome variables: 1. Average duration of TTD 2. Average time from injury to actual return to work 3. Average cost of PPD per PPD case 4. Average impairment rating per PPD case B. Management information Outcome variables: 1. Time lag in reporting injuries 2. Average time lag in payment of initial benefits	A. Medical Parameters and outcome variables: 1. Total medical payments (aggregated) 2. Distribution of medical payments by medical only and lost time cases a. New b. Old cases 3. Distribution of medical payments by ICDA codes 4. Average medical cost per claim 5. Average number of medical visits by ICDA code or body part code 6. Average cost per medical visit by primary care provider and specialty provider Orthopedic surgery Physical medicine Neurosurgery 7. Rate of hospitalization per lost-time case 8. Percentage of claims with inpatient surgery by major ICDA coding 9. Average cost per day of hospitalized patient 10. Percentage of claims with physical therapy 11. Percentages of claims with chiropractor B. Environmental Parameters and outcome variables: 1. Environmental abatement projects 2. Cost per environmental abatement project 3. Budget for health, safety and environmental services 4. Cost per employee of health, safety and environmental services 5. Waste generation by class (biologic, chemical, radiation) in pounds 6. Waste minimization (recycling, incineration) in pounds	A. Litigation Parameters and outcome variables: 1. Proportion of cases involving disputes 2. Denial rate 3. Rate of attorney involvement 4. Dispute resolution requests per 100 indemnity (lost-time) cases 5. Percentage of claims that are are occupational diseases 6. Percentage of claims that are cumulative injuries 7. Hearing cost per contested claim 8. Number of appeals 9. Attorney costs as a percentage of premium 10. Dispute resolution outcomes per 100 indemnity claims Informal level Formal level 11. Time from filing to dispute resolution B. Fines and citations 1. Number of inspections by federal, state, or local agencies 2. Number of fines or citations leveled by inspecting agencies 3. Monetary payouts for fines or citations per year	A. Employee satisfaction Parameters and outcome variables: 1. Timeliness of contact 2. Average waiting time to see physician 3. Access to information about the system 4. Timeliness of indemnity payments 5. Environmental or ergonomic assessment conducted 6. Postinjury safety inspection of work area B. Employer satisfaction Parameters and outcome variables 1. Access to coverage 2. Level of loss prevention services 3. Satisfaction with claims service 4. Communication regarding nature and extent of injury performed immediately postinjury and when appropriate thereafter

NCCI, National Council on Compensation Insurance; ICDA, International Classification of Diseases.

Bureau of Labor Statistics, American Hospital Association, National Safety Council, and the medical and safety literature.

THE JOHNS HOPKINS INSTITUTIONS HEALTH, SAFETY, AND ENVIRONMENTAL PROGRAM

There are three basic requirements for an occupational health, safety, and environmental program to meet its safety and regulatory goals. There are two more requirements if this program is to be delivered in an efficient manner. The requirements are as follows:

1. Hazards, regulatory issues, and abatement procedures are well delineated.
2. The organization possesses the technical expertise and financial resources necessary to identify and abate these problems.
3. The organizational framework that allows the safety and health effort to meet its objectives has been formalized.
4. The health and safety organization has critical mass in terms of population and risk to allow adequate staffing and efficient delivery of services.
5. If critical mass cannot be achieved internally or through consolidation of programs in contiguous or adjacent health care institutions, the necessary economies of scale can be achieved by offering health and safety services to outside clients, increasing the population and the risk base.

The Johns Hopkins Institutions health, safety, and environmental program is an example of how these requirements were addressed in one program that serves two large corporate entities with multiple independent subunits. It is presented primarily for the reader to visualize how a number of separate entities can initiate and maintain a health and safety organization that addresses the health, safety, and environmental problems and regulatory concerns of each entity but do so at less cost than if each organization were to initiate and manage its own program. The discussion encompasses the rationale for setting up the program, the organizational structure, an example to illustrate how the various units within the program interact with each other, and the parameters used to gauge the effectiveness of the program in meeting its goals.

In 1990, the safety committees of the various Johns Hopkins Institutions realized that safety, health, and environmental issues were not being optimally addressed within the Hopkins community. The issues included newly implemented OSHA regulations regarding HIV, hepatitis B, and hepatitis C exposures among health care and laboratory workers. The need to act on this problem appeared to be most acute on the medical campus, which includes the Johns Hopkins Hospital, the School of Medicine, the School of Hygiene and Public Health, and the School of Nursing, collectively called the Johns Hopkins Medical Institutions. At the beginning of 1991, the decision was made to consolidate all occupational safety and health activities into one office serving the entire Hopkins community. The office was called the department of health and safety, later called health, safety, and environment. This brought together a group of departments—office of workers' compensation, occupational health services, office of safety and environmental health, and employee assistance program—that were formerly housed in four separate and distinct organizations within the hospital and university structure. A director was recruited to manage the new department and serve as chair of the hospital and university safety committees, which were later consolidated into a joint committee to serve both the hospital and the university. These actions incorporated the responsibility of developing and implementing health, safety, and environmental policies for both the hospital and the university and the management of the entire program into the portfolio of one person and committee. The objective of the unified committee and department structure was the management of (a) risk related to noncompliance with federal and state regulations, (b) risk related to workers' compensation losses, and (c) risk related to working in a potentially hazardous environment.

As shown in Fig. 26-1, the joint committee on health, safety, and environment reports to

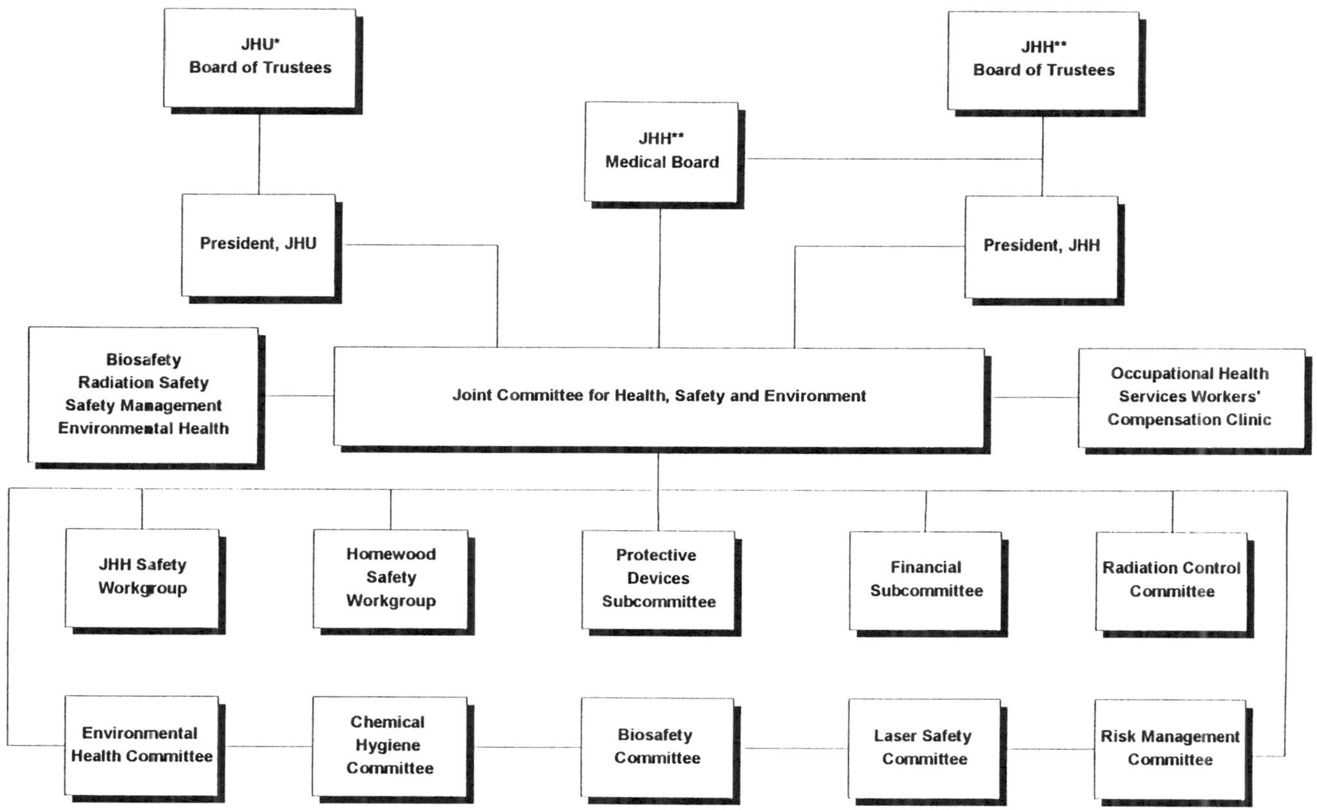

* Johns Hopkins University
** Johns Hopkins Hospital

FIG. 26-1. The Johns Hopkins health, safety, and environmental governance.

the presidents of the Johns Hopkins health system and the university and through them to the boards of trustees of both institutions and the medical board of the Johns Hopkins Hospital. As shown in Fig. 26-2, the administrative activities of the joint committee are performed by nine separate departments that report to the chair of the joint committee. These departments are safety management, biosafety, radiation safety, environmental health services, workers' compensation office (a self-insured and self-administered workers' compensation program), workers' compensation clinic, faculty and staff assistance program (an employee assistance program), occupational health services—Homewood campus, and occupational health services–East Baltimore campus.

As shown in Table 26-3, the activities of the department encompass all safety-related activities, including prevention of occupational injuries and illnesses, management of injuries and illnesses among workers, prevention and correction of environmental hazards, and payment and adjustment of claims related to workplace injuries. Reporting to the chair, who also serves as a division director within the department of medicine, is the center for occupational and environmental health, the entity that serves corporate clients throughout Maryland. The reporting relationship for the division of occupational medicine is the traditional academic structure: division director to department chair to dean of medicine to president. The activity of this unit also is shown in Table 26-3.

The safety governance structure at Johns Hopkins is provided in Fig. 26-1. The committees that report to the joint committee are the Johns Hopkins Hospital and Homewood safety workgroups, the protective devices subcommittee, the radiation control committee, the environmental health committee, chemical hygiene committee, biosafety committee, and laser safety committee. The composition and function of these committees are described in detail in Table 26-4.

The components of this organizational structure interact to allow maximum efficiency in preventing injuries and illnesses while reducing costs. An example is the reorganization and management of the Johns Hopkins self-insured workers' compensation program (37–42).

The Johns Hopkins self-insured workers' compensation program (JHWCP) was established in 1969 to provide an integrated claims management service for the Johns Hopkins Institutions. The JHWCP is staffed by an administrator, three clerks, a part-time adjuster, and a part-time attorney supplemented by two outside attorneys. The program contracts with a large law firm to reserve its cases and represent it at the workers' compensation commission and appellate court. The services of the program initially were limited to claims processing, adjustment, and adjudication and payment of incurred workers' compensation claims. In 1992, the program was reorganized and expanded to include the management of medical care and duration of disability of all employees insured under the program. The JHWCP initially covered the Johns Hopkins Hospital. The Johns Hopkins University, a separate corporation, was added in July of 1980, and by 1984 all of the independent entities owned by the Johns Hopkins Health System (parent corporation of The Johns Hopkins Hospital) and schools of the university were integrated into the program.

At the beginning of 1992, occupational physician staffing was changed from outside contractors to a preceptor and occupational medicine resident coverage. An in-house preferred provider organization (PPO) was established to deliver specialty care. The PPO network consisted of full-time Johns Hopkins University faculty physicians credentialed by the Johns Hopkins Hospital from the departments of medicine (occupational medicine), orthopedics, neurosurgery, and physical medicine and rehabilitation of the Johns Hopkins University School of Medicine who volunteered to participate. Medical management guidelines and indications and return to work protocols were constructed and used by the PPO physicians. The management guidelines are an aggregation of practice parameters used

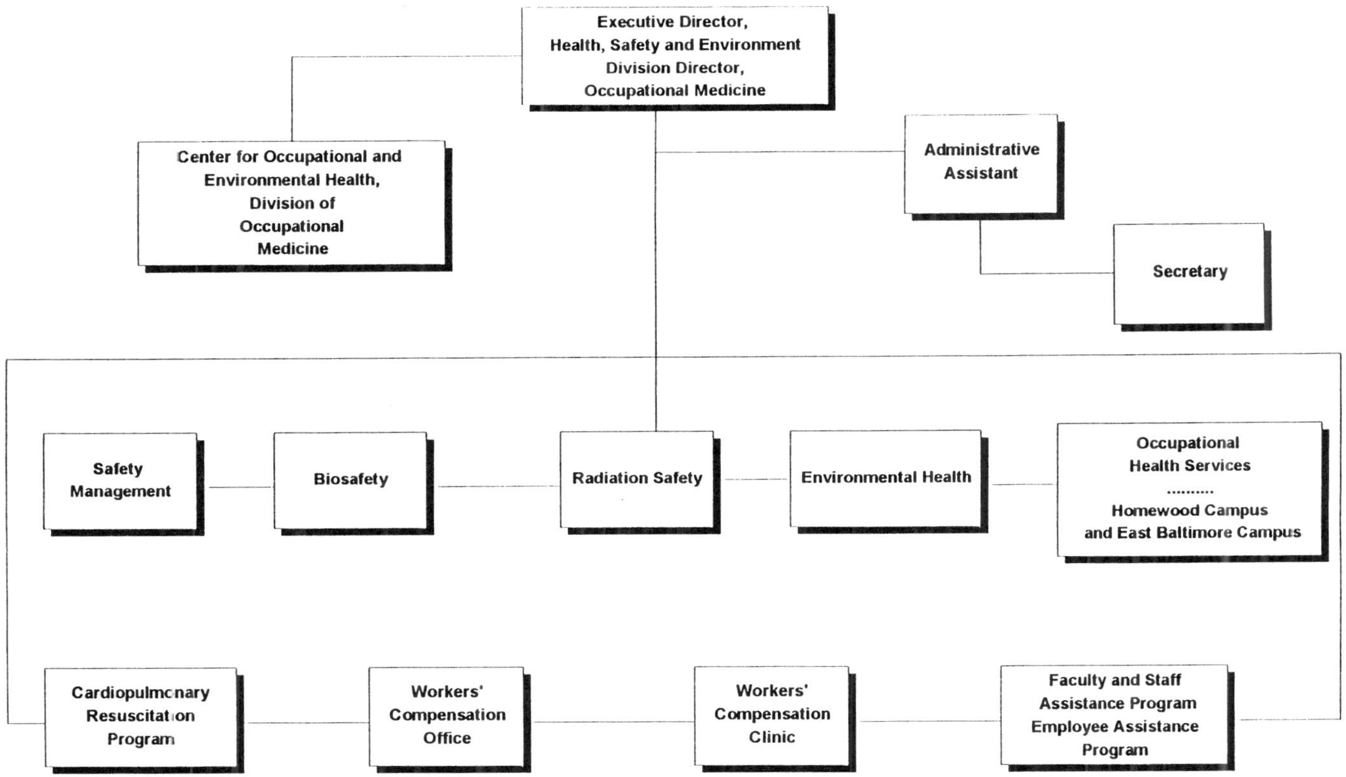

FIG. 26-2. The Johns Hopkins health, safety, and environment departmental reporting mechanism.

TABLE 26-3. *Health, safety, and environment activities by division*

- Safety management
  - Conducts periodic facility surveys and laboratory safety inspections
  - Performs incident investigations and record-keeping functions
  - Conducts job hazard analyses
  - Reviews facilities designs for compliance with federal, state, and local fire prevention and life safety codes
  - Monitors compliance with insurance carrier requirements and recommendations
  - Conducts fire prevention and safety training
  - Responds to fire and other emergency situations
  - Monitors fixed and portable fire suppression equipment
  - Conducts emergency response drills
  - Surveys all hospital areas for compliance with regulatory standards and public health practices
  - Accompanies licensing and regulatory agencies during facility inspections
  - Designs and implements safety control programs
  - Reviews facility design and work practices
  - Investigates complaints
  - Monitors food-service facilities
  - Monitors pest control programs
  - Conducts training in sanitation and public health
- Environmental health (industrial hygiene and ergonomics)
  - Identifies and controls chemical hazards
  - Monitors and administers hazardous chemical waste disposal program
  - Develops and conducts hazard communication program
  - Reviews facility and laboratory practices
  - Consults on design of containment facilities
  - Conducts environmental sampling and monitoring
  - Responds to chemical spills and accidents
  - Investigates complaints related to workplace exposures
  - Conducts training in the use, control, and disposal of hazardous chemicals
- Biologic safety
  - Registers recombinant DNA investigators and activities
  - Inspects biohazard laboratories
  - Registers biologic agent usage and personnel involved
  - Consults on design of containment laboratories and laboratory practices
  - Responds to emergency situation involving biologic agents
  - Coordinates maintenance and certification of biohazard control equipment
  - Conducts training in laboratory practices and control and disposal of biohazardous wastes
- Radiation control
  - Conducts periodic facility surveys with licensing and regulatory agencies
  - Performs monitoring of personnel and radiation sources
  - Conducts training concerning radionuclides
  - Reviews facilities designs for compliance with federal, state, and local guidelines
  - Conducts calibration of monitoring equipment
  - Maintains licenses for radioactive materials and registrations for x-ray–producing equipment
  - Orders, receives, inspects inventories and delivers radioactive materials to nuclear medicine, radiation oncology, and special chemistry
  - Monitors patients who have received therapeutic administrations of radioactive materials and determines radiation safety restrictions, visitor limitations, date when patient may be released, and when room may be reassigned
  - Inspects quarterly all areas were radioactive materials are stored or used
  - Tests semiannually cesium brachytherapy sources for leakage
  - Inspects semiannually gamma irradiators
  - Monitors exhaust stacks for emission of radioactive materials
  - Collects, processes, stores, and disposes of radioactive waste
  - Supervises necessary action in emergencies to minimize problems and assure quick recovery
  - Investigates radiation accidents or radioisotope contamination and provides technical expertise to accomplish decontamination when required
  - Investigates and reports patient misadministrations involving radiopharmaceuticals or radiation therapy
  - Inspects x-ray machines that are not in radiology and electron microscopes
- Occupational health services
  - Conducts preemployment health screening (hepatitis B, varicella, rubella, rubeola, hematocrit, serologic test for syphilis, urinalysis, vision, blood pressure, drug screen, health assessment, tuberculosis testing)
  - Performs immunizations (hepatitis B, rubella, rubeola, tetanus, rabies, smallpox, MMR)
  - Conducts flu vaccine program (immunization of employees, faculty, and staff)
  - Conducts izoniazid evaluations with evaluation and treatment as necessary for tuberculin converters
  - Conducts health screenings
  - Performs return-to-work clearance (any employee absent from work for more than 7 days, any employee who reports off with a communicable or contagious disease, any employee injured in a non–job-related accident)
  - Performs health evaluations (employees about to enter the disciplinary process are referred by supervisors to rule out health problems)
  - Performs tuberculosis surveillance (screening of employees annually for exposures and as required by regulations)

TABLE 26-3. *Continued.*

- Performs hearing testing (scheduling, reviewing, interviewing all exposed employees)
- Conducts respiratory program (medical assessment including pulmonary function testing of all employees identified as needing to wear a respirator in their job assignment)
- Conducts laser use surveillance (scheduling and evaluation of all employees with laser exposure)
- Conducts ethylene oxide surveillance (periodic testing of employees as necessary)
- Conducts physician immunization program (review of records, immunizations as necessary)
- Conducts Americans with Disabilities Act compliance (job assessments, employee assessments for accommodation, accessible parking as necessary)
- Evaluates communicable disease exposures (evaluation and treatment of all employees identified as being exposed to patients with communicable or contagious diseases, e.g., varicella, meningitis, pertussis)
- Maintains records (maintenance and update of all employee health records for employment plus 30 years)
- Performs drug testing (random and for cause drug testing of employees referred by supervisors or substance abuse counselors)

Workers compensation clinic
- Performs assessment and treatment of work-related injury and illness
- Conducts management after exposure to blood borne pathogens (HIV, HBV, HCV)
- Conducts early detection and intervention ergonomics program (in cooperation with safety and rehabilitation medicine)
- Conducts case management of workers' compensation claims in cooperation with preferred provider organization physicians, human resources, safety management, and industrial hygiene

Workers' compensation office
- Pays workers' compensation claims
- Adjusts workers' compensation cases
- Arranges for legal defense of workers' compensation claims
- Performs all administrative responses and filings for state workers' compensation commission

Employee assistance program
- Evaluates all employees requesting assistance for a drug or mental illness problem
- Evaluates employees suspected of having a mental illness or drug abuse problem affecting performance
- Performs mental health counseling
- Performs substance abuse counseling
- Performs financial counseling and facilitation of loans

Center for occupational and environmental health
- Provides clinical evaluation and treatment
- Administers workers' compensation preferred provider network (WCPPN)
- Performs employer outreach and training
- Provides 24-hour, toll-free, injury notification hotline for WCPPN
- Coordinates care and case management for WCPPN
- Provides nurse case management and monitoring for WCPPN
- Provides on-site medical assessment and management for WCPPN
- Provides disability management
- Conducts medical bill audits and repricing
- Performs preplacement and return-to-work and fitness for duty examinations
- Performs exposure-specific medical surveillance examinations
- Performs Department of transportation (DOT) medical clearance examinations
- Performs Federal Aviation Administration (FAA) medial clearance examinations
- Performs DOT-mandated and non-DOT urine drug screening
- Performs DOT-mandated and non-DOT alcohol testing
- Provides medical review officer services
- Conducts hearing conservation program
- Conducts blood borne pathogens program
- Conducts tuberculosis infection control program
- Conducts mobile and on-site testing
- Performs independent medical examinations
  - Impairment evaluations
  - Worsening of condition
  - Causal connection
  - Second opinion
  - Need for additional treatment
  - Work capacity assessment
  - Chart reviews
- Provides general occupational medical consulting
- Evaluates worksite hazards and monitors industrial hygiene
- Provides ergonomics services, workplace and process redesign
- Monitors OSHA and EPA compliance
- Provides guaranteed insurance for small to midsize employers
- Third-party administration
- Underwriting and risk management
- Network of casualty agents and bookers

TABLE 26-4. *Health, safety, and environment activities by committee, Johns Hopkins Medical Institutions*

1. Joint Committee for Health, Safety and Environment		
	Functions:	Develop policy for the Johns Hopkins University (JHU) and Johns Hopkins Hospital (JHH) on all matters related to health, safety, and environment
		Insure compliance with all applicable federal and state health, safety, and environmental regulations
		Insure compliance with guidelines promulgated by federal and state accrediting organizations in the area of health, safety, and environmental affairs
		Review and approve budgets for departments that compose the Johns Hopkins Medical Institutions (JHMI) Department of Occupational Health and Safety
		Oversee the management of the JHMI department of occupational health and safety
		Report quarterly to the governing bodies of the JHU and JHH regarding activities in the areas of health, safety and the environment. Evaluate annually the efficacy of all JHU and JHH health, safety, and environmental programs.
		Evaluate on a monthly basis the status of hazardous materials, waste monitoring, environmental monitoring, and incident reporting programs
		Evaluate all Plans of Correction submitted to correct identified safety deficiencies and develops Plans of Correction for safety deficiencies that are beyond the technical and financial scope of individual departments
		Prepare periodic reports on safety activities for the presidents of the JHU and the JHH
		Report on a monthly basis, to the medical board of the JHH
	Membership:	JHH, School of Public Hygiene and Public Health, Homewood, School of Medicine, nursing, purchasing, human resources, Occupational Safety and Environmental Health (OSEH), infection control, legal department, security
2. JHH Safety Workgroup		
	Functions:	Evaluate mechanism to investigate equipment incidents
		Monitor employee injury trends
		Review of employee health programs; vaccination; medical surveillance
		Evaluate visitor's injury claims
		Evaluate environmental monitoring (hazard analysis) surveys
		Review and/or develop safety policy and procedure
		Review activity of case management protective devices subcommittee
		Discuss pertinent infection control, waste management, facilities issues
	Membership:	Clinical engineering, materials management, security, nursing, pathology, Johns Hopkins Outpatient Center, legal department, infection control, human resources, environmental services, occupational health, union representatives, facilities, workers' compensation clinic
3. Homewood Safety Workgroup		
	Functions:	Assess ongoing programs relative to safety on the Homewood Campus
	Membership:	Risk manager, facilities, human resources, purchasing, legal department, housekeeping, student health/activities, academics, OSEH, security, occupational health
4. Protective Devices Subcommittee		
	Functions:	Assess occupational exposures
		Coordinate evaluation of protective devices
		Recommend devices for approval by joint committee
		Monitor implementation of approved devices
	Membership:	OSEH, workers' compensation clinic, nursing, materials management, infection control, purchasing
5. Financial Subcommittee of the Joint Committee		
	Functions:	Review and approve OSEH budget
		Membership: Selected from joint committee membership
6. Radiation Control Committee		
	Functions:	Monitors and insures compliance with federal and state radiation safety regulations
	Membership:	Radiation safety, radiology, nuclear medicine, radiation oncology, OSEH, nursing, School of Medicine, School of Hygiene and Public Health
7. Environmental Health Committee		
	Functions:	Recommend control procedures to reduce chemical and physical hazards.
		Monitor JHMI compliance with federal and state environmental regulations, particularly health-monitoring aspects
	Membership:	OSEH, nursing, infection control, workers' compensation clinic, clinical departments, occupational health services

TABLE 26-4. *Continued.*

Committee		
8. Chemical Hygiene Committee		
	Functions:	Insure compliance with Occupational Safety and Health Administration (OSHA) laboratory safety standard
	Membership:	OSEH, facilities, nursing, occupational health services, infection control, workers' compensation clinic, clinical departments
9. Biosafety Committee		
	Functions:	Monitor control of biologic hazards at the JHMI
	Membership:	OSEH, nursing, infection control, workers' compensation clinic, clinical departments, School of Medicine, School of Hygiene and Public Health
10. Laser Committee		
	Functions:	Evaluate new applications of laser technology at the JHMI Insure compliance with all federal and state regulations related to laser safety
	Membership:	Radiation safety, nursing, occupational health, clinical engineering, anesthesiology, cardiology, chemistry, homewood, dermatology, ophthalmology
11. Risk Management Committee		
	Functions:	Reduce the financial risk associated with errors and omissions in medical practice
	Membership:	Legal department, nursing, clinical engineering, environmental services, infection control, clinical departments

within the Johns Hopkins University limited to conditions normally funded under the workers' compensation system (e.g., carpal tunnel syndrome, epicondylitis, regional low-back pain). The return to work protocols are an average of the original PPO members' predicted durations of disability for conditions contained in the management guidelines.

A multidisciplinary medical management workgroup consisting of nurse case managers and primary and specialty physicians was established when the PPO was formed. The group meets twice a month to develop a coordinated treatment plan for each worker. The workers' compensation claims management workgroup also was established at that time. This workgroup consists of nurse case managers, safety professionals, human resource specialists, administrators, and an adjustor. This group meets once a month to formulate a plan for each employee who has lost time because of an occupational injury. Special emphasis is placed on returning the employee to work as soon as possible through liberal use of restricted or modified duties.

The claims adjudication workgroup was formed in fall of 1993 for the purpose of planning each workers' compensation case scheduled for a hearing at the Maryland Workers' Compensation Commission. Its members consist of attorneys, administrators, an adjustor, and nurse case managers and meets once per month. In addition to case planning, the group reviews statistics on the number of open and closed cases and the appropriateness of the reserves set for each lost-time workers' compensation case.

Occupational medicine physicians provide the primary medical care and with nurse case managers act as liaisons with the PPO physicians and therapists. The nurse case manager makes referrals for ergonomic assessment or safety evaluation of the workplace when indicated. Once an injury is identified as possibly arising from an unfavorable environmental ergonomic condition, the workplace is inspected by one of the department's industrial hygienists or safety professionals. A formal workplace assessment is followed by recommendations and follow-up evaluation of abatement measures. An additional mechanism for follow-up evaluation of workplace hazards is provided by the claims management workgroup when human resources representatives are informed of the problem work areas by the safety manager or industrial hygienist. The industrial hygienist or safety professional and human resources specialists follow up with supervisors who have not enacted recommended remedial efforts.

What did this reorganization and integration of services achieve? Between 1992 and

1997 per capita workers' compensation losses were reduced by 39%, from $241 in 1992 (the year before integration) to $146 in 1997 (37–42) (Table 26-5). In 1992, there were 22 lost-time cases per 1,000 employees, whereas the number of lost-time cases in 1997 was 8 per 1,000 employees (42). Although the purpose of this program was to integrate all safety-related activities to achieve a reduction in losses, the ultimate outcome of the program was marked reduction in both the injury and severity rates. In 1996, at Johns Hopkins Hospital, for example, the average number of lost workday cases per 100 employees was 3.15; nationally it was 4.20 (see Table 26-5). The number of lost workdays per 100 employees at the Johns Hopkins Hospital in 1996 was 33.41 versus 81.00 nationally (8), or less than half the national average. What is more important, the 1996 rates are significantly less than the rates at the Johns Hopkins Hospital in 1992 (see Table 26-5).

Perhaps the most visible outcome measure of the integrated program was seen with respect to the JCAHO surveys of the Johns Hopkins Hospital in 1992 and 1995. In the 1995 survey, the Johns Hopkins Hospital had only three minor supplemental environment of care recommendations levied against it. No type I recommendations were made. This is stark contrast to the 1992 JCAHO survey in which 25 type I recommendations five supplemental recommendations were made. As seen in Table 26-5, substantial changes and economies of scale have been documented in other programs. The number of needle-stick injuries per 1,000 nurses dropped from 92 to 41 between 1992 and 1997, and these rates were markedly less than reported in the literature (43). The percentage of Hopkins employees trained in mandated programs (e.g., hazard communication, fire safety, and blood-borne pathogens) increased from approximately 38% in 1992 to 95% in 1997 (see Table 26-5).

In 1992, before consolidation of the safety program, the aggregate expenses of the health and safety operations at the various Johns Hopkins Institutions, exclusive of workers' compensation costs serving an employee population of 21,000, was approximately $8 mil-

TABLE 26-5. *Health, safety, and environment key performance measurements by year*

Performance measurements	Hopkins		National	
	1992	1996 or 1997	1992	1996
Number of JCAHO type I recommendations (JHH)	25	0	NA	NA
Workers' compensation cost[a] per employee (JHU, JHHS)	$241	$167	NA	NA
Lost workday cases per 100 employees (JHH)	5.89	3.15	4.20	4.40
Days lost per 100 employees (JHH)	73.81	33.41	81.60[b]	81.50[b]
Cost[a] of safety-related services per employee (JHU, JHHS)	$380	$185	NA	NA
Hazardous waste and radioactive waste storage in landfills (JHU, JHHS)	1,252 cu ft	71 cu ft	NA	NA
JHH needle-stick injury rate per 1,000 employees (nursing JHH)	92	41	92.6	NA
Number of employees treated in occupational health clinics (JHH, JHU)	25,269	45,000[c]	NA	NA
Percentage of employees attending mandated training sessions (JHH, JHU)	38%	95%	NA	NA
Income from external corporate clients (Center for Occupational & Environmental Health)	NA	$1.4 million[c]	NA	NA

[a]Not adjusted for inflation.
[b]1994 rate reported by the Bureau of Labor Statistics.
[c]Fiscal Year 1998 (July 1, 1997–June 30, 1998)
JCAHO, Joint Commission on the Accreditation of Healthcare Organizations; JHH, Johns Hopkins Hospital (6,758 employees); NA, not applicable; JHU Johns Hopkins University (13,500 employees); JHHS Johns Hopkins Health System (12,513 employees).

lion, or $380.00 per employee (see Table 26-5). Expenses in 1997 for all safety-related operations were $5.0 million for a population of approximately 27,000 individuals, or $185.00 per employee (see Table 26-5). In fiscal year 1998 (July 1, 1997 through June 30, 1998), the income generated by the center for occupational and environmental health for the Johns Hopkins University for serving a statewide client base of approximately 200 with a population of approximately 74,000 employees, was $1.4 million with expenses of $1.2 million (45) (see Table 26-5).

CONCLUSION

The establishment of an occupational health, safety, and environmental program in the health care setting must be based on a need to address the hazards and regulatory concerns of the particular institution. This chapter provides guidance on establishing and managing these programs. How these services are delivered and at what cost must be an integral part of managing that program. Occupational health and safety programs like all other programs in a hospital or other health care setting are under extreme cost pressures—pressures placed on the industry by managed care organizations and government agencies in their efforts to reduce medical costs. From the example presented, a health care institution can cost-effectively protect the lives of employees and the environment. The key is to continuously identify risk, prioritize risk-control procedures, monitor performance, and constantly look for opportunities that can reduce the unit costs of occupational health, safety, and environmental services.

REFERENCES

1. US Department of Commerce, Economics and Statistics Administration, Bureau of the Census. Statistical abstract of the United States: the national data book, 115th ed. Washington, DC: US Government Printing Office, 1995.
2. Committee on Medical Center Employee Occupational Health, American Occupational and Environmental Medical Association. Guidelines for employee health services in health care institutions. *J Occup Environ Med* 1986;28:7:518–523.
3. Emmett EA, ed. *Health problems of health care workers in occupational medicine: state of the art reviews.* Philadelphia: Hanley & Bellfus, 1987:ix–xv, 617–648,
4. Patterson WB, Craven DE, Schwartz DA, Nardell EA, Kasmer J, Noble J. Occupational hazards to hospital personnel. *Ann Intern Med* 1985;102:658–680.
5. US Department of Health, Education and Welfare. Hospital occupational health services' study, VII: study and conclusions. Washington, DC: National Institute for Occupational Safety and Health, 1976.
6. Strickoff RS, Walters DB. *Handbook of laboratory health and safety,* 2nd ed. New York: Wiley, 1995:3–23.
7. National Research Council. Prudent practices in the laboratory: handling and disposal of chemicals. Washington, DC: National Academy Press, 1995.
8. National Safety Council. Accident facts, 1996: Bureau of Labor Statistics estimates of non-fatal occupational injury and illness rates for selected industries. Itasca, IL: National Safety Council, 1996.
9. National Council on Compensation Insurance. Workers' compensation claims distribution, 1994. Boca Raton, FL: National Council on Compensation Insurance, 1994.
10. Employee benefits: survey data from benefit year 1994. Washington, DC: US Chamber of Commerce, 1995: 8–20.
11. Colligan MJ, Smith MJ, Hurrell JJ Jr. Occupational incidence rates of mental health disorders. *J Human Stress* 1977;3:36.
12. Eaton WW, Anthony JC, Mandel W, Garrison R. Occupations and the prevalence of major depressive disorder. *J Occup Med* 1990;32:1079–1087.
13. Keeve JP. Physicians at risk, some epidemiologic considerations of alcoholism, drug abuse and suicide. *J Occup Med* 1984.26:7:503–508.
14. Steppacher RC, Mausner JS. Suicide in male and female physicians. *JAMA* 1974.228:3:323–328.
15. Grosch JW, Duffy KG, Hessink. Employee assistance programs in higher education: factors associated with program usage and effectiveness. *Emp Asst Q* 1996; 11:4:43–57.
16. US Department of Labor, Occupational Safety and Health Administration. The bloodborne pathogens standard. 29CFR 1910.1030. Washington, DC: US Government Printing Office.
17. US Department of Labor, Occupational Safety and Health Administration. The occupational exposures to hazardous chemicals in laboratories standard. 29CFR 1910. Washington, DC: US Government Printing Office.
18. Department of Health and Human Services. Draft guidelines for preventing the transmission of tuberculosis in healthcare facilities, 2nd ed. *Federal Register* 1993;558:52810–52854.
19. US Environmental Protection Agency. Resource conservation and recovery act (RCRA); 42 USC 6901 et seq.
20. US Environmental Protection Agency. Comprehensive environmental response, compensation and liability act (CERCLA); 42 USC 9601 et. seq.
21. US Environmental Protection Agency. Superfund amendments and reauthorization act (SARA); 42 UCS 9601 et seq, 42 USC 11000 et seq.
22. US Environmental Protection Agency. Land disposal restrictions, summary of requirements; 53 CFR 31138 article 268.11, June 1989.

23. US Environmental Protection Agency. Guidance to hazardous waste generators on the elements of a waste minimization program. May 28, 1993.
24. US Department of Commerce. Report to congress: management of hazardous wastes from educational institutions. April 1989.
25. US Office of Technology Assessment. Low-level radioactive waste policy act of 1980. United States Code, vol. 42, sections 2021 (b) to 2021 (j). Washington, DC: US Government Printing Office, 1989.
26. US Nuclear Regulatory Commission. Title 10 CFR 35, January, 1993.
27. Guidelines for protecting the safety and health of health care workers; DHHS, Public Health Service, Centers for Disease Control, NIOSH publication no. 88-119. Cincinnati, OH: National Institute for Occupational Safety and Health, 1988.
28. US Department of Labor. Framework for a comprehensive health and safety program in the hospital environment, 1993.
29. Joint Commission on Accreditation of Healthcare Organizations. *Comprehensive accreditation manual for hospitals.* Oakbrook Terrace, IL, 1996:321–380.
30. Felton JS. Occupational medical management: a guide to the organization and operation of in-plant occupational health services. Boston: Little, Brown, 1990.
31. Silver, RR. *Basic occupational medicine: a guide to developing delivery systems.* Boca Raton, FL: CRC Press, 1991.
32. McCunney RJ, ed. *A manager's guide to occupational health services.* Beverly, MA: OEM Health Information, 1996.
33. Lang P, ed. *Accident prevention manual for business and industry.* Itasca, IL: National Safety Council, 1992.
34. Plog BA, ed. *Fundamentals of industrial hygiene*, 4th ed. Itasca, IL: National Safety Council, 1996.
35. Occupational health services: a guide to program planning and management. American Health Professions Institute, 1989.
36. Schwartz BS, Pransky G, Lashley D. Recruiting the occupational and environmental medicine physicians of the future: results of a survey of current residents. *J Occup Environ Med* 1995.37:6:739–743.
37. McGrail MP, Tsai SP, Bernacki EJ. A comprehensive initiative to manage the incidence and cost of occupational injury and illness: report of an outcomes analysis. *J Occup Environ Med* 1995.37:11:1263–1268.
38. Bernacki EJ, Tsai SP. Managed care for workers' compensation: three years experience in an "employee choice" state. *J Occup Environ Med* 1996.38:11: 1091–1097.
39. Wise D. How providing more case costs less. *Business Health* April 1994;12:67–68.
40. McKenzie JG, Parkerson J, Bernacki EJ. Comparison of workers' compensation costs for two cohorts of injured workers before and after the introduction of managed care. *J Occup Environ Med* 1998;40:568–572.
41. Bernacki EJ, Guidera JA. The effect of managed care on surgical rates among individuals filing for workers' compensation. *J Occup Environ Med* 1998;40:623–631.
42. Bernacki, EJ, Health, Safety and Environment Annual Report FY 96/97, Activities of the Joint Committee on Health, Safety and Environment [Unpublished]. Baltimore: Johns Hopkins University, 1998.
43. McCormick RD, Maki DG. Epidemiology of needlestick injuries in hospital personnel. *Am J Occup Med* 1981;70:919–932.
44. Tan CC. Occupational health problems among nurses. *Scand J Work Environ Health* 1991;27:221–30.
45. Annual Report of the Center for Occupational and Environmental Health, Fiscal Year 1998 [Unpublished]. Baltimore: Johns Hopkins University, 1999.

Medical Center Occupational Health and Safety,
edited by Robert J. McCunney.
Lippincott Williams & Wilkins, Philadelphia

27

Psychologic Hazards in the Health Care Profession

Kevin C. Staudinger and *Michael A. Mueller

Occupational Medicine Clinics, Baptists Health Center, Birmingham, Alabama 35243;
**Division of Occupational and Environmental Medicine,*
University of Alabama at Birmingham School of Medicine, Birmingham, Alabama 35205

Psychologic hazards in the workplace are increasingly recognized as a component of occupation-related mental and physical illness. Over the past few decades, medicine has increased its emphasis on treating the whole patient, and particular focus has been placed on the associations between emotions and disease (1). Stress has come to be recognized as one of the most pervasive health hazards in the work environment. Several studies have shown that approximately 15% of every workforce has at least one episode of psychosocial disability each year (2). Job-related stress can have serious consequences for both individuals and the organizations in which they work (3). Stress resulting from work-related difficulties may cause job dissatisfaction, absenteeism, mental health problems, somatic problems, and reduced productivity.

Increasing attention has been focused on health professionals and the stress they encounter in their daily duties. Work-related frustrations and stress are especially prevalent within health-oriented professions that require constant and intense involvement with people (4). Muldary (5) found that stress "associated with the delivery of health care services can have various adverse effects on providers and ultimately on the quality of health care." Research findings suggest that protracted job stress among health care workers may be a leading determinant of poor delivery of health service (4).

The health care profession possesses a unique mix of rewards and stresses not found in other occupations. The unique tasks, organization, and nature of health care provides an environment in which risk for the development of stress-related disorders is especially high. In a study conducted by the National Institute for Occupational Safety and Health (NIOSH) on the incidence of mental health problems within 130 occupations, health care workers represented a significant portion of the groups at high risk. Six of the 12 occupations with the highest incidence rates were found to be within health care (6). Specific factors have been identified as psychologic hazards to health care workers, including work content, physical and mental work overload, work control, role ambiguity, role conflict, work scheduling, and poor social support. The contributions of these individual factors to the overall stress perceived by individuals within different disciplines in the health care profession—physicians, physicians' assistants, nurses, and others—are not necessarily equivalent. The effects of stress on an individual within a specific discipline may vary considerably depending on the unique coping strategies of the particular person. Nonetheless, certain occupations in health care have characteristic stressors with potential for inducing physical and psychologic adverse effects. The result of unmediated job stress typically is burnout, a phenomenon resulting from the cumulative effects of stress in the work environment (7). Maladaptive coping responses of persons who experience high levels of work-related stress may include depression, alcoholism, substance abuse, and suicide.

With the increased recognition of stress as a cause of disability in nearly all compensation jurisdictions, stress-related health effects represent considerable economic cost. In a 13-state study conducted in 1985 (8) 11% of all occupational disease claims were estimated to be related to stress. Workers' compensation claims that attribute disability to work-related stress have increased over 30% in the past decade (9). Estimates of the annual direct and indirect medical costs associated with occupational stress in the United States have ranged from $80 billion to $150 billion; loss of productivity costs were not estimated (8). The costs of indemnity payments and medical benefits for stress claims are approximately twice the average of all injury claims (10).

To more fully elucidate the inherent psychologic hazards in the health care profession, a review of the concept of stress and its representative models and specific health effects is delineated. A discussion of burnout is followed by a review of the psychologic hazards unique to various disciplines in health care. Abnormal coping responses and suggestions for prevention are considered briefly.

STRESS

The concept of stress is difficult to define and to quantify. Selye, as cited by Evanoff and Rosenstock (8), defined stress as the nonspecific response of the body to any demand made on it; stressors are the actual demands or stimuli that elicit stress. Selye described a general adaptation syndrome as a three-stage process that occurs when an organism is exposed to protracted stress-provoking environmental demands, ultimately resulting in alarm, adaptation, and exhaustion. The final stage, exhaustion, called *strain* by some authors, is induced by chronic stress. Psychologic strain occurs when psychosocial resources such as work control and social support are not sufficient to buffer psychologic stressors such as work demands and time pressures (8). For example, lack of control or autonomy within one's workplace combined with increased workload and time pressure increases perceived stress for most persons.

Stress is not necessarily detrimental if encountered in moderate amounts; it can be motivating. As Selye, cited by Sutherland and Cooper (10), suggested, stress is necessary for motivation, growth, and development. Stress can become deleterious if the duration or intensity of these demands overwhelms a person's ability to control it and causes a sense of disharmony or strain. Each person has a capacity to tolerate a level of stress regardless of its source. When that level is exceeded, physical and psychologic difficulties may be manifested.

A consistent relation between stress and productivity has been demonstrated in occupational stress research. Each occupation within the health care profession has unique characteristics with respect to level of responsibility and degrees of authority, autonomy, and ambiguity. The stress curve is a useful representation of this relation. The curve shows that either extreme in any characteristic (too much or too little responsibility, authority, autonomy, or ambiguity) can produce varying levels of stress and therefore affects productivity (Fig. 27-1) (11). As stress increases, productivity rises to a critical point, and additional stress causes a corresponding decrease in level of productivity. For example, a neurosurgeon (very high level of responsibility) may have the same level of perceived stress as a patient care technician (very low level of responsibility) and have a similar effect on productivity.

Psychologic stressors respect no occupational boundaries, unlike physical and chemical hazards. Potential exposures to these stressors is ubiquitous, and multiple factors being identified as potential contributors to an individual's psychologic and physical well-being

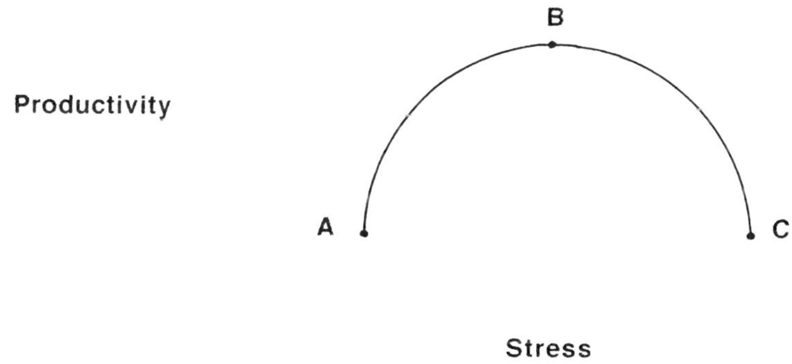

FIG. 27-1. Relation between productivity and stress. **A:** Stress is too low, therefore productivity is low. **B:** Optimum stress and productivity. **C:** Stress is too high, therefore productivity is low. (From ref 10, with permission.)

(12). Most health care professionals, despite extensive training, have never had any formal education in the prevention and management of job-related stress. They are no more protected from its adverse effects than those in other occupations, and in the view of some researchers, they are much more susceptible to the effects (5).

MODELS OF STRESS

Stress models attempt to integrate individual and environmental factors into a working scheme of how stress is generated. A particular model attempts to explain why certain stress events among different individuals cause varying degrees of stress or pathologic events. The central question is whether stress results primarily from the nature of the stimulus, the manner in which the stimulus is perceived, or the way in which the individual responds to the stimulus (13).

The findings on occupational stress have been governed by two perspectives: the person-environment-fit model and the job demands-control or job strain model (14). The person-environment-fit model focuses on the individual's *subjective* interaction with the environment. The demand-control model centers on *objective* features of the work environment and the extent to which a worker may modify a stress response (13,14).

Person-Environment-Fit Model

In the person-environment-fit model, stress is derived from the subjective person-environment fit, which is mediated principally by the individual's perception of self and the environment (13). The effect of a particular stressor depends on the individual's perception and subsequent response to particular environmental conditions, not on the conditions themselves. An unsuitable fit between person and environment can cause varying degrees of perceived stress and risk for resultant physical and mental illness. For example, role conflict, excessive job demands, and poor relationships between supervisors and workers have been found to be associated with adverse health effects (6).

Job Demand-Control Model

The main premise of the demand-control model is that the generation of stress is caused by an imbalance between demands on the worker and the worker's ability to modify those demands (work control) (Fig. 27-2) (13). Karasek, as cited by Schnall and Landsbergis (14), described the development of job strain in occupations characterized by high psychologic workload demands combined with low decision latitude. Psychologic demands measure work pace and scope, and decision latitude measures control. Decision lat-

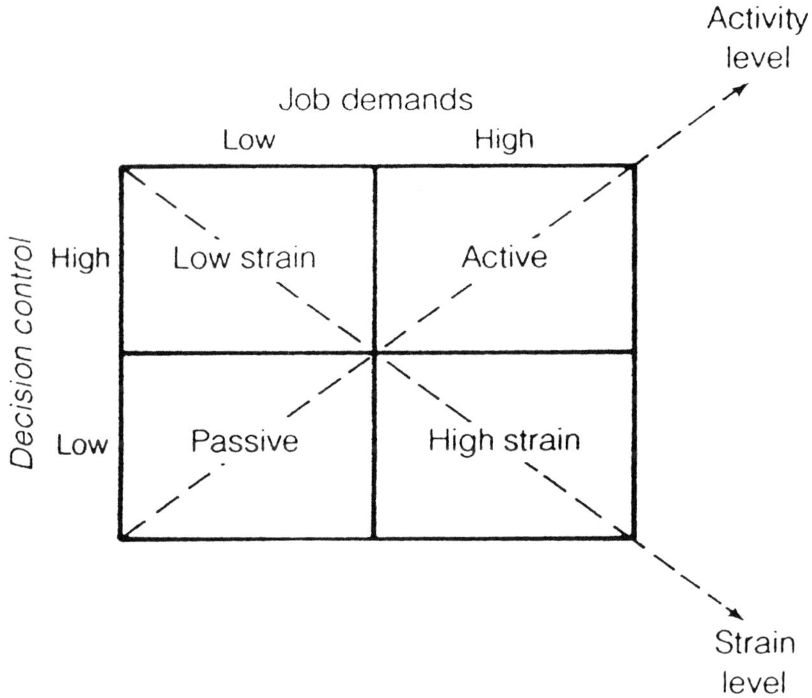

FIG. 27-2. The job-demand control model shows the effects of job demands and decision latitude on strain. (From Baker DB. The study of stress at work. *Annu Rev Public Health* 1985;6:367–381, with permission.)

itude is further subdivided into intellectual discretion and authority over decision. Decision latitude represents the worker's potential to influence work practices and modify stress (7). Workers who can modify work demands by increasing their job decision-making authority may lower their degree of stress. Different occupations in health care have varying degrees of job control and thus distinct levels of job-related stress.

Both Models

Both models of stress focus on some form of imbalance between the individual and the environment and allow certain predictions concerning occupations that are most stressful. The person-environment-fit model emphasizes the importance of individual differences in ability for any given profession. The demand-control model accentuates interaction of potential stressors (job demands and job control). Each model allows for adverse consequences depending on ability to cope with or control the situation (6). Baker, as cited by Schnall and Landsbergis (14), evaluated evidence for these two models and concluded that the job-strain model has greater predictive power than the person-environment-fit model.

In addition to work demands and work control over job tasks, a number of studies have suggested that hazardous effects of psychosocial stress on health are modified by social support both on and off the job (6,8). The buffering effect of social support has been found to improve the effect of perceived stress and job strain (15). Recognizing these important effects of social support, some researchers invoke a demands-control-support model (8).

MEASUREMENT OF STRESS

A methodologic problem in stress research is difficulty measuring exposures and outcomes. Job stress generally is measured by means of subjective responses to interviews and self-administered questionnaires, both of which suffer from insufficient validation and standardization. Confounded relations may be found in studies that principally rely on self-reports of workload, stressors, and health outcomes. Despite these difficulties, several studies have shown strong associations between occupational stress and various adverse health effects (8).

STRESS EFFECTS

Acute Stress Effects

Effects of acute stress exposure are characterized by activation of the sympathetic nervous system and secretion of adrenal medullary and adrenal cortical hormones. This reaction increases heart rate, blood pressure, peripheral vascular resistance, extrasystole, and muscle tension. This symptom complex may aggravate other medical conditions such as asthma or angina (8).

Chronic Stress Effects

Cardiovascular Effects

Multiple studies have reported associations between illnesses, such as hypertension, atherogenic risk profiles, and myocardial infarction, and high-strain jobs, those with high demands and low control. The cardiovascular relation represents the strongest evidence linking chronic job stress to adverse health outcome (8). Excessive workload has been associated with increased rates of myocardial infarction rates. Job satisfaction also has been shown to exhibit an inverse relation with the prevalence of cardiovascular disease (13). Between 1981 and 1993, results of 36 studies were published; most showed a significant positive relation between job strain and cardiovascular disease or cardiovascular risk factors such as hypertension (14). The mechanism involved in promoting the development of cardiovascular disease is thought to be multifactorial in origin. In addition to the physiologic effects of stress, behavioral responses such as smoking and dietary changes may contribute to increasing risk for cardiovascular disease. It has been postulated that high-strain jobs may select higher-risk personality types (8).

Gastrointestinal Effects

The correlation between gastrointestinal disorders and protracted occupational stress is well known. Persons in occupations with a high level of responsibility, such as health care professionals and air traffic controllers, have been found to have an increased incidence of peptic ulcer disease (13). Acute symptoms resulting from increased gastric secretion and changes in motility are common during exposure to stressors (8). Controlled studies have demonstrated that stress management may be effective for irritable bowel syndrome, a disorder believed to be stress-related (16). It has been found that the incidence of ulcer disease may be modified by good social support both at work and at home (13).

Musculoskeletal Effects

Epidemiologic findings increasingly suggest that psychosocial work factors may play an important role in a variety of work-related musculoskeletal diseases. High perceived workload, time pressure, monotonous work, low job control, and low social support have been related to musculoskeletal dysfunction (8). Skov et al. (17) found that many dimensions of the demand-control-support model were associated with musculoskeletal symptoms, but only one personality characteristic (tendency to feel overworked) significantly influenced the prevalence of musculoskeletal symptoms.

Immunologic Effects

Evidence is available that immune system responses may mediate some of the relations between stress and disease. Studies with animals have demonstrated that exposure to experimentally induced stressors increases the incidence of certain tumors and susceptibility to a variety of infectious agents (12). Stress has been postulated to induce changes in levels of circulating antibodies, lymphocyte cytotoxicity, and lymphocytic proliferation (12). Psychoneuroimmunology is a burgeoning field that relates disease to this biopsychosocial model (18). Research findings have shown that the interrelation of nervous and endocrine systems with the immune system appears to be influenced by behavior and psychosocial stress (19).

Psychologic Effects

Higher rates of depression, exhaustion, and medication use have been associated with high-strain jobs in many studies. It is difficult, however, to obtain unbiased measures of association between job strain and psychologic symptoms. The presence of psychologic symptoms, such as anxiety or depression, may affect a worker's perception of any of the elements of the demand-control-support model, a common problem in cross-sectional studies (8).

STRESS-REDUCING MEASURES

Reduction of job stress begins with recognition that the stress is present. Approaches to management and further prevention may be at the individual or organizational level (13). Using the conceptual framework that emphasizes the subjective element of stress, a large number of studies of stress reduction have focused on individual rather than organizational modifications. An individual-based approach to reduction of job stress involves imparting specific skills to improve the person's ability to respond to stressful stimuli. These skills can be classified into stress management and stress reduction techniques. Stress management techniques focus on methods to mitigate physiologic and psychologic reactions to stress (Table 27-1). Stress reduction techniques involve interpersonal strategies directed at the abatement of work-related stress (Table 27-2).

TABLE 27-1. *Stress management techniques*

Autogenic training
Biofeedback
Deep breathing
Exercise
Leisure activities
Massage
Meditation
Progressive relaxation exercise
Social support
Yoga

From ref. 13, with permission.

Although modification at the level of the individual may be more easily implemented, consideration of organizational redesign as a method of stress reduction seems advantageous because it focuses on reducing or eliminating the source of the problem and results in improving the relationship between person and environment (12). An important conclusion from stress research is that improving psychosocial work conditions may be the most effective means of motivating people to engage in healthful behavior in their daily lives (8). Organizational strategies reduce stressors caused by the organization itself. Specific organizational strategies for reducing job stress include peer support groups, quality circles, open communication channels, clear job descriptions, comprehensive job training to reduce job ambiguity, and job redesign to reduce demands and increase control). It is clear that the demand-control-support model emphasizes the benefits of change at the organizational level (12). Looking at

TABLE 27-2. *Stress reduction techniques*

Assertiveness training
Conflict resolution
Decision making and problem solving
Goal and priority setting
Interpersonal skills training
Time management
Psychotherapy
Psychopharmacologic treatments

(From ref. 13, with permission.)

job-related stress from the perspective of both the person-environment-fit model and the demand-control-support model, it seems evident that an integrated approach addressing the problem at both the individual and organizational levels would be most beneficial.

STRESS, BURNOUT, AND THE HEALTH CARE PROFESSIONAL

Health care professionals are generally considered to be at high risk for job stress and subsequent burnout because of a unique set of job stressors and because of unrealistic expectations of the caregivers on the part of patients and the caregivers themselves. For health care professionals, as for any professional group, one can compile a long list of work-related stressors, including extended hours, client neediness, excessive demands, public misunderstanding of the nature of the work, inadequate job training, and insufficient resources (20). Health care professionals may be more predisposed to stress and subsequent burnout than other professionals because of their excessive focus on the person being served. Health care workers have been characterized as persons with a particularly strong need to make a difference in other people's lives, a situation that lends to intense stress if efforts fail (5). If this stress is unmediated, burnout occurs.

Burnout is a multidimensional problem that can present itself in a multitude of ways (Table 27-3). Although not synonymous with job stress, burnout is frequently used as a measure of job stress. The phenomenon known as burnout was originally described by Freudenberger approximately two decades ago and also has been called caregiver's fatigue (21) and professional stress syndrome (22). Freudenberger, as cited by Fischer (23), related that this syndrome occurred among people who where overly committed and excessively dedicated, typically ignored their own discomfort and preferences, used their jobs as a substitute for social life, and spent their free time on the job. People who make their work their entire life have been found to be significantly more vulnerable to burnout than those who do not (24).

TABLE 27-3. *Signs and symptoms of burnout*[a]

Early
Eagerness to work overtime or shifts that disrupt one's life
Unrealistic standards of care
Belief of being immune to burnout
Middle
Irritability, restlessness, fatigue, boredom
Depression, anxiety or somatic symptoms (headaches, backaches, gastrointestinal symptoms)
Insomnia
Skipping lunch or other breaks
Excess worry about work
Talking excessively about the job
Use of alcohol or drugs
Late
Cynicism, apathy, use of gallows humor
Referring to patients in a dehumanizing way
Callousness, loss of empathy
Feelings of loneliness, despair, isolation from colleagues
Loss of control (physical or emotional); verbal abuse is a dangerous sign, and physical abuse (shaking or striking a patient or staff member) is an emergency
Impulsively fleeing the clinical setting
Extreme psychologic manifestations (panic attacks, severe depression, guilt, rumination); some caregivers may become suicidal, particularly when abusing drugs

[a]These signs occur on a continuum and may overlap at any stage.
(From ref. 52, with permission.)

Freudenberger, as cited by Nordhaus-Bike (25), explained that burnout is gradual, occurring in phases over several years. The burnout syndrome is a highly variable complex of signs, symptoms, and manifestations. Somatic symptoms, psychologic effects, or work performance difficulties may be expressed solely or in combination (5). With regard to the health care professional, the manner in which burnout is manifested depends on personality characteristics, coping styles, premorbid mental health, and the inherent stresses of medical care (26). Coping is an adaptation or series of adaptations that enable persons to minimize their responses to a stressor. Examples of positive coping strategies include using support groups or time management skills. Maladaptive coping strategies include alcoholism, substance abuse, and suicide (7).

Maslach (27) found that burnout among professionals is characterized by the loss of all concern and emotional feeling for those being treated, ultimately resulting in delivery of treatment in a detached or dehumanized way. One of the more widely known models of burnout is that proposed by Maslach, who identified three major elements of the syndrome—emotional exhaustion, depersonalization of others, and feelings of reduced accomplishment (cited in 28). Emotional exhaustion is caused by excessive psychologic and emotional demands that overwhelm the individual over a protracted period of time. Depersonalization is an attitude that may arise as a means of protection against further emotional depletion. Although some degree of emotional detachment is appropriate for continued effective performance and interaction, depersonalization eventually is manifested as callousness and cynicism. The final dimension, lowered feelings of personal accomplishment, is reflected by a worker's feelings of inefficacy and diminished competence (29). Maslach, as cited by Scott and Jaffee (30), called burnout the cost of caring and suggested it originated from a desire to make a difference coupled with the inability to achieve these results. Impractical expectations are a fundamental element in the appearance of professional exhaustion and subsequent burnout (31).

A large portion of the literature on stress among health care professionals has focused on physicians. Multiple factors have been suggested as contributing to the development of stress and subsequent burnout. Some authors believe this process starts in medical school, where the technical aspects of care are highly emphasized (29). Hales (32) refers to the high pressures of residency programs as a possible nidus for later burnout. Role ambiguity, periods of transition, responsibilities beyond one's capabilities, social isolation, and sleep deprivation are characteristic stressors of postgraduate training (33). Other authors focus attention on the unique demands and constant stressors related to patient care. Many physicians share a common set of assumptions that add to the stress of their work, including the assumption that one should always be available to patients and always be able to produce the desired outcome (30). McCue (33) emphasized that physicians encounter daily stressors that are an intrinsic part of medical practice. These stressors include dealing with highly emotional aspects of care (suffering, fear, sexuality, and death), handling problem patients, and the need for certainty when current medical knowledge allows only approximation (33,34).

Although the intrinsic stresses associated with provision of medical care are well described, today's turbulent health care environment exposes physicians to a number of external pressures as well (35). Additional stressors include fear of litigation, increased managed care intervention, increased competition within specialties, decreased third-party payments, and projected physician surpluses. It has been suggested that a physician's job is more stressful than many other forms of work (36). This observation is borne out by studies that have estimated that 30% to 40% of physicians suffer from a degree of burnout sufficient to affect their personal or professional performance (35).

It is generally agreed that stressors have increased within the medical profession, and lower job satisfaction is a consequence. Much of the dissatisfaction can be traced to revolutionary changes in health care and concomitant erosion of a physician's latitude in decision making (37). Hospitals are becoming more competitive, and mergers are not unusual. As health care systems continue to downsize, personnel experience changes in positions and possibly termination (38). Managed care has been growing and likely will increase its market share with marked alterations in the number and specialty distribution of physicians (39). The current trends threaten job security and establish an atmosphere of uncertainty, which adds to the inherent stress of this occupation.

SPECIFIC SOURCES OF STRESS FOR THE HEALTH CARE PROFESSIONAL

A wide variety of stressors in health care have been described, including work content, workload, work control, role ambiguity, contact with patients, and hardiness (5,40). Workers in each discipline may perceive varying degrees of stress depending on the presence of particular stressors that characterize the occupation. Nurses, for example, may perceive more stress than physicians with respect to the same job demands considering their characteristically lower degree of latitude in decision making. To best manage stress in the workplace of health care professionals, the predominant stressors within the various disciplines should be acknowledged. The following review outlines research findings regarding causes of job-related stress in health care.

Work content has been found to be the primary reason for selection of the medical profession in a variety of studies of nurses and physicians in training. From a person-environment-fit perspective, the greater the fit between the worker's ability and the demands of the job, the more likely are job satisfaction and psychologic well-being (6). Although studies have shown that residents experience adverse emotions and attitudes, it is not known whether they continue to experience these throughout their residencies. Girard et al. (41) reviewed internal medicine residents' emotions and attitudes and found increased career satisfaction and emotional states as they progressed in seniority. Part of the increased job satisfaction may be the result of lessening role ambiguity as the years progressed.

Fields et al. (42) conducted a population-based survey to determine the prevalence of burnout among pediatric intensive care specialists across a variety of practice settings. For practicing critical care pediatricians, this survey demonstrated that 50% of intensive care specialists were at risk or burned out. Burnout was significantly associated with feelings by the respondents that their work was not valued, indicating poor job satisfaction. These findings support the premise that factors in the work environment other than physical demands are associated with burnout.

Deckard et al. (35) studied the occurrence and distribution of the three dimensions of the burnout syndrome among infectious disease physicians. Statistical analyses of the data from a written study revealed that approximately 44% of the sample reported high scores for emotional exhaustion and that 40% scored high on depersonalization. Nearly 92% reported high personal accomplishment despite increased levels in the other two dimensions. The highest percentage of burnout was found among physicians in private practice (55%) followed by government settings (39%) and academia (37%).

The practice of oncology requires daily interaction with patients with terminal illnesses. To a great extent, treatment offered by physicians is primarily palliative. Whippen and Canellos (43) reviewed the extent of burnout in the practice of oncology in a random survey of oncologists. Statistical analysis of questionnaire data revealed that 56% of the respondents reported burnout at some time in their professional careers. Significant differences were found between the type of practice and incidence of burnout; university-based oncologists reported a lower incidence of burnout (47%) versus all other types of practice (66%). Frustration or a sense of failure was the most frequently chosen description of burnout (56%).

Johnson et al. (44) reviewed the extent of burnout among head and neck surgical oncologists and found that 34% of respondents felt burned out, as opposed to 56% of medical oncologists in the previously described study (43). The principal sources of stress cited by the head and neck surgeons was the government and the changing socioeconomic climate. The medical oncologists (43) indicated a sense of failure and insufficient personal time. This difference might relate to some disparity in the patient populations of the two groups.

Work overload is consistently found to be an important stressor among health care professionals. The research of Caplan et al. (45) on job demands has shown that physicians report the highest workloads, the greatest responsibility for other people, and the highest levels of job complexity. Linn et al. (46) conducted a study with a large number of physicians and found that time pressure was the most frequent stressor and indicated the conflict between workload and time constraints. Lewis et al. (47) found that workload was the major contributing factor to both stress and burnout among dialysis nurses. Dewe (48) in a study of nurses in New Zealand found that work overload, difficulties relating to staff, critical care involvement, and interaction with difficult patients were potential stressors.

Women physicians typically have more domestic responsibilities than their male counterparts and have resultant time pressures that affect workload (36). Researchers agree that the principal source of stress for women physicians with families is conflict between personal life and work. This role strain is always present but is likely to be at a maximum when young children and elderly relatives are most dependent (49).

Deckard et al. (29) reviewed the assessment of burnout among physicians in two health maintenance organization settings and examined the relation between burnout and personal, professional, and organizational factors. The survey results found that nearly 60% of the physicians reported high scores in emotional exhaustion. The strongest predictors of emotional exhaustion were found to be organizational measures, including workload and scheduling factors and the amount of input or influence an individual perceived about work. The organizational structure within which physicians work has important effects on the personal satisfaction of its members.

Sutherland and Cooper (10) attempted to identify sources of job stress as predictors of psychologic ill-health and job dissatisfaction among a large sample of general practitioners in the United Kingdom after an enforced change in medical practice. Job satisfaction levels were significantly lower than when measured in 1987. The main predictors of job dissatisfaction were job demands, patients' expectations, and administrative work.

Work control, or the authority over work-related decisions including work pace and scheduling, have been shown to be important in work stress perceptions. In a large study of NIOSH nurses in which those who worked on a rotating shift schedule were compared with those who worked on a permanent shift, shift work was associated with greater psychosomatic disorders, family disruptions, and fatigue (6). Glass et al. (50) analyzed depression, burnout, and perceived job control among nurses and found that perceptions of uncontrollability in the workplace were significantly related to higher levels of depression and burnout.

Ramirez et al. (51) evaluated the effects of stress and satisfaction at work by means of a questionnaire for four different groups of consultants, gastroenterologists, surgeons, radiologists, and oncologists. Two of the groups had on-call responsibilities (gastroenterologists and surgeons), one had considerable exposure to dying patients (oncologists), and one provided a clinical support service (radiologists). Radiologists reported the lowest scores on stress but also reported the most burnout in terms of low job satisfaction. Surgeons generally had the highest scores for both stress and satisfaction and were thought to be protected from burnout in part by the considerable control and discretion they had over their work. Radiologists, who reported low job satisfaction, had work schedules determined more by the needs of their colleagues. The experience of the surgeons illustrates Karasek's job strain model that high demands can be offset by a greater degree of personal work control.

Multiple studies have identified that the greatest sources of stress for emergency physicians are related to lack of work control. Lack of control over patient volume, emergency department pace, type of patient seen, and predictable time breaks have all been cited as stressors. It has been postulated that stress related to emergency department practice may prevent many doctors from working long term without becoming functionally impaired (52). In 1991, the American College of Emergency Physicians conducted a survey that indicated about 23% of current emergency physicians intended to leave practice within the ensuing 10 years. Although most experienced some work satisfaction, 60% reported emotional exhaustion, and 78% identified depersonalization as a principal factor affecting their decision whether to continue practicing in the field (53).

A study by Whitely et al. (54) of work-related stress and depression among emergency medicine physicians in the United States, United Kingdom, and Australia provided evidence that stress effects and depression cross national boundaries. The study also indicated that women and unmarried physicians in training in emergency medicine experience higher levels of work-related stress and more frequent symptoms of depression than men or married physicians in training.

Johnson et al. (55) examined the relation between the psychosocial work environment and cross-sectional job dissatisfaction and prospective psychiatric distress in a cohort of medical school graduates in midcareer. A job content questionnaire was constructed with five scales—psychologic job demands, patient demands, work control, physician resources, and coworker support. In multiple regression analysis, the strongest and most consistent findings suggested that the presence of both greater work control and social support, independently and additively, serve to decrease job dissatisfaction and psychiatric distress among physicians.

Wolfgang (3) administered a standardized questionnaire to measure stress among physicians, registered nurses, and pharmacists. Nurses reported significantly more stress than pharmacists or physicians. Nurses' higher scores may reflect the lack of control they often encounter with respect to their daily job demands.

Kandolin (56) used the Maslach burnout inventory to measure burnout and psychologic stress among nurses engaged in two- and three-shift work. The aim of the study was to determine whether burnout is more common among nurses whose shift schedule includes night work compared with the situation for nurses who work on an only-daytime schedule. A schedule of rotating work shifts is a common stressor that has been shown to have consequences for mental and physical well-being (13). Night shift workers are more likely to suffer from insomnia and difficulty staying awake at work, ultimately resulting in decreased total sleep time and a chronically sleep-deprived condition (11). In this study, male nurses experienced the same amount of stress symptoms and burnout in two- and three-shift work, whereas female nurses in three-shift work reported more stress symptoms than their counterparts. For men, work conditions were cited as being responsible for burnout and stress symptoms; female workers found both working conditions and shift schedule to be responsible for burnout and stress. The dual role of women who combined work and household duties was not reflected in this study as producing a higher level of stress.

Among organizational stressors, role ambiguity has been identified as a correlate of burnout. The more ambiguous a role is perceived to be, the more likely are stress and burnout. Firth et al. (57) found that role ambiguity correlated positively with burnout among nurses. Nursing burnout does not seem to be related to direct time spent with patients or to work on specific nursing units (40).

A well-described individual characteristic denoted as hardiness has been found to be protective against stress. Hardy persons are those who exhibit attitudes toward life such an openness to change (challenge), a capacity of obligation in whatever they undertake (commitment), and a feeling of command in varying situations (control). Linn and Zeppa (58) examined the role of stress in career choice among physicians and suggested that those who are less vulnerable to stress (more hardy) may self-select to the more stressful residency training programs.

MALADAPTIVE COPING RESPONSES

Responses to stress among health care professionals vary depending on the magnitude of the stressors themselves, the individual's personality (hardiness), coping strategies, and available social support. Maladaptive coping efforts can lead to alcoholism, substance abuse, and suicide among persons subjected to high levels of stress. Drug addiction and alcohol abuse among physicians have been recognized for several decades and may be grossly underreported and underestimated (59). Chemical dependency has been cited as the single most frequently disabling illness among medical professionals (60).

Estimates of the lifetime occupational prevalence of chemical dependency among physicians (the percentage who experience dependency during their working careers) are 13% to 14%, figures only slightly in excess of those found among the general population. Results of a longitudinal study by Bissell and Haberman as cited by Talbott and Wright (60) suggested that addiction frequencies among nurses and physicians are similar. Increased access to drugs may play a role in the slightly higher proportion among health care professionals.

Alcohol and drugs are involved in a large percentage of cases requiring disciplinary action against health care professionals. State boards of nursing have reported that about two thirds of disciplinary actions against nurses' licenses are related to the use, abuse, or misuse of alcohol or controlled substances (61). More important than the precise number of health care professionals affected is the estimate of the damage done to the professionals themselves, their interpersonal relationships, and subsequent quality of medical care (60).

Physician impairment due to substance abuse contributes to patient morbidity, malpractice claims, and loss of physician licenses. Health care professionals suffer the same devastating emotional, legal, and financial sequelae of chemical dependency as the rest of the population. In addition, loss of clinical judgment and reliability of an impaired provider because of substance abuse can adversely affect quality of medical care (62). Associated with the high rates of addiction is the risk for suicide.

A review by Boxer et al. (63) of research with regard to suicide and occupation provides insight into the prevalence of suicide among physicians. Although the results of studies of physician suicide are not entirely consistent, the weight of evidence supports the conclusion that both male and female physicians have elevated rates of suicide and that women are at higher risk. Most well-designed studies show that the suicide rate among male physicians is about three times that of the general U.S. population but comparable with that of white men older than 25 years. The suicide rate among female physicians is about equal to that of male physicians but is at least three times that of women in the general population. Physician knowledge of anatomy and toxicology and access to drugs may increase the likelihood that an impulsive suicide attempt is lethal. No firm conclusions can be drawn regarding variation in suicide risk according to physician specialty. Conflicts between family and career and obstacles to career advancement have been proposed as stressors that contribute to the higher risk of suicide among female physicians.

RECOGNITION AND MANAGEMENT

In the last two decades, medical societies have called for improved training of physicians in the evaluation of psychosocial aspects of care (64). Many also have made valid cases for occupational physicians to become social scientists with a strong voice in the planning and implementation of programs to promote a healthy quality of work life (65). Psychosocial competence among occupational physicians, which should include stress recognition and management, is critical for the prevention of stress-related illness.

Recognition of the early effects of stress and a multidimensional management approach are the mainstays of the prevention of burnout. Such recognition begins with heightened awareness on the part of the health care professional. Denial, quite prevalent among physicians, effectively prevents stressed professionals from heeding early warning symptoms of burnout. Maladaptive behavior may be the first sign (53). For this reason, it is not unusual for colleagues to notice that a worker is stressed before it becomes evident to the affected health care professional.

Occupational medicine physicians should be aware of the possible indicators of burnout (see Table 27-3) including long work hours, regular overtime, social isolation, multiple somatic disorders, changing attitudes toward patients and colleagues, and frequent absences from work. Should the stressed health care professional be on the receiving end of a medical encounter (preplacement or because of injury or illness), a few pointed questions with regard to job satisfaction may provide clues to stress-related disorders. Once alerted to possible psychosocial factors, the clinician should take primary responsibility for helping the worker gain insight into the problem and recommend treatment. Methods for managing stress-related disorders vary with the symptom complex and may involve both individual and organizational approaches.

On an individual level, it is imperative that health care professionals realize that they are people first and that medicine is their special interest (66). Tactfully pointing out signs of burnout in a colleague may be a method of helping the person recognize the problem and understand the need for further management. Helping a coworker identify the specific sources of stress, both occupational and nonoccupational, is necessary for treatment.

With early symptoms, stress management and reduction techniques such as time management, relaxation, regular exercise, and the development of avocational interests are effective antidotes. Reducing work hours, taking time off, and moderating self-inflicted pressure to achieve are other measures to consider. If concerns are widespread, initiating physician or nurse support groups can be of great benefit.

Symptoms of end-stage burnout, including depression, loss of control with patients or staff, and alcohol or drug abuse, necessitate professional assistance and treatment. Rather than covering for impaired colleagues, health care professionals should consider direct confrontation and appropriate referral. In these circumstances, consultation with a psychiatrist or psychologist can enable individuals to regain their perspective. A therapist can help identify stressors and facilitate the use of medication or coping strategies appropriate for the situation (52). For some in the health care profession, leaving clinical work completely may be a healthy alternative and may be followed by adjustment into nonclinical medical opportunities such as hospital administration, university teaching, medical publishing, or physician executive pursuits.

Burnout and dysfunctional stress may not necessarily be reduced with individual techniques alone. Organizational factors that tend to promote stress may have to be modified for optimal results. The health care setting should be redesigned to promote staff well-being with facilitation by the occupational medicine physician. Organizational intervention to reduce stress includes techniques such as periodic surveys of problem and tension areas in the workplace; flexible self-care leave and part-time work options; quality circles focused on improving the work environment; and institutional policies promoting wellness, including a reward system for healthful behavior (30). Such primary prevention strategies increase workers' self-awareness and stress-resistance skills and reduce the incidence of stress-related disorders.

Once symptoms of stress and burnout develop, several types of organizational programs should be made available. Employee assistance programs, the coordinated efforts of a variety of counseling and psychologic services, assist employees who have emotional problems that interfere with their work. Employee assistance programs are becoming more available within many hospitals today. They are often staffed by mental health personnel with the intent of allowing troubled employees easier access to care. A comprehensive employee assistance programs should include primary counseling services and appropriate resources for referral because of alcoholism and drug abuse (11) and provide confidentiality, employee education, individual evaluation, and stress reduction (67).

Stress management for emergency personnel can be accomplished with a technique known as critical incident stress debriefing (CISD). This approach, a formalized and systematic method developed for the reduction of critical incident stress (fatal fire or line-of-duty death), consists of debriefing within 24 to 72 hours of the event and offers affected employees an opportunity to talk about their feelings over what has occurred (68). CISD teams consist of well-trained health care professionals and peer-support personnel. The main objective of the CISD is to mitigate the impact of a critical incident to hasten the return of personnel to routine function (67).

SUMMARY

The prevention and management of occupational stress is a formidable challenge for occupational medicine physicians. Regardless of precipitating factors, the effects of stress and burnout are a concern in the health care field. The structure of the health care system today is such that stressors are embedded in the various occupations themselves. Health care professionals are exposed to a number of work-related stressors that place them at risk for adverse psychologic sequelae (6). It is ironic that the hardest working and best-intentioned health care professionals are typically at highest risk for burnout (52). This affects the personal and professional lives of health care professionals, and patient care suffers.

The belief that one's status and role as a physician is sufficient to provide automatic expertise in life's complex daily scheme is a grandiose delusion that ultimately leads to burnout. Nowhere in physicians' training are they taught to deal with stress. Before physicians can advise others on psychologic hazards, it is necessary to have their own psyches in order (69). Various individual and organizational methods involve recognition and management of stress-related effects among health care workers. For occupational medicine physicians, increased awareness and early intervention are the mainstays of treatment. It is becoming more apparent that the ability to work in the medical environment and consistently promote high-quality care is only as good as health care professionals' ability to care for themselves.

REFERENCES

1. Lerner BH. Can stress cause disease? revisiting the tuberculosis research of Thomas Holmes, 1949–61. *Ann Intern Med* 1996;124:673–680.
2. Warslaw LJ. Occupational stress. *Occup Med* 1988;3: 587–593.
3. Wolfgang AP. Job stress in the health professions: a study of physicians, nurses, and pharmacists. Behav Med 1988;14:43–47.
4. Rewcki DA, May HJ, Whitely T. Reliability and validity of the work-related stress inventory among health professionals. *Behav Med* 1991;3:111–120.
5. Muldary TW. *Burnout and health professionals: manifestations and management.* Norwalk, CT: Appleton-Century-Crofts, 1983.
6. Celentano DD, Johnson JV. Stress in health care workers. *Occup Med* 1987;2:593–608.
7. Crawford SL. Job stress and occupational health nursing. *AAOHN J* 1993;41:522–528.
8. Evanoff BA, Rosenstock L. Psychophysiologic stressors and work organization. In: Rosenstock L, Cullen MR, eds. *Textbook of clinical occupational and environmental medicine*. Philadelphia: WB Saunders, 1994: 717–728.
9. Harlow K, Johnson R, Callen P. Comparison of physical health benefits utilization: mental and physical health claimants. *J Occup Med* 1993:35:275–281.
10. Sutherland VJ, Cooper CL. Identifying distress among general practitioners: predictors of psychological ill-health and job dissatisfaction. *Soc Sci Med* 1993:37: 575–581.
11. Holland PJ. Psychiatric aspects of occupational medicine. In: McCunney RJ. *A practical approach to occupational and environmental medicine,* 2nd ed. Boston: Little, Brown, 1994:265–278.
12. Hurrell JJ, Murphy LR. Psychological job stress. In: Rom WN. *Environmental and occupational medicine*, 2nd ed. Boston: Little, Brown, 1992:675–684.
13. Seward JP. Occupational stress. In: Ladou J. *Occupational medicine.* Norwalk: Appleton & Lange, 1990:467–480.
14. Schnall PL, Landsbergis PA. Job strain and cardiovascular disease. *Annu Rev Public Health* 1994;15:381–411.
15. Lavandero R. Nurse burnout: what can we learn? *J Nurs Adm* 1981:11:17–23.
16. Whitehead WE. Behavioral medicine approaches to gastrointestinal disorders. *J Consult Clin Psychol* 1992; 60:605–612.
17. Skov T, Vilhelm B, Orhede E. Psychosocial and physical risk factors for musculoskeletal disorders of the neck, shoulders, and lower back in salespeople. *Occup Environ Med* 1996;53:351–356.
18. Justice B. Critical life events and the onset of illness. *Compr Ther* 1994;20:232–238.
19. Bergsma J. Illness, the mind, and the body: cancer and immunology—an introduction. *Theor Med* 1994;15: 337–347.
20. Farber FA. Introduction: a critical perspective on burnout. In: Farber FA. *Stress and burnout in the human service professions.* New York: Pergamon Press, 1983.
21. Joinson C. Coping with compassion fatigue. *Nursing* 1992;22:116–120.
22. Gardner ER, Hall RC. The professional stress syndrome. *Psychosomatics* 1981;22:672–680.
23. Fischer HJ. A psychoanalytic view of burnout. In: Far-

ber FA. *Stress and burnout in the human service profession.* New York: Pergamon Press, 1983.
24. Horner AJ. Occupational hazards and characterological vulnerability: the problem of "burnout." *Am J Psychoanal* 1993;53:137–42.
25. Nordhaus-Bike AM. The battle against burnout. *Hosp Health Netw* 1995;5:36–40.
26. Hawk J, Scott CD. A case of family medicine: Sources of stress in residents and physicians in practice. In: Scott CD, Hawk J, eds. *Heal thyself: the health of health care professionals.* New York: Brunner/Mazel, 1986:71–85.
27. Maslach C. Burned out. *Can J Psychiatr Nurs* 1979;20: 5–9.
28. Piedmont RL. A longitudinal analysis of burnout in the health care settings: the role of personal dispositions. *J Pers Assess* 1993;61:457–473.
29. Deckard G, Meterko M, Field D. Physician burnout: an examination of personal, professional, and organizational relationships. *Med Care* 1994;32:745–754.
30. Scott CD, Jaffee DT. Managing occupational stress associated with HIV infection. *Occup Med* 1989;4:85–93.
31. Marquis, S. Death of the nursed: burnout of the provider. *Omega* 1993;27:17–33.
32. Hales RE. Physician burnout. *Am Med News* 1981;24:3.
33. McCue JD. The effects of stress on physicians and their medical practice. *N Engl J Med* 1982;306:458–463.
34. May HJ, Revicki DA. Professional stress among family physicians. *J Fam Pract* 1985;20:165–171.
35. Deckard GJ, Hicks LL, Hamory BH. The occurrence and distribution of burnout among infectious diseases physicians. *J Infect Dis* 1992;165:224–228.
36. Simpson LA, Grant L. Sources and magnitude of job stress among physicians, *J Behav Med* 1991;14:27–42.
37. Emmett EA, Baetz JH. Health in the health care industries? *Occup Med* 1987;2:9–15.
38. Moore S, Kuhrick M, Kuhrich N, Katz B. Coping with downsizing. *Nurs Manage* 1993;27:28–30.
39. Politzer RM, Gambel SR, Cultice JM, Bazell CM, Rivo ML, Mullan F. Matching physician supply and requirements: testing policy recommendations. *Inquiry* 1996; 33:181–194.
40. Duquette A, Kerouac S, Sandhu BK, Beaudet L. Factors related to nursing burnout: a review of empirical knowledge. *Issues Ment Health Nurs* 1994;15:337–358.
41. Girard DE, Hickam DH, Gordon GH, Robeson RO. A prospective study of internal medicine residents' emotions and attitudes throughout their training. *Acad Med* 1991;66:111–114.
42. Fields AI, Cuerdon TT, Brasseux CO, et al. Physician burnout in pediatric critical care medicine. *Crit Care Med* 1995;23:1425–1429.
43. Whippen DA, Canellos GP. Burnout syndrome in the practice of oncology: results of a random survey of 1,000 oncologists. *J Clin Oncol* 1991;9:1916–1920.
44. Johnson JT, Wagner RL, Bueger RM, Goepfert H. Professional burnout among head and neck surgeons: results of a survey. *Head Neck* 1993;15:557–560.
45. Caplan RD, Cobb S, French JRP. Job demands and worker health; 1975; DHEW publication no. (NIOSH)75-160.
46. Linn LS, Yager J, Cope D. Health status, job satisfaction, job stress and life satisfaction among academic and clinical faculty. *JAMA* 1985;254:2775–2782.
47. Lewis SL, Campbell MA, Becktell PJ, Cooper CL, Bonner PN, Hunt WC. Work stress, burnout, and sense of coherence among dialysis nurses. *ANNA J* 1992;19: 545–553.
48. Dewe PJ. Identifying the cause of nurses' stress: a survey of New Zealand nurses. *Work and Stress* 1987;1: 15–24.
49. Bynoe G. Stress in women doctors. *Br J Hosp Med* 1994;51:267–269.
50. Glass DC, McKnight JD, Valdimarsdotter H. Depression, burnout and perceptions of control in hospital nurses. *J Consult Clin Psychol* 1993;61:147–155.
51. Ramirez AJ, Graham J, Richards MA, Cull A, Gregory WM. Mental health of hospital consultants: the effects of stress and satisfaction at work. *Lancet* 1996;347: 724–728.
52. Dwyer B. Surviving the ten-year ache: emergency practice burnout. *Emerg Med Rep* 1991;23:S1–S8.
53. Keller KL, Koenig WJ. Management of stress and prevention of burnout in emergency physicians. *Ann Emerg Med* 1991;18:42–47.
54. Whitley TW, Allison EJ, Gallery ME, et al. Work-related stress and depression among practicing emergency physicians: an international study. *Ann Emerg Med* 1994;23:1068–1071.
55. Johnson JV, Hall EM, Ford DE, et al. The psychosocial work environment of physicians. *J Occup Environ Med* 1995;37:1151–1159.
56. Kandolin I. Burnout of female and male nurses in shiftwork. *Ergonomics* 1993;36:141–147.
57. Firth H, McIntee J, McKeown P, Britton P. Burnout and professional depression related concepts. *J Adv Nurs* 1986;11:633–641.
58. Linn BS, Zeppa R. Does surgery attract students who are more resistant to stress? *Ann Surg* 1984;200:638–643.
59. Keeves JP. Physicians at risk. *J Occup Med* 1984;26: 503–508.
60. Talbott GD, Wright C. Chemical dependency in health care professionals. Occup Med 1987;2:581–591.
61. Tirrell CD. Psychoactive substance disorders among health care professionals. *Plast Surg Nurs* 1994:14:1 69–172.
62. Schwartz RP, White RK, McDuff DR, Johnson JL. Four years experience of a hospital's impaired physician committee. *J Addict Dis* 1995;14:13–21.
63. Boxer PA, Burnett C, Swanson N. Suicide and occupation: a review of the literature. *J Occup Environ Med* 1995;37:442–452.
64. Kushnir T, Malkinson R, Ribak J. Teaching stress management skills to occupational and environmental health physicians and practitioners. *J Occup Med* 1994;36:1335–1340.
65. Block DL. How will we be remembered? C. O. Sapping Memorial Lecture. *J Occup Med* 1987;29;605–609.
66. Pfifferling JH. How to cope with the stresses of practice. Mich Med 1993;92:17–22.
67. Fontanarosa PB. Occupational considerations for the prehospital care provider. *Emerg Med Clin North Am* 1990:8:119–133.
68. Colon K. Running on empty. *Minn Med* 1996;79:12–20.
69. Koltonow SH. Who's stressing whom? *Ann Emerg Med* 1989;18:103–104.

Medical Center Occupational Health and Safety,
edited by Robert J. McCunney.
Lippincott Williams & Wilkins, Philadelphia © 1999.

28

Internet Resources for Medical Center Occupational Health

Geoffrey A. Kelafant

Sarah Bush Lincoln Occupational Health, Mattoon, Illinois 61938

THE INTERNET: A BRIEF SUMMARY

Once upon a time, understanding how the Internet worked really mattered. As recently as the mid 1990s it was a text-only universe populated with colorfully named programs such as Pine, Elm, Lynx, Gopher, Archie, and Veronica. It was important to know about Telnet and File Transfer Protocol. Logging on from home or office required considerable resourcefulness and patience—once the appropriate software had been painstakingly assembled.

All this software was necessary to perform three basic functions: send and receive e-mail, transfer files between computers, and control a remote computer. The explosive growth in Internet use is due to the development of software programs, called browsers, that allow quick and easy Internet access. Browsers seamlessly integrate a number of functions and obviate even minimal technical knowledge regarding the Internet.

The Internet is a worldwide network of computers that have the capability to access each other at varying levels of sophistication. There is no place or organization that is "the Internet." Home users become part of the Internet when they dial in and sign on and leave the Internet when they sign off. Other computers are connected to the Internet continuously, allowing round-the-clock access to information.

Almost all new computers and modems are capable of connecting to the Internet. Users with older computers should check the hardware requirements of the software programs they intend to use. Multimedia applications with sound and graphics may require special hardware. A connection program and browser also are required; these often are provided free by the Internet service provider. The most popular browsers can be used to send and receive e-mail and carry out other Internet functions. There are several features to evaluate when choosing software. The program should be compatible with the existing platform and any other resident programs. The program should be easy to use; most time should be spent on the Internet not learning how to get there. Because connection time or availability sometimes is limited, the ability to view and manipulate files off-line, especially mail and newsgroup items, is important for some users. The constantly evolving language of the Internet, Hypertext Markup Language (HTML), allows a great deal of flexibility in terms of actual implementation. A particular World Wide Web site may take on different looks depending on the browser used, because HTML is interpreted slightly differently by each browser. These differences usually have minimal effect on text content.

Because the Internet is not really a place, there is no unique way to access it. Thousands of Internet service companies provide access over phone lines (dial-up connection) or through dedicated high-speed connections. For most home and casual and many business users, an Internet connection means a dial-up connection. With this type of connection a modem is used to dial an access number, which connects the user's computer to a another computer, which connects to the Internet. Hanging up the modem terminates the connection. Many businesses and universities have dedicated high-speed Internet connections.

Internet service providers (ISPs) provide no frills dial-up access to the Internet, and many provide free software. Commercial on-line services such as CompuServe and America Online offer Internet access, database access, shopping, and games not freely available on the Internet. The pricing is competitive with that of ISPs, and usually the first month is free. Connection software can be found in many computer magazines or preinstalled on most new computers.

FINDING INFORMATION

There is no shortage of information on the Internet. Finding professionally helpful information, however, presents a considerable challenge. Fortunately, the technology allows simple ways to find relevant data. Search engines are one of the most fascinating and popular tools on the Internet. They allow users to search through millions of pages and billions of words on computers that compose the Internet. This is made possible by software robots or spiders that roam the Internet incessantly and catalog everything they find. Each browser uses a different search and retrieval strategy, which means searching a topic or word with ten engines yields ten different sets of results.

Although search engines are helpful for many inquiries, they are less helpful when searching for occupational and environmental medicine information. An extreme example is that a search for information on lead (the mineral) would produce millions of "hits" that include the word *lead,* which has a multitude of meanings. There is certainly no harm in trying, especially if the topic or word is highly specialized. If the search results are overwhelming or simply not pertinent, a directory or site that specializes in the area of interest may be helpful.

A directory allows searches by topic or subject. Because a directory is compiled by real people and not by automated software, there are generally far fewer choices to consider, and the information tends to be more relevant. Many directories involve a review process, and sites are not included unless they are genuinely useful or interesting. The largest and oldest such directory is Yahoo (http://www.yahoo.com) which has extensive health and medicine listings. Other directories are medicine-specific and are listed at many of the sites discussed herein.

The easiest way to find information is to begin at an index site or site specializing in the subject area of interest. Index sites contain extensive listings of sites and resources pertaining to specific subject areas. For medicine in general, good places to start are the following:

- National Library of Medicine (http://www.nlm.nih.gov). Provides easy access to a vast amount of government-generated health information and free Medline and Toxnet searches.
- Karolinska Institute (http://www.mic.ki.se/Diseases/index.html). Provides links to medical information around the world classified in both Medical Subject Heading (MeSH) and non-MeSH terminology.
- Martindale's Virtual Medical Library (http://www.sci.lib.uci.edu/hsg/hsguide.html). Links to thousands of medical sites around the world by specialty and type of resource. This virtual library is a subset of the vast Martindale's Virtual Science Library, one of the premier sites for all kinds of scientific information.
- Others listed at Occupational and Environmental Medicine Resources (http://www.occenvmed.net). Although dedicated specifically to occupational and environmental medicine, this site maintains links to a number of popular medical starting points.

There are sites restricted to health care professionals. Such sites require registration (input of minimal demographic and personal information to check professional status) to enable access to basic services. Some of the sites are entirely free and some allow free access for basic services and charge only for premium services. The services available include Medline searching, Toxline searching, full-text references from selected journals, and some disease and drug databases. Examples are as follows:

- Medical Matrix (http://www.medmatrix.org/index.asp)—free registration, many free services
- Medscape (http://www.medscape.com)—free registration, many free services
- Others listed at Occupational and Environmental Medicine Resources (http://www.occenvmed.net/)—listing of many more physician-specific services.

The best places to start are the following sites dedicated to occupational and environmental medicine:

- Occupational and Environmental Medicine Resources (http://www.occenvmed.net/). Maintains hundreds of links to useful occupational and environmental medicine sites and special sections dedicated to Department of Transportation and Federal Highway Administration issues, medical center occupational health, and occupational and environmental medicine mailing lists.
- Duke University Occupational and Environmental Medicine (http://152.3.65.120/oem/). Home of the occupational and environmental medicine mailing list. Closely tracks and archives and links to documents from Environmental Protection Agency (EPA), Centers for Disease Control and Prevention (CDC), Occupational Safety and Health Administration (OSHA), NIOSH, and other sources.
- Canadian Centre for Occupational Health and Safety (http://www.ccohs.ca/): Large collection of resources and links to occupational and environmental medicine resources from North America and around the world.

EVALUATING INFORMATION

Few believe everything they read in the printed media, which makes it all the more amazing so many believe everything they read on line. Millions of files are available on the Internet, and finding useful, accurate information can be difficult. Publishing and selling a newspaper or magazine is a complex operation compared with publishing a document on the Internet, a task that takes a few seconds and a couple of mouse clicks.

Linking to a page deep within a Web site should cause one to question as to the source of the information. Navigating back to the home page or index of the site can be helpful in identifying the source. Controversial or hot topics, such as multiple chemical sensitivities, therapy for human immunodeficiency virus infection or acquired immunodeficiency syndrome, and latex allergy may have thousands of sites containing scientifically unsound information, novel theories, someone's personal agenda, or pure speculation. Other sites may have good information regarding the same topics. A good strategy is to start at a reliable and familiar site and follow links from there.

Even if a site appears to be reliable, one needs to evaluate the accuracy and timeliness of the information. If the site has not been updated in two years, think about visiting somewhere else. If familiar topics are available, review those to evaluate the overall reliability of the new site. The Internet is chaotic compared with the staid world of academia and refereed journals. Standards are evolving, but any professional venture onto the Internet should be undertaken with caution.

MAILING LISTS

Mailing lists are nothing more than a clever way to use e-mail. These lists are automated systems by which users can send (or post) messages to everyone who has subscribed to a list and automatically receive any messages or replies posted to the list. Some lists have the capability to search past postings to the list. Replies can be sent to the entire list or privately to the author. Mailing lists offer an efficient way to query hundreds of colleagues quickly and easily. Feedback may take as little as a few minutes; in a few days an amazing amount of advice and information can be accumulated.

The Medical Center Occupational Health (MCOH) list is dedicated to medical center occupational health issues. List and subscription information for the MCOH list and dozens of other mailing lists can be found at http://www.occenvmed.net/. The oldest and most widely subscribed occupational and environmental medicine list is the Occupational and Environmental Medicine List (OEM-L). List and subscription information can be found at http://152.3.65.120/oem/.

GUIDELINES FOR EMPLOYEE HEALTH CARE SERVICES IN HEALTH CARE FACILITIES

These guidelines were first published on the Internet (http://www.occenvmed.net/ehsg) in late 1997 as part of an ongoing project sponsored by the medical center occupational health section of the American College of Occupational and Environmental Medicine. Written in HTML, it contains hundreds of links to helpful resources, such as CDC, NIOSH, and OSHA documents pertinent to medical center occupational health. Because of the everchanging nature of many aspects of medical center occupational health, no printed version is available. The guidelines are frequently revised and updated to reflect best practice and address new areas of concern. Existing links are checked for accuracy, and new links are added as appropriate. Reader feedback is welcome. The guidelines represent the single best place to start for both an overview of medical center occupational health issues and links to relevant Internet resources.

USEFUL SITES FOR MEDICAL CENTER AND HEALTH CARE FACILITY OCCUPATIONAL HEALTH AND SAFETY

The following sites are intended to be starting points only. There are dozens of other useful sites, most of which can be accessed from one or more of the selected sites listed.

Centers for Disease Control and Prevention (http://www.cdc.gov)

This site contains a wealth of resources, including the *Morbidity and Mortality Weekly Report,* hospital infections program, division of tuberculosis elimination, and the hepatitis branch.

Occupational Safety and Health Administration (http://www.osha.gov/)

This site provides on-line access to all OSHA regulations, letters of interpretation, memos, technical manuals, special initiatives, pending legislation, and other documents.

National Institute of Occupational Safety and Health (http://www.cdc.gov/niosh/)

NIOSH has made great strides in providing on-line versions of both recent and past criteria documents, alerts, and other materials, some of which are pertinent to medical center issues. Unfortunately, NIOSHTICS and RTECS are not accessible here.

Occupational and Environmental Medicine Resources (http://www.occenvmed.net/)

This site is the home of the MCOH mailing list, the Medical Center Occupational Health Home Page, and Guidelines for Employee Health Services in Health Care Facilities (described earlier). It also has hundreds of links to useful occupational and environmental medicine resources.

Duke University Occupational and Environmental Medicine (http://152.3.65.120/oem/)

This site has current information and documents from many government and regulatory agencies, links to useful occupational and environmental medicine resources, and is the home of the Occupational and Environmental Medicine mailing list.

National Library of Medicine (http://www.nlm.nih.gov/)

This site provides free Medline and Toxnet searching and access to many health-related medical documents.

SUMMARY

The best way to learn about the Internet is to explore the Internet. The worst way to learn is to buy a pile of books and read about it. Anyone familiar with computer programs written in the last few years already has the intuitive capability to use the Internet. The technology and nature of the Internet are evolving so quickly it is virtually impossible for traditional printed media to stay current. One distinct advantage of the Internet is the opportunity for immediate feedback and questions. All of the sites listed herein provide links to send e-mail to those responsible for maintaining the sites. Questions regarding this chapter or using the Internet for occupational and environmental medicine should be directed to the author at kelafant@occenvmed.net.

REFERENCES

The dynamic nature of the Internet virtually guarantees any current printed reference will be badly dated by the time this book is published. If a written reference is important, the best strategy is to browse the computer section at a bookstore and find a book that suits the user's needs and level of sophistication. Most ISPs and on-line services have links to many useful resources. The Internet itself is the best place to learn and ask questions.

Subject Index

Page numbers followed by *f* indicate figures; those followed by *t* indicate tabular material.

C